Guidelines
for Women's
Health Care

A Resource Manual

Fourth Edition

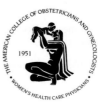

The American College of
Obstetricians and Gynecologists
WOMEN'S HEALTH CARE PHYSICIANS

Guidelines for Women's Health Care: A Resource Manual, Fourth Edition, was developed under the direction of the Editorial Committee for *Guidelines for Women's Health Care* (2009–2014):

Abraham Lichtmacher, MD, Chair
Monica G. Adams, MS, PA-C
Sarah L. Berga, MD
Ann J. Davis, MD
Mitchell I. Edelson, MD
Roxanne M. Jamshidi, MD
Rebecca A. Lehman, PA-C
Jeffrey F. Peipert, MD, PhD
Johanna F. Perlmutter, MD
Holly E. Richter, MD, PhD
Mark D. Walters, MD
Catherine T. Witkop, MD, MPH

The American College of Obstetricians and Gynecologists' Staff:
Gerald F. Joseph Jr, MD
Mary F. Mitchell
Nancy O'Reilly, MHS
Alyssa Politzer, MA
Chuck Emig, MA

RA
564.85
.G85
2014

Library of Congress Cataloging-in-Publication Data

Guidelines for women's health care : a resource manual. -- Fourth edition.
    p. ; cm.
Includes bibliographical references and index.
ISBN 978-1-934984-37-6
I. American College of Obstetricians and Gynecologists, issuing body.
[DNLM: 1. Women's Health Services--standards--United States--Guideline. 2. Ambulatory Care Facilities--organization & administration--United States--Guideline. 3. Genital Diseases, Female--therapy--United States--Guideline. WA 309]
RA564.85
362.198002'1873--dc23
                            2014006171

Copies of *Guidelines for Women's Health Care: A Resource Manual*, Fourth Edition, can be ordered by calling toll free 800-762-2264.

12345/87654

CONTENTS

Appendixes

PREFACE

This fourth edition of *Guidelines for Women's Health Care: A Resource Manual* is a concise reference that encompasses the full spectrum of current policy and management issues relating to women's health care. The book was developed under the direction of the Editorial Committee for *Guidelines for Women's Health Care*, a diverse group of obstetrician-gynecologists and women's health care providers that represent academic and private practice, as well as general and subspecialty medicine. Although some of the information in *Guidelines for Women's Health Care* is specific to obstetrician–gynecologists, much of the information covered in this volume is equally appropriate for others involved in the delivery of women's health care, such as nursing staff, physician assistants and other allied health care providers, health care administrators, and health plan decision makers.

Guidelines for Women's Health Care provides a digest of clinical information, with particular emphasis on information not readily found in current textbooks. This volume is not intended to be a comprehensive guide to women's health, but rather aims to consolidate useful information from a variety of topics in a single place. The book draws extensively on recommendations from the American College of Obstetricians and Gynecologists' (the College) Committee Opinions, Practice Bulletins, and Policy Statements as well as guidelines from other governmental and professional organizations. The College will continue to update the guidance presented in this edition through these periodic recommendation statements, particularly with regard to rapidly evolving areas of clinical practice. Readers are encouraged to visit www.acog.org for the most up-to-date recommendations from the College. Recommendations and legal considerations are by no means inclusive, and other requirements may apply in certain situations or jurisdictions.

The book's subtitle *A Resource Manual* emphasizes the book's usefulness as a guide to relevant resources for health care providers and patients from the College as well as other organizations. A topic-specific resource list is included at the end of each section to provide readers with sources of additional information. Referral to resources and web sites is provided for information only and does not imply the endorsement of the College. Resource lists are not meant to be comprehensive; the exclusion of a site or resource does not reflect the quality of that site or resource. Web sites and URLs are subject to change without warning.

Guidelines for Women's Health Care is a companion volume to *Guidelines for Perinatal Care*, which is a joint publication with the American Academy of Pediatrics that provides information on obstetric and neonatal care. As a set, *Guidelines for Women's Health Care* and *Guidelines for Perinatal Care* provide a thorough overview of all aspects of women's health care.

There are significant changes in this fourth edition, including new and updated clinical guidance and resources and the addition of many new boxes, tables, and illustrations designed for quick reference. Also, the organization of the book has been changed; it now includes four parts: 1) Governance and Administration, 2) Organization of Services, 3) Well-Woman Care, and 4) Gynecologic Care. Each part is divided into sections with their own Bibliography and Resources list. Additional information and resources can be found in the book's 12 appendixes.

Part 1, "Governance and Administration," provides updated and expanded guidance for the establishment of systems of governance, credentialing, quality improvement, patient safety, risk management, regulatory compliance, human resources, and ethics.

Part 2, "Organization of Services," provides guidance on the physical environment—ambulatory and inpatient—in which women's health care is provided. This part contains practical information about facilities and equipment, ancillary services, and practice management issues. The "Infection Control" section includes guidance for protecting patients and health care providers from infectious disease transmission and offers recommendations on how to manage infected health care workers. The

"Information Management" section has been expanded with updated guidance on the use of electronic health records as well as electronic communication media, including social media, for exchanging medical information among patients and health care providers.

Part 3, "Well-Woman Care," focuses on routine screening and preventive care. In addition, there are individual sections that address adolescent health care and pediatric gynecologic care. A wealth of new information is provided, including new sections on health care access and complementary and alternative medicine; updated clinical guidance on cardiovascular disease, diabetes, and osteoporosis; revised breast cancer and cervical cancer screening guidelines; expanded information on preconception care, including new information on interconception care; and expanded information on family planning, including the Centers for Disease Control and Prevention's *Medical Eligibility Criteria for Contraceptive Use, 2010* and the *U.S. Selected Practice Recommendations for Contraceptive Use, 2013*.

Part 4, "Gynecologic Care," deals with selected women's health topics that may go beyond the depth of cases seen by the typical generalist. This part includes updated guidelines on the diagnosis and management of abnormal uterine bleeding, abnormal cervical cytology, and common cancers in women; new sections on vulvar skin disorders and chronic gynecologic pain; and new information on premenstrual dysphoric disorder, with diagnostic criteria from the fifth edition of the *Diagnostic and Statistical Manual of Mental Disorders*.

Guidelines for Women's Health Care is the result of the efforts of many individuals who contributed their time and expertise. The Editorial Committee and the College wish to extend their thanks to the following individuals for their review and revision of particular sections:

David L. Eisenberg, MD, MPH ("Sexually Transmitted Infections" in Part 3)

Tessa Madden, MD, MPH ("Transgender Individuals" in Part 3)

Laura Meints, MD, MBA ("Abuse" in Part 3)

Joyce M. Peipert, MMSc, RDN, LD ("Fitness" in Part 3)

Zevidah Vickery, MD ("Sexual Function and Dysfunction" in Part 4)

Members of the Editorial Committee for *Guidelines for Women's Health Care* include Abraham Lichtmacher, MD, Chair; Monica G. Adams, MS,

PA-C; Sarah L. Berga, MD; Ann J. Davis, MD; Mitchell I. Edelson, MD; Roxanne M. Jamshidi, MD; Jeffrey F. Peipert, MD, PhD; Johanna F. Perlmutter, MD; Holly E. Richter, MD, PhD; and Catherine T. Witkop, MD, MPH. Special thanks are extended to past members, Rebecca A. Lehman, PA-C, and Mark D. Walters, MD, for their contributions to this edition.

GOVERNANCE AND ADMINISTRATION

The delivery of high-quality women's health care requires an organizational framework of governance and administration. Effective management of staff increases the efficiency of these systems and results in improved patient care. This part offers general principles to adapt, as appropriate, for the provision of quality women's health care services, regardless of the setting. The following sections provide guidance for the establishment of systems of governance, credentialing, quality improvement, patient safety, risk management, regulatory compliance, human resources, and ethics.

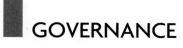

GOVERNANCE

To provide effective and efficient women's health care, a well-defined organizational structure must be in place. The organizational structure will facilitate compliance with operational, regulatory, risk management, and ethical guidelines. Although organizational structure tends to be thought of as applying only to hospitals, all facilities that provide women's health care need a clearly delineated structure. The structure of the department of obstetrics and gynecology may serve as a model for other facilities, such as ambulatory surgical centers and offices. This section provides general guidelines for the hospital setting that may be adapted, as appropriate, to other facilities.

The Department of Obstetrics and Gynecology

Open communication and a multidisciplinary approach to problem solving facilitate the growth and development of obstetric and gynecologic services within an institution, which enables it to better meet the needs of patients and the community. Administration and departmental leadership should strive to maintain such an approach in the management of these services. The departmental organization should fulfill the following functions:

- Clarify issues of accountability.
- Provide departmental representation in institutional policy-making decisions.
- Provide a system of governance for clinicians who provide obstetric and gynecologic services within an institution.
- Foster collaborative practice with other allied personnel engaged in the care of women (eg, certified nurse–midwives, nurses, physician assistants, nurse practitioners, technicians, therapists, clergy and others providing spiritual support, support personnel, clerical workers, and administrators).
- Foster collaborative practice with other medical specialists.

The ultimate goal of a department of obstetrics and gynecology is to provide a mechanism that ensures the best possible patient care and treatment outcome. Each aspect of the department's organization, structure, and function should be directed toward that goal.

The department of obstetrics and gynecology should be organized as an independent unit. In addition to ensuring the provision of quality patient care, the department also should address the prudent use of medical resources, liability issues, and equitable treatment of departmental members, and it should be responsive to the needs and policies of the parent institution. It should be responsible for education and research and should ensure regulatory compliance. At the same time, it should maintain a relationship with the community. A sound organizational plan encourages the prevention of problems, monitors quality of care, and supports quality improvement. The plan should include processes for the early identification of problems and, using evidence-based medicine, address issues in a fair and nonpunitive manner as a teaching and learning experience. Errors and problems, once identified, should be dealt with quickly. A department's structure should be evaluated in terms of improving the outcome of patient care.

The functional responsibility of the department of obstetrics and gynecology is delegated by the institution's governing board. The duties, expectations, and authority of the department chair (and other departmental leadership, if any) should be delineated clearly. The chair is responsible for communicating and ensuring compliance with hospital and departmental policies and procedures. All individuals who are granted privileges in a department should be subject to the policies and procedures of that department and should respect them. When physicians accept leadership positions, such as a chief medical officer, chief of staff, or department chair, their primary purpose is to establish an environment in which quality improvements can thrive. As a corollary to the physician's time commitment, the hospital should consider providing a stipend for these leadership positions.

The size and type of institution, together with the bylaws of the medical staff, determine the type of organization appropriate for the department of obstetrics and gynecology. The Joint Commission requires bylaws to address the medical staff's self-governance and its accountability to the governing board for the quality and safety of patient care and recognizes that the governing board, medical staff, and administration must collaborate to achieve this goal. The organizational needs of a department in an institution devoted exclusively to patient care may differ from those of a department with teaching and research responsibilities. Regardless, there are some basic components and key alliances that provide an organizational approach to quality patient care.

OFFICERS

Each department should have a designated head or chair, who may be elected or appointed. That individual should be chosen on the basis of professional ability, experience, management skills, and commitment to continued improvement of patient care.

The responsibilities and authority of the department leadership should be defined in writing by the medical staff and institution administration. They should be consistent with the general structure of the medical staff bylaws and other accepted external standards established for such facilities. Responsibilities of the department head generally include the following:

- Make recommendations on the appointment, reappointment, promotion, or suspension of staff.
- Make recommendations to grant or withdraw privileges as mandated in the institution's bylaws.
- Periodically evaluate, in writing, the professional performance of each member of the department, and maintain confidential documents appropriately.
- Delineate clinical privileges.
- Provide a system whereby substandard performance of any department member can be identified and corrected.
- Develop, institute, and oversee the quality assessment and quality improvement programs for the department.
- Integrate the department's quality assessment and improvement activities with those of the institution.

- Establish committees with clear charges regarding purpose, tenure, and reporting responsibilities.
- Appoint committee members.
- Provide a mechanism for appointing committee chairs.
- Recommend and approve members of the department for appointment to institutional committees.
- Provide a continuing education program for department members, and maintain records of attendance.
- Establish and monitor policies, procedures, and protocols.
- Collaborate with other professional health care providers when appropriate.
- Serve as a consultant or arbitrator for unresolved differences of opinion regarding patient care or questions of policy.
- Make recommendations regarding policies for any obstetric or gynecologic care needed by women admitted to other services within the institution.
- Establish responsibilities of all department health care providers for teaching and patient care, and ensure that a schedule of assignments is established to carry out such activities.
- When responsible for medical student or resident education, ensure that standards for content, quality, and needs for supervision are met in accordance with the Liaison Committee on Medical Education and the Accreditation Council for Graduate Medical Education.
- Serve as a voting representative of the department on the medical staff executive committee.
- Participate in any institutional planning for further development or changes that may affect the department.

Members of the department should be involved in the formulation of policies to improve the quality of patient care. A consensus should be achieved on these policies when possible, and they should apply to all members of the department. The department head should review all policies and procedures and ensure that they meet the standard of care.

Mechanisms by which these policies are formally adopted and reported should be established. When decisions made within the department of obstetrics and gynecology have an effect on other departments, on patients of other departments, or on the institution as a whole, those departments should be consulted.

If there is a department staff fund, it is necessary to maintain accurate records of the use of that fund and to obtain an external audit at least annually. If the fund's size justifies it, a treasurer may be elected; alternatively, a departmental advisory committee can be made responsible for overseeing the fund. Access to, and management and disbursement of, department funds must conform to the standards set by the department, the institution, and generally accepted accounting principles.

COMMITTEES

The purpose of a committee is to address specific issues that relate to patient care. The extent to which a department will have committees for certain functions will depend on the size and complexity of the institution and the department. In some instances, the institution's organizational structure may fill some of those needs and require only departmental participation. When an institution-wide committee performs any of these functions, the department of obstetrics and gynecology should have active membership on that committee.

The department head should be familiar with the institution's committee structure. Certain institutional committees make decisions that have substantial effects on patient care within the department of obstetrics and gynecology (see Box 1-1). The department should have representation on these committees. The representatives should report on the activities of these committees and convey their significance and importance to the other members of the department.

All department members should be strongly encouraged to participate in the activities of the department, including serving on committees. Such involvement encourages a better understanding of how the department functions and maintains the interest of the members. Assignments usually are made by the department head. All committee members should understand their responsibility, authority, tenure, and reporting requirements. The department may have different committees that focus on a variety

---

Box 1-1. Items for Committee Review

The institutional governance structure should ensure, at a minimum, the ongoing function of the following activities:

- Medical staff credentials review
- Reappraisal and reappointment
- Medical records review
- Bylaws, rules, and regulations review
- Quality assessment and improvement and patient safety
- Infection and environmental control evaluation
- Pharmacy and therapeutics control
- Laser safety control
- Risk management review
- Hospital admissions and complications review
- Continuing education and performance standards review of all members of the health care team
- Operating room and tissue review
- Ethics review

---

of objectives, such as finance, managed care, and education. At least one committee should focus on assessment and improvement of the quality of patient care (see also the "Quality Improvement" section later in Part 1).

Committees may be ad hoc or standing. Ad hoc committees are established for a limited purpose and a limited duration. Standing committees are required to carry out basic departmental functions. The department head should appoint members of ad hoc committees. These committees should have the broadest representation possible to include individuals who might be affected and those who can contribute. An ad hoc committee should have a specific charge and should be given specific time requirements for reporting. When the ad hoc committee has achieved its goal and submitted its report, it should be disbanded formally unless there is a compelling reason to continue its function or to convert it to a standing committee.

In departments with large numbers of staff members, an executive or advisory committee is desirable to expedite the decision-making process and to provide representation for all members of the staff. There should be appropriate representation from full-time, part-time, and volunteer staff in departments that have such a configuration.

MEETINGS

Regular meetings and conferences of the department should be held. A level of acceptable attendance for continued maintenance of privileges should be established. An agenda should be developed for each meeting. The number and complexity of these meetings will vary with the size and intricacy of the department:

- An administrative and business focus may address needs, changes, or problems within the department.
- Committee reports can keep the department members informed.
- Quality assessment, risk management, and quality improvement activities should be summarized and discussed when appropriate and are helpful in improving patient care.
- Minutes of departmental meetings should be documented. They provide continuity in the activities of the department and help keep the medical staff administration informed. Information and policy decisions that are applicable to the department should be distributed to all staff members.
- Quality assessment and quality improvement activities are privileged and should have legal protection under state or federal laws. Legal counsel should be sought in establishing and maintaining such committees. Records of such activities are confidential and should be filed separately from the business minutes of the department in a secure location.

EDUCATION AND RESEARCH

In addition to regular business meetings of the department, educational conferences should be held. These conferences should include continuing education activities provided by the members of the department, the institution, or visiting lecturers. Such activities create an opportunity to provide current information about evidence-based approaches to patient management, technological advances, and new technological developments in the field. These conferences also can be used to discuss global issues identified in the quality assessment process.

Education is of key importance in all institutions. The medical staff and other health care providers achieved their degrees, certifications, and licensure through a formal education process. Continuing education is required to maintain and update these skills and knowledge. It is a responsibility of the institution and each department to have an organized educational program appropriate to its needs. The medical and nursing staff who provide gynecologic care at any level should become knowledgeable about current practices through in-service training programs. Such educational programs should be sensitive and responsive to any deficiencies that have been identified by either the institution or the department. These programs are an excellent forum for introducing new technology and treatment methods.

An educational program provides the opportunity to exchange useful information with others, including clinicians, risk managers, ethicists, or guest speakers. The sponsorship of guest speakers should be reviewed to avoid any actual or implied impropriety by linking program financing to sales of drugs or equipment (see also the "Human Resources" section later in Part 1).

Educational programs must take into account ethical obligations to the patient. Specific consent should be obtained for some procedures included in such programs, such as pelvic examinations under anesthesia for educational purposes. Although alternatives to using patients under anesthesia to teach pelvic examination exist, such as the use of professional patients, the examination of actual patients under anesthesia before surgery allows for increased relaxation of the pelvic floor muscles, which may be beneficial to the education process. Because this examination offers no personal benefit to the patient, it should be performed only with the patient's specific informed consent (see also the "Ethical Issues" section later in Part 1, the "Information Management" section in Part 2, and Appendix A.)

Only certain institutions have active research programs. Most of these institutions are teaching hospitals, which also offer residency programs for specialty training. Research experience is a special requirement for residents, as defined by the Residency Review Committee for Obstetrics and Gynecology. When research is clinical and affects patients, institutional rules should be in place to protect the welfare of each patient. In general, this function is best served by an institutional review board (IRB), which reviews research proposals and has the authority to approve or reject them based on their implications for patients' rights and safety. The role of an IRB is to review and monitor biomedical research involving human participation, with the goal of ensuring the protection of the rights and welfare of the participants. Federal guidelines have been established for research conducted, supported, or otherwise regulated by the federal government (see Resources). The IRB should have written policies that are consistent with federal guidelines. Its members should be selected to reflect expertise in science, ethics, and the sensitivities of the community. Research that affects patients must not be done without such review and written approval. An IRB review is required for all clinical investigations. Additionally, many journals require IRB review as a condition of publication, even for studies that would not otherwise need IRB review.

In the recruitment of participants for research, women should be presumed eligible for all studies except those that solely target the health concerns of men. Female participants should be included in sufficient numbers so that the analysis of data is valid for both sexes and so that sex differences can be detected. In addition, research on women should conform to general scientific standards and requires informed consent, without inducements to influence participation. It is appropriate for investigators and sponsors, with the approval of the IRB, to require a negative pregnancy test result and effective birth control measures for women of reproductive capacity as criteria for participation in research when the research may pose more than minimal risk to the fetus. The health care needs of the woman always take precedence over research interests.

Involvement of adolescent participants in research is important to improve adolescent health care and to aid in health policy decisions. Researchers should be familiar with, and adhere to, current federal regulations and federal and state laws that affect research. They include laws regarding age of majority and emancipation, minor consent statutes, confidentiality, and reporting of abuse, as well as a federal educational law that governs certain research conducted in schools (see also the "Human Resources" section later in Part 1 and the "Adolescents" section in Part 3). More detailed guidance is available to assist researchers in understanding these laws and in determining when parental permission is required and when it may be waived (see Resources).

Ambulatory Surgical Facilities

A freestanding ambulatory care surgical facility should have a governing board similar to a hospital's board of trustees. This governing board should have final authority and responsibility for the following:

- Patient care
- Facilities
- Services
- Appointment of the medical staff
- Delineation of clinical privileges
- Administrative regulations

A policy similar to that used in a hospital must be established for granting privileges. A hospital-based facility usually functions under the hospital's governing board. Hospital regulations determine the staff privileges for such a facility.

Some ambulatory surgical facilities offer a wide variety of procedures, whereas other facilities limit their services to a particular surgical specialty. If obstetric and gynecologic services are provided, obstetrician–gynecologists should be included in the process of developing policies related to overall operations, quality assessment activities, and patient care. Physicians should check state and federal laws and regulations on self-referral prohibitions before referring a patient for health care services in which the physician or a member of the physician's immediate family has a financial interest. These laws and regulations continue to evolve, and current requirements should be reviewed (see also the "Human Resources" section later in Part 1).

Offices

Medical office practices, especially any facility in which outpatient surgical procedures are performed, should have a designated medical director. In a solo practice, the physician should assume the role of medical director. In a group practice, one of the partners should be designated as medical director. In very large practices, other individuals may assume some of the responsibilities (eg, Director of Quality Assurance, Director of Credentialing). The medical director verifies the qualifications and safety of people, equipment, space, and supplies, which requires a full understanding of all the elements necessary for the safe completion of any planned procedure. Involving the collective efforts of all stakeholders should help ensure a safe environment for the delivery of care. Stakeholders include all participants: the patient, the receptionist, nursing staff, physicians, mid-level health care providers, and outside participants, such as laboratory, pathology, and vendor services.

Regular meetings should be held for all office staff. These meetings can be useful in improving staff communication and in exploring ways to enhance patient relations and communication. The office staff meeting is the ideal setting to discuss quality assessment issues and risk management and provide continuing medical education for clinical and nonclinical staff members. Staff should be encouraged to make suggestions for improving office procedures.

Office staff should be reminded periodically of the need for maintaining strict confidentiality of all patient contacts, treatment, and records, including those that pertain to adolescents. A written personnel policy should exist that states that any violation of patient confidentiality is grounds for employee dismissal (see also the "Compliance With Government Regulations" section later in Part 1). Specific policies (eg, sexual harassment, conflict of interest, grievances and complaints, and faculty leave) should be established, and all personnel should be made aware of them. Discussion with staff should include the use of chaperones when either male or female health care providers perform physical examinations (see also the "Human Resources" section later in Part 1).

Bibliography

American College of Obstetricians and Gynecologists. Guidelines for adolescent health care [CD-ROM]. 2nd ed. Washington, DC: American College of Obstetricians and Gynecologists; 2011.

Definition of "experimental procedures." Practice Committee of the American Society for Reproductive Medicine. Fertil Steril 2009;92:1517.

Professional responsibilities in obstetric-gynecologic medical education and training. Committee Opinion No. 500. American College of Obstetricians and Gynecologists. Obstet Gynecol 2011;118:400–4.

Research involving women. ACOG Committee Opinion No. 377. American College of Obstetricians and Gynecologists. Obstet Gynecol 2007;110:731–6.

Santelli JS, Smith Rogers A, Rosenfeld WD, DuRant RH, Dubler N, Morreale M, et al. Guidelines for adolescent health research. A position paper of the Society for Adolescent Medicine. Society for Adolescent Medicine. J Adolesc Health 2003; 33:396–409.

Resources

Accreditation Association for Ambulatory Health Care. 2014 Accreditation handbook for ambulatory health care. 2014 ed. Skokie (IL): Accreditation Association For Ambulatory Health Care; 2014.

American College of Obstetricians and Gynecologists. Code of professional ethics of the American College of Obstetricians and Gynecologists. Washington, DC: American College of Obstetricians and Gynecologists; 2011. Available at: http://www.acog.org/~/media/Departments/National%20Officer%20Nominations%20Process/ACOGcode.pdf?dmc=1&ts=20130715T1226302728. Retrieved July 15, 2013.

American Medical Association. Organized Medical Staff Section: helpful resources. Available at: http://www.ama-assn.org/ama/pub/about-ama/our-people/member-groups-sections/organized-medical-staff-section/helpful-resources.page?. Retrieved July 10, 2013.

American Medical Association. Physician's guide to medical staff organization bylaws. 5th ed. Chicago (IL): AMA; 2012.

CONSORT Group. Consolidated Standards of Reporting Trials (CONSORT) Statement. Available at: http://www.consort-statement.org. Retrieved July 10, 2013.

Food and Drug Administration. Information sheet guidance for institutional review boards (IRBs), clinical investigators, and sponsors. Available at: http://www.fda.gov/ScienceResearch/SpecialTopics/RunningClinicalTrials/GuidancesInformationSheetsandNotices/ucm113709.htm. Retrieved July 10, 2013.

Institutional review boards. 21 C.F.R. part 56 (2013). Available at: http://www. gpo.gov/fdsys/pkg/CFR-2013-title21-vol1/pdf/CFR-2013-title21-vol1-part56.pdf. Retrieved September 20, 2013.

MedPage Today. Guide to biostatistics. New York (NY): MedPage Today; 2007. Available at: http://www.medpagetoday.com/lib/content/Medpage-Guide-to-Bio statistics.pdf. Retrieved July 10, 2013.

Partner consent for participation in women's reproductive health research. ACOG Committee Opinion No. 307. American College of Obstetricians and Gynecologists. Obstet Gynecol 2004;104:1467–70.

Protection of human subjects. 45 C.F.R. part 46 (2012). Available at: http://www. gpo.gov/fdsys/pkg/CFR-2012-title45-vol1/pdf/CFR-2012-title45-vol1-part46.pdf. Retrieved September 20, 2013.

The Joint Commission. Comprehensive accreditation manual for ambulatory care: CAMAC. Oakbrook Terrace (IL): The Commission; 2014.

The Joint Commission. Comprehensive accreditation manual for hospitals: CAMH. Oakbrook Terrace (IL): The Commission; 2014.

EVALUATING CREDENTIALS AND GRANTING PRIVILEGES

Evaluating credentials and granting privileges are essential to ensure that high-quality, safe care is provided. During the initial application for staff membership at a hospital or other institution, the applicant is responsible for demonstrating his or her qualifications. After an applicant's credentials have been verified, it becomes the institution's responsibility to determine which privileges should be granted. Standards for granting privileges should be established by the institution's governing board and applied uniformly within a specialty and across specialties. Documented successful completion of training should allow any practitioner, regardless of specialty, to meet the criteria for privileges in a specific area of practice but not necessarily for all procedures. Therefore, credentialing and granting of privileges are activities that should be based on training, experience, and demonstrated current clinical competence.

Medical Staff Appointments and Credentialing

The institution is responsible for verifying the information in the applicant's credentials from the primary source, whenever feasible. This documentation should include, but may not be limited to, the following information:

- Education and current curriculum vitae
- Residency and subspecialty training
- Status of American Board of Obstetrics and Gynecology certification or equivalent
- Technical experience and verification of competence and delineation of privileges from previous facilities
- State licensure and history of any disciplinary action either by medical staff or by the state licensing board

- Current cover letter for professional liability insurance indicating limits of coverage
- Letters of recommendation assessing professional judgment and behavior as well as perceived skill levels and clinical competence
- Drug Enforcement Administration certificate
- Any special certificates held (eg, laser)
- Signature sheets for institutional policies (eg, Health Insurance Portability and Accountability Act, compliance program, Code of Conduct, and patient safety)

A credentialing system also should require notification of any material changes in the credentialed health care provider's status at any other facilities where the health care provider holds privileges. For instance, if the health care provider's privileges are limited at another local hospital or surgical center, this should be reported. Likewise, a health department investigation of a complaint resulting in anything other than full exculpation needs to be reported.

Information should be obtained directly from the practitioner's liability insurance company and, as required by law, the National Practitioner Data Bank (NPDB) (see Box 1-2). Hospitals must query the NPDB when a health care provider applies for medical staff appointment (courtesy or otherwise) or for clinical privileges at the hospital. This process is ongoing, and the data bank must be queried for all health care providers on the medical staff and those who have clinical privileges at new appointment, every 2 years at the time of reappointment, and at any time within the 2-year cycle if new privileges are requested. Inquiries regarding the training, privileges, behavioral issues, and any negative actions should be directed to any institution where the health care clinician has practiced. Verification also may rely on accepted secondary sources, such as web sites of the American Medical Association (AMA), or even state health departments and national resources, such as the Office of the Inspector General.

For recredentialing, it is reasonable to forego outside peer assessments if the health care provider does enough activity for the institution's quality assurance and risk management system to oversee the quality of the health care provider's work. These ongoing peer review data should be considered

---

Box 1-2. The National Practitioner Data Bank

PO Box 10832
Chantilly, VA 20153-0832
800-767-6732
http://www.npdb-hipdb.hrsa.gov

The National Practitioner Data Bank (NPDB) was established by the Health Care Quality Improvement Act of 1986. The NPDB is an information repository that includes reports of medical malpractice payments and disciplinary actions against physicians, dentists and, in some cases, other licensed health care providers regarding licensure, clinical privileges, and professional society standing.

Practitioners can query the NPDB regarding information about themselves. All queries require payment of a fee. Hospitals are required by law to query the NPDB; other entities that may be eligible to query the NPDB include state boards of medical examiners or state licensing boards, professional societies that follow a formal peer review process, and entities that provide health care services and follow a formal peer review process. Practitioners who are the subject of a report receive notification when a report is submitted. These practitioners may add a statement to a report, dispute the report, or contact the reporting entity to make corrections to a report.

The NPDB Help Line number listed provides recorded information 7 days a week, 24 hours a day. Information specialists are available at the same number weekdays from 8:30 AM to 6:00 PM (5:30 PM on Fridays) Eastern time. The web site also provides detailed information.

---

in recredentialing decisions. Current standards from The Joint Commission require hospitals to evaluate physicians on an ongoing basis, rather than just a periodic peer review. This process is referred to as an "ongoing professional practice evaluation." The Joint Commission has left it up to each hospital to develop the process and determine which indicators to use.

Many institutions require medical specialty board certification for membership and often accept certification from other countries. A physician may be either board certified or an active candidate, which indicates that the individual has passed the written examination and has not exceeded the limitations of eligibility for the oral examination. Once this period of eligibility has passed without successful completion, the physician is no longer an active candidate and should no longer use this terminology.

As mandated by the American Board of Medical Specialties, all physicians with time-limited board certification must participate in maintenance of certification. The four-part maintenance of certification process for obstetrics and gynecology is described in Box 1-3.

Beginning in 2001, all new certificates issued by the American Board of Obstetrics and Gynecology (ABOG) were 6 years in duration. Beginning in 2008, all newly board-certified obstetrician–gynecologists automatically began the annual maintenance of certification process. In addition, as the certifications expire for those physicians with time-limited certification, they too will begin maintenance of certification.

Institutions may decide that certified nurse–midwives (CNMs), nurse practitioners (NPs), and physician assistants (PAs) should be credentialed using the same process as that used for physicians, although the criteria may be different. This process will allow these individuals to function to the full extent of their educational preparation and legal scope of practice. They must be licensed properly and certified by their state, and they should conform to legal requirements and hospital bylaws regarding professional liability insurance.

Institutions also should be aware of the board certification equivalents for other health care providers, such as CNMs (American Midwifery Certification Board) and PAs (National Commission on Certification of Physician Assistants). Nurses and NPs have multiple options for certification. The National Certification Corporation awards certification to NPs in the obstetric, gynecologic, and neonatal nursing specialties as well as various certificates for nurses, physicians, and other licensed health care personnel. Certification also is awarded to nurses and NPs in specialties, such as family, nurse executive, high-risk perinatal, maternal–child, pediatric, or perinatal, through the American Nurses Credentialing Center. Institutions should ensure that the certification from any accredited certification board is appropriate to the responsibilities and privileges of the respective staff position (see also the "Practice Management" section in Part 2).

Credentialing of noncertified physicians and other health care providers should be performed using the same rigorous standards as those used for physicians. The education and experience of these individuals should be reviewed carefully to determine whether institutional standards are met.

Box 1-3. Maintenance of Certification

Annual Maintenance of Certification

All obstetrician–gynecologists newly certified by the American Board of Obstetricians and Gynecologists (ABOG) and physicians with time-limited certificates are required to participate in maintenance of certification to continue ABOG certification. Maintenance of certification is a four-part program to be completed over each 6-year maintenance-of-certification cycle:

- Part 1: Professional Standing—Each physician's license is reviewed by ABOG annually.

- Part 2: Lifetime Education (formerly known as annual board certification, or "ABC")—Each physician must complete annual article reviews and questions.

- Part 3: Cognitive Expertise—Each physician is required to pass a written examination. The examination was offered for the first time in 2012. Each physician must complete the examination by the end of the 6-year maintenance-of-certification cycle.

- Part 4: Practice Performance and Self-Assessment/Continuous Quality Improvement—Each physician must complete five self-assessment modules by the end of the 6-year maintenance-of-certification cycle.

Voluntary Recertification

- Voluntary recertification applies only to those diplomates whose certification occurred before 1986 (in general obstetrics and gynecology) or 1987 (in the subspecialties). These individuals have no time limitation on their certificates. Not participating in maintenance of certification will not affect their board certification.

- Even though ABOG does not require these physicians to participate in maintenance of certification, many state licensing boards and hospitals do require them to do so. Requirements vary by state and institution, so individuals in this category need to confirm that they are in compliance.

- Voluntary recertification can be obtained only through the maintenance-of-certification program. Physicians seeking voluntary recertification should contact ABOG.

Data from American Board of Obstetricians and Gynecologists (ABOG). Available at: www.abog.org. Retrieved January 3, 2014.

Delineation of Privileges

The authority for granting privileges, including special, temporary, or other appointments, is established by the governing board of an institution or the chief medical officer of the office practice and should be delineated in the institution and medical staff bylaws. Although the criteria and process by which clinical privileges are granted should be outlined in the medical staff bylaws, the actual privileges that may be granted should be stated in the medical staff rules and regulations, where they can be amended more easily. The rules and regulations should delineate which procedures or operations or operative approaches require proctoring and the number of cases that must be proctored before full independence privileges can be granted. The rules and regulations should stipulate who can proctor and whether proctoring must entail consecutive cases.

Privileges should be granted based on the individual's training, experience, and demonstrated current clinical competence. The department head, after a careful review of the application and all supporting data, should make recommendations for the initial granting of privileges, the renewal of privileges, and the addition or denial of new privileges. The recommendations of the department head regarding appointments and privileges often are reviewed and acted on by designated institutional staff (eg, credentials and medical executive committees) who forward their recommendations to the institution's governing board. The ultimate responsibility for the quality of medical care rests with the governing board of the institution or chief medical officer of the office practice, with the medical staff responsible for effective self-governance. Privileges should be granted only for treating illnesses or performing procedures that can be supported properly by the facilities and the staff.

After an applicant's credentials have been verified, the specific privileges that have been requested should be considered carefully. Physicians who are trained appropriately, have sufficient experience, and have demonstrated current clinical competence should be granted privileges accordingly. Assessment for granting privileges may vary according to the type of procedure and the risks associated with it. For example, the assessment for dilation and curettage privileges will require less observation and preceptor time than the assessment for laparoscopic hysterectomy. New technology and procedures require training and demonstration of competence before privileges are granted. Also essential to this review is the capacity of the institution to meet the requirements for the privileges granted.

Blanket approval for all aspects of patient care under the designation "obstetric and gynecologic privileges" fails to recognize the reality of tertiary care issues and variations in training in technical procedures. The institution should have in place a policy that allows for differentiation of privileges. There are various approaches to differentiating privileges, including the following:

- "Laundry list"—An applicant can specifically request procedures and conditions from a checklist.

- Categorization—Major procedures or treatment areas are identified and classified based on complexity or the level of training.

- Descriptive—An applicant describes the requested privileges in narrative form.

- Delineation by codes—Privileges are requested based on diagnoses codes (from the current edition of the *International Classification of Diseases, Clinical Modification* system), current procedural terminology codes, or diagnosis-related group codes.

- Combination—A hybrid of two or more of the methods previously described.

Core privileging, an alternative to the methods previously described, groups together privileges that might require similar education, training, or skill to be performed. Privileges also can be related by organ systems, pathophysiology, diagnostic or therapeutic principles, anatomic relationships, or surgical approach and technologies (eg, robotic surgery or assisted reproduction). This method assumes that anyone who has completed an approved residency has sufficient knowledge and technical skills to perform competently within the specialty. Procedures or privileges that require special training, such as radical hysterectomy, would be listed separately, not in a core group. A sample list of specific procedures for which privileges may be granted as a group follows:

- General core privileges in obstetrics and gynecology
- Maternal–fetal medicine

- Gynecologic oncology
- Major surgical procedures
- Reproductive endocrinology and infertility
- Assisted reproduction
- Operative laparoscopy
- Robotic surgery
- Urogynecologic procedures
- Pelvic floor reconstructive surgery
- Diagnosis and treatment of breast disease

Cosmetic procedures (eg, laser hair removal, tattoo removal, and liposuction) are not considered gynecologic procedures. As with other surgical procedures, privileging for cosmetic procedures should be based on education, training, experience, and demonstrated competence.

Privileges often are formatted by levels (eg, Level I, Level II, and Level III gynecologic privileges) as shown in Appendix B. As new technologies evolve, processes for granting privileges for them will need to be formulated. Appendix C includes a sample application for privileges, which outlines such areas as the provisional period, emergency situations, and the performance of new procedures.

Whether licensed or not, residents ordinarily do not have independent admitting privileges. Fellows (eg, those in subspecialty training who usually have completed basic specialty requirements) may have admitting privileges if allowed by the institution's bylaws; however, their privileges and appointments should be regarded as time limited for the term of training. Institutions should develop specific policies governing dual employment (moonlighting) for residents that adhere to state requirements. The institution's policy regarding dual employment should be articulated clearly in residents' contracts.

Certified nurse–midwives and NPs are licensed independent practitioners and may have delineated clinical privileges or may function under a job description. In either case, specific requirements established by The Joint Commission and state regulatory and licensing authorities govern the scope and independence of their practice. Physician assistants are regarded as supervised clinical practitioners, whereas the requirements for CNM and NP collaboration with physicians vary by state. Certified nurse–midwives and NPs generally operate under guidelines, developed collaboratively and subject to institutional approval, that define their roles in the institution and protocols that govern their practice. These documents should define conditions that require referral and include guidelines for physician collaboration and supervision.

Institutions initially may grant medical staff membership to physicians and licensed independent practitioners for a limited period with the understanding that at the end of that time, privileges may be withdrawn or reduced. Periods requiring proctoring, probationary periods, temporary privileges, as well as any combination of these are also common.

TEMPORARY PRIVILEGES

On occasion there arises a need to provide access to the facilities for a practitioner who, although fully qualified, is not a member of the institution's medical staff. The reasons for providing temporary access should be reviewed for appropriateness and to ensure that they serve the best interests of patient care, the medical staff, and the community. The practitioner's credentials and qualifications and the adequacy of the practitioner's professional liability insurance, if required, should be verified before privileges are granted. The institution's bylaws should specify who has authority to award such privileges, which should be granted for a period not to exceed 120 days.

PROVISIONAL STATUS

An initial appointment to the medical staff should be based on a thorough review of the individual's credentials and proctoring. The classification of privileges should be designated and the provisional period limited. Medical staff bylaws may provide for an extension of the provisional period if the volume of work or the opportunity for observation has not been sufficient to satisfy the requirements for active staff eligibility.

At the end of the provisional period, an appointee found to be professionally competent and ethical should be granted active staff membership with an appropriate classification of privileges. If, however, at the end of or during the provisional period there is objective and documented evidence that the individual is not professionally competent or ethical, the department head should make a recommendation to the appropriate committee and the institution's governing board that privileges be restricted or denied. There should be detailed documentation of the problems and difficulties to support such a recommendation. Any such action is subject to the provisions of applicable medical staff bylaws. Professional review actions based on reasons related to professional competence or conduct that adversely affect clinical privileges of a physician for a period longer than 30 days must be reported to the state licensing board and the NPDB.

Itinerant Surgeons

Surgeons who occasionally commute as needed to perform surgery (eg, to rural areas) often are referred to as itinerant surgeons. Itinerant surgeons sometimes can provide a community with services it would not otherwise have. If the services of itinerant surgeons are used, the hospital should follow its own policy to verify the physicians' credentials. In addition, when itinerant surgery is an appropriate option for the community and the patient, the physician should provide the following:

- A written and complete preoperative workup
- A written plan for postoperative care

The hospital should provide the following:

- Regular review of the medical records and outcomes
- Appropriate preoperative and postoperative support services for safe patient care
- Appropriate technical support and equipment

Added Skills or Qualifications

Physicians may request privileges for new skills or emerging technology that has been introduced subsequent to an individual's residency or fellowship training. New equipment or technology usually improves health care, provided that practitioners and other hospital staff understand the proper indications for usage. Problems can arise when staff perform duties or use equipment for which they are not trained. Privileges for new skills should only be granted when the appropriate training has been completed and documented and the competency level has been achieved with adequate supervision. Proof of attendance at a postgraduate training course in a new technology or procedure is not sufficient evidence to demonstrate competence in the performance of such procedures. In addition, the NPDB must be queried whenever physicians request new privileges outside of the normal reappointment credentialing process.

Each physician requesting additional privileges for new equipment or technology should be evaluated by answering the following questions:

- Does the hospital have a mechanism in place to ensure that necessary support for the new equipment or technology is available?

- Has the physician been adequately trained, including hands-on experience, to use the new equipment or to perform the new technology?

- Has the physician adequately demonstrated an ability to use the new equipment or perform the new technology?

Institutional departments should establish documented requirements for assessing competence in performing new procedures or technologies, and these requirements should be forwarded ultimately to the governing board. This may require that the physician undergo a period of proctoring, supervision, or both. If no one on staff can serve as a proctor, the hospital may either require reciprocal proctoring at another hospital or grant temporary privileges to someone from another hospital to supervise the applicant. Specifically, if the procedures for which new privileges are requested were not included in residency training, the applicant must do the following:

- Complete a preceptorship with a physician already credentialed to perform the procedures of that skill level; the preceptorship should require the applicant to perform the designated surgery, with the preceptor acting as first assistant.

- Provide a list of cases satisfactorily completed under supervision at each skill level, as defined by the local institution.

- Submit a letter from the preceptor documenting that the procedures were completed in a satisfactory manner and that the applicant is competent to perform the procedures independently at the designated skill level.

If there is no experienced surgeon on the hospital staff who is able to serve as a preceptor for advanced or new surgical procedures, a supervised preceptorship must be arranged. This may be done by scheduling a number of cases from physicians who require privileging and inviting a credentialed surgeon from another institution to serve as a surgical consultant.

AFTER A PERIOD OF INACTIVITY

The AMA defines physician reentry as "a return to clinical practice in the discipline in which one has been trained and certified following an extended period of inactivity." Inactivity that results from disciplinary action or impairment is addressed later in this section.

There are several reasons why a physician might take a leave of absence from clinical practice, such as family leave (maternity and paternity leave and childrearing); personal health reasons; career dissatisfaction; alternative careers, such as administration; military service; academic pursuits; or humanitarian leave. Traditionally, women were more likely to experience career interruptions; however, recent research shows that younger cohorts of male physicians also take on multiple roles and express intentions to adjust their careers accordingly.

It is extremely important for physicians considering a leave of absence or major change in practice activities to think in advance about options should they wish to return. At a minimum, licensure and continuing medical education activities should be maintained. Working at least part-time during an absence to maintain competency should be considered.

When physicians request reentry after a period of inactivity, a general guideline for evaluation would be to consider the physician as any other new applicant for privileges. This would include evaluation of the following:

- Demonstration that a minimum number of hours of continuing medical education has been earned during the period of inactivity. It is also important to meet any board certification requirements (ie, maintenance of certification) during the absence.

- In accordance with the medical staff bylaws, supervision by a proctor (who evaluates and documents proficiency) appointed by the department head for a minimum number and defined breadth of cases during the provisional period.
- A time-sensitive, focused review of cases as required by the departmental quality and safety improvement committee may be completed as appropriate.

The area of skills assessment may prove challenging if the proctored supervision and review of cases are not felt to be adequate. The Joint Commission also requires a focused professional practice evaluation for all physicians who initially request privileges and those existing practitioners who request new privileges. Options to consider are as follows:

1. Residency training programs
   Benefits: More locations are available, providing structured didactic programs and implementing competency assessment. Participating in these programs can provide a source of manpower to help compensate for restricted residency work hours.
   Drawbacks: Many hospitals with residency programs have only a limited number of cases available for training. Reentry programs must not negatively affect the residency training program (ie, if someone is being brought into a reentry program in an institution that has a residency program, the Residency Review Committee must be notified with an explanation of why it will not negatively affect the residents).

2. Simulation centers
   Benefits: These centers can help supplement hands-on clinical experience and may be more geographically accessible. The use of simulation centers for reentry into practice is a new concept. This training may precede and supplement proctored clinical experience.
   Drawbacks: Currently there are few functioning simulation centers, although this number continues to increase. Cost is another drawback.

3. Physician reentry program
   Benefits: Well-designed physician reentry program systems should be consistent with the current continuum of medical education and meet the needs of the reentering physician.

Drawbacks: Only a few physician reentry program systems are offered nationally; thus, cost and location are considerable obstacles in using these programs. An underlying assumption is that physicians do not necessarily lose competence in all areas of practice with time. Competencies such as patient communication and professionalism may not decline. Therefore, a reentry program should target those areas in which physicians are more likely to have lost relevant skills or knowledge or in which skills and knowledge need to be updated.

Evaluation for Continuing Competence

The performance of each staff member and documentation of continuing competence should be reviewed continuously (more than annually) through a clearly defined process as required by The Joint Commission Standards for Ongoing Professional Practice Evaluation (which can be found in The Joint Commission publication, *Credentialing and Privileging Your Hospital Medical Staff*, Second Edition; see Resources). Institutions should establish objective criteria for evaluation of care that can be equally applied to all licensed independent practitioners, including CNMs, NPs, family physicians, and obstetrician–gynecologists. Evaluation criteria may include the following:

- Additional medical education for new skills
- Continuing education
- Professional recognition
- Untoward outcomes and cases reviewed by the quality and safety improvement committee
- Professional behavior
- Maintenance of certification for board-certified physicians
- Results of ongoing departmental assessment of quality of care

The ongoing quality improvement program requires data collection based on objective criteria (eg, measure specifications) and should delineate which outcomes of clinical practice will be monitored for each practitioner. This delineation of areas to be monitored often is referred to as a "dashboard" of indicators and should be transparent to credentialed physicians being monitored. The standards require an evaluation of all practitioners, not just those with performance issues. This evaluation may include periodic chart review; direct observation; monitoring of diagnostic and treatment techniques; and discussion with other individuals involved in the care of each patient, including consulting physicians, nurses, and administrative personnel.

The quality improvement process should be designed to detect variations from the established or recommended patterns of care for clinical practice in areas that are considered important aspects of care. The process should determine, in each instance, whether a variation is acceptable or unacceptable. Unacceptable variations are considered deficiencies. A deficiency found through this process should be entered in the credentials file for each practitioner. When a pattern is identified, it should be reviewed by a quality assessment committee or similar body. The absence of unacceptable variations based on preselected indicators for any practitioner is not sufficient to meet the requirement for performance data on every practitioner. The Joint Commission requires hospitals to evaluate physicians on an ongoing basis rather than just a periodic peer review, using these indicators deemed appropriate by the respective facility.

If a practitioner's performance profile indicates that the standards of the department have not been met, corrective action may need to be instituted and documented. The severity of the problem will dictate the steps that need to be taken. Remedial action and its outcome, if necessary, also should be recorded. This information forms an important basis for the recommendations made for the renewal of privileges.

Established policies and procedures should be followed, in consultation with legal counsel whenever privileges are to be modified, restricted, or revoked. When a negative action is recommended, all applicable bylaw procedures must be followed. The final authority for such action resides with the institution's governing board. Professional review actions based on reasons related to professional competence or conduct that adversely affect clinical privileges of a physician for a period longer than 30 days must be reported to the state licensing board and the NPDB. If a physician voluntarily surrenders or restricts his or her privileges while under investigation (or to avoid it), this information also must be reported. These actions may be, but are not required to be, reported when taken against practitioners who are not physicians.

Reappraisal of privileges should occur at least every 2 years and include verification of current licensure and proof of professional liability coverage. Information regarding professional performance, including clinical and technical skills and information from hospital performance improvement activities, also should be considered. A decision should be made as to whether privileges are to be continued in full, modified, restricted, or revoked. Expansion of privileges should come through formal application and appropriate review.

Impairment and Disruptive Behavior

The following discussion provides practical guidance for the management of physicians and licensed independent practitioners who abuse substances or who exhibit disruptive behavior.

IMPAIRMENT

Impairment presents a sensitive problem in all settings in which physicians and licensed independent practitioners practice, including hospitals, clinics, and medical groups. Practitioners are considered impaired if they are unable to practice medicine with reasonable skill and safety because of physical or mental illness (including alcohol or other chemical drug dependencies) and mood disorders. Any condition that may affect decision-making capabilities, medical judgment, and competence—including diseases of an organic nature—may contribute to impairment. (For information on the ethical obligations of impaired physicians and their colleagues, see also the "Human Resources" section later in Part 1.)

Early recognition of chemical dependency or other impairment can be difficult. Denial is common. The following are some of the manifestations of impairment:

- Failure to monitor patients appropriately
- Poor quality of medical care
- Incomplete or poor-quality medical records
- Frequent absences

- Increased isolation from colleagues and other staff members
- Self-prescribing of drugs

To assist in the management of a health care provider who may be impaired, consider the following:

- Is there evidence of impaired ability to practice?
- Is there imminent danger to patients?
- Is there a history of previous treatment for impairment?
- Is the practitioner motivated to enter a treatment program for impairment?
- Should privileges be suspended?

It is often difficult to deal directly with an impaired physician. However, there is a responsibility to recognize, assess, and report impairment. The department head or other responsible person should be informed and should consult personally with the health care provider involved. In an emergency situation, physicians should know whom they should ask to address a problem related to an impaired colleague. The chief medical officer and on-call administrator often are the designated authorities, but staff members should know who the appropriate on-call contact person is for all types of health care providers at an institution.

Legal requirements applicable to the impaired physician vary from state to state. It is important to consult the institution's legal counsel before initiating any disciplinary or other type of action regarding an impaired physician. Each state has specific laws that outline the reporting requirements to the respective licensing board. The institution's legal counsel should have information on the individual state's "duty to report" laws, and departmental members should be aware of the content of these laws. Many states have programs that allow for anonymous reporting.

Intervention as soon as impairment is suspected or before professional performance is impaired is encouraged. If intervention is to succeed, the following steps are important:

- Obtain specific, well-documented evidence. The hospital's committee on physician well-being (or the group serving this function) should be involved from the beginning, and bylaws addressing impairment should be followed.

- Consider using a group approach for the intervention. This group should include respected peers, a representative of the county or state physician diversion program, and a family member, if possible.

- Use a nonjudgmental and direct approach. This approach may result in an admission of impairment by the health care provider. Less direct efforts are more likely to result in denial.

An impaired health care provider should be obligated to enter a treatment program, with the specific type of program dependent on state legal requirements, the requirements of the state licensure board, and the preferences of the impaired practitioner. Impaired physician or diversion programs, usually operated through the state medical licensing board, are an excellent source of information regarding the evaluation and treatment of impaired health care providers and any applicable legal requirements. Most state medical societies have a committee on physicians' health that serves as an advocate and referral resource for physicians at risk of alcohol and drug dependence. Successful treatment plans, either inpatient or outpatient, must address the type and severity of the problem.

The voluntary entrance of an impaired practitioner into a rehabilitation program is not reportable to the NPDB if no professional review action was taken and the practitioner did not relinquish clinical privileges. Furthermore, when a health care provider takes a leave of absence and clinical privileges have not been taken away, no report to the NPDB is required. However, if a professional review action requires an impaired physician to enter a rehabilitation program involuntarily, that review action is reportable to the NPDB if it is based on the physician's competence or professional conduct and adversely affects the physician's clinical privileges for more than 30 days. Throughout the process, it is important to respect the physician's right to privacy and confidentiality wherever possible.

The AMA has recommended that institutions develop a policy on reporting and investigating suspected impairment. In addition, The Joint Commission has specific requirements regarding the institution's method for identifying and managing matters of individual health for licensed independent practitioners, including physicians (see Resources).

DISRUPTIVE BEHAVIOR

Physicians exhibiting disruptive behavior pose special problems. According to the AMA, disruptive behavior may be defined as personal conduct, whether verbal or physical, that affects or that may affect patient care negatively. The AMA suggests that "each medical staff should develop and adapt bylaw provisions or policies for intervening in situations where a physician's behavior is identified as disruptive." Hospitals may consider adopting a code of conduct with which all medical staff members agree to comply. Conduct that poses imminent danger to patient safety should be referred to the department chair or appropriate leader for immediate action. Offenses of a less serious nature may be referred to the hospital's committee on physician well-being or a similar group. In either case, a mechanism for reporting disruptive behavior should be in place, and medical staff members should be aware of the procedures. It is important to remember that the ultimate goals for any intervention regarding a clinician with impairment or disruptive behavior are to help (rather than discipline), restore the practitioner to optimal professional functioning, and protect patients.

Revoking Privileges

Revoking privileges, including summary suspension, is an extreme step ordinarily not taken unless all other measures have failed or the behavior of the health care provider is so egregious that the safety of patients is jeopardized. The legal implications of such action require that the processes identified in the institution's administrative documents be reviewed carefully by legal counsel and followed with precision. Such actions must be taken in accordance with the institution's bylaws and applicable legal requirements. Careful documentation is of critical importance. Due process procedures must be documented in the medical staff bylaws before initiating the review process that could result in disciplinary action.

A follow-up evaluation of the practitioner's quality of care is necessary to document the effectiveness of the actions. The findings, actions, and outcomes of the quality improvement process should be reported in a timely manner to the appropriate institutional governing board. When the initial intervention does not result in the anticipated improvement, the problem must be reassessed. A second effort should be made to provide a solution, and the result of this effort must be evaluated. Results should be recorded in the individual's quality improvement file and reported to the institution's governing board, as appropriate. If the second attempt does not result in the anticipated improvements, further steps may be necessary. The department head and the quality improvement committee may need to recommend disciplinary action against a practitioner who fails to comply or improve. Because such action has important legal ramifications, it is critical that legal counsel, usually provided by the institution, be consulted in advance.

Bibliography

American College of Obstetricians and Gynecologists. Certification and procedural credentialing. College Statement of Policy 84. Washington, DC: American College of Obstetricians and Gynecologists; 2012.

American College of Obstetricians and Gynecologists. Midwifery education and certification. College Statement of Policy 82. Washington, DC: American College of Obstetricians and Gynecologists; 2011.

American College of Obstetricians and Gynecologists. The role of the obstetrician-gynecologist in cosmetic procedures. College Statement of Policy 85. Washington, DC: American College of Obstetricians and Gynecologists; 2012.

American Medical Association. Physician reentry. Report 6 of the Council on Medical Education (A-08). Chicago (IL): AMA; 2008. Available at: http://www.ama-assn.org/ama1/pub/upload/mm/377/cmerpt_6a-08.pdf. Retrieved July 10, 2013.

American Medical Association. Physicians with disruptive behavior. In: Code of medical ethics of the American Medical Association: current opinions with annotations. 2012–2013 ed. Chicago (IL): AMA; 2012. p. 339–40.

Cairns CS. Core privileges: a practical approach to development and implementation. 3rd ed. Marblehead (MA): HCPro; 2005.

Disruptive behavior. Committee Opinion No. 508. American College of Obstetricians and Gynecologists. Obstet Gynecol 2011;118:970–2.

Identifying impaired physicians: how to address problem physicians quickly. Jt Comm Perspect Patient Saf 2006;6(1):1, 2, 8.

Leape LL, Fromson JA. Problem doctors: is there a system-level solution? Ann Intern Med 2006;144:107–15.

Mark S, Gupta J. Reentry into clinical practice: challenges and strategies. JAMA 2002;288:1091–6.

Re-entering the practice of obstetrics and gynecology. Committee Opinion No. 523. American College of Obstetricians and Gynecologists. Obstet Gynecol 2012;119:1066–9.

Resources

Accreditation Council for Graduate Medical Education. Policies and procedures. Chicago (IL): ACGME; 2013. Available at: http://www.acgme.org/acgmeweb/Portals/0/PDFs/ab_ACGMEPoliciesProcedures.pdf. Retrieved July 10, 2013.

American Board of Obstetrics and Gynecology, American College of Obstetricians and Gynecologists. Maintenance of Certification (MOC) Part 4 Modules. Washington, DC: American College of Obstetricians and Gynecologists; 2013. Available at: https://moc.acog.org/. Retrieved July 16, 2013.

American College of Obstetricians and Gynecologists. Guidelines for implementing collaborative practice. Washington, DC: ACOG; 1995.

American College of Obstetricians and Gynecologists. Quality and safety in women's health care. 2nd ed. Washington, DC: American College of Obstetricians and Gynecologists; 2010.

The Joint Commission. Behaviors that undermine a culture of safety. Sentinel Event Alert No. 40. Oakbrook Terrace (IL): Joint Commission; 2008. Available at: http://www.jointcommission.org/assets/1/18/SEA_40.pdf. Retrieved July 10, 2013.

The Joint Commission. Comprehensive accreditation manual for ambulatory care: CAMAC. Oakbrook Terrace (IL): The Commission; 2014.

The Joint Commission. Comprehensive accreditation manual for hospitals: CAMH. Oakbrook Terrace (IL): The Commission; 2014.

The Joint Commission. Credentialing and privileging your hospital medical staff: examples for improving compliance. 2nd ed. Oakbrook Terrace (IL): Joint Commission Resources; 2010.

The Joint Commission. The medical staff handbook: a guide to Joint Commission standards. 3rd ed. Oakbrook Terrace (IL): Joint Commission Resources; 2011.

QUALITY IMPROVEMENT

Many organizations, including the American College of Obstetricians and Gynecologists and The Joint Commission, have promoted quality improvement in hospitals and other health care organizations for many years. Quality improvement starts from the premise that although most medical care is good, it always can be better. As shown in Figure 1-1, the goal is to reduce unwarranted variation in care and improve performance. Quality improvement accepts that good care depends on more than just the judgment of the individual.

In its report, "Crossing the Quality Chasm," the Institute of Medicine set forth a list of performance characteristics that, if addressed and improved, would lead to better health and function for the people of the United States. There are six specific qualities of good care, which can be helpful in designing a quality improvement program:

1. Safe—avoids injuries to patients from care that is intended to help them

2. Effective—provides services based on scientific knowledge to all who could benefit and refrains from providing services to individuals not likely to benefit (avoiding underuse and overuse)

3. Patient centered—provides care that is respectful of and responsive to individual patient preferences, needs, and values, and ensures that patient values guide all clinical decisions

4. Timely—reduces waiting times and sometimes harmful delays for those who receive and those who give care

5. Efficient—avoids waste, in particular waste of equipment, supplies, ideas, and energy

6. Equitable—provides care that does not vary in quality because of personal characteristics, such as gender, ethnicity, geographic location, and socioeconomic status

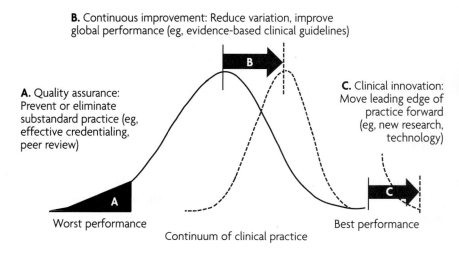

B. Continuous improvement: Reduce variation, improve global performance (eg, evidence-based clinical guidelines)

A. Quality assurance: Prevent or eliminate substandard practice (eg, effective credentialing, peer review)

C. Clinical innovation: Move leading edge of practice forward (eg, new research, technology)

Worst performance

Best performance

Continuum of clinical practice

Fig. 1-1. Approaches to quality: clinical improvement strategies. (Reprinted with permission from ProMedica.)

Quality care focuses on the following aspects of care: structure, process, and outcomes. To provide the structure, there must be adequate space, equipment, and staffing. The process refers to the use of these resources, policies and procedures, the provision of medical care, data collection, and continuous chart and record review. Finally, even with adequate structures and an efficient process, quality care requires that the desired outcomes be achieved. Any or all of these three components—structure, process, or outcome, with an emphasis on patient safety—may be the focus of a quality improvement program.

Quality Improvement in the Inpatient Setting

An institutional quality improvement program evaluates the systems, processes, and outcomes of care, including those that are not under the direct control of health care providers. Because the process is meant to be continuous, there must be a way to assess the effectiveness of changes that are made. These findings can be a major mechanism for future quality improvement.

Quality measurement should determine whether the care provided to a single patient or population of patients achieved good outcomes (outcomes measurement) or represented those processes that are thought or known to be associated with achievement of good outcomes (process measurement). All physicians have the professional and ethical responsibility to participate in quality improvement, peer review, and proctoring activities appropriate to their skills and qualifications. Their active roles in the quality improvement process can be rotated to distribute the burden of uncompensated time and effort. Hospitals or outpatient practices may choose to offer incentives to physicians who actively volunteer to take part in this process as long as it does not create a conflict of interest for participating physicians.

LEADERSHIP

A quality improvement program requires both openness to feedback and a willingness to change existing practices. Because of this characteristic, a quality improvement program requires effective, responsive leadership in the department of obstetrics and gynecology, with support from the chief executive officer, the medical executive committee, and the governing board. The establishment of effective leadership is essential in developing a quality improvement program. The head of the department is responsible for overseeing quality improvement activities. In some cases, heads of departments or chief medical officers also may delegate specific quality improvement responsibilities to other physicians, such as patient safety officers, peer review committee chairs, or physician champions. When physicians accept leadership positions, such as a chief medical officer, chief of staff, or department chair, one of their primary responsibilities is to establish an environment in which quality improvements can thrive. As a corollary to the physician's time commitment, the hospital should consider providing a stipend for these leadership positions.

QUALITY IMPROVEMENT COMMITTEE

The quality improvement process should be multidisciplinary in nature and involve participation of all practitioners who provide care at the hospital, group, and private practice levels. A departmental quality improvement committee may include the following members, with consideration given to the vice chair of the department serving as the committee chair:

- Representative physicians with varying levels of clinical experience (junior and senior staff) within the department
- Representative licensed independent practitioners, physician assistants, and other health care providers
- A house staff member, when appropriate
- The department head (ex officio)

Participants in case reviews must be sensitive to potential conflicts of interest and scrupulously adhere to a consistent and unbiased process. When appropriate, physicians (including those from other specialties), physician assistants, certified nurse–midwives, nurse practitioners, registered nurses, pharmacists, hospital administrative and quality control personnel, social workers, or other health care providers may need to form a multidisciplinary task force to address specific issues identified during the quality improvement review process. These individuals also may be invited to the regular quality improvement committee meetings, as appropriate. At all times, confidentiality must be maintained. Minutes of previous meetings in which peer review activities are documented should be circulated only during the meetings themselves. Cases should be referenced by patient number to preserve confidentiality in accordance with the Health Insurance Portability and Accountability Act regulations.

The rules and regulations of the department should outline the responsibilities of the quality improvement committee and provide information on committee size, composition of membership, term of office, and method of appointment. Meeting guidelines also should be established. Part of the role of this committee and the department head is to create an atmosphere whereby clinicians and other members of the department are able to raise quality issues in a confidential manner. Committee meetings should be scheduled at regular intervals, often monthly, to allow sufficient time for concurrent and retrospective case analysis.

DEPARTMENT MEETINGS AND COMMUNICATION

Regular departmental meetings can be used to educate practitioners about improvement of quality of care. These meetings can be a good forum to discuss the importance of documentation; errors in documentation, such as failure to include a treatment plan or failure to sign and date all notes in the record; and making corrections in the record. Regular meetings of the department also can be used to address specific clinical issues. Some of the typical formats for discussing these topics include the following:

- Presentations by a team member of problem cases or near misses, including a discussion of the issues and a review of the literature and the methods that have been used by others to resolve the problems

- Presentations by outside guest experts

- Discussion of which practice guidelines can and should be incorporated into the department and how to implement those changes. This method of teaching reinforces the need to improve processes at a departmental level rather than addressing problems on an individual basis.

- Presentations that review complicated cases or difficult situations that were handled appropriately. These cases serve to identify which methods and treatments work well and can be used as the basis for protocols and improvement of care.

- Use of variances identified through the ongoing quality improvement process to determine topics for continuing education programs, such as grand rounds and morbidity and mortality conferences

Meetings can be organized into distinct sessions. Quality improvement can be discussed with a broader committee audience to allow for more collaborative exploration of processes. Case review can be attended by a more limited membership that will promote a more thorough and confidential discussion of the items presented.

Feedback is an essential part of quality improvement. Periodic presentation of morbidity and other departmental statistics helps department members see how they, as a department and individually, are doing. Staff members thus can understand the importance of what they are doing and how the changes they have instituted have had an effect on quality of care.

Staff also can be informed about changes and new protocols through staff letters or departmental e-mails. Reminders about quality of care, trends in the department, and the need for documentation can be included regularly. Electronic communications can be used to reinforce education and teaching. This technology allows new information to be disseminated more rapidly and efficiently. The staff can be informed quickly about a newly identified problem, the recall of drugs, or defective instruments. The medical staff office should maintain a database that includes contact information, and the contact information should be regularly verified and updated to ensure that physicians and other practitioners receive information that needs to be communicated and disseminated.

Reducing Variation

Experts suggest that substantial improvements in quality can be achieved by eliminating unnecessary variation in treatment plans. This standardization can be accomplished by drafting a protocol or algorithm or by using an existing protocol to address the issue. The department may choose to apply or develop clinical pathways or protocols for high-volume, resource-intensive, or costly procedures. Protocols may take the form of a multidisciplinary plan of care or a simple decision tree. As appropriate, national evidence-based guidelines should provide the basis for the development of clinical protocols. Deviations from the finalized protocol may occur, but documentation should reflect an awareness of the protocol and include the rationale for not following the standard procedure. All disciplines involved in providing care under a protocol should be involved in the design and implementation of the protocol.

Quality Measurement

Quality improvement programs must focus on measurable dimensions of care to identify areas in need of improvement and should evaluate the department as a whole, as well as individual physicians. A department should consider the dimensions of care when selecting indicators to track (see Box 1-4). Cases identified by one of these indicators may not necessarily indicate substandard care but do require careful review by physicians. Quality measurement should determine whether the care provided to a single patient or population of patients achieved good outcomes (outcomes measurement) or represented those processes that are thought or known to be associated with achievement of good outcomes (process measurement).

Box 1-4. Examples of Gynecologic Clinical Quality Indicators

- Unplanned readmission within 14 days
- Admission after a return visit to the emergency department for the same problem
- Cardiopulmonary arrest, resuscitated
- Infection that was not present on admission
- Unplanned admission to special (intensive) care unit
- Unplanned return to the operating room for surgery during the same admission
- Ambulatory surgery patient admitted or retained for complication of surgery or anesthesia
- Failure to administer appropriate deep vein thrombosis prophylaxis for gynecologic surgery
- Gynecologic surgery, except radical hysterectomy, cytoreductive surgery, or exenteration, using 2 or more units of blood, or postoperative hematocrit of less than 24% or hemoglobin of less than 8 g
- Wrong site, wrong patient, or wrong surgical procedure
- Unplanned removal, injury, or repair of organ during operative procedure
- Initiation of antibiotics more than 24 hours after surgery
- Discrepancy between preoperative diagnosis and postoperative tissue report
- Removal of uterus that weighs less than 280 g for leiomyomas
- Removal of follicular cyst or corpus luteum of ovary
- Hysterectomy performed on women younger than 30 years except for malignancy
- Prolonged hospitalization (more than two standard deviations from the mean stay for that diagnosis)
- Unanticipated death

Modified from American College of Obstetricians and Gynecologists. Quality and safety in women's health care. 2nd ed. Washington, DC: American College of Obstetricians and Gynecologists; 2010. p.17.

The methods used to determine quality or efficiency of care are called by many different names, such as rates, instruments, elements, standards, indicators, or measures. Although differences in definitions are nuanced depending on the audience, for this section, they will simply be referred to as indicators or measures.

Quality Indicators

The primary purpose of quality indicators is to stimulate discussion (and action if needed) around improving the care of and services for patients. Quality indicators are defined as follows*:

> ...specific and measurable elements of practice that can be used to assess the quality of care. They are usually derived from retrospective reviews of medical records or administrative claims and enrollment data. Measures are also being incorporated into and between electronic health records and data registries. Some authorities differentiate "quality" from "activity" or "performance" indicators. The important issue is that a good quality indicator should define care that is attributable and within the control of the person who is delivering the care.

It is important to note that indicators are not direct measures of quality; quality is multi-dimensional, and many different measurements must be made before it can be fully assessed. Quality indicators are best used as a means of improving a system of care, not judging performance or being used solely as a management tool.

Quality indicators may focus on structural elements, process components, or outcomes in the health care system or setting under study. Except for the most common outcomes, there are multiple technical and practical difficulties in assessing outcomes. As a result, quality is most often measured in the form of process indicators. It is important to note, however, that process indicators do not signify quality until their relationship to the desirable outcome is validated. Process indicators are particularly helpful when quality improvement is the goal of the assessment process, when

---

*Source: Marshall M, Campbell S, Hacker J, Roland M, editors. Quality indicators for general practice: a practical guide for health professionals and managers. London (UK): Royal Society of Medicine Press; 2002.

short time frames for measurement are needed, or when tools to adjust or stratify for patient factors are not available.

Evidence-based clinical indicators can be developed by following a six-step system:

1. Identify the outcome of interest.
2. Form a measurement team to provide an overview of existing evidence and practice.
3. Choose quality indicator(s) on the basis of research evidence.
4. Determine the standard of quality being sought.
5. Design a reliable and valid system of measurements that can be applied consistently.
6. Conduct preliminary testing for reliability and validity.

Several sources of benchmarks of quality indicators are available for individual health care providers or practices, such as *Healthy People 2020*, National Committee for Quality Assurance Healthcare Effectiveness Data and Information Set (also known as HEDIS) data, and the Agency for Healthcare Research and Quality National Healthcare Quality Report (see Resources).

Indicators may be monitors of sentinel events, such as retained foreign objects; if so, every case should be reviewed frequently on an expedited basis. Indicators may monitor specific rates, such as with excess blood loss. If the frequency of a rate-based indicator exceeds the departmental threshold or there are changes in frequency over time, an in-depth review may be needed. Indicators may be positive and desirable, such as detection and treatment of chlamydial infection, or negative, such as an unplanned return to the operating room.

Indicators should be clearly and specifically defined so that they can be benchmarked and the results can be compared with regional or national norms. Risk-adjustment methods (eg, body mass index, comorbidities, diabetes, and hypertension) should be used when possible. Deviations from the norm can then be readily identified. Physician profiles also may be developed so that an individual's practice pattern for each indicator can be compared with department and national or regional benchmarks. Such profiles will form part of the database used to make decisions on granting or renewing clinical privileges and can be used to show improvement over time. Deviations from the norm do not necessarily indicate inappropriate care. Use of a clinical indicator may flag cases managed by a particular physician that, when peer reviewed, appear to show plausible reasons for the variations. However, continued monitoring over time (referred to as trending) may demonstrate that this physician has a much higher rate of variation than the department as a whole. Therefore, trending data may suggest a problem, such as surgical technique, that an individual case review does not identify.

Institutions may wish to define acceptable levels of care (ie, thresholds) for different indicators. A threshold is a data point that, when reached or crossed, signals an outlier that needs further investigation and evaluation. Using thresholds is a method for deciding when an issue should be addressed and where first to look for possible problems without requiring peer review of all records. The threshold level chosen as the standard for the institution should be supported by the best available clinical and quality improvement literature. Information on local and national rates of complications may be obtained from the respective state health data organization, the National Center for Health Statistics, or the Agency for Healthcare Research and Quality. Hospital departments also may participate in data registries, such as the National Surgical Quality Improvement Programs through the American College of Surgeons or the U.S. Department of Veterans Affairs, for risk-adjusted benchmarks. Thresholds may need to be changed as new technology evolves and treatments improve.

Performance Measures

Performance measures are designed to guide physicians in their evaluation, reporting, and delivery of quality care to patients. Although they may measure different components of quality, they should ultimately be linked in a meaningful way to outcomes. Currently, the major obstacle to improving the quality of health care in the United States is the lack of a coherent and consistent system for assessing and reporting on the performance of the health care system. Regardless, stakeholders want more information about how the health care system is performing, and they want to know that health care delivery actually is improving health outcomes. The Institute of Medicine report on performance measures, payment, and performance improvement noted that current performance measurement systems are limited because it is not always clear that the criteria being measured are truly or solely responsible for improvements that may be seen (see Bibliography).

Types of Performance Measures. Performance measures include measures of the health care process (eg, hemoglobin A_{1C} testing for patients with diabetes), health outcomes (eg, surgical-site infections), perceptions of care (eg, patient satisfaction with physician interactions), and organizational structure and systems (eg, electronic order entry). Standardized performance measures have detailed specifications; they may require risk adjustment or stratification of results across key subgroups. A key element of any performance measurement system is ensuring that data for performance measures are reported accurately.

Performance measures should be designed to be used as a guide by physicians in their evaluation, reporting, and delivery of quality care to patients. They should be linked in a meaningful way to outcomes, but they do not necessarily have to measure outcomes. Performance measures and process measures may have some fundamental advantages over outcomes measures:

- Reduce case mix bias—Performance measures use opportunity for error rather than the number of patients treated as the denominator.

- Avoid stigma—Performance measures are more likely to be perceived as suggestions for improvement, rather than criticisms of performance.

- Prompt wider action—Process measures encourage action at every level of the organization, not just by a few individuals or the outliers.

- Evaluate delayed events—Process measures are more useful for evaluating events that may take longer to appear.

Process measurements can be precisely defined and are often very specific; hence, they are not usually subject to risk adjustment. They are ideal measures to include as performance measures, but only if there is an evidence-based link to quality improvement. It is not practical to set the threshold for measurement at 100%—too many exclusion criteria would need to be incorporated and result in increased data burdens on health care providers—but levels may be based on aggregate national data.

Data for Performance Measurement. There are three main sources of data for performance measurements: 1) administrative claims and enrollment data, 2) medical records (paper and electronic) and registries, and 3) surveys. Administrative claims systems are not designed to be specific and reliable tools for quality measurement and reporting. Paper medical record abstraction of data is time consuming and expensive, and electronic medical records are in their infancy in regards to interoperability, standardization, and use. Surveys of patient perception of patient care are attributed to a specific practice because either the patient identified one of the health care providers as her primary care provider or computerized algorithms based on claims designate a practitioner as the primary care provider. All of these approaches are subject to error.

QUALITY MEASUREMENT TOOLS

A quality improvement program also requires tools to assess and determine overall performance. Failure mode and effects analysis and root cause analysis are tools that may be used in the process of setting up systems or procedures in order to evaluate these systems for possible errors. They also may be used for continued surveillance of ongoing systems and procedures to effect change and corrective actions designed to make them safer.

Failure Mode and Effects Analysis

Failure mode and effects analysis is a prospective risk assessment tool that is used to analyze proposed systems, production lines, or processes for possible unanticipated faults, defects, and errors. This tool generally is used during the planning or organizing process for these systems or procedures. The potential errors or faults are identified and rated by levels of severity or potential harm that they may cause. This tool also assesses the effect of these errors on the system or procedure that is being considered.

Failure mode and effects analysis initially was used by the military and in aerospace development. It is widely used in manufacturing industries in various phases of production. Medical device and drug delivery systems have added failure mode and effects analysis procedures as a means to understand the potential risks and defects that may not be considered by individual designers. Failure mode and effects analysis is now increasingly finding use in the service industry, and hospitals also have begun to use this technique to prevent the possibility of process errors and mistakes, which lead to incorrect surgery or medication administration. This use is driven by The Joint Commission.

Failure mode and effects analysis allows a team of individuals to review the design or process at key points in its development and make comments and changes to the design of the system or process well in advance of actually experiencing the failure. The U.S. Food and Drug Administration has recognized failure mode and effects analysis as a design verification method for drugs and medical devices.

In a failure mode and effects analysis, failures and errors are prioritized according to how serious their consequences are, how frequently they occur, and how easily they can be detected. This analysis also documents and updates current knowledge about the process being monitored and is used as a tool for continuous improvement. Failure mode and effects analysis begins during the earliest conceptual stages of design of a process or system and then continues throughout the life of that system. It is used during the design stage with an aim to avoid future potential or actual complications and errors. Later it is used for monitoring and modification before and during ongoing operation of the process.

The Department of Veterans Affairs National Center for Patient Safety developed a hybrid prospective risk analysis system, Healthcare Failure Mode and Effect Analysis, which includes a five-step process that uses an interdisciplinary team to proactively evaluate a health care process. The team uses process flow diagramming, a Hazard Scoring Matrix, and the Healthcare Failure Mode and Effect Analysis Decision Tree to identify and assess potential vulnerabilities. Information on this system is publicly available through the National Center for Patient Safety (see www.patient safety.va.gov/).

Root Cause Analysis

Root cause analysis is a group of problem-solving methods aimed at identifying the underlying causes of problems or events. The theory of root cause analysis is that problems are best solved by correcting or eliminating root (underlying) causes of the problem and not merely addressing the obvious symptoms. Root cause analysis is a tool used to identify process and system failures that result in sentinel events, medical error, or near misses. A root cause analysis should identify the reason for the presence of a defect or problem that, if eliminated, would prevent recurrence. There is recognition that complete prevention of recurrence of an error by a single intervention is not always possible, and as a result, a root cause analysis often is considered to be an iterative process and viewed as a tool of continuous improvement.

There are several general principles that apply to a root cause analysis. The process is a retrospective tool that is applied systematically. It is also an interdisciplinary tool and is performed with the ultimate goal of concentrating on the systems and processes rather than the performance of individuals. It is a learning tool that is used to promote teamwork, facilitate open communication, prevent similar errors in the future, and enhance patient safety and quality of care. Relevant data and literature must be used in drawing conclusions that are evidence based. There is frequently more than one root cause for any given problem. This tool looks into determining human factors as well as related processes and systems.

Performing a root cause analysis often is triggered as a requirement of The Joint Commission. The Joint Commission requires that specific sentinel events that trigger a root cause analysis include an evaluation of very specific processes as part of the root cause analysis. In addition to The Joint Commission, there may be other state and local regulatory agencies that could require a root cause analysis in response to a medical error or some other poor outcome. In some cases, a professional liability carrier might require a root cause analysis as a result of a poor patient outcome that could potentially increase a liability exposure for the carrier and its clients. Hospitals should incorporate the root cause analysis and its resultant monitoring into the ongoing quality improvement process.

DATA COLLECTION AND ANALYSIS

The quality improvement process requires accurate collection and analysis of meaningful data. Data collection is important not only to formulate the problem statement, but also to support the team's belief that a planned change will result in improvement. Initial data collection is key for problem identification. Data also are critical for demonstrating that changes will result in system improvement. This is particularly helpful because not all change results in improvement. It may not be necessary to collect volumes of data before effecting change. For example, sampling can be used to demonstrate the change being tested. Another suggestion is to use both qualitative and quantitative data. Process and outcome measures also may be used to help determine whether a change has led to improvement.

Historically, data have been collected by retrospective chart review. Quality improvement ideally includes concurrent data collection as well. Clinical indicators should guide the abstraction of data by trained individuals. Cases identified through application of the indicators should be reviewed by physicians with judgment and experience in the clinical issues and the peer review process.

The data obtained by this process also can be used for educational purposes:

- To inform all staff members of the performance of the unit as a whole

- To inform individual clinicians how their care compares with that of their peers

- To update staff about current techniques to improve outcomes

The ultimate objective is to encourage behavioral changes, system changes, or both to reduce unwarranted variation and improve patient safety. Results may be shared through departmental meetings, quarterly summaries of trends, and letters directed at the medical staff. Continuing medical education should focus on correcting deficiencies in knowledge or unexplained variations in care identified through the quality improvement process.

Although screening medical records for indicators can aid in identifying practice variations that might indicate the need for further review, documentation, or justification, more often than not, cases that are identified through this process have no quality of care issues. Peer review can determine whether such variations are appropriate. Therefore, identified cases should be reviewed by physicians with the knowledge, experience, and judgment to assess the clinical appropriateness of practice variations.

PEER REVIEW

Small departments face a variety of challenges to conduct effective peer review because of several factors, which might include the following:

- Competitive interests
- Fear of reprisal
- Conflict of interest
- Lack of objectivity
- Personal relationships
- Lack of qualified reviewers

These factors may have a real or perceived effect on the efficacy of the review. Therefore, it may be helpful to develop a relationship with another hospital to conduct peer review. An alternative would be to use the services of an outside, independent reviewer. In either case, it is important to remember that responsibility for peer review and quality improvement rests with the hospital medical staff and, ultimately, the governing board.

Departments of any size may face these challenges and consider developing a relationship with another hospital or an outside peer review organization. A specialty-specific program that can assist with issues related to quality assessment and peer review is the Voluntary Review of Quality of Care Program of the American Congress of Obstetricians and Gynecologists (see Box 1-5).

Both federal and state laws provide some protection for physician peer review. The Health Care Quality Improvement Act, passed by the U.S. Congress in October 1986, grants immunity from damages under federal and state laws (including antitrust provisions) to health care providers engaged in good faith peer review. Most states also have adopted laws to encourage and protect physician peer review, although the type of immunity offered and the class of individuals protected from personal liability for participating in peer review vary from state to state.

Most states safeguard the confidentiality of records used in peer review actions. Again, the extent of the protection varies from jurisdiction to jurisdiction, and anyone engaged in peer review should know the laws of his or her state. For example, some states recognize confidentiality only for the

---

Box 1-5. Voluntary Review of Quality of Care

The Voluntary Review of Quality of Care (VRQC) program of the American Congress of Obstetricians and Gynecologists is available to assist hospitals and physicians in assessing the quality of care provided in their departments of obstetrics and gynecology as well as the quality improvement process within the department. The VRQC peer review teams consist of five reviewers: three obstetrician–gynecologists, one nurse, and one medical writer. When requested, these review teams also can include individuals with expertise in midwifery, anesthesiology, and family medicine. The reviews are conducted over 4 days and include one-on-one interviews, chart reviews, an introductory entrance conference as well as an exit conference, and a detailed report that includes an analysis of data submitted by the hospital, the VRQC review team's findings, and recommendations for improvement based on the American Congress of Obstetricians and Gynecologists' guidelines.

For more information about the VRQC Program, send an email to vrqc@acog.org, call (800) 266-8043, or visit www.acog.org/goto/vrqc.

American Congress of Obstetricians and Gynecologists. VRQC program overview. Available at: http://www.acog.org/About_ACOG/ACOG_Departments/VRQC_and_SCOPE/VRQC_Program_Overview. Retrieved July 10, 2013.

---

peer review records of a hospital review committee, whereas others protect all information reported to the committee. In some states, the information is not admissible as evidence in a trial but may be discoverable in pretrial proceedings. To ensure the maximum protection of records, individuals formulating a hospital's quality review program should seek legal advice.

CORRECTING A DEFICIENCY

When a quality improvement process identifies deficiencies in the quality of care provided by a specific individual, the department head or other responsible person has the responsibility, and should have the authority, to take steps to correct the deficiency. The identification of the problem, how it was addressed, and what action was instituted should be documented. This documentation should include a statement of the expectations for change, the means by which change will be measured, and if appropriate, a time line. Most opportunities for improvement can be handled under the authority of the department head or other responsible person. When the recommended action requires the involvement of the appropriate institutional governing board, established procedures should facilitate necessary decision making. When the action required involves a reduction or revocation of privileges, it is critical to have legal consultation to ensure that the process is handled appropriately.

Timely discussion and counseling with the practitioner always should be the first step in the process. In certain circumstances it may be all that is required. The following are other possible actions that may be instituted:

- Observation of the practitioner's skills. Observation is either by the department head or by a designated staff member who may have the skills required to assess a particular procedure or treatment.

- Trending. Continued monitoring over time can determine whether the physician has a much higher rate of variation than the department as a whole. Trending data may identify a problem, such as surgical technique, that an individual case review does not identify.

- Remedial education. This education may take the form of special programs focused on need. Remedial education may be necessary because of an identified deficiency in care, in which case a remedial program for the individual may be provided or obtained elsewhere. When a deficiency involves several staff members, it is more appropriate to direct the education toward the unit as a whole. This process, along with resulting findings, should be reported to the institutional quality improvement committee.

- Proctoring. Proctoring requires the direct observation of an individual's practice by a peer or a chart review of current or recently treated patients to ensure that the deficiencies are being corrected.

- External peer review. This action may be used when there is interpersonal conflict, disagreement as to the appropriate action, or a lack of comparable skill within the department.

When the quality improvement process or other mechanisms have identified unwarranted variation, a specific problem, an opportunity to improve care, concerns about patient safety, or individual performance problems, a plan should be formulated. When data gathered suggest that change will lead to improvement, the changes then can be implemented in a systemwide manner.

When the deficiency is considered more serious, privileges may be reduced. Reducing privileges requires formal proceedings, which should be prescribed in the medical staff bylaws and may be subject to reporting to the National Practitioner Data Bank (see also the "Evaluating Credentials and Granting Privileges" section earlier in Part 1).

Quality Improvement in the Office

The medical office or clinic is well suited to modern methods of quality improvement, and programs and resources that address quality improvement in the office continue to evolve. Ideally, a written quality management plan should be established. In the outpatient setting, whether in a solo office practice or a multispecialty ambulatory surgery center, a physician should be designated as the chief medical officer to be responsible for the patient safety and quality improvement initiatives. As with hospitals, outpatient settings should consider providing a stipend for these leadership positions. The office staff (including clinicians and administrative staff) should meet periodically as a team to discuss methods of measuring and improving the quality of the care administered by the office. Larger practices may want to designate an interdisciplinary quality management team.

Each office should establish a simple, reliable tracking and reminder system to improve patient safety and quality of care and to minimize missed diagnoses. The use of an electronic health record may be used as a real-time, evidence-based support tool that can help obstetrician–gynecologists improve the quality of care they provide through improved care coordination, communication, and documentation.

The office can develop specific indicators to evaluate one or more systems (see Box 1-6). Quality management activities within the medical office may concentrate on assessing and improving function in one specific system at a time. Once that function has improved to a level of quality acceptable to the practice, the quality management team can move to another system for review. Several systems may be monitored optimally by regular tracking (eg, patient complaints or complications of office procedures). Medical practices also may wish to evaluate the quality of care

Box 1-6. Examples of Systems to Monitor for Quality Improvement in the Office

Medical Records and Information Systems
- Legibility
- Organization
- Documentation—general (including problem list)
- Lost medical records
- Misfiled medical records
- Breach of confidentiality
- List of current medications
- Health Insurance Portability and Accountability Act compliance

Appointments and Scheduling—Patient Flow
- Acceptable waiting time for appointments
- Appropriate waiting time in office to see clinician

Billing
- Precertification
- Timeliness
- Accurate coding

Patient Communications
- Method of informing patients of a delayed or rescheduled appointment
- Monitoring of appropriateness of method of terminating patient–practitioner relationship

Telephone Communications
- Excessive busy signals (data are available from telephone company)
- Excessive holding time
- Documentation of telephone contact in medical records, with disposition documented
- Monitoring of telephone prescription refills for doctor approval
- Monitoring of "dropped" or lost calls

(continued)

Box 1-6. Examples of Systems to Monitor for Quality Improvement in the Office *(continued)*

Personnel Management
- Employee morale
- Absenteeism
- Periodic employee performance assessment
- Maintenance of patient confidentiality

Equipment and Drugs
- Periodic equipment check for proper function
- Maintenance logs of equipment repair
- Security system for controlled drugs
- Security system for syringes and needles
- Method of monitoring drugs for expiration dates (including samples)

Patient Safety and Medical Error Reduction
- Tracking systems for laboratory, radiology, and cytology results
- Safe medication use
- Wound infections
- Delayed complications from hospitalized patients
- Equipment failure

administered by their practitioners in the hospital setting separate from the hospital's quality management program. These issues may include continuity of care, consistency of care, cross-coverage, and communication.

Efforts made to improve quality and patient safety also will have positive effects on risk reduction; therefore, the two programs may be carried out in tandem. An example of a program that can assist with issues related to quality assessment and peer review in the outpatient setting is the Safety Certification in Outpatient Practice Excellence program of the American Congress of Obstetricians and Gynecologists (Box 1-7). Professional liability carriers also may have useful tools for improving quality and patient safety.

Box 1-7. Safety Certification in Outpatient Practice Excellence

The Safety Certification in Outpatient Practice Excellence (SCOPE) for Women's Health program of the American Congress of Obstetricians and Gynecologists is a voluntary, comprehensive, patient safety review program available to medical practices in which obstetric services, gynecologic services, or both are provided. Through the two-step application and site-review process, the SCOPE for Women's Health program assesses the implementation and use of patient safety concepts and techniques in an individual office setting. For more information about the SCOPE for Women's Health program, send an e-mail to scope@acog.org, call (800) 266-8043, or visit www.scopeforwomenshealth.org.

American Congress of Obstetricians and Gynecologists. Safety Certification in Outpatient Practice Excellence (SCOPE). Available at: http://www.scopeforwomens health.org. Retrieved July 10, 2013.

There are a number of challenges to developing a performance measurement framework for physician practices. Listed are questions to consider at the beginning of the development process:

- What will be the specific purposes of the measurement system?

- How should the specific aspects of performance (for which individual physicians or physician organizations will be held accountable) be measured?

- What specific information should be part of the performance measurement system and included in the reporting system? What are the optimal formats for disseminating performance information?

- How will performance measures for physicians or physician practices be implemented in an ongoing and feasibly sustainable way? Who will bear the costs?

Meaningful reporting at the practice level is a challenge. For example, the challenges for measuring performance in small practices include lack of infrastructure, lack of health information technology, lack of support staff, and increased burden of data collection. A 2003 survey found that less than 24% of physicians were able to compare their performance with their peers either within their specialty or within health plans. Only 11% were able to meet the benchmark of physicians nationally.

Public and private payor data must be pooled to yield meaningful information for small practice settings. Individual insurers do not account for a large enough share of a practice's population to provide meaningful measures of performance. Some aspects of practice performance are quite difficult to assess; this is particularly true if a practitioner sees a low volume of patients, in which case there will not be enough data to provide meaningful or valid assessments of performance. When sample sizes are small, there are problems with risk adjustment and bias, and although these issues may be dealt with, there is currently no mechanism for pooling data across purchasers. Whereas all health care providers involved in the care of a patient share in the responsibility for providing quality care, designing measurement systems that accurately reflect the degree of influence and responsibility of each practitioner is problematic at best.

Bibliography

Berwick DM. Continuous improvement as an ideal in health care. N Engl J Med 1989;320:53–6.

DeRosier J, Stalhandske E, Bagian JP, Nudell T. Using health care Failure Mode and Effect Analysis: the VA National Center for Patient Safety's prospective risk analysis system. Jt Comm J Qual Improv 2002;28:248–67.

Institute of Medicine (U.S.). Health literacy: a prescription to end confusion. Washington, D.C.: The National Academies Press; 2004.

Institute of Medicine (U.S.). Performance measurement: accelerating improvement. Washington, D.C.: National Academies Press; 2006.

Institute of Medicine (U.S.). Priority areas for national action: transforming health care quality. Washington, D.C.: National Academies Press; 2003.

Institute of Medicine (U.S.). Crossing the quality chasm: a new health system for the 21st century. Washington, D.C.: National Academy Press; 2001.

Kongnyuy EJ, Uthman OA. Use of criterion-based clinical audit to improve the quality of obstetric care: A systematic review. Acta Obstet Gynecol Scand 2009;88: 873–81.

Marshall M, Campbell S, Hacker J, Roland M, editors. Quality indicators for general practice: a practical guide for health professionals and managers. London (UK): Royal Society of Medicine Press; 2002.

Patient safety and the electronic health record. Committee Opinion No. 472. American College of Obstetricians and Gynecologists. Obstet Gynecol 2010; 116:1245–7.

Standardization of practice to improve outcomes. Committee Opinion No. 526. American College of Obstetricians and Gynecologists. Obstet Gynecol 2012;119:1081–2.

Tracking and reminder systems. Committee Opinion No. 546. American College of Obstetricians and Gynecologists. Obstet Gynecol 2012;120:1535–7.

Resources

ABIM Foundation. Choosing Wisely: Five things physicians and patients should question. Available at: http://www.choosingwisely.org/doctor-patient-lists. Retrieved July 10, 2013.

Agency for Healthcare Research and Quality. National healthcare quality and disparities reports. Available at: http://www.ahrq.gov/research/findings/nhqrdr/index.html. Retrieved July 10, 2013.

American College of Obstetricians and Gynecologists. Quality and safety in women's health care. 2nd ed. Washington, DC: American College of Obstetricians and Gynecologists; 2010.

Audet AJ, Doty MM, Shamasdin J, Schoenbaum SC. Physicians' views on quality of care: findings from the Commonwealth Fund National Survey of Physicians and Quality of Care. New York (NY): The Commonwealth Fund; 2005. Available at: http://www.commonwealthfund.org/Publications/Fund-Reports/2005/May/Physicians-Views-on-Quality-of-Care--Findings-From-The-Commonwealth-Fund-National-Survey-of-Physicia.aspx. Retrieved July 10, 2013.

Department of Health and Human Services. Healthy People 2020. Available at: http://www.healthypeople.gov/2020/default.aspx. Retrieved July 10, 2013.

National Committee for Quality Assurance. HEDIS and performance measurement. Available at: http://www.ncqa.org/tabid/59/Default.aspx. Retrieved July 10, 2013.

PATIENT SAFETY

Patient safety shares many characteristics with a well-designed quality improvement model. However, patient safety emphasizes a systems analysis of medical errors and minimizes individual blame and retribution while still maintaining individual accountability. Patient safety is an explicit principle that must be embraced as a core value in patient care. This is an ongoing process that requires health care providers to continually strive to learn from problems, identify system deficiencies, redesign processes, and implement change in their daily practice. Patient-centered care, open communication, and teamwork provide the foundation for optimal patient care and safety.

National Patient Safety Goals

The Joint Commission recognizes the importance of patient safety. In 2003, it created the first set of National Patient Safety Goals. These goals, derived from Sentinel Event Alerts and other sources, are designed to be explicit, evidence based, and measurable. Each year, The Joint Commission modifies existing goals based on public comment and the experience of its reviewers, and new goals are added. In this way, over time, The Joint Commission will develop a compendium of recommended practices that will improve patient safety (see www.jointcommission.org/standards_information/npsgs.aspx).

Patient Safety Principles

The American College of Obstetricians and Gynecologists (the College) continues to emphasize its longstanding commitment to quality improvement and patient safety by codifying a set of objectives to improve patient care and reduce medical errors. The College encourages all obstetrician–gynecologists to promote the following principles in all practice settings:

- Develop a commitment to encourage a culture of patient safety.
- Implement recommended safe medication practices.
- Reduce the likelihood of surgical errors.
- Improve hand hygiene.
- Improve communication with health care providers and patients.
- Make safety a priority in every aspect of practice.

DEVELOP A CULTURE OF PATIENT SAFETY

A culture of patient safety (see Box 1-8) continuously evolves and should be the framework for every effort to reduce medical errors. Patient safety focuses on systems of care, not individuals. Confidential reporting and analysis of errors and near misses will reveal areas that require system changes, not individual punishment, to improve patient safety. State and

---

Box 1-8. A Culture of Patient Safety

Although an exact definition of a culture of patient safety does not exist, a recurring theme in the literature is that organizations with effective safety cultures share a constant commitment to safety as a top-level priority, which permeates the entire organization. Noted components include the following:

- Acknowledgment of the high-risk nature of an organization's activities and the determination to achieve consistently safe operations
- A blame-free environment where individuals are able to report errors or near misses without fear of reprimand or punishment
- Encouragement of collaboration across ranks and disciplines to seek solutions to patient safety problems
- Organizational commitment of resources to address safety concerns

Data from Agency for Healthcare Research and Quality. Patient safety primers: Safety Culture. Available at: http://psnet.ahrq.gov/primer.aspx?primerID=5. Retrieved October 28, 2013.

federal laws may have an effect on the level of confidentiality and the manner of reporting.

A culture of patient safety starts at the top with strong leadership that provides the necessary human and financial resources to maximize patient safety. Additionally, a culture of patient safety recognizes the importance of team function in optimizing individual performance. Essential to this team effort is effective leadership, communication, collaboration, situational awareness, and mutual respect. Associated with a safety culture is the concept of a "just culture," which recognizes that competent professionals make mistakes and acknowledges that even competent professionals may develop unhealthy norms, such as shortcuts or routine rule violations, but has zero tolerance for reckless behavior.

IMPLEMENT RECOMMENDED SAFE MEDICATION PRACTICES

Medication errors are one of the most common types of preventable adverse events. Automated systems for prescribing and dispensing medication can reduce, but will not eliminate, these errors; however, many "low-tech" solutions can be implemented rapidly, with minimal costs:

- Improve the legibility of written orders.
- Ensure the completeness of medical orders, including the name of the drug, dose, route of administration, frequency or rate, reason or conditions under which the drug should be administered (if prescribing with directions to take as required), and patient's weight and age (if relevant to dosing).
- Avoid nonstandard abbreviations, as recommended by The Joint Commission (see Table 1-1).
- Always use a leading 0 for doses less than 1 unit (eg, 0.1, not .1), and never use a trailing 0 after a decimal point (eg, 1 mg, not 1.0 mg): "Always lead, never follow."
- Provide the reasons for giving the medication or the parameters for giving a pro re nata (p.r.n.) dose. This is particularly helpful in preventing errors with medications that sound alike and look alike or for medications that are to be given on an as-needed basis (eg, p.r.n. for moderate-to-severe cramping, rather than simply p.r.n.).

- Ensure that all verbal orders are written by the individual receiving the order and then read back to the prescriber. Verbal orders should be limited to urgent situations in which written or electronic orders are not feasible. Because many drugs have soundalike names, it is also helpful to include the indication for the drug in verbal medication orders.

Table 1-1. The Joint Commission's Official "Do Not Use" Abbreviations List*

Do Not Use	Potential Problem	Use Instead
U, u (unit)	Mistaken for "0" (zero), the number "4" (four), or "cc"	Write "unit"
IU (International Unit)	Mistaken for IV (intravenous) or the number 10 (ten)	Write "International Unit"
Q.D., QD, q.d., qd (daily)	Mistaken for each other	Write "daily"
Q.O.D., QOD, q.o.d., qod (every other day)	Period after the Q mistaken for "I" and the "O" mistaken for "I"	Write "every other day"
Trailing zero (X.0 mg)†	Decimal point is missed	Write "X mg"
Lack of leading zero (.X mg)	Decimal point is missed	Write "0.X mg"
MS	Can mean morphine sulfate or magnesium sulfate	Write "morphine sulfate"
MSO_4 and $MgSO_4$	Confused for one another	Write "magnesium sulfate"

*Applies to all orders and all medication-related documentation that is handwritten (including free-text computer entry) or on preprinted forms.

†Exception: A "trailing zero" may be used only where required to demonstrate the level of precision of the value being reported, such as for laboratory results, imaging studies that report size of lesions, or catheter and tube sizes. It may not be used in medication orders or other medication-related documentation.

Copyright The Joint Commission, 2013. Reprinted with permission. The Joint Commission. Facts about the official "Do Not Use" List. Oakbrook Terrace (IL): Joint Commission; 2013. Available at: http://www.jointcommission.org/assets/1/18/Do_Not_Use_List.pdf. Retrieved July 10, 2013.

REDUCE THE LIKELIHOOD OF SURGICAL ERRORS

In 2003, The Joint Commission published "Universal Protocol for Preventing Wrong Site, Wrong Procedure, Wrong Person Surgery" (see www.jointcommission.org/standards_information/up.aspx). This protocol complements the World Health Organization Surgical Safety Checklist, last revised in 2009 (see Fig.1-2).

The Universal Protocol involves the completion of three principal components before initiation of any surgical procedure:

1. Preprocedure verification process. The health care team ensures that all relevant documents and studies are available before the procedure starts; are correctly identified, labeled, and matched to the patient's identifiers; and are reviewed and are consistent with the team's understanding of the intended patient, procedure, and site. The team must address missing information or discrepancies before starting the procedure.

2. Marking the operative site. Procedures that require marking of the incision or insertion site include those in which there is more than one possible location for the procedure or when performing the procedure in a different location would negatively affect quality or safety. Although The Joint Commission does not require a specific site-marking method, each facility should be consistent in the method it uses to ensure that the mark is unambiguous. Only the correct site should be marked; an "X" or "No" should never be used on the wrong side.

3. Performing a "time out" before the procedure. The operative team (anesthesia personnel, surgeons, and nurse) conducts a final assessment to verify that the correct patient, site, and procedure are identified; admittedly, this is problematic in emergency situations.

An essential element of this overall process is the formal enlistment of active involvement by the patient to avert errors in the operative arena. Involving the patient in this manner requires personal effort by the surgeon to educate the patient during the preoperative evaluation process. The patient, who has the greatest stake in avoiding errors, thus becomes integrally involved in helping ensure that errors are avoided.

Surgical Safety Checklist

Before induction of anesthesia → **Before skin incision** → **Before patient leaves operating room**

Before induction of anesthesia

(with at least nurse and anesthetist)

Has the patient confirmed her identity, site, procedure, and consent?
- ☐ Yes

Is the site marked?
- ☐ Yes
- ☐ Not applicable

Is the anesthesia machine and medication check complete?
- ☐ Yes

Is the pulse oximeter on the patient and functioning?
- ☐ Yes

Does the patient have a:

Known allergy?
- ☐ No
- ☐ Yes

Difficult airway or aspiration risk?
- ☐ No
- ☐ Yes, and equipment/assistance available

Risk of >500 mL blood loss (7 mL/kg in children)?
- ☐ No
- ☐ Yes, and two IVs/central access and fluids planned

Before skin incision

(with nurse, anesthetist, and surgeon)

- ☐ **Confirm all team members have introduced themselves by name and role.**
- ☐ **Confirm the patient's name, procedure, and where the incision will be made.**

Has antibiotic prophylaxis been given within the past 60 minutes?
- ☐ Yes
- ☐ Not applicable

Anticipated critical events

To surgeon:
- ☐ What are the critical or nonroutine steps?
- ☐ How long will the case take?
- ☐ What is the anticipated blood loss?

To anesthetist:
- ☐ Are there any patient-specific concerns?

To nursing team:
- ☐ Has sterility (including indicator results) been confirmed?
- ☐ Are there equipment issues or any concerns?

Is essential imaging displayed?
- ☐ Yes
- ☐ Not applicable

Before patient leaves operating room

(with nurse, anesthetist, and surgeon)

Nurse verbally confirms:
- ☐ The name of the procedure
- ☐ Completion of instrument, sponge, and needle counts
- ☐ Specimen labeling (read specimen labels aloud, including patient name)
- ☐ Whether there are any equipment problems to be addressed

To surgeon, anesthetist, and nurse:
- ☐ What are the key concerns for recovery and management of this patient?

Fig. 1-2. World Health Organization's surgical safety checklist. Abbreviation: IV, intravenous. This checklist is not intended to be comprehensive. Based on the WHO Surgical Safety Checklist, URL http://whqlibdoc.who.int/publications/2009/9789241598590_eng_Checklist.pdf. Copyright World Health Organization 2009. All rights reserved.

New techniques and new equipment are important components for developing and delivering the best quality care in the operating room, but they also represent sources of potential surgical error. A surgeon who is performing a new surgical technique should be assisted or supervised by a colleague more experienced in the technique until competency has been satisfactorily demonstrated. In some circumstances, however, a technique may be so innovative that no other surgeon at that locale has more experience. In such situations, it may be wise to arrange for extra support staff or surgical backup to be available should difficulties arise. The surgeon involved should have already documented skills and experience in the related surgical arena and should have solicited and received the advice and support of other experienced surgeons. Using a simulator to assess expertise with new techniques and equipment also may be helpful with this process.

When new equipment is introduced, all members of the surgical team must be trained on and practice with the new equipment as appropriate for the extent of their involvement; additionally, all personnel involved must be aware of all device safety features, warnings, and alarms. Any manuals or operating instructions provided by the manufacturer should be reviewed carefully by the principal users and should be familiar to anyone using the equipment. Stickers attached to the device or plastic cards summarizing instructions for proper use may be helpful.

IMPROVE HAND HYGIENE

It is estimated that approximately 90,000 hospital patient deaths per year are related to nosocomial infections. Many of these infections are considered preventable with proper attention to standard infection control guidelines and proper hand hygiene. An effective program of routine hand hygiene before and after every patient encounter and appropriate glove use for all caregivers is a critical component of a culture of safety (see also the "Infection Control" section in Part 2). Effective infection control programs have been introduced in institutions around the country and have been proven to reduce the incidence of nosocomial infections and to be cost-effective. However, many institutions nationwide have been frustrated in their inability to establish a routine of hand hygiene for all physicians and nursing staff, despite evidence of the success of such programs.

Proper infection control programs, including hand hygiene guidelines, have become a requirement for The Joint Commission hospital accreditation. The Joint Commission standard IC.01.04.01 requires a policy for improving adherence to hand hygiene guidelines. In addition, The Joint Commission's National Patient Safety Goal 7 requires adherence to current World Health Organization or Centers for Disease Control and Prevention hand hygiene guidelines. Other organizations have endorsed effective hand washing guidelines, including the American Medical Association, the American Academy of Family Physicians (four principles of hand awareness), Agency for Healthcare Research and Quality, the Institute for Healthcare Improvement, and the College. The critical importance of proper hand hygiene, especially for prevention of methicillin-resistant *Staphylococcus aureus*, is well known and documented throughout the medical literature.

Numerous suggestions have been found to help improve hand hygiene campaigns in hospitals across the country. A hand hygiene awareness program may include posters, buttons, lapel pins, stickers, posted signs at every sink, and frequent reminders for all members of the health care team. Some institutions have encouraged patient involvement with information in every patient care area asking patients to remind caregivers to cleanse their hands before and after each patient contact, especially with systems of "gel in, gel out" that utilize convenient hand sanitizer dispensers in every patient care location.

IMPROVE COMMUNICATION WITH HEALTH CARE PROVIDERS AND PATIENTS

Physicians should be aware that complete and accurate communication of medical information is imperative for reducing preventable medical errors. Improving communication skills merits the same attention as improving surgical skills. According to information gathered from The Joint Commission in collecting sentinel event information, the most common cause of preventable adverse outcomes is communication error. Additionally, patient–physician communication problems may increase professional liability actions. Optimal communication to improve patient safety has many dimensions, including the following:

- Communication with patient and family
- Communication among all individuals caring for the patient
- Availability of information necessary for coordination of care

Communication With Patients

The key to a good patient–clinician relationship is the ability to listen, explain, and empathize. The U.S. Preventive Services Task Force defines shared decision making as a process in which the patient and clinician share information, participate in the decision-making process, and agree on a course of action. Patients who are involved in making their health care decisions have better outcomes than those who are not. Patients should be encouraged to ask questions about medical procedures, the medications they are taking, and any other aspect of their care.

According to an Institute of Medicine report, "nearly half of all American adults—90 million people—have difficulty understanding and acting upon health information." To have a meaningful discussion with an individual about her health care, it is imperative that one recognize and address her level of understanding and knowledge. Consider the following options to improve communication, elevate the level of understanding, and improve health literacy:

- Listen to the patient and understand her concerns and issues.
- Ask open-ended questions using the words "what" or "how" to start the sentence. (For example: "What questions do you have for me?" rather than "Do you have any questions?")
- Use familiar language and avoid jargon. (For example, "You may have itching" instead of "You may experience pruritus.")
- Have patients bring a family member or friend when difficult and crucial discussions are held.
- Check for comprehension by asking patients to restate the health information given in their own words. (For example: "Tell me how you are going to take this medication.") This is particularly useful during the informed consent process.

- Limit the amount of information provided.
- Use visual aids such as drawings or models for key points. Make sure the visual messages are culturally relevant.
- Do not rush encounters. Take as much time as is needed for patient comprehension.

A very important part of patient–physician communication is when and how to disclose medical errors. The Joint Commission requires that accredited hospitals inform patients of adverse events. When an error contributed to the injury, the patient and the family or representative should receive a truthful and compassionate explanation about the error and the remedies available to the patient. They should be informed that the factors involved in the injury will be investigated so that steps can be taken to reduce the likelihood of similar injury to other patients. The improvement of the disclosure process through policies, programmatic training, and available resources will enhance patient satisfaction, strengthen the patient–physician relationship, potentially decrease litigation, and most importantly promote higher quality health care.

Cultural Sensitivity and Awareness

Cultural sensitivity and awareness in the delivery of health care can improve patient communication and care. Cultural competency encompasses gender, sexual orientation, socioeconomic status, faith, profession, tastes, disability, age, as well as race and ethnicity. Physicians should be sensitive to the unique needs of women in the communities they serve. Sensitivity to patients' reactions and possible behavioral differences will alert clinicians to ask appropriate questions and take appropriate actions. The National Standards for Culturally and Linguistically Appropriate Services in Health Care, published by the U.S. Department of Health and Human Service's Office of Minority Health, provide a framework for all health care organizations to best serve the nation's increasingly diverse communities. These standards and their guide for implementation (known as The Blueprint) offer guidance on how to advance health equity, improve quality, and help eliminate health care disparities under three main areas: 1) governance, leadership, and workforce; 2) communication and language assistance; and 3) engagement, continuous improvement, and accountability.

In general, family and friends should not be used to provide interpretation services. For those who do not speak English, efforts should be made to provide assistance, such as offering medically trained interpreters and written translations of forms and patient education materials. In some circumstances, federal and state laws and regulations impose responsibilities on health care providers to accommodate individuals with limited English proficiency. Appropriate measures for overcoming communication barriers will depend on the circumstances of the individual practice and patient population. Various options may be available, including hiring bilingual staff for clerical or medical positions, using appropriate community resources, or using translation telephone services. Because patients interact with many individuals in the office and hospital, it is important to educate the front desk, billing, nursing, and ancillary medical staff in cultural sensitivity.

The Americans With Disabilities Act requirement to provide "auxiliary aids and services" includes a responsibility of making aurally delivered materials accessible for hearing disabled patients. This may be accomplished through multiple means, including qualified interpreters, note taking, written materials, and telecommunications devices for deaf individuals. The Americans With Disabilities Act does not mandate the use of interpreters in every instance. The health care provider can choose alternatives to interpreters, as long as the result is effective communication.

Communication With Health Care Providers

A culture of patient safety fosters open communication and welcomes input from team members at every level. Care must be taken to ensure that hierarchical systems do not hamper free communication among clinicians. Good communication promotes and fosters better medical care. It requires that all members of the team work in concert. A successful team includes the administrative staff and clinicians. Open communication, collaboration, mutual respect, and trust are necessary to provide quality patient care. As noted in the Code of Professional Ethics of the American College of Obstetricians and Gynecologists, "The obstetrician–gynecologist's relationships with other physicians, nurses, and health care providers should reflect fairness, honesty, and integrity, sharing a mutual respect and concern for the patient" (see also Appendix A). There should be an established policy to resolve conflicts.

Patient Handoffs and Coordination of Care

Physician-to-physician handoff of patient information is one of the most important factors to focus on to prevent discontinuity of care, eliminate preventable errors, and provide a safe patient environment. Competing clinical demands, interruptions, and distractions are inherent in clinical practice. Specific effort is needed to ensure that issues are understood and that meaningful information is transferred. Certain clinical communications should be verified, such as reading back medication orders. Relevant communications should be documented appropriately.

Make Safety a Priority in Every Aspect of Practice

The discipline of obstetrics and gynecology has a long tradition of leadership in quality improvement activities, which have been associated with an increase in patient safety.

Patient safety is an explicit principle that must be embraced as a core value in patient care. This ongoing process requires health care providers to strive continually to learn from problems, identify system deficiencies, redesign processes, and implement change in their daily practice. Opportunities to improve patient safety should be used whenever identified. Emphasizing compassion, communication, teamwork, and patient-focused care will aid in creating a culture of excellence and provide the foundation for optimal patient care and safety.

Bibliography

Agency for Healthcare Research and Quality. Patient safety primers: Safety Culture. Available at: http://psnet.ahrq.gov/primer.aspx?primerID=5. Retrieved on October 28, 2013.

American College of Obstetricians and Gynecologists. Code of professional ethics of the American College of Obstetricians and Gynecologists. Washington, DC: American College of Obstetricians and Gynecologists; 2011. Available at: http://www.acog.org/~/media/Departments/National%20Officer%20Nominations%20Process/ACOGcode.pdf?dmc=1&ts=20130715T1226302728. Retrieved July 15, 2013.

American College of Obstetricians and Gynecologists. Quality and safety in women's health care. 2nd ed. Washington, DC: American College of Obstetricians and Gynecologists; 2010.

Communication strategies for patient handoffs. Committee Opinion No. 517. American College of Obstetricians and Gynecologists. Obstet Gynecol 2012; 119:408–11.

Cultural sensitivity and awareness in the delivery of health care. Committee Opinion No. 493. American College of Obstetricians and Gynecologists. Obstet Gynecol 2011;117:1258–61.

Department of Health and Human Services, Office of Minority Health. National standards for culturally and linguistically appropriate services (CLAS) in health and health care. Available at: https://www.thinkculturalhealth.hhs.gov/pdfs/ EnhancedNationalCLASStandards.pdf. Retrieved September 26, 2013.

Department of Health and Human Services, Office of Minority Health. National standards for culturally and linguistically appropriate services in health and health care: a blueprint for advancing and sustaining CLAS policy and practice. Rockville (MD): OMH; 2013. Available at: https://www.thinkculturalhealth.hhs.gov/pdfs/ EnhancedCLASStandardsBlueprint.pdf. Retrieved September 26, 2013.

Disclosure and discussion of adverse events. Committee Opinion No. 520. American College of Obstetricians and Gynecologists. Obstet Gynecol 2012;119:686–9.

Effective patient-physician communication. Committee Opinion No. 587. American College of Obstetricians and Gynecologists. Obstet Gynecol 2014;123:389–93.

Fatigue and patient safety. Committee Opinion No. 519. American College of Obstetricians and Gynecologists. Obstet Gynecol 2012;119:683–5.

Health literacy. Committee Opinion No. 585. American College of Obstetricians and Gynecologists. Obstet Gynecol 2014;123:380–3.

Informed consent. ACOG Committee Opinion No. 439. American College of Obstetricians and Gynecologists. Obstet Gynecol 2009;114:401–8.

Partnering with patients to improve safety. Committee Opinion No. 490. American College of Obstetricians and Gynecologists. Obstet Gynecol 2011;117:1247–9.

Patient safety and the electronic health record. Committee Opinion No. 472. American College of Obstetricians and Gynecologists. Obstet Gynecol 2010; 116:1245–7.

Patient safety in obstetrics and gynecology. ACOG Committee Opinion No. 447. American College of Obstetricians and Gynecologists. Obstet Gynecol 2009; 114:1424–7.

Patient safety in the surgical environment. Committee Opinion No. 464. Obstet Gynecol 2010;116:786–90.

Improving medication safety. Committee Opinion No. 531. American College of Obstetricians and Gynecologists. Obstet Gynecol 2012;120:406–10.

Shekelle PG, Wachter RM, Pronovost PJ. Making health care safer II: an updated critical analysis of the evidence for patient safety practices. Evidence report/technology assessment; number 211 AHRQ publication; no. 13-E001-EF. Rockville (MD): Agency for Healthcare Research and Quality, U.S. Department of Health and Human Services; 2013.

Sheridan SL, Harris RP, Woolf SH. Shared decision-making about screening and chemoprevention. a suggested approach from the U.S. Preventive Services Task Force. Shared Decision-Making Workgroup of the U.S. Preventive Services Task Force. Am J Prev Med 2004;26:56–66.

The Joint Commission. Comprehensive accreditation manual for hospitals: CAMH. Oakbrook Terrace (IL): The Commission; 2014.

The Joint Commission. Introduction to the universal protocol for preventing wrong site, wrong procedure, and wrong person surgery. Comprehensive accreditation manual for hospitals: CAMH. Oakbrook Terrace (IL): The Commission; 2014. p. NPSG-18-NPSG-24.

Weinstein RA. Nosocomial infection update. Emerg Infect Dis 1998;4:416-20.

Resources

Agency for Healthcare Research and Quality. Health literacy universal precautions toolkit. AHRQ Publication No. 10-0046-EF. Rockville (MD): AHRQ; 2010. Available at: http://www.ahrq.gov/professionals/quality-patient-safety/quality-resources/tools/literacy-toolkit/healthliteracytoolkit.pdf. Retrieved July 10, 2013.

Agency for Healthcare Research and Quality. Medications at transitions and clinical handoffs (MATCH) toolkit for medication reconciliation. Rockville (MD): AHRQ; 2012. Available at: http://www.ahrq.gov/professionals/quality-patient-safety/patient-safety-resources/resources/match/match.pdf. Retrieved September 26, 2013.

American College of Obstetricians and Gynecologists. Report of the presidential task force on patient safety in the office setting: appendix G. Quality and safety in women's health care. 2nd ed. Washington, DC: American College of Obstetricians and Gynecologists; 2010. p. 91–108.

Boyce JM, Pittet D. Guideline for Hand Hygiene in Health-Care Settings. Recommendations of the Healthcare Infection Control Practices Advisory Committee and the HICPAC/SHEA/APIC/IDSA Hand Hygiene Task Force. Society for Healthcare Epidemiology of America/Association for Professionals in Infection Control/Infectious Diseases Society of America. Healthcare Infection Control Practices Advisory Committee; HICPAC/SHEA/APIC/IDSA Hand Hygiene Task Force. MMWR Recomm Rep 2002;51(RR-16):1–45, quiz CE1–4.

Institute of Medicine (US). Crossing the quality chasm: a new health system for the 21st century. Washington, D.C.: National Academy Press; 2001.

The Joint Commission. Facts about the official "Do Not Use" List. Oakbrook Terrace (IL): Joint Commission; 2013. Available at: http://www.jointcommission.org/assets/1/18/Do_Not_Use_List.pdf. Retrieved July 10, 2013.

World Health Organization. Surgical safety checklist. Geneva: WHO; 2009. Available at: http://whqlibdoc.who.int/publications/2009/9789241598590_eng_Checklist.pdf. Retrieved July 10, 2013. Copyright WHO, 2009.

RISK MANAGEMENT

Risk management is an approach that aims to minimize the risk of patient injury and subsequent lawsuits through the following actions:

- Developing algorithms, policies, and procedures to decrease medical error
- Changing practice patterns to obtain quality care
- Showing clinicians how to document records properly to include all events that occurred

Risk management cannot always prevent a lawsuit. However, it often can protect a clinician against nonmeritorious claims and help improve the outcome of professional liability litigation.

The goal of risk management is quality medical practice. For the practitioner, risk management involves excellent communication skills, attention to the process of informed consent, and thorough documentation practices. Risk management is also a team effort, and all participants, including staff members, must understand that the acts of one individual reflect on the entire team and easily can lead to liability for everyone. Communication breakdown among team members can be a major source of patient injury.

Risk Reduction

A program of risk management should be developed and maintained, with an emphasis on patient safety. This program should have the following elements:

- A person responsible for the risk management program and, if applicable, the risk management committee
- Periodic review of clinical records and clinical care policies

- Education in risk management activities for all staff within the institution or office
- Methods to identify incidents and adverse occurrences that arise in the practice setting

The risk management program should address important clinical care issues, which may include, but are not limited to, the following:

- Procedures for communicating with patients about confidentiality issues, follow-up of abnormal tests or other results, and missed appointments
- Procedures for communicating with other physicians, hospitals, laboratories, and diagnostic imaging facilities to ensure efficient handling and follow-up of clinical information
- Methods for maintaining a realistic patient schedule and allowing for emergencies
- Periodic review for legal and medical accuracy of any forms used for informed consent
- Review of all incidents and complaints reported by employees, visitors, and patients
- Review of all deaths, trauma, or adverse outcome events
- Procedures for disclosure and discussion of adverse outcome events with patients and family members
- Periodic review of patient office records
- Periodic review of liability insurance policy coverage and exclusions in comparison to clinical activities performed
- Procedures for how and when to communicate with the professional liability insurance carrier
- Review of obligations under managed care contracts to ensure that proper procedures are followed
- Procedures for complying with applicable state and federal laws and regulations

- Procedures for addressing relationships with competing health care organizations so as to avoid antitrust and restraint of trade concerns
- Procedures for dealing with inquiries from government agencies, attorneys, consumer advocate groups, and the media
- Procedures for transfer of medical information at the patient's request to other health care providers
- Procedures by which a patient may be dismissed from care or refused care
- Periodic performance reviews of employees and allied health personnel
- Procedures for managing situations in which a physician becomes acutely incapacitated during a medical or surgical procedure
- Identification and management of the impaired or disruptive health care providers
- Procedures for complying with contractual agreements
- Procedures for the prevention of unauthorized prescribing and the use of drugs
- Protocols for introducing the use of new technologies, devices, or medications

Practice Coverage and Referrals

PRACTICE COVERAGE

Practice coverage outside normal business hours should be established and documented. Covering physicians should have the same privileges as the treating or attending physician. Any coverage arrangements need to comply with hospital requirements and the managed care plan requirements applicable to a given patient. The covering physician must have adequate and appropriate professional liability insurance coverage.

When a physician is not available for any reason, a qualified substitute practitioner should be identified and made available to patients. The office staff, hospital, and answering service need to be advised of the treating physician's absence, along with the name and contact information for the covering physician.

REFERRALS

The obstetrician–gynecologist often serves as a primary medical resource and counselor to the patient and her family for a wide range of medical conditions. However, all clinicians, regardless of the extent of their training, have limitations to their knowledge and skills and should seek consultation at appropriate times for reproductive and nonreproductive care.

Physicians may be reluctant to obtain a consultation and refer patients to a specialist for the following reasons:

- Unrealistic perception of one's own level of expertise
- Belief that training is adequate to treat the patient's condition
- Lack of recognition of limits of knowledge
- Lack of understanding of limits of skills
- Belief that knowledge base is sufficient to answer all questions personally
- Pressure from managed care plans not to refer patients
- Limited patient finances
- Concern that patient will leave the practice
- Physician's moral beliefs or religious convictions

Once a physician is aware that a patient's medical needs may fall outside the realm of his or her expertise or present a conflict of conscience, appropriate care should be arranged. The physician should discuss the situation with the patient and make a referral to a competent specialist. Responsibilities for referrals and consultations are outlined in the "Human Resources" section later in Part 1. The patient should be made aware of the diagnosis, the reason for the referral, and the urgency with which she should seek consultation. The physician should pay attention to the needs of the patient and ensure that she does not perceive the consultation as abandonment. The consultant has the obligation to keep the primary care physician and the referring physician apprised of the patient's progress. If consultation is recommended and the patient refuses or fails to adhere to the recommendation, that fact should be documented clearly in the patient's record. In some situations, the physician might wish to obtain a written statement from the patient acknowledging that the risk of refusal was fully explained.

RETIREMENT OR OFFICE CLOSURE

Patients should be given adequate notice that a medical practice is closing. The period that constitutes adequate notice may vary from state to state. Usually, 30–60 days' notice is sufficient. Patients should be given the names of other obstetrician–gynecologists or the telephone number of the local medical society. To expedite the transfer of care and reduce inconvenience to the patient, an authorization form to transfer copies of the medical record to the patient's physician of choice, which is compliant with the Health Insurance Portability and Accountability Act, can be included with the letter of notification. The original record, all correspondence, and all authorization forms should be retained by the original physician. In general, only copies of records are transferred.

Considerations regarding how long to maintain medical records include the obligation to make records available for the patient's future medical care, requirements of the Centers for Medicare & Medicaid Services, state rules for retaining business records, and state statutes of limitation for malpractice actions that involve adults and minors. The longest of these retention requirements should be followed. The physician should consult his or her attorney, county medical society, or liability insurance carrier for record retention guidance.

Billing

A billing system should be established to ensure reimbursement for services rendered. Payment and reimbursement requests should comply with all third-party payers and meet federal and state standards and guidelines. Physicians should develop a program to ensure that office visits, consultations, inpatient visits, and procedures are coded and billed accurately. Unpaid accounts should be reviewed before referral to a collection agency.

Federal scrutiny of Medicare claims has increased. To reduce the possibility of an allegation of fraud and abuse, it is wise to develop a compliance plan. Compliance plans are not currently required for physician practices by the U.S. Department of Health and Human Services. However, establishing and following a compliance plan could reduce the anxiety and possible acrimony that can be associated with a federal audit.

Adverse Events, Litigation Stress, and Physician Behavior

Among the many stressors encountered by physicians in clinical practice is the constant threat of adverse outcome events, with or without subsequent medical professional liability litigation. Common responses to both adverse events and medical liability litigation include feelings of shock, denial, anger, anxiety, guilt, shame, and despair. These distressing emotions can disrupt relationships with patients and colleagues and potentially increase risk of error. Because a professional liability case in obstetrics and gynecology can take several years to resolve, coping is an ongoing, complex process in which physicians often must struggle to regain a sense of personal identity, professional mastery, and control of their clinical practices. Residents, as young physicians in training, may be particularly vulnerable to this psychologic and emotional upheaval. A program of risk management should include education about the potential effect of adverse events and litigation stress on physician behavior and practice. Physicians should be made aware of resources and supportive mechanisms available to them.

Bibliography

American College of Obstetricians and Gynecologists. Coding responsibility. ACOG Committee Opinion 249. Washington, DC: ACOG; 2001.

American College of Obstetricians and Gynecologists. Professional liability and risk management: an essential guide for obstetrician-gynecologists. 2nd ed. Washington, DC: ACOG; 2008.

Coping with the stress of medical professional liability litigation. ACOG Committee Opinion No. 551. American College of Obstetricians and Gynecologists. Obstet Gynecol 2013;121:220–2.

Disclosure and discussion of adverse events. Committee Opinion No. 520. American College of Obstetricians and Gynecologists. Obstet Gynecol 2012; 119:686–9.

Informed consent. ACOG Committee Opinion No. 439. American College of Obstetricians and Gynecologists. Obstet Gynecol 2009;114:401-8.

Professional liability and gynecology-only practice. Committee Opinion No. 567. American College of Obstetricians and Gynecologists. Obstet Gynecol 2013; 122:186.

Seeking and giving consultation. ACOG Committee Opinion No. 365. American College of Obstetricians and Gynecologists. Obstet Gynecol 2007;109:1255-60.

Resources

Accreditation Association for Ambulatory Health Care. 2014 Accreditation handbook for ambulatory health care. 2014 ed. Skokie (IL): Accreditation Association for Ambulatory Health Care; 2014.

American College of Obstetricians and Gynecologists. From exam room to courtroom: navigating litigation and coping with stress [CD-Rom]. Washington, DC: ACOG; 2006.

American Congress of Obstetricians and Gynecologists. Healing our own: adverse events in obstetrics and gynecology [DVD]. Washington, DC: American Congress of Obstetricians and Gynecologists; 2012.

Hartnett J, Ginsburg K. Closing down a medical practice: guidelines and considerations. Washington, DC: American College of Obstetricians and Gynecologists; 2009. Available at: http://www.acog.org/About_ACOG/ACOG_Departments/ Practice_Management_and_Managed_Care/Closing_a_Practice. Retrieved July 16, 2013.

Office of Inspector General. Self-disclosure information. Available at: http://oig.hhs. gov/compliance/self-disclosure-info/index.asp. Retrieved August 13, 2013.

OIG compliance program for individual and small group physician practices. Office of Inspector General. Fed Regist 2000;65:59434-52.

OIG supplemental compliance program guidance for hospitals. Office of Inspector General. Fed Regist 2005;70:4858-76.

Publication of the OIG compliance program guidance for hospitals. Office of Inspector General. Fed Regist 1998;63:8987-98.

COMPLIANCE WITH GOVERNMENT REGULATIONS

State and federal government regulations have a substantial effect on the health care workplace. Practitioners and managers of medical offices and clinics should recognize the regulations that affect the office and clinic setting and properly implement the procedures required by law. The following regulations have the most substantial effect:

- Occupational Safety and Health Administration (OSHA) Regulations on Occupational Exposure to Bloodborne Pathogens (Appendix D)
- Clinical Laboratory Improvement Amendments of 1988 (CLIA) (Appendix E)
- Emergency Medical Treatment and Labor Act (EMTALA) (Appendix F)
- Americans With Disabilities Act (Appendix G)
- Title VI of the Civil Rights Act (Appendix H)
- Health Insurance Portability and Accountability Act (HIPAA) (Appendix I)
- Mammography Quality Standards Act (MQSA)

The Patient Protection and Affordable Care Act passed by Congress in 2010 also may produce additional requirements on physician practices. There are ongoing federal and state implementation efforts around many of these provisions, which make it important for obstetrician–gynecologists to stay abreast of new developments (see Resources).

Occupational Exposure to Bloodborne Pathogens Standard

In 1991, OSHA issued regulations designed to minimize the transmission of human immunodeficiency virus (HIV), hepatitis B virus (HBV), and other potentially infectious materials in the workplace. The regulations went into effect in 1992 and were last revised in 2001. They are meant to protect all employees who work in any health-related facility from "reasonably anticipated" contact or exposure to blood and other potentially infectious materials. The regulations require a control plan to minimize employees' exposure to all bloodborne pathogens. The plan must contain the following components:

- Personal protective equipment for employees exposed to blood and other body fluids
- Adoption of healthy work practices (eg, hand-washing)
- Adequate equipment for hand-washing
- Proper disposal of needles
- Appropriate handling and storage of specimens
- Adequate housekeeping to clean contaminated areas
- Provision of HBV vaccination to employees
- Postexposure evaluation and follow-up procedures
- Employee training
- Use of warning labels
- Record-keeping requirements

These requirements are enforced by OSHA or, in the case of states that have OSHA-approved comparable job safety and health plans, by state agencies. Violations are punishable by fines.

In 1999, OSHA issued a revised compliance directive for the bloodborne pathogens standard. This directive clarifies the standard and emphasizes that employers must use readily available technology in their safety and health programs. For example, employers must ensure that their exposure review plans are reviewed annually and reflect consideration and use of commercially available safer medical devices, such as shielded needles. The directive also includes the Centers for Disease Control and Prevention guidelines on vaccinations to prevent HBV and on postexposure evaluation and follow-up for HIV and hepatitis C virus. It requires employee training on new and safer medical devices. As mandated by the Needlestick Safety and Prevention Act in 2001, OSHA again revised its bloodborne pathogens standard to clarify the need for employers to select safer needle devices as they become available. Employees must be involved in identifying and choosing the devices. Employers also are required to maintain a sharps injury log. Several states have enacted needlestick laws, and many more are considering such legislation. Practitioners can expect this standard to continue to evolve. For detailed information on the OSHA bloodborne pathogens standard, see Appendix D.

Clinical Laboratory Improvement Amendments

In 1988, Congress enacted the CLIA in response to growing public concerns regarding the quality and accuracy of laboratory testing. There have been updates and revisions to these regulations (see Bibliography).

Under CLIA, federal oversight is required for all nonresearch laboratories, including physician offices, which perform tests on human specimens for the health assessment, prevention, diagnosis, or treatment of any disease. All laboratories and offices that conduct these tests must register with the Centers for Medicare & Medicaid Services and receive appropriate certification. The certification depends on the complexity and type of testing done. There are no exceptions. Even an office that is performing minimal testing (eg, urine pregnancy tests, wet mount procedures, and dipstick urine tests) must obtain the appropriate certificate for the level of laboratory testing it is performing. There are three levels of test categories based on the complexity of the testing:

1. Waived tests, eg, urine pregnancy tests, blood glucose tests (over-the-counter)

2. Tests of moderate-level complexity—These include provider-performed microscopy procedures (eg, microscopic analysis of urinary sediment) and most of the testing performed in clinical laboratories

3. Tests of high-level complexity—These include tests that are the most difficult to perform or are the most subject to error. They usually are performed by a large clinical laboratory and are subject to the Centers for Medicare & Medicaid Services survey. Examples include nonautomated procedures, such as histopathologic tests.

The level of testing determines the type of certificate a laboratory or office is issued. There are five types of certificates: 1) Certificate of Waiver, 2) Certificate for Provider-Performed Microscopy Procedures, 3) Certificate of Registration, 4) Certificate of Compliance, and 5) Certificate of Accreditation. Each category of testing has different regulatory requirements; the more complex the category of testing, the more stringent the regulations. Most obstetrician–gynecologists' offices conduct only waived tests or provider-performed microscopy procedures, a subset of the moderate complexity tests. Appendix E provides basic information on these two categories of tests and the CLIA regulations governing these procedures.

When a laboratory office initially applies for a Certificate of Compliance or a Certificate of Accreditation, to conduct tests of moderate-level or high-level complexity, it is issued a registration certificate. This certificate authorizes the laboratory or office to conduct moderate-complexity testing, high-complexity testing, or both until it is verified through either an on-site survey or a nonprofit accreditation program that the laboratory meets all requirements. After the laboratory is found to be in compliance with CLIA, the laboratory is either issued a Certificate of Compliance (after an on-site survey) or a Certificate of Accreditation (after a private nonprofit accreditation program), which authorizes performance of designated tests.

Emergency Medical Treatment and Labor Act

The EMTALA contains specific federal legal requirements that apply to patient screening in emergency departments, the transfer of patients by Medicare-participating hospitals, and the care of pregnant women. It is essential that institutions and health care providers understand their obligations under the law. All Medicare-participating hospitals must provide an appropriate medical screening examination for any individual who seeks medical treatment at an emergency department, and EMTALA places strict requirements on the transfer of these patients. Even hospitals that are not capable of handling high-risk deliveries or high-risk infants and have written transfer agreements must meet all the screening, treatment, and transfer requirements before transferring a patient.

An ongoing education program should be developed to inform users about the interhospital transfer service. The institutions that refer and receive should understand the clinical capabilities and special resources available. Periodic updates should be used to inform all participants involved in the transport program about new changes or procedures. For detailed information about the EMTALA requirements, see Appendix F.

Health Insurance Portability and Accountability Act

When Congress passed HIPAA in 1996, the law was known primarily for its provisions that provide stronger health insurance protection for people leaving jobs and people with preexisting medical conditions. Over time, however, regulations have been developed to protect the privacy and security of certain health information. If a physician's practice stores or transmits patient health information electronically, it must comply with the HIPAA regulations. More detailed information about HIPAA can be found in Appendix I.

Mammography Quality Standards Act and Program

In 1992, Congress enacted the MQSA in response to concerns about breast cancer and the quality of mammography services in the United States. To operate lawfully after 1994, all mammography facilities, including physician offices, must be certified by the U.S. Food and Drug Administration (FDA) as providing quality mammography services. This regulation applies even if an office has only one mammography unit and the film is processed and interpreted elsewhere. A facility must be certified either by the FDA or by an approved state certification agency as capable of providing quality mammography. In addition, a facility's clinical images and mammography equipment must be reviewed periodically, and the facility must employ specially trained personnel to obtain the mammograms and interpret data, be inspected annually, and meet federally developed standards. Comprehensive regulations govern the requirements for mammography personnel, quality control, record keeping, and medical audits.

It is required that all women be sent a lay summary of their mammography results directly from the facility. Physicians who refer patients to mammography facilities still receive the examination report.

For more information, go to the MQSA home page (see Bibliography), which has a searchable Policy Guidance Help System. The National Cancer

Institute Cancer Information Service (see Bibliography) also can assist callers in finding a mammography facility certified by the FDA.

Bibliography

American Congress of Obstetricians and Gynecologists. HIPAA regulations and requirements explained. Washington, DC: American Congress of Obstetricians and Gynecologists; 2013. Available at: http://www.acog.org/About_ACOG/ACOG_Departments/HIPAA. Retrieved July 16, 2013.

Americans with Disabilities Act, 42 U.S.C. §12101 (2011). Available at: http://www.gpo.gov/fdsys/pkg/USCODE-2011-title42/pdf/USCODE-2011-title42-chap126.pdf. Retrieved September 20, 2013.

Bloodborne pathogens, 29 C.F.R. part 1910.1030 (2013). Available at: http://www.gpo.gov/fdsys/pkg/CFR-2013-title29-vol6/pdf/CFR-2013-title29-vol6-sec1910-1030.pdf. Retrieved September 20, 2013.

Certification of laboratories, 42 U.S.C. § 263a (2011). Available at: http://www.gpo.gov/fdsys/pkg/USCODE-2011-title42/pdf/USCODE-2011-title42-chap6A-subchapII-partF-subpart2-sec263a.pdf. Retrieved September 20, 2013.

Civil Rights Act, 42 U.S.C. §2000d-2000d1 (2011). Available at: http://www.gpo.gov/fdsys/pkg/USCODE-2011-title42/pdf/USCODE-2011-title42-chap21-subchapV.pdf. Retrieved September 20, 2013.

Department of Health and Human Services, Office of Population Affairs. Affordable Care Act. Available at: http://www.hhs.gov/opa/affordable-care-act/index.html. Retrieved September 26, 2013.

Examination and treatment for emergency medical conditions and women in labor, 42 U.S.C. § 1395dd (2011). Available at: http://www.gpo.gov/fdsys/pkg/USCODE-2011-title42/pdf/USCODE-2011-title42-chap7-subchapXVIII-partE-sec1395dd.pdf. Retrieved September 20, 2013.

Food and Drug Administration. Mammography quality standards act and program. Available at: http://www.fda.gov/Radiation-EmittingProducts/Mammography QualityStandardsActandProgram/default.htm. Retrieved July 10, 2013.

Forming a just health care system. Committee Opinion No. 456. American College of Obstetricians and Gynecologists. Obstet Gynecol 2010;115:672–7.

Health Insurance Portability and Accountability Act of 1996, Pub. L. No. 104-191, 100 Stat. 1936. Available at: http://www.gpo.gov/fdsys/pkg/PLAW-104publ191/pdf/PLAW-104publ191.pdf. Retrieved September 20, 2013.

National Cancer Institute. Cancer Information Service. Available at: http://www.cancer.gov/aboutnci/cis. Retrieved July 10, 2013.

Resources

American Congress of Obstetricians and Gynecologists. Government relations and outreach. Washington, DC: American Congress of Obstetricians and Gynecologists; 2013. Available at: http://www.acog.org/About_ACOG/ACOG_Departments/ Government_Relations_and_Outreach. Retrieved July 16, 2013.

American Congress of Obstetricians and Gynecologists. Health system reform: the law, your practice, your patients. Washington, DC: American Congress of Obstetricians and Gynecologists; 2010. Available at: http://www.acog.org/About_ACOG/ ACOG_Departments/Health_Care_Reform. Retrieved July 16, 2013.

American Congress of Obstetricians and Gynecologists. Practice management and managed care. Washington, DC: American Congress of Obstetricians and Gynecologists; 2013. Available at: http://www.acog.org/About_ACOG/ACOG_ Departments/Practice_Management_and_Managed_Care. Retrieved July 16, 2013.

HUMAN RESOURCES

The successful delivery of women's health care depends on the people directly and indirectly involved with providing that care. For this reason, issues of human resources management must be addressed at all levels of health care delivery, including health systems, hospitals, surgical centers, and offices.

Human resources encompasses practical matters of hiring, managing, and evaluating, and—when necessary—terminating employment of staff. Equally important, however, is an understanding of the principles that drive these personnel management decisions and an understanding of what constitutes professional and unprofessional behavior. Human resources issues vary depending on the type of institution, scope of practice, union regulations, and staff needs.

Personnel

Regardless of the setting, certain elements constitute effective personnel management in the delivery of health care services. Written job descriptions should exist for each staff position, and these descriptions should be reviewed periodically to ensure that staff members function at an appropriate level and do not perform tasks beyond those they are licensed and trained to do. Written policies that indicate specific responsibilities of personnel should be prepared, approved by the medical staff, and reviewed periodically. Previous employment references should be checked for all new employees. Current licensure verification is mandatory for all licensed personnel. A system for credentialing of personnel should be in place and reviewed at least every 2 years (see also the "Evaluating Credentials and Granting Privileges" section earlier in Part 1).

The human resources operations in health care institutions are governed by the policies and procedures of that institution. The leadership of the women's health component should have extensive knowledge of and a collegial working relationship with the institutional human resources unit.

At the office practice level, human resource needs also must be addressed. An office-based medical practice or clinic should have an office manager or other key staff member assigned to personnel management. A personnel manual should be created for the entire office staff. Issues of preemployment screening, benefits, employee assistance programs, and performance reviews should be considered for inclusion in the manual.

Professional Behavior

It is vitally important in providing health care services that all staff be aware of what constitutes professional and unprofessional behavior. Such behavior can be outlined in codes of ethics, such as the codes developed by the American Medical Association (AMA) and the American College of Obstetricians and Gynecologists (the College) (see Bibliography, Resources, and Appendix A). The behavior that institutions expect of staff may be summarized in a personnel manual or similar guide. Certain situations in the practice of women's health care merit special attention from an ethical perspective and are addressed here. Institutional ethics committees, ethics consultants, and ethics consultation services are valuable resources in determining the appropriate resolution of these situations and others (see also the "Ethical Issues" section later in Part 1).

Academic institutions, professional corporations, hospitals, and other health care organizations should have policies and procedures by which alleged violations of professional behavior can be reported and investigated. Also, it is necessary for these institutions to adopt policies on legal representation and indemnification for their employees or others acting in an official capacity who, in discharging their obligations relative to unethical or illegal behavior of individuals, are exposed to potentially costly legal actions. The College agrees with the position of the American Association of University Professors that institutions should "ensure effective legal and other necessary representation and full indemnification in the first instance for any faculty member named or included in lawsuits or other extra-institutional legal proceedings arising from an act or omission in the discharge of institutional or related professional duties or in the defense of academic freedom at the institution."

CODE OF PROFESSIONAL ETHICS OF THE AMERICAN COLLEGE OF OBSTETRICIANS AND GYNECOLOGISTS

Obstetrician–gynecologists (and other clinicians caring for women) have ethical responsibilities to patients, society, and other health care providers. The College has developed a code of professional ethics to provide guidance to its Fellows (see Appendix A). Many of the ethical considerations described also apply to other health care providers who provide care to women.

This code of ethics describes the ethical foundations for professional activities in women's health care and summarizes the rules of ethical conduct built on these foundations. Noncompliance with this code may affect an individual's initial or continuing Fellowship in the College. The code is an excellent guide for other individuals or organizations to evaluate the ethical appropriateness of an individual's practice, behavior, or both. The fundamental code of ethics is supported by Committee Opinions issued by the College's Committee on Ethics, which comment upon other timely ethical issues relevant to the practice of obstetrics and gynecology. Some, but not all, of the ethics Committee Opinions are referenced in the code of ethics.

CONFIDENTIALITY

Clinicians who provide women's health care should respect the rights of patients, colleagues, and others and safeguard patient information and confidences within the limits of the law. Maintaining confidentiality is intrinsic to respect for patient autonomy and promotes the free exchange of information between patient and physician relevant to medical decision making (see also the "Ethical Issues" section later in Part 1). Additionally, in certain situations, maintaining confidentiality is critical to ensure a woman's safety from retaliatory actions by an abusive family member or partner.

Institutions should have policies in place to safeguard patient information from inadvertent or inappropriate breaches of confidentiality. Federal regulations detailed in the Health Insurance Portability and Accountability Act (HIPAA) also set rules for what information may be shared with other practitioners and agencies with and without an individual's permission (see also the "Compliance With Government Regulations" section earlier in Part 1). In addition, jurisdictions vary in their laws and regulations regarding reporting, disclosure, and breach of confidentiality. For example, the results of human immunodeficiency virus (HIV) testing may need to be recorded and stored differently than other medical information. Laws and regulations for documenting HIV testing vary by state, and clinicians should become familiar with the legal requirements that exist in their communities.

There has been substantial growth in the variety of methods of communication. Patient information may be stored not only on a paper record but also electronically. Patient information may be transmitted over the telephone (including wireless cellular telephones), facsimile machines, and e-mail. By whatever means a patient's health information is stored or exchanged, the same ethical principles of confidentiality apply. Health information technology systems should be compatible with the requirements of HIPAA and flexible enough to accommodate state privacy laws, a particular concern for adolescent care, assisted reproductive technology, and genetic testing. Health information technology systems must integrate these various rules.

Moreover, in 2003 and in subsequent amendments, the U.S. Department of Health and Human Services implemented compulsory privacy rules under HIPAA that sought to create assurances that all patient account handling, billing, and medical records protect the confidentiality and privacy of patient information. These rules apply to health care plans, health care clearinghouses, and practitioners, including hospitals and physicians, and they carry substantial penalties for violations. These laws enforce the patient's right to confidential and private medical information in all settings.

Tests that may have multiple medical or psychosocial ramifications require nondirective counseling and comprehensive explanation of the process, goals, and implications. The patient should be informed of pertinent policies regarding the use of information resulting from tests and the legal requirements that relate to the release of information before she grants her consent. She should be aware of what information might be communicated and to whom and the potential implications of reporting the information. For example, if a urine test for illicit drugs is requested and a positive result mandates reporting to a social services agency, a patient should understand this requirement and its implications in advance.

Situations may arise in which a clinician has competing obligations: on the one hand to protect the patient's confidentiality and on the other hand to disclose test results to prevent harm to a third party. In these situations, the clinician first should explore every avenue of communication in discussions with the patient about rights and responsibilities. Consultation with an institutional ethics committee or a medical ethics specialist may help the clinician decide whether to disclose the information. In some rare situations, it may be appropriate to disclose confidential information, though it may be prudent to seek legal advice before doing so.

Practitioners and patients consistently cite confidentiality as a major obstacle to the delivery of health care to minors. Although ensuring confidentiality is relatively simple when providing services to adults, providing the same degree of confidentiality to minors can be less straightforward. The legal status of a minor, requirements for parental consent or notification before the provision of medical services, and economic considerations often encumber the patient–physician relationship. The AMA has reaffirmed a policy that supports confidential care of adolescents as critical to their health care and encourages practitioners to allow emancipated and mature minors to give informed consent for medical, surgical, and psychiatric procedures within state and federal law. Clinicians should be familiar with current state statutes on the rights of minors to consent to health care services and the laws that affect confidentiality. All states require consent for the treatment of a minor from a person legally entitled to authorize such care. Exceptions to this requirement for consent vary by state. State medical societies may provide information about local regulations. The AMA provides links to all state medical society web sites (see Bibliography). For further discussion of confidentiality specific to adolescents, see the "Adolescents" section in Part 3.

CHAPERONES

Local practices and expectations differ with regard to the use of chaperones, but the presence of another staff member in the room during the physical examination can confer benefits for the patient and the clinician, regardless of the sex of the clinician. Chaperones can provide reassurance to the patient about the professional context and content of the examination and the intention of the clinician, and they can offer witness to the actual events taking place should there be any misunderstanding. The request by either a patient or a health care provider to have a chaperone present during a physical examination should be accommodated regardless of the health care practitioner's sex. In addition to any staff chaperone, patients may find it helpful to have a family member present.

The presence of a third party in the room, however, may cause some embarrassment to the patient and limit her willingness to talk openly with the clinician. If a chaperone is present during the examination, the clinician may need to provide a separate opportunity for private conversation. If the chaperone is an employee of the practice, the clinician must establish clear rules about respect for privacy and confidentiality. In addition, some patients (especially, but not limited to, adolescents) may consider the presence of a family member as an intrusion. Family members should not be used as chaperones unless specifically requested by the patient, and then only in the presence of an additional chaperone who is not a family member.

REFERRAL

Relationships with other health care providers should reflect fairness, honesty, integrity, mutual respect, and concern for the patient. Clinicians may best fulfill their obligations to patients through referral to other professionals who have the appropriate skills and expertise to address the situation. Therefore, clinicians should consult, refer to, or cooperate with other professionals and institutions to the extent necessary to serve the patients' best interests. In cases of conscientious objection, in which a clinician declines to provide requested care to a patient for moral or religious reasons, transfer of primary clinical responsibility to another clinician is in the patient's best interest.

With respect to referrals, the role of the referring clinician is to identify the most appropriate resources and qualified consultants. Physicians should be aware of potential conflicts of interest and be sure that referrals cannot be construed as inappropriate or otherwise prohibited by state or federal law.

In the current health care climate, however, clinicians may find barriers to making appropriate referrals. Managed care plans or other systems may limit referrals or stipulate referral to a defined panel of specialists. Physicians who believe that a patient's health is jeopardized by these policies should consider appealing to the plan or medical director (see "Conflict of Interest" later in this section).

It is in the best interest of everyone—primary care physicians, consultants, patients, and health care plans—that consultation criteria are mutually agreed upon in clearly stated policies. At times a consultant may be called on unexpectedly, inconveniently, and sometimes inappropriately to be involved in or to assume the care of a patient. In these situations, a physician is only ethically obligated to provide consultation or assume the care of the patient if there is a contractual agreement or a preexisting patient–physician relationship or if there is a severe medical emergency in which there is no reasonably available alternative caregiver. Whether the specialist assumes ongoing care of the patient or functions as a consultant should be established clearly by mutual agreement of the consultant, the referring practitioner, and the patient.

EXPERT WITNESSES

Clinicians have a continuing responsibility to society as a whole and should support and participate in activities that enhance the community. As professionals and members of medical or nursing societies, they are required to uphold the dignity and honor of their professions. One way health care providers can do so is through serving as expert witnesses on behalf of defendants, the government, or plaintiffs.

The moral and legal duty of health care providers who testify before a court of law is to do so in accordance with their expertise. This duty implies adherence to the strictest code of personal and professional ethics. Truthfulness is essential. Misrepresentation of one's personal clinical opinion as the only right or wrong treatment option for the patient may be harmful to individual parties and to the profession at large. Health care providers who serve as expert witnesses should have experience and knowledge in the areas of clinical medicine that enable them to testify about the standards of care that applied and the scientific evidence that existed at the time of the occurrence that is the subject of the legal action. Their review of the facts should be thorough, fair, and impartial and should not exclude any relevant information. It should not be biased in favor of the defendant, the plaintiff, or the government. The role of an expert witness should be to provide testimony that is complete, objective, and helpful to a just resolution of the proceeding.

Testimony should evaluate performance in light of generally accepted standards, neither condemning performance that falls within generally accepted standards nor endorsing or condoning performance that falls below these standards. The expert witness should distinguish clearly between medical malpractice and medical maloccurrence and should make every effort to assess the relationship of the alleged substandard practice to the outcome. Deviation from a practice standard is not always substandard care or causally related to a bad outcome. Expert witnesses should be prepared to have the testimony they have given in any judicial proceeding subjected to peer review by an institution or professional organization to which they belong.

Fees for testifying should not be greatly disproportionate to fees customary for professional services. It is clearly unethical for health care providers to accept compensation that is contingent on the outcome of litigation.

IMPAIRED CLINICIANS

Impairment in providers of patient care is common; the lifetime prevalence of alcohol or drug dependence is reported to be 8–15% among physicians. This fact carries responsibility for impaired clinicians and their colleagues. As noted in the "Code of Professional Ethics of the American College of Obstetricians and Gynecologists" (see also Appendix A):

- The obstetrician–gynecologist should not practice medicine while impaired by alcohol, drugs, or physical or mental disability. The

obstetrician–gynecologist who experiences substance abuse problems or who is physically or emotionally impaired should seek
appropriate assistance to address these problems and must limit his
or her practice until the impairment no longer affects the quality of
patient care.

- The obstetrician–gynecologist should strive to address through the
appropriate procedures the status of those physicians who demonstrate questionable competence, impairment, or unethical or illegal
behavior. In addition, the obstetrician–gynecologist should cooperate with appropriate authorities to prevent the continuation of such
behavior.

Physicians and other clinicians are considered impaired when their
ability to practice is limited or altered by mental illness, a physical illness
or condition, or misuse of alcohol or other drugs and medications. An
impaired health care provider should be obligated to enter a treatment program, with the specific type of program dependent on state legal requirements, the requirements of the state licensure board, and the preferences
of the impaired practitioner. Obviously, there is considerable advantage
to the impaired practitioner, the practitioner's family, the department, the
medical staff, the institution, and the public when a colleague's suspicion
leads to early identification and successful rehabilitation.

In many states, it is mandatory to report a physician or advanced-
practice health care clinician who is reasonably believed to be impaired.
Conditions that are reportable include, but are not limited to, impairment
by alcohol, drugs, physical disability, or mental instability; practice misconduct; practicing medicine fraudulently; gross incompetence; or gross
negligence. The failure of a colleague to take action or any action taken to
shield the impaired clinician from disclosure, although understandable,
can result in serious consequences for individuals who should have recognized the situation.

Practitioners who have developed a degree of chemical dependency or
inappropriate behavior that causes stress within their families and in their
personal lives but that has not impaired their medical practice should not
be ignored and may still require intervention. A colleague's ability to identify a health care provider in this state carries with it the responsibility to

make an effort to personally help the individual or to guide the individual to competent help. This helps the troubled colleague and prevents his or her problems from having a detrimental effect on patients in the future. Ignoring the issue is a disservice to the affected practitioner.

Other personal, medical, or family problems may negatively affect a practitioner's professional functioning. Such problems ordinarily are not included under the term impaired practitioner, but they should not be ignored. The department head or other responsible person should be informed and should consult personally with the health care provider involved. In an emergency situation, physicians should know whom they should ask to address a problem related to an impaired colleague. The chief medical officer and on-call administrator often are the designated authorities, but staff members should know who the appropriate on-call contact person is for all types of health care providers at an institution. (Practical guidance regarding the management of impaired and disruptive clinicians can be found in the "Evaluating Credentials and Granting Privileges" section earlier in Part 1.)

INFECTIOUS DISEASE PREVENTION

Another factor that may impair a health care provider's ability to practice is the presence of an infectious disease. The welfare of the patient is central to all considerations in the patient–provider relationship. For this reason, health care institutions and health care providers share a responsibility to avoid causing harm to patients by taking reasonable steps to reduce the risk of transmission of vaccine-preventable or other infectious diseases. The Centers for Disease Control and Prevention (CDC) recommends that health care facilities and organizations have vaccine programs in place, review health care provider vaccination and immunity status at the time of hire and on a regular basis (ie, at least annually), and offer needed vaccines in conjunction with routine annual disease-prevention measures (eg, seasonal influenza vaccination or tuberculin testing). In addition, it is recommended that health care providers follow standard precautions for patient care to prevent transmission of a vaccine-preventable or other infectious disease.

Vaccinations

Health care providers are obligated to serve their patients' best interests by following authoritative guidance on vaccination for patients and clinicians, where medically appropriate and based on the best evidence. To avoid their own contribution to the spread of disease, College Fellows have an ethical obligation to be vaccinated themselves and to follow recommendations and other safety policies put into place by their local or national public health authorities, such as the CDC and the College. Any perceived burdens or potential risks to clinicians from vaccination do not supersede their responsibility to limit the spread of potentially harmful infectious disease.

Despite the evidence pointing to the benefit of vaccination, compliance with voluntary vaccination programs for health care providers has been disappointing. Mandatory vaccination of health care providers may be an ethically justified strategy in cases in which the harm to patients and the general population is believed to outweigh the autonomy of individual physicians. Mandates should be put in place only if supported by valid data about the efficacy and safety of the vaccine. In addition, public health plans that include mandatory vaccination will be most beneficial if they are developed in cooperation with key stakeholders and consider the needs of individual practitioners, institutions, and communities. Any vaccine mandates should include recognized exceptions for medical contraindications as well as an active opt-out mechanism for those physicians who profess conscientious objections to vaccination. Practitioners should be reminded that there is a high standard applied to the qualification of conscientious objections.

The CDC recommends that all health care providers be immunized against the following diseases: hepatitis B virus (HBV), influenza, measles, mumps, rubella, pertussis, and varicella. In addition, there are certain diseases, such as meningococcal disease, typhoid fever, and polio, for which vaccination of health care providers might be indicated in certain circumstances (ie, health care providers with certain health conditions or who are at risk of work-related exposure). The CDC advises that all health care providers who perform exposure-prone procedures (eg, hysterectomy) or who are otherwise at risk of HBV infection should receive prevaccination testing for chronic HBV infection. The CDC also recommends postvaccination serologic HBV antibody testing 1–2 months after the final dose of HBV vaccine is administered for all health care providers who are recently vaccinated or have recently completed HBV vaccination and who are at risk of occupational blood or body fluid exposure.

Vaccinations against hepatitis C virus (HCV) and HIV are not available. Although routine HCV and HIV testing is not recommended specifically for health care workers, the CDC recommends that all individuals born from 1945 to 1965 undergo one-time HCV testing to enable early diagnosis and treatment, and the CDC and the U.S. Preventive Services Task Force recommend that adults be screened routinely for HIV infection.

During an influenza pandemic, disruption of critical services can pose as much of a threat to the public's health as influenza itself, which justifies prioritizing key workers—such as essential health care workers—in an effort to protect critical services. To meet the ethical objectives of promoting public health, especially during a pandemic, strategies should be implemented to increase vaccination rates among clinicians and prevent contact between symptomatic clinicians and patients. In the event of a bioterrorism attack that uses an infectious agent (such as smallpox), other immunizations may be recommended for the preservation of the health care workforce. Clinicians should seek accurate and timely information from appropriate sources, including the CDC (see Bibliography and Resources) and professional organizations.

Immunization policies and practices should be individually tailored for patients and clinicians, as well as the unique infectious agent. During a public health emergency, access to care and resources should be based on women's clinical needs rather than the type of insurance, if any, that they have or their prior relationship to a clinic or other health care institution. Some infectious agents, such as influenza, affect pregnant women disproportionately, and clinicians should advocate for appropriate allocation of vaccines to this high-risk population. To adequately protect pregnant women, pandemic preparedness efforts should include clinical research specifically designed to address the safety and efficacy of treatment interventions or prevention strategies used by pregnant women. Live vaccines should not, in general, be administered to pregnant women. Clinicians who treat pregnant patients or women with compromised immune systems may wish to receive an inactivated vaccine rather than a live vaccine to minimize the risk of unintentional transmission of the infectious agent.

Other Preventive Measures

In the absence of effective immunization against infectious agents, such as HIV and HCV, health care providers should follow standard precautions for patient care to minimize the risk of transmission from patient to health care provider. It appears that health care providers who follow recommended infection-control procedures are at little risk of acquiring HIV while caring for HIV-infected patients. The risk of acquiring HCV appears to be lower than the risk of acquiring HBV and higher than the risk of acquiring HIV. Although routine screening for HIV and HCV is not recommended for health care workers, clinicians who have reason to believe that they are infected with these or other serious infectious agents that might be transmitted to patients should be tested voluntarily for the protection of their patients. Guidance on the management of health care workers exposed to blood or body fluids, such as through a needlestick, is found in the "Infection Control" section in Part 2.

Health care providers who have influenza or other acute, nonchronic infectious diseases that are easily transmitted to patients, staff, and others should refrain from working until they are no longer infectious. Clinicians infected with a bloodborne virus must make a decision as to which procedures they can continue to perform safely. This decision will depend on the category of clinical activity and the circulating viral burden (see also the "Infection Control" section in Part 2).

CONFLICT OF INTEREST

Potential conflicts of interest are inherent to the practice of medicine. Clinicians are expected to recognize them and to maintain patient care and welfare as a priority. If there is a possible substantial conflict of interest, the clinician should attempt to resolve the issue. Consultation with colleagues or an institutional ethics committee may be sought. If a conflict of interest cannot be resolved, the clinician should disclose his or her concerns to the patient and take steps to withdraw from her care.

Clinicians may feel pressure from regulatory bodies and managed care organizations (which may seek to limit or otherwise direct the care that is provided) and from the health care industry (which urges the use of its procedures and products through advertising and promotions). Both situations can present conflicts of interest.

Participation in managed care organizations and care directed by regulatory bodies may create potential conflicts of interest for women's health care providers in fulfilling their primary duty to their patient. Financial and administrative constraints may create disincentives to treatment otherwise recommended by the obstetrician–gynecologist. Clinicians should serve as the patient's advocate and exercise all reasonable means to ensure that the most appropriate care is provided to the patient. Practitioners who believe, based on clinical evidence, that a patient's health is jeopardized by the policies, coverage limits, or utilization restrictions of a plan should consider an appeal to the plan or medical director. Health care providers are encouraged to become actively involved with the policy-making boards of managed care or other plans in which they participate with the goal of improving patient welfare, and they should contribute to the quality improvement processes that result in plan guidelines.

Conflict of interest also may arise through patenting or restrictive licensing of medical procedures, diagnostic tests, or predictive tests. In addition to raising problems of efficacy and safety, the patenting of medical procedures and tests may jeopardize patients' interests by delaying the rapid transmission of new scientific knowledge and adding costs to a procedure or test that might put it out of reach of patients. Academic health care providers should be aware of the powerful incentives placed on them by their universities to maximize extramural revenues and should urge that such policies not encourage patenting arrangements that restrict use by other researchers or clinicians.

Physicians also may be faced with conflicts of interest in the conduct of clinical trials in which a treating clinician is also a principal investigator of a trial. At a minimum, the principal investigator should disclose financial relationships with the trial sponsor to the patient or research participant before her enrollment in the trial. In addition, the physician–investigator should ensure that publication of results of the trial is not contingent on a positive outcome for the sponsor. Clinical investigators also should participate actively in the writing of manuscripts that bear their name, not merely sign a "ghostwritten" manuscript.

The College has provided guidance for Fellows interacting with the health care industry and recommends that physicians set guidelines for themselves and their office staff for interaction with representatives. As the practice environment of medicine evolves, interactions with pharmaceutical and device industries necessarily change. The College guidelines summarized in the following paragraphs are subject to continual review and update, and the most recent version can be accessed at www.acog.org/Resources_And_Publications/Committee_Opinions_List.

Clinicians should choose diagnostic procedures and treatments on the basis of medical considerations and patient needs, regardless of any direct or indirect interest in the health care industry that they may have or any benefits they receive from that industry. Clinicians have an obligation to seek the most accurate, up-to-date, evidence-based, and balanced sources of information about new products that they contemplate using. They should not base decisions solely or primarily on information provided by the products' marketers. When any product promotion leads to inappropriate or unbalanced medical advice or recommendations to patients, an ethical problem exists.

Clinicians should understand that gifts tied to promotional information, even small gifts and meals, are designed to influence health care provider behavior. The acceptance of any gift, even of nominal value, tied to promotional information is strongly discouraged. The acceptance of cash donations, trips, and services directly from industry by individual physicians raises clear conflicts and is not ethical.

Although the provision of pharmaceutical samples offers potential benefits to patients, particularly for those who are uninsured or for whom purchase of medications otherwise represents a burden, such samples also may influence prescribing behavior inappropriately. Physicians may choose to provide samples or vouchers but should be aware that providing samples may promote patients' ongoing use of a particular medication, when other potential alternatives exist. When vouchers or samples are dispensed, consideration should be given to providing them preferentially to those patients with a true need and dispensing a supply sufficient for a full course of therapy.

Limitations on commercial support of continuing medical education (CME) have been published by the Accreditation Council for Continuing Medical Education, the Council of Medical Specialty Societies, and the AMA (see Resources). The gift of special funds to permit medical students, residents, and fellows to attend carefully selected educational conferences may be permissible as long as the selection of the attendees is made by the academic or training institution or by the accredited CME provider with the full concurrence of the academic or training institution. Subsidies from industry should not be accepted directly to pay for the costs of travel, lodging, or other personal expenses of clinicians who are attending the conferences, nor should subsidies be accepted to compensate for the clinician's time.

When new medical devices are approved or cleared by the U.S. Food and Drug Administration (FDA), access to training on those devices may be tightly regulated by the FDA and may require training by the manufacturer. The company may require physicians to travel to non-CME seminars designed to familiarize the physician with the new equipment. This presents an ethical difficulty for the physician. Training in proper use of devices encountered in the practice of obstetrics and gynecology is ideally provided through professional societies with CME accreditation. When training is not available from an accredited CME provider, or industry training is mandated by the FDA, and industry offers appropriate education, the obstetrician–gynecologist may participate if the training is focused on the safe, medically relevant, and FDA-cleared or FDA-approved indications for use of the equipment or device in the shortest possible time.

BILLING FRAUD

Practitioners should understand billing and coding requirements thoroughly or have staff on whom they can rely for this expertise (see also the "Practice Management" section in Part 2). Even honest mistakes have caused clinicians difficulties in this area. Dishonest billing is illegal and is an abdication of the clinician's responsibilities to society. This statement applies even when deceptive practices are meant to benefit the patient. For example, if the annual gynecologic examination is not covered under the insurance plan, the clinician may opt to code for vaginitis or menopausal syndrome instead of the routine examination. However, as well intentioned as such strategies may be, they introduce dishonesty into the patient–practitioner relationship, and the insurance companies will consider it fraud.

SEXUAL HARASSMENT

Sexual harassment is a form of sex discrimination prohibited under Title VII of the Civil Rights Act of 1964. Unwelcome sexual advances, requests for sexual favors, and other verbal or physical conduct of a sexual nature constitute sexual harassment. The following conditions apply to sexual harassment:

- A term or condition of an individual's employment or academic success is predicated on submission to such conduct. These overtures may be explicit or implicit.

- The basis for employment or academic decisions or advancement is reliant on submission to or rejection of such behavior.

- An individual's work or academic performance is affected because of this behavior, which creates an intimidating, hostile, or offensive working environment.

Men and women can be victims of sexual harassment. Institutions and other facilities should have policies on sexual harassment, and all personnel should be made aware of these policies. Guidance should be offered to all employees, students, residents, and supervisors who report these incidents. All complaints should be investigated and have follow-up.

SEXUAL MISCONDUCT

The practice of obstetrics and gynecology includes interaction at times of intense emotion and vulnerability for the patient and involves sensitive medical and social histories, physical examinations, and diagnoses. Children and adolescents are particularly vulnerable to emotional conflict and damage to their developing sense of identity and sexuality when roles and role boundaries with trusted adults are confused.

Sexual misconduct is not a new issue in the practice of medicine. It has been reevaluated in terms of current medical ethics to give additional consideration to respect for the rights of individuals, the unequal power relationship between a professional and a patient, and the potential for abuse of that power.

The College's Committee on Ethics agrees with the AMA's Council on Ethical and Judicial Affairs statement on this issue (see Bibliography). The AMA council provided the following guidelines, which the College's Committee on Ethics first affirmed in 1994 and continues to affirm:

- Mere mutual consent is rejected as a justification for sexual relations with patients because the disparity in power, status, vulnerability, and need makes it difficult for a patient to give meaningful consent to sexual contact or sexual relations.
- Sexual contact or a romantic relationship concurrent with the patient–physician relationship is unethical.
- Sexual contact or a romantic relationship with a former patient may be unethical under certain circumstances. The relevant standard is the potential for misuse of physician power and exploitation of patient emotions derived from the former relationship.
- Education on ethical issues involved in sexual misconduct should be included throughout all levels of medical training.
- Physicians have a responsibility to report offending colleagues to disciplinary boards.

Although the AMA and College statements were developed specifically in reference to physicians, sexual misconduct by any health care provider is an abuse of professional power and a violation of patient trust. Regardless of societal changes, rigid conformance to ethical principles in this regard is considered essential.

Bibliography

American Association of University Professors. Institutional responsibility for legal demands on faculty. AAUP policy documents and reports. 10th ed. Baltimore (MD): The Johns Hopkins University Press; 2006. p. 129.

American College of Obstetricians and Gynecologists. Code of professional ethics of the American College of Obstetricians and Gynecologists. Washington, DC: American College of Obstetricians and Gynecologists; 2011. Available at: http://www.acog.org/~/media/Departments/National%20Officer%20Nominations%20Process/ACOGcode.pdf?dmc=1&ts=20130715T1226302728. Retrieved July 15, 2013.

American College of Obstetricians and Gynecologists. Coding responsibility. ACOG Committee Opinion 249. Washington, DC: ACOG; 2001.

American Medical Association. Code of medical ethics of the American Medical Association: current opinions with annotations. 2012–2013 ed. Chicago (IL): AMA; 2012.

American Medical Association. State medical society websites. Available at: http://www.ama-assn.org/ama/pub/about-ama/our-people/the-federation-medicine/state-medical-society-websites.page. Retrieved September 26, 2013.

CDC guidance for evaluating health-care personnel for hepatitis B virus protection and for administering postexposure management. National Center for HIV/AIDS, Viral Hepatitis, STD, and TB Prevention, Centers for Disease Control and Prevention. MMWR Recomm Rep 2013;62:1–19.

Centers for Disease Control and Prevention. Recommendations for routine testing and follow-up for chronic hepatitis B virus (HBV) infection. Available at: http://www.cdc.gov/hepatitis/HBV/PDFs/ChronicHepBTestingFlwUp-BW.pdf. Retrieved September 26, 2013.

Ethical issues in pandemic influenza planning concerning pregnant women. Committee Opinion No. 563. American College of Obstetricians and Gynecologists. Obstet Gynecol 2013;121:1138–43.

Ethical issues with vaccination for the obstetrician–gynecologist. Committee Opinion No. 564. American College of Obstetricians and Gynecologists. Obstet Gynecol 2013;121:1144–50.

Expert testimony. ACOG Committee Opinion No. 374. American College of Obstetricians and Gynecologists. Obstet Gynecol 2007;110:445–6.

Human immunodeficiency virus. ACOG Committee Opinion No. 389. American College of Obstetricians and Gynecologists. Obstet Gynecol 2007;110:1473–8.

Immunization of health-care personnel: recommendations of the Advisory Committee on Immunization Practices (ACIP). Centers for Disease Control and Prevention. MMWR Recomm Rep 2011;60 (RR-7):1–45.

Patient safety and the electronic health record. Committee Opinion No. 472. American College of Obstetricians and Gynecologists. Obstet Gynecol 2010;116: 1245–7.

Patient testing: ethical issues in selection and counseling. ACOG Committee Opinion No. 363. American College of Obstetricians and Gynecologists. Obstet Gynecol 2007;109:1021–3.

Pearson ML, Bridges CB, Harper SA. Influenza vaccination of health-care personnel: recommendations of the Healthcare Infection Control Practices Advisory Committee (HICPAC) and the Advisory Committee on Immunization Practices (ACIP). MMWR Recomm Rep 2006;55 (RR-2):1–16.

Professional relationships with industry. Committee Opinion No. 541. American College of Obstetricians and Gynecologists. Obstet Gynecol 2012;120:1243–9.

Seeking and giving consultation. ACOG Committee Opinion No. 365. American College of Obstetricians and Gynecologists. Obstet Gynecol 2007;109:1255–60.

Sexual misconduct in the practice of medicine. Council on Ethical and Judicial Affairs, American Medical Association. JAMA 1991;266:2741–5.

Sexual misconduct. ACOG Committee Opinion No. 373. American College of Obstetricians and Gynecologists. Obstet Gynecol 2007;110:441–4.

Smith BD, Morgan RL, Beckett GA, Falck-Ytter Y, Holtzman D, Teo CG, et al. Recommendations for the identification of chronic hepatitis C virus infection among persons born during 1945-1965. Centers for Disease Control and Prevention. MMWR Recomm Rep 2012;61 (RR-4):1–32.

Updated CDC recommendations for the management of hepatitis B virus-infected health-care providers and students. Centers for Disease Control and Prevention. MMWR Recomm Rep 2012;61(RR-3):1–12.

Resources

Accreditation Council for Continuing Medical Education. Standards for commercial support: standards to ensure independence in CME activities. Available at: http://www.accme.org/requirements/accreditation-requirements-cme-providers/standards-for-commercial-support. Retrieved July 10, 2013.

Accreditation Council for Graduate Medical Education. Principles to guide the relationship between graduate medical education, industry, and other funding sources for programs and sponsoring institutions accredited by ACGME. Chicago (IL): ACGME; 2011. Available at: http://www.acgme.org/acgmeweb/Portals/0/PFAssets/PublicationsPapers/pp_GMEGuide.pdf. Retrieved August 12, 2013.

American College of Obstetricians and Gynecologists. Expert witness affirmation. Washington, DC: ACOG; 2002. Available at: http://www.acog.org/~/media/Depart ments/Members%20Only/Professional%20Liability/ExpertWitnessAffirmation.pdf ?dmc=1&ts=20130716T1446303966. Retrieved July 16, 2013.

American College of Obstetricians and Gynecologists. Qualifications for the physician expert witness. Washington, DC: ACOG; 2003. Available at: http://www. acog.org/~/media/Departments/Members%20Only/Professional%20Liability/ ExpertWitnessQualifications.pdf?dmc=1&ts=20120727T1351476623. Retrieved July 16, 2013.

American Congress of Obstetricians and Gynecologists. Social media and professionalism in the medical community (DVD). Washington, DC: American Congress of Obstetricians and Gynecologists; 2013.

American Medical Association. Clarification of Opinion 8.061: gifts to physicians from industry. Code of medical ethics of the American Medical Association: current opinions with annotations. Council on Ethical and Judicial Affairs. 2012–2013 ed. Chicago (IL): AMA; 2012. p. 257–65.

American Medical Association. Gifts to physicians from industry. Code of medical ethics of the American Medical Association: current opinions with annotations. Council on Ethical and Judicial Affairs. 2012-2013 ed. Chicago (IL): AMA; 2012. p. 252–7.

Centers for Disease Control and Prevention. Occupational HIV transmission and prevention among health care workers. Atlanta (GA): CDC; 2013. Available at: http://www.cdc.gov/hiv/pdf/risk_occupational_factsheet.pdf. Retrieved September 26, 2013.

Centers for Disease Control and Prevention. Vaccines and immunizations. Available at: http://www.cdc.gov/vaccines. Retrieved July 16, 2013.

Council of Medical Specialty Societies. Code for interactions with companies. Chicago (IL): CMSS; 2011. Available at: http://www.cmss.org/codeforinteractions. aspx. Retrieved July 16, 2013.

The impaired surgeon. Diagnosis, treatment, and reentry. Committee on the Impaired Physician, American College of Surgeons Board of Governors. Bull Am Coll Surg 1992;77:29–32, 39.

Morreale MC, Stinnett AJ, Dowling EC, editors. Policy compendium on confidential health services for adolescents. 2nd ed. Chapel Hill (NC): Center for Adolescent Health & the Law; 2005.

Vawter DE, Garrett JE, Gervais KG, Prehn AW, DeBruin DA, Tauer CA, et al. For the good of us all: ethically rationing health resources in Minnesota in a severe influenza pandemic. St. Paul (MN): Minnesota Department of Health; 2010. Available at: http://www.health.state.mn.us/divs/idepc/ethics/ethics.pdf. Retrieved September 26, 2013.

World Health Organization. Ethical considerations in developing a public health response to pandemic influenza. Geneva: WHO; 2007. Available at: http://www.who.int/csr/resources/publications/WHO_CDS_EPR_GIP_2007_2c.pdf. Retrieved September 26, 2013.

ETHICAL ISSUES

Medical knowledge and technology offer an increasing array of options for managing reproductive processes. Assisted reproductive technologies, maternal–fetal surgery, and interventions at the end of life raise questions that cannot be addressed by physicians or by the field of medicine alone. Decisions in these areas depend on thoughtful consideration of the values, desires, and goals of those involved. For clinicians to achieve an ethical approach to confronting difficult problems, they must address certain fundamental issues:

- Clinicians should explicitly understand their own value system and the ways in which personal judgments influence clinical decision-making and the care of patients.
- Clinicians should have general knowledge of the discipline of ethics.
- The process by which clinicians make and implement ethical decisions should be systematic, logically consistent, and consistent with accepted frameworks of ethics.

Ethics is the formal study of behavior in which moral obligations are analyzed in terms of recognized methods. After critical reflection, an attempt is made to determine which of a number of commonly held assumptions are justifiable. In applying ethical frameworks to the analysis of human action, the discipline of ethics does not identify any particular moral view as the correct one. It serves instead as a framework for systematically analyzing different points of view and rationally justifying one course of action over another, based on consideration of recognized principles and accepted values.

Ethical principles and practices are important in a broad variety of areas in obstetrics and gynecology. They are the foundation of professional behavior (see also the "Human Resources" section earlier in Part 1) and underpin actions taken to protect the interests and autonomy of patients.

A basic understanding of ethical principles and practices will aid in decision making. Institutions and individuals should be ethically guided in policy making, and institutional ethics committees may be helpful in determining the appropriate course of action.

Ethical Foundations

Several methods exist for ethical decision making in medicine. In recent decades, medical decision making has been dominated by principle-based ethics; several alternative approaches have been promoted, including virtue-based ethics, the ethic of care, feminist ethics, communitarian ethics, and case-based approaches. Each of these methods has merits and limitations. These methods, when put into practice, can promote understanding of common ethical practices regarding informed consent, honesty, and confidentiality.

PRINCIPLE-BASED ETHICS

In principle-based ethics, four principles are used to identify, analyze, and address ethical dilemmas. They are 1) respect for autonomy, 2) beneficence, 3) nonmaleficence, and 4) justice.

Autonomy (literally, "self-rule") refers to a person's freedom to establish personal norms of conduct and to choose a course of action voluntarily based on personal beliefs and values. Respect for a patient's autonomy acknowledges an individual's right to hold views, make choices, and take actions based on these beliefs and values. Respect for autonomy is important, but it cannot be regarded as absolute. At times it may conflict with other principles or values and sometimes must yield to them. A clinician may consider a particular course of treatment to be best for a patient, and respect for autonomy provides a strong moral foundation for informed consent; once a patient has been adequately informed about her medical condition and the available therapies, she freely chooses, based on her values and beliefs, specific treatments or nontreatment.

Beneficence is the obligation to promote the well-being of others. The related principle of nonmaleficence obliges an individual to avoid doing harm. With roots in the Hippocratic tradition, beneficence and nonmaleficence also are fundamental to the ethical practice of medicine. These two principles, taken together, are operative in almost every treatment decision because every medical or surgical procedure has both benefits and risks, which must be balanced knowledgeably and wisely. These principles, therefore, are the source of a clinician's obligation to act with due care. In balancing beneficence with respect for autonomy, the clinician should define the patient's "best interests" as objectively as possible. Attempting to override patient autonomy to promote what the clinician perceives as a patient's best interests is called paternalism. The opposite end of the spectrum is the informative model. In this model, the physician is a provider of objective and technical information regarding the patient's medical problem and its potential therapeutic solutions. The drawback of this model is the loss of the physician's perspective, concern, and medical expertise in the decision-making process. In addition, at times it may be difficult to achieve objectivity with this model. A middle ground between these models is the interpretive model. The physician helps the patient clarify and integrate her values into the decision-making process while acting as an information source regarding the technical aspects of any given medical procedure.

Justice is the principle of rendering what is due to others. Justice has been defined as a complex and important concept that requires medical professionals and policymakers to treat individuals fairly and requires the provision of medical services to individuals to be nondiscriminatory. Some theories of justice determine distribution of benefits and burdens based on criteria such as need, effort, contribution, or merit. Other theories specify that all benefits and burdens be distributed equally (distributive justice). It is important that criteria to be used are determined in advance and selected in a manner consistent with accepted moral rules and principles; criteria also should be relevant to the benefits and burdens being assigned. In the United States, for example, race, gender, and religion are not considered to be morally legitimate criteria for the distribution of benefits such as employment and housing. Justice generates an obligation to treat equally individuals who are alike according to whatever criteria are selected. Patients with identical needs should receive equal treatment unless it is demonstrated that they differ from others in a way that is relevant to the treatment in question.

Although competing claims for care or services may have appeared equal when resources were ample, scarcity of resources may require clinicians and policymakers to reevaluate the criteria used for distribution of benefits and burdens. Different criteria must then be chosen as a result of this scarcity, and selection of these criteria is in itself a moral decision.

VIRTUE-BASED ETHICS

Virtue-based medical ethics relies on health care providers possessing qualities in character that dispose them to make choices and decisions that achieve the well-being of others. These qualities of character include honesty, trustworthiness, prudence, fairness, fortitude, temperance, integrity, self-effacement, empathy, and compassion. Virtues complement rather than replace principles because they are necessary to interpret and apply methods in medical ethics with moral sensitivity and judgment.

ETHIC OF CARE

The ethic of care raises the importance of dimensions of moral experience generally excluded from traditional moral theories and is concerned primarily with obligations that arise from relationships with others rather than the impartiality that traditional ethics demands. The moral foundations underlying the ethic of care are not rights and duties, but commitment, empathy, compassion, caring, and love. The application of the ethic of care requires attention to context and particularity rather than abstraction. An ethic of care overlaps with a virtue ethic in emphasizing the caregiver's orientation and qualities. In this ethical approach, care represents the fundamental orientation of obstetrics and gynecology as well as much of medicine and health care. It indicates the direction and rationale of the relationship between health care providers and those who seek their care.

FEMINIST ETHICS

Feminist ethics compels us to recognize that gender roles and power differentials between the genders in our culture may distort traditional ethical analyses. Ethical decisions about women's health care may be biased by attitudes and traditions about gender that are embedded in our culture.

Historically, gender-entrenched associations regarding men and women contribute to the tendency in traditional moral theory to view "feminine" perspectives or emotions as irrelevant or distorting. Appropriate emotion and empathy are indispensable to moral reasoning in the ethical conduct of medical care. Feminist ethics challenges gender-based and sex-based presuppositions and their consequences, including the relative societal value of men and women.

COMMUNITARIAN ETHICS

Communitarian ethics challenges the primacy often attributed to respect for autonomy in principle-based ethics. It emphasizes shared values, ideals, and goals and suggests that the needs of the larger community may take precedence, in some cases, over the rights and desires of individuals, as in the case of vaccination.

CASE-BASED REASONING

Case-based reasoning is ethical decision making based on precedents set in specific cases, analogous to the role of case law in jurisprudence. An accumulated body of influential cases and their interpretation provide moral guidance. Case-based reasoning asserts the priority of practice over theory, rejects the primacy of principles, and recognizes the emergence of principles from a process of generalization from the analysis of cases.

Ethics in Practice

Several ethical norms can be derived from the application of theory to practice. These norms or concepts are important because they influence many of the decisions made in obstetrics and gynecology. An understanding of these concepts will facilitate ethical decision making and the ethical practice of medicine.

INFORMED CONSENT

Informed consent is the process during which a patient makes a voluntary choice regarding a medical intervention after appropriate explanation and disclosure by the clinician of the nature of the intervention and its risks and benefits as well as the risks and benefits of alternatives. The primary purpose of the consent process is the exercise of patient autonomy. Informed consent also has been associated with health care quality and safety. A patient's right to make her own decisions about medical issues extends to the right of informed refusal—the right to refuse recommended medical treatment. By encouraging ongoing and open communication about relevant information, the health care provider enables the patient to exercise personal choice. This sort of communication is central to the patient–clinician relationship. Specific requirements for informed consent of U.S. research participants have been codified in the Code of Federal Regulations. They are addressed in the "Governance" section earlier in Part 1.

Ethically and legally, adult patients are presumed to be capable of making health care choices. At times, however, a patient's capacity to comprehend and process the medical information presented to her may be in doubt. In such cases, the health care provider, through consultation and further discussion with the patient, should attempt to clarify and improve the patient's ability to provide consent. The attempt to clarify is based on disclosure of information and the interpretation of its meaning. The adequacy of the information disclosed has been judged by various criteria, which may include the following:

- The common practice of the profession
- The reasonable needs and expectations of the ordinary individual who might be making a particular decision
- The unique needs of the individual patient faced with a given choice

If a patient is unable to provide consent, a substitute decision maker should be sought. A surrogate decision maker should be identified to provide a "substituted judgment" (a decision based on what the patient would want, assuming some knowledge of what the patient's wishes and values would be). If the patient has previously executed an advance directive, that document should guide the selection of a surrogate decision maker, the specific decisions made by the surrogate, or both depending on the nature of the advance directive. If a patient who lacks decision-making capacity has not designated a surrogate, state law may dictate the order in which relatives should be asked to serve in this role. In rare occasions, a court will determine the decision maker.

If a patient does not have decision-making capacity, the appropriate decision-maker to provide authorization for health care should be determined before the initiation of an examination or procedure. In doing so, it is important to ascertain whether the patient is capable of understanding findings and recommendations or whether this information needs to be transmitted to an identified guardian or caregiver. This process should not preclude including the patient in counseling and determining the degree to which she may participate in decisions.

It is important to emphasize that informed consent is a process. In some minds, it has become synonymous with the informed consent forms used to document that the informed consent process has taken place. Documenting the informed consent process, of course, is important from a medical–legal perspective, but completion of a written document is never a substitute for the communication needed to have an informed and voluntary consent.

For certain types of medical procedures, such as hysterectomy and sterilization, additional elements that affect informed consent bear mentioning. The clinician should be familiar with any federal and state laws and regulations that may constrain sterilization (even as a result of hysterectomy), such as limitations on the patient's age and requirements for the consent process. For example, when a sterilization procedure will be covered under Medicare, Medicaid, or other U.S. Public Health Service programs, 30 days must elapse after the consent form has been signed before the procedure can be performed (except in emergencies). Additionally, the patient must be 21 years of age or older and mentally competent, and she may not be institutionalized.

Women may be vulnerable to various forms of coercion in their medical decision making. Laws, regulations, and reimbursement restrictions concerning sterilization have been created to protect vulnerable individuals, including those with mental disabilities and other specific populations, from abuse. However, regulations intended to protect vulnerable individuals may in some cases serve as barriers to care. Women should not be denied access to care they choose to have (eg, a sterilization procedure) simply because they also may be members of vulnerable populations or have common characteristics with such populations. Clinicians caring for patients who request or require procedures that result in sterilization may find themselves in a dilemma when legal and reimbursement restrictions interfere with a patient's choice of treatment. Rigid timing and age requirements can restrict access to good health care and result in unnecessary risk. Clinicians are encouraged to seek legal or ethical consultation whenever necessary in their efforts to provide care that is most appropriate to individual situations.

Acknowledgment of the importance of respect for patient autonomy and increased patient access to information has prompted some patients to request surgery or other interventions that their physicians may view as not in the patients' best interests. An example may be requests for prophylactic oophorectomy by women at low risk to reduce their risk of ovarian cancer. When patients request surgical interventions that are not traditionally recommended, physicians should make sure that their counseling about specific risks and benefits is based on current evidence. Determining an appropriate course of treatment for individual patients who request such a surgical intervention requires particularly careful communication. The goal should be to reach a decision in partnership between the patient and physician. Depending on the context, agreeing to a request for a surgical option that is not traditionally recommended can be ethical. Decisions should be based on strong support for patients' informed preferences and values; be understood in the context of an interpretive conversation; and be consistent with considerations of safety, cost-effectiveness, and attention to effects on the health care system of expanded choice. After the physician has provided information and careful counseling, the patient and physician often will reach a mutually acceptable decision. If the patient and physician cannot reach an agreement, then referral or second opinion may be appropriate.

CONSCIENTIOUS OBJECTION

There are limits to which appeals to conscience may justifiably guide decision making. Professional ethics requires that health care be delivered in a way that is respectful of patient autonomy, timely and effective, evidence based, and nondiscriminatory. When, as a matter of conscience, physicians plan to deviate from standard practices, including abortion, sterilization, and provision of contraceptives, they must provide potential patients with accurate and prior notice of their personal moral commitments and should not use this opportunity to argue or advocate their positions. When conscientious refusals conflict with moral obligations that are central to the ethical practice of medicine, ethical care requires either that the physician provide care despite reservations or that there be resources or a referral system in place to allow the patient to gain access to care in the presence of conscientious refusal.

Providing complete and scientifically accurate information about options for reproductive health is fundamental to respect for patient autonomy. Those who choose the profession of medicine are obligated to act in good faith to protect patients' health, particularly to the extent that a patient's health interests may conflict with a physician's personal beliefs or self-interests. In the case of interventions performed during pregnancy, the physician should respect the woman's autonomous decisions on the very rare occasions when the interest of the fetus and woman diverge. Pregnancy does not obviate or limit the requirement to obtain informed consent.

In resource-poor areas, access to safe and legal reproductive services should be maintained. A health care provider with moral or religious objections should either practice in proximity to individuals who do not share his or her views or ensure that referral processes are in place so that patients have access to the service that the physician does not wish to provide. Rights to withdraw from caring for an individual should not be a pretext for interfering with patients' rights to health care services.

HONESTY

The principle of respect for autonomy requires that a patient be given complete and truthful information about her medical condition and about any proposed treatment. Only with such information is she able to exercise her right to make choices about health care. If complete information is not available, existing uncertainty should be shared with the patient. The perception that a health care provider has concealed the truth or has engaged in deception will weaken patient trust and undermine the patient–clinician relationship. This statement is true regardless of the intent of the clinician; for example, improper diagnostic coding to allow insurance coverage of a service the clinician judges to be medically indicated is nonetheless deceptive and fraudulent.

CONFIDENTIALITY

A patient's right to make decisions about health care includes a right to decide how and to whom personal medical information will be communicated. The principle of respect for autonomy underlies a health care provider's duty to respect patient confidentiality. As is the case with dishonesty, breaches of confidentiality threaten the patient's trust and may destroy the patient–clinician relationship. Ethically, breaches of confidentiality may be justified in rare cases to protect others from serious harm. Physicians must weigh a patient's claims of confidentiality against risks to others. How the health care provider's responsibility to respect confidentiality plays out in daily practice, including in the care of minors, is addressed in the "Human Resources" section earlier in Part 1 and the "Adolescents" section in Part 3. Guidance on setting up systems to maintain confidentiality is detailed in the "Information Management" section in Part 2.

Patient Protection

A variety of mechanisms have been put in place to help ensure that patients' rights are respected and that patients are protected from harm. A patient's bill of rights outlines the rights and, sometimes, responsibilities of a patient who receives care at a health care facility. All patients who receive care, including those who participate in research studies and receive experimental interventions, should receive the same protection. In fact, there are usually special policies that provide protection for research participants, which are overseen by the institutional review board.

Patients can exercise their autonomy by making an advance directive. This may be an instructional directive ("living will") or the identification of a surrogate with power of attorney. Physician orders for life-sustaining treatment (POLST; also known as medical orders for life-sustaining treatment) are available once a patient develops serious, progressive, chronic illnesses that may require standing medical orders. (For more information on advance directives and end-of-life decision making, see the "End-of-Life Considerations" section in Part 3.)

The intent of a patient's bill of rights is to outline the rights and responsibilities of a patient within the health care system. Several organizations (the American Hospital Association, the American Medical Association, and The Joint Commission) have developed various versions. The contents usually include the following rights for patients:

- The right to adequate health care
- The right to considerate and respectful care
- The right to relevant, current, and understandable information concerning their condition
- The right to be involved in all aspects of their care
- The right to provide informed consent
- The right to refuse care
- The right to know the identity of their caregivers
- The right to be informed of institutional policies, including those that could affect patient choice
- The right to all appropriate treatments or procedures
- The right to make an advance directive and have it respected (see also the "End-of-Life Considerations" section in Part 3)
- The right to privacy and confidentiality except when otherwise mandated by law
- The right to review their own medical records
- The right to know about the institution's charges and payment methods
- The right to know about potential conflicts of interest, including business relationships among institutions and health care providers that may affect patient care
- The right to consent to or decline participation in research studies
- The right to a full explanation of potential risks and benefits of research studies, procedures to be followed, and alternative services available

- The right to the most effective care the institution can provide if participation in a research protocol is refused
- The right to reasonable continuity of care, when appropriate
- The right to know about resources available for resolving conflicts and grievances
- The right to quality and safe care in a health care system designed to minimize medical errors

The idea that all people have a right to some level of health care has developed since the end of World War II. The United Nations and the World Health Organization support this right. The issue of access to care has engendered much discussion in recent years. The President's Advisory Commission on Consumer Protection and Quality in the Health Care Industry echoed this call in its patients' bill of rights (see Resources). The 2010 Patient Protection and Affordable Care Act provides a number of health care benefits, including providing many preventive services with no co-payments or cost-sharing, allowing parents to cover on their health plans their children who are younger than 26 years, providing new coverage options for those with preexisting conditions, and increasing funding for community health centers. As of 2014, most individuals who can afford it will be required to obtain basic health insurance coverage or pay a fee to help offset the costs of caring for uninsured Americans. If affordable coverage is not available to an individual, he or she will be eligible for an exemption.

A just health care system provides universal coverage in the form of affordable and effective health care for all residents of the United States regardless of citizenship or employment status. The American College of Obstetricians and Gynecologists (the College) calls for quality health care appropriate to every woman's needs throughout her life and for ensuring that a full array of clinical services are available to women without costly delays or the imposition of geographic, financial, attitudinal, or legal barriers. When health care institutions have policies that limit patients' reproductive options, including contraception, sterilization, or infertility services, patients should be advised of those policies openly and as early as possible.

The College and its membership represent expert voices in the social process of health care reform and creating and sustaining a just health care system, and they have a wide range of opportunities to advocate for and advance the goal of just health care. Fellows of the College should exercise their responsibility to improve the health status of women. They can do so in traditional patient–physician relationships and by working within their community and at the state and national levels to ensure access to high-quality programs that meet the health needs of all women. Involvement in the community may extend to nonmedical areas, such as building safe housing or donating food or clothing, that directly or indirectly improve women's health.

Patients rightfully share responsibility for their care. Thus, patients should be encouraged to do the following:

- Ask questions about medical treatments they do not understand in order to make informed choices about their care.
- Follow through with collaboratively developed care decisions.
- Keep scheduled physician's appointments, including follow-up appointments, and notify the office in a timely manner if they need to reschedule.
- Provide insurance information for reimbursement, and pay for services themselves if not covered by insurance.
- Provide accurate information necessary for appropriate diagnosis and treatment planning (including lifestyle factors, sexual practices, and religious or cultural beliefs).
- Maintain a complete list of medications, including herbal supplements and nonprescription medications, and provide this information to health care personnel.

Ethical Decision Making and Institutional Ethics Committees

In most cases, there is minimal conflict among the patient, family, health care provider, and health care facility in selecting the most appropriate health care option even though more than one course of action may be morally and ethically justifiable. Sometimes parties may disagree about the most appropriate choice. If the risk–benefit relationship is not optimal, no course of action will seem acceptable.

Although the key to ethical decision making is the patient–clinician relationship, the involvement of individuals with a variety of backgrounds and perspectives can be useful, especially if an impasse has been reached. Through establishment of institutional review boards and use of institutional ethics committees, ethics consultants, or ethics consultation services, health care facilities can support the protection of patient rights and assist in ethical decision making in difficult situations (see also the "Governance" section earlier in Part 1).

Changes in medical technology and social structure have moved the site of much medical decision making from the home to health care facilities. Decisions once made privately and confidentially now are more openly discussed, with wide social, economic, and ethical consequences. Moreover, nonmedical decision making (eg, third-party payer contracts, institutional purchasing, and cancellation of services that were not fiscally sound) is having a greater influence on patient care. Accordingly, patients, practitioners, and health care administrative personnel need a forum for discussion and education. The Joint Commission requires all U.S. hospitals to have a process that allows staff, patients, and families to address ethical issues or issues prone to conflict. An institutional ethics committee can provide such a forum, or hospitals may seek support in addressing ethical issues from an ethics consultant or an ethics consultation service. Whatever the process, it needs to be readily accessible to patients and their surrogate decision makers as well as staff, physicians and other licensed independent practitioners, and managers.

Ethics committees typically have the following functions:

- To foster awareness of ethical issues and create an environment of sensitivity
- To establish educational programs regarding ethical principles, biomedical ethics literature, and relevant legal decisions
- To act as an expert informational resource concerning clinical ethics in the institutional setting

- To offer counsel on ethics for individual cases and organizational issues
- To help create, promote, and audit a code of ethical behavior for the entire institution
- To develop organizational policies that support ethical principles

Most committees serve in advisory, rather than decision-making, capacities. In general, the committee may aid the patient, health care provider, and institution by serving as a resource for education, conflict resolution, support, and institutional quality improvement. The committee also can serve as a forum for the discussion of unresolved biomedical issues, such as the application of new reproductive technologies. Mechanisms other than institutional ethics committees exist within health care institutions to enforce institution policies and standards and to assume appropriate legal responsibility for practices within the institution (see also the "Human Resources" section earlier in Part 1).

Institutional ethics committees and bioethics consultants also can assist in ensuring that the processes of informed consent and decision making are followed with patients or their proxies. Consent for acceptance or refusal of treatment should be based on accurate and current medical information that presents all reasonable options. The committee should establish programs to promote this goal. The committee also should determine that the institution has systems to ensure that the patient has the capacity to choose and that appropriate decision makers are identified when the patient does not have this capacity.

The use of institutional ethics committees is an evolving technique for helping with difficult decisions. Continuing appraisal of the form and function of these committees is important. They are not meant to supplant other good techniques that have been found effective in the institution.

Bibliography

Beauchamp TL, Childress JF. Principles of biomedical ethics. 7th ed. New York (NY): Oxford University Press; 2013.

Charo RA. The celestial fire of conscience—refusing to deliver medical care. N Engl J Med 2005;352:2471–3.

Community involvement and volunteerism. ACOG Committee Opinion No. 437. American College of Obstetricians and Gynecologists. Obstet Gynecol 2009; 114:203–4.

Department of Health and Human Services. Key features of the Affordable Care Act by year. Available at: http://www.hhs.gov/healthcare/facts/timeline/timeline-text. html. Retrieved July 16, 2013.

Dickens BM, Cook RJ. Conflict of interest: legal and ethical aspects. Int J Gynaecol Obstet 2006;92:192–7.

Elective surgery and patient choice. Committee Opinion No. 578. American College of Obstetricians and Gynecologists. Obstet Gynecol 2013;122:1134–8.

Emanuel EJ, Emanuel LL. Four models of the physician-patient relationship. JAMA 1992;267:2221–6.

Ethical decision making in obstetrics and gynecology. ACOG Committee Opinion No. 390. American College of Obstetricians and Gynecologists. Obstet Gynecol 2007;110:1479–87.

Forming a just health care system. Committee Opinion No. 456. American College of Obstetricians and Gynecologists. Obstet Gynecol 2010;115:672–7.

Informed consent. ACOG Committee Opinion No. 439. American College of Obstetricians and Gynecologists. Obstet Gynecol 2009;114:401–8.

Little MO. Why a feminist approach to bioethics? Kennedy Inst Ethics J 1996;6:1–18.

National Quality Forum. Improving patient safety through informed consent for patients with limited health literacy: an implementation report. Washington, DC: 2005. Available at: http://www.qualityforum.org/Publications/2005/09/Improving_ Patient_Safety_Through_Informed_Consent_for_Patients_with_Limited_Health_ Literacy.aspx. Retrieved September 26, 2013.

Schyve PM. Leadership in healthcare organizations; a guide to Joint Commission leadership standards. San Diego (CA): The Governance Institute; 2009. Available at: http://www.jointcommission.org/assets/1/18/wp_leadership_standards.pdf. Retrieved September 27, 2013.

Sterilization of women, including those with mental disabilities. ACOG Committee Opinion No. 371. American College of Obstetricians and Gynecologists. Obstet Gynecol 2007;110:217–20.

The limits of conscientious refusal in reproductive medicine. ACOG Committee Opinion No. 385. American College of Obstetricians and Gynecologists. Obstet Gynecol 2007;110:1203–8.

The uninsured. ACOG Committee Opinion No. 416. American College of Obstetricians and Gynecologists. Obstet Gynecol 2008;112:731–4.

Resources

American College of Obstetricians and Gynecologists. Access to women's health care. College Statement of Policy 64. Washington, DC: ACOG; 2009.

American College of Obstetricians and Gynecologists. Code of professional ethics of the American College of Obstetricians and Gynecologists. Washington, DC: American College of Obstetricians and Gynecologists; 2011. Available at: http://www.acog.org/~/media/Departments/National%20Officer%20Nominations%20Process/ACOGcode.pdf?dmc=1&ts=20130715T1226302728. Retrieved July 15, 2013.

American Congress of Obstetricians and Gynecologists. Health System Reform: the law, your practice, your patients. Washington, DC: American Congress of Obstetricians and Gynecologists; 2010. Available at: http://www.acog.org/About_ACOG/ACOG_Departments/Health_Care_Reform. Retrieved July 16, 2013.

American Medical Association. Code of medical ethics of the American Medical Association: current opinions with annotations. 2012-2013 ed. Chicago (IL): AMA; 2012.

American Medical Association. Virtual Mentor: American Medical Association Journal of Ethics. Available at: http://virtualmentor.ama-assn.org. Retrieved July 16, 2013.

American Society for Bioethics and Humanities. Improving competencies in clinical ethics consultation: an education guide. Glenview (IL): ASBH; 2009.

American Society for Reproductive Medicine. Ethics Committee documents. Available at: http://www.asrm.org/EthicsReports. Retrieved July 16, 2013.

Empathy in women's health care. Committee Opinion No. 480. American College of Obstetricians and Gynecologists. Obstet Gynecol 2011;117:756–61.

Institutional review boards. 21 C.F.R. part 56 (2013). Available at: http://www.gpo.gov/fdsys/pkg/CFR-2013-title21-vol1/pdf/CFR-2013-title21-vol1-part56.pdf. Retrieved September 20, 2013.

Jonsen AR, Siegler M, Winslade WJ. Clinical ethics: a practical approach to ethical decisions in clinical medicine. 7th ed. New York: McGraw-Hill Medical; 2010.

Lynch HF. Conflicts of conscience in health care: an institutional compromise. Cambridge, Mass.: MIT Press; 2008.

National Center for Ethics in Health Care. Available at: http://www.ethics.va.gov/. Retrieved July 16, 2013.

Presidential Commission for the Study of Bioethical Issues. Available at: http://www.bioethics.gov/. Retrieved July 16, 2013.

President's Advisory Commission on Consumer Protection and Quality in the Health Care Industry. Quality first: better health care for all Americans. Available at: http://archive.ahrq.gov/hcqual/final/. Retrieved July 16, 2013.

Snyder L. American College of Physicians Ethics Manual: sixth edition. American College of Physicians Ethics, Professionalism, and Human Rights Committee. Ann Intern Med 2012;156:73–104.

The Hastings Center. Available at: http://www.thehastingscenter.org/. Retrieved September 18, 2012.

The Joint Commission. Comprehensive accreditation manual for hospitals: CAMH. Oakbrook Terrace (IL): The Commission; 2014.

ORGANIZATION OF SERVICES

The delivery of high-quality obstetric and gynecologic care requires the establishment of efficient systems that can fulfill certain functions regardless of whether the care is provided in a hospital or an ambulatory setting. Such systems should support health care providers with essential human and material resources and foster interdisciplinary collaboration. How practitioners define their scope of practice will affect how their office is organized and managed. In many cases, the structure and systems of the department of obstetrics and gynecology may serve as a model for other facilities, such as an ambulatory surgical center or an office.

Common to all medical practices are certain principles and processes necessary to maintain an efficient and safe atmosphere in which to provide services. The following sections review principles of management for the organization of facilities and equipment, infection control procedures, support services, and information and practice management systems may be applied regardless of the size of the office or clinic or the scope of women's health care to be administered.

FACILITIES AND EQUIPMENT

The facilities in which gynecologic care is provided—regardless of whether the setting is an office, an outpatient surgical facility, or an inpatient hospital—should be safe, efficient, and conducive to the compassionate delivery of health care to all women. The following section describes many requirements necessary for all facilities that deliver gynecologic care, as well as some of the most important ones for specific settings.

General Requirements

Whether the facility in question is an office, an ambulatory surgical facility, or a hospital, there are certain requirements for optimal delivery of gynecologic care. Building codes are city, county, and state specific. Facilities should adhere to all applicable codes.

Specific plans and procedures should be established for the health and safety of patients and personnel. These should include the following:

- Disaster Plans and Procedures
  — Mechanisms to minimize the risk of hazards from electrical and mechanical failure, explosion, fire, and loss of refrigeration
  — Training in and knowledge of the proper use of safety, emergency, and fire-extinguishing equipment
  — Facility evacuation plans for patients and personnel
- Medical Emergencies
  — Management of medical emergencies that arise from services rendered
  — Mechanism to transfer patients to backup hospital when necessary
  — Training of personnel in cardiopulmonary resuscitation
  — Proper preparation and administration of drugs

- Facilities
  - Control and disposal of sharps (eg, needles, syringes, glass, and knife blades), and contaminated material
  - Proper storage of medications and drugs
  - Accessibility to individuals with disabilities (ie, safety and absence of barriers)
  - Adequate maintenance and cleanliness of facilities

In addition, violence against physicians and other health care workers has raised concerns about personal safety in health care settings. The following are suggestions to enhance the safety of physicians, staff, and patients:

- Establish a relationship with the local police force and other security personnel.
- Obtain a security audit of the office or institution.
- Review emergency plans periodically.
- Restrict after-hours access.
- Improve lighting at entrances and in parking areas.
- Install security cameras, mirrors, and panic buzzers.
- Install deadbolt or electronic locks.
- Restrict access to all doors except the main entrance.
- Preprogram 911 (emergency telephone number) into all telephones.
- Enclose and secure reception areas.
- Develop an emergency notification system.

Electrical, lighting, air quality, and temperature systems need to function appropriately and safely. A program for regular maintenance should be in place and may require the services of an environmental engineer. Standards for electrical outlets and electrical equipment have been developed by The Joint Commission (see Resources).

Medical and other equipment should be well maintained and inspected at regular intervals for proper functioning and safety as specified by the manufacturer's operations manual. This may require the assistance and services of a mechanical engineer, a biomedical technician, or both. A log should be maintained of routine checks, repairs, and service calls on medical equipment. Only properly trained and qualified personnel should operate medical equipment.

Emergency equipment and supplies should be readily available and maintained. All personnel in an office should know the location of critical emergency equipment. Personnel should be instructed periodically in the proper use of safety, emergency, and fire-extinguishing equipment. Plans should be developed for emergency situations, including assisting individuals with special needs. Drills should be conducted regularly to ensure preparedness. Alternate sources of power should be available and adequate for staff to manage patients in the event of an emergency.

One of the primary concerns is the safety of the patient and any accompanying individuals. There should be proper lighting and flooring to minimize accidents. Avoid small rugs or rugs with loose edges; these are hazardous to everyone, particularly those with mobility issues. Examination rooms, restrooms, and other patient areas should be handicap accessible.

Safety extends to those accompanying the patient. As women often have young children with them, attention should be given to childproofing all reception and clinical areas. Move dangerous instruments and solutions to cabinets out of reach of small children, install childproof locks on cabinet doors, keep sharps containers away from the edge of countertops, and cover waste containers. Toys should be carefully evaluated for safety issues: avoid those with small parts that can be swallowed by infants and toddlers.

Specific Physical and Supply Requirements

The specific physical and supply requirements for basic care in the office, ambulatory, and hospital setting will depend greatly on the type of practice and patients served. Box 2-1 lists basic equipment and supplies that should be available for gynecologic care.

Rooms should be designed to provide patient privacy at all times during the visit. Patient names on charts, specimens, and daily visit records should not be visible to other patients.

Box 2-1. Basic Equipment and Supplies for Gynecologic Care

- Patient drapes and examination table covers
- Sharps disposal containers
- Vaginal specula of various sizes
- Supplies for cervical cytology tests, wet mounts, and cultures, if performed in the setting
- Instruments for suture, staple, and clip removal
- Instruments for minor surgical procedures (eg, biopsies of the endometrium, cervix, and vulva or insertion of implants and intrauterine devices)
- Cleaning and sterilization equipment, unless this is provided by an external service

---

Policies and procedures to keep the environment healthy and avoid potential hazards should be established:

- Ban smoking on the premises.
- Minimize or eliminate hazards that might result in accidents, electrical shock, or trauma.
- Minimize sources and dissemination of infections.
- Assess adequacy of the infection control program periodically (see also the "Infection Control" section later in Part 2).
- Ensure that there are systems in place for the identification, safe handling, and disposal of hazardous materials and waste (see also the "Practice Management" section later in Part 2).
- Minimize radiation exposure.
- Reduce or eliminate exposure risks to latex-sensitive individuals.

LATEX PRODUCTS

Latex products, particularly gloves, are ubiquitous in the medical setting, and many consumer products (eg, condoms and diaphragms) are made of latex. Allergy to natural latex rubber is a serious health risk for many health care workers and patients. Manufacturers of medical devices are required to label products that include natural rubber latex or dry natural rubber.

The prevalence of latex sensitivity in the general population has been estimated to be less than 1%, but it may be higher. Individuals who are at high risk include the following:

- Health care workers
- Patients with spina bifida
- Patients who have had multiple surgical procedures
- Individuals subject to occupational exposure
- Individuals who have a history of atopy
- Individuals who have food allergies, especially those allergic to avocados, bananas, chestnuts, kiwifruit, or passion fruit

Allergic reactions to latex range from mild skin reactions and mild swelling of the lips to systemic reactions, such as asthma and anaphylaxis, which may result in chronic illness, disability, career loss, hardship, or death.

Antigen avoidance is the cardinal principle in the management of latex allergy. Facilities should establish a protocol for achieving this goal and train all staff accordingly. For those individuals who have latex allergy, a latex-free environment should be provided, if feasible. Latex-allergic workers should use only nonlatex gloves, and others in the same environment should use nonlatex gloves or powder-free, low-protein gloves to minimize airborne latex exposure. Symptom reduction has been documented with the use of powder-free gloves, which enables some sensitized workers to return to the workplace.

REPROCESSING SINGLE-USE MEDICAL DEVICES

Reprocessing single-use devices involves reusing instruments that were designed and sold for single-use only. The reprocessing and reuse of single-use instruments has become increasingly common. Current law requires that the institutions or companies that reprocess single-use devices for repeat use be held to the original manufacturing specifications for the single-use instrument. Devices must be clearly labeled as manufactured by the reprocessor. Although there are limited data on reprocessed single-use devices, existing studies have found a significant rate of physical defects, performance issues, or improper decontamination. There are currently no data in the medical literature of studies that evaluate the cost-effectiveness of reprocessed single-use devices in gynecologic surgery. Studies on the safety, quality, and cost-effectiveness of reprocessed single-use devices in gynecologic surgery are needed.

The use of a reprocessed single-use device provides no direct benefit to an individual patient or her physician. Physicians should be informed whether the instruments used in surgery are original or reprocessed, and adverse events should be reported to improve the safety information about reprocessed single-use devices. (For more information, refer to MedWatch, the U.S. Food and Drug Administration safety information and adverse event reporting program, which can be accessed at www.fda.gov/Safety/MedWatch/default.htm.)

Office and Other Ambulatory Settings

The office or clinic, no matter how small or how large, should be well organized and clean. The reception area should be comfortable and should have adequate seating capacity to accommodate patients. Current general-interest reading material that is consistent with promotion of healthy lifestyles and patient education materials should be available. The reception area should be separate from, yet visible to, the receptionist. Patients in the reception area should not be able to overhear telephone conversations or business conducted by the receptionist. Restrooms and a patient changing area should be available.

The facility should have a utility area, which should be separate from the examination rooms. It should be equipped with work counters, closed cabinets for storage, locked medicine cabinets, a refrigerator, and facilities for sterilization and hand washing. There should be a comfortable, private area for discussing confidential information and for interviewing and counseling the patient and her family.

The physician's office may serve as a consultation room; however, depending on the size of the office or clinic, separate rooms, other than the physician's office and examining rooms, are desirable for use by nurses, social workers, health educators, or other members of the health care team. The number of examination rooms, consultation rooms, and interview rooms will depend on the patient profile and the size of the practice. In general, a minimum of two examination rooms per practitioner is desirable.

Some obstetrician–gynecologists provide mammography screening in their offices. Mammography equipment is subject to regulation by the U.S. Food and Drug Administration. (For further details, refer to the "Compliance With Government Regulations" section in Part 1.)

An increasing number of invasive and potentially harmful procedures are moving from the more highly regulated surgery center of hospital surgery units into the office setting. Once patients have been invited into an office setting for procedures, they have the right to expect the same level of patient safety that occurs in the more regulated hospital setting. Any facility that performs outpatient surgery should have a designated medical director. The "Report of the Presidential Task Force on Patient Safety in the Office Setting" of the American College of Obstetricians and Gynecologists contains important checklists for the office setting, including the office setup checklist, preoperative checklist, intraoperative checklist, and postoperative checklist (see Bibliography).

Surgical Facilities

A freestanding surgical facility should be organized and equipped as a multidisciplinary unit. This includes the provision of preoperative, intraoperative, and postoperative care and arrangement for the transfer of a patient if an emergency arises. To ensure that high-quality care is maintained, periodic assessment of care as well as review of practice procedures, governance, and outcome should be conducted. Patient safety should be incorporated into all aspects of patient care and is the hallmark for all care that is provided. The American College of Obstetricians and Gynecologists has been reluctant to mandate specific requirements for surgical care in the office or other ambulatory surgical settings because each facility is unique. General recommendations and guidance about office-based surgery and ambulatory surgical care are provided in the "Ambulatory Gynecologic Surgery" section in Part 4. Further information on minimal requirements is available from the American College of Surgeons (see Resources).

The appropriate physical design for an ambulatory surgical facility depends on the number and types of surgical procedures to be performed. The facility should provide a comfortable, safe environment with minimal architectural barriers. The requirements of the Occupational Safety and Health Administration, as well as state and local requirements, should be met. Traffic flow should be convenient and efficient. A multilevel facility should have elevators that can accommodate gurneys. The facility also should include adequate space for the following functions:

- Reception and waiting
- Administrative activities, such as patient admission, record storage, and business affairs
- Patient dressing and locker storage
- Preoperative evaluation, including physical examination, laboratory testing, and preparation for anesthesia
- Performance of surgical procedures
- Preparation and sterilization of instruments
- Radiographic capability (eg, to check for instruments, needles, and sponges when counts at the end of a procedure are not correct)
- Storage of equipment, drugs, and fluids
- Postanesthesia recovery
- Staff activities
- Janitorial and utility support

Inpatient Facilities

Inpatient hospital, emergency, and urgent care settings should include a private, secure examination room appropriate for gynecologic examinations. The room should be of adequate size with a door that locks from the inside or a curtain to pull across the doorway. It should be adequately equipped for a gynecologic examination (see also "Specific Physical and Supply Requirements" earlier in this section). Counter space or a tray stand should be available to hold the supplies needed for the examination. In essence, this room should be similar in size and layout to, and be equipped like, an examination room in an outpatient office.

High-quality care is more easily attained in a specialty service. When hospital size permits, the gynecologic inpatient service should be consolidated in one designated area. In smaller hospitals, where the number of patients may not justify the establishment of a separate area, gynecologic patients may be treated in either a medical or surgical area. Gynecologic patients who do not have transmissible infections may be treated in the obstetric area, provided that hospital policy permits and their care does not interfere with the operation of the obstetric unit.

Bibliography

AAAAI and ACAAI Joint Statement concerning the use of powdered and non-powdered natural rubber latex gloves. Ann Allergy Asthma Immunol 1997;79:487.

American College of Obstetricians and Gynecologists. Report of the presidential task force on patient safety in the office setting. Washington, DC: American College of Obstetricians and Gynecologists; 2010.

Preparing for clinical emergencies in obstetrics and gynecology. Committee Opinion No. 590. American College of Obstetricians and Gynecologists. Obstet Gynecol 2014;123:722–5.

Reprocessed single-use devices. Committee Opinion No. 537. American College of Obstetricians and Gynecologists. Obstet Gynecol 2012;120:974–6.

User labeling for devices that contain natural rubber, 21 C.F.R. part 801.437 (2013). Available at: http://www.gpo.gov/fdsys/pkg/CFR-2013-title21-vol8/pdf/CFR-2013-title21-vol8-sec801-437.pdf. Retrieved September 20, 2013.

Resources

American College of Surgeons. Guidelines for optimal ambulatory surgical care and office-based surgery. 3rd ed. Chicago (IL): ACS; 2000.

American Congress of Obstetricians and Gynecologists. HIPAA regulations and requirements explained. Washington, DC: American Congress of Obstetricians and Gynecologists; 2013. Available at: http://www.acog.org/About_ACOG/ACOG_Departments/HIPAA. Retrieved July 16, 2013.

American Society of Anesthesiologists. Standards, guidelines, statements and other documents. Available at: http://www.asahq.org/For-Members/Standards-Guidelines-and-Statements.aspx. Retrieved July 16, 2013.

Association of periOperative Registered Nurses. Perioperative standards and recommended practices. 2013 ed. Denver, CO: AORN; 2013.

Ethical considerations for performing gynecologic surgery in low-resource settings abroad. Committee Opinion No. 466. American College of Obstetricians and Gynecologists. Obstet Gynecol 2010;116:793–9.

Facilities Guidelines Institute. Guidelines for design and construction of health care facilities. 2014 ed. Chicago (IL): American Society for Healthcare Engineering of the American Hospital Association; 2014.

Food and Drug Administration. Reprocessing of single-use devices. Available at: http://www.fda.gov/MedicalDevices/DeviceRegulationandGuidance/Reprocessing ofSingle-UseDevices/default.htm. Retrieved July 16, 2013.

National Institute for Occupational Safety and Health. Occupational latex allergies. Available at: http://www.cdc.gov/niosh/topics/latex. Retrieved July 16, 2013.

National Institute for Occupational Safety and Health. Preventing allergic reactions to natural rubber latex in the workplace. Available at: http://www.cdc.gov/niosh/docs/97-135/pdfs/97-135.pdf. Retrieved July 16, 2013.

Occupational Safety and Health Administration. Compliance assistance/outreach. Available at: https://www.osha.gov/dcsp/compliance_assistance/index.html. Retrieved September 26, 2013.

Occupational Safety and Health Administration. Latex allergy. Available at: https://www.osha.gov/SLTC/latexallergy/index.html. Retrieved July 16, 2013.

Recommendations for development of an emergency plan for in vitro fertilization programs: a committee opinion. Practice Committees of American Society for Reproductive Medicine and the Society for Assisted Reproductive Technology. Fertil Steril 2012;98:e3–5.

Sussman G, Gold M. Guidelines for the management of latex allergies and safe latex use in health care facilities. Arlington Heights (IL): American College of Allergy, Asthma and Immunology; 1996. Available at: http://www.acaai.org/allergist/aller gies/Types/latex-allergy/Pages/latex-allergies-safe-use.aspx. Retrieved July 16, 2013.

The Joint Commission. Comprehensive accreditation manual for ambulatory care: CAMAC. Oakbrook Terrace (IL): The Commission; 2014.

INFECTION CONTROL

All women's health care facilities need effective infection control procedures to protect patients and staff. The following recommendations—for hand hygiene; cleaning, disinfecting, and sterilizing patient care equipment; isolation and standard precautions; management of occupational exposures and of infected health care workers; and cleaning and disinfecting the environment of care—provide an infection control framework for all health care facilities. For guidance on the prevention of infectious disease in health care professionals, see the "Human Resources" section in Part 1.

Hand Hygiene

Hand antisepsis is the single most important means of reducing health care–associated infections, a concept first introduced by the Hungarian obstetrician Ignaz Semmelweis in 1847. Improved adherence to hand hygiene has been shown to terminate outbreaks of infection in health care facilities, to reduce transmission of antimicrobial-resistant organisms (eg, methicillin-resistant *Staphylococcus aureus*), and to reduce overall infection rates. It is a key part of patient safety efforts (see also the "Patient Safety" section in Part 1).

The term hand hygiene refers to either hand washing with soap and water or the use of alcohol-based gels or foams that do not require water. The introduction of alcohol-based products has made hand hygiene much easier to perform and less time consuming, which leads to improved compliance with guidelines. The widespread placement of gel or foam dispensers in all patient care areas has increased compliance. Alcohol-based hand rubs are more effective at killing bacteria and less irritating to the skin than soap and water. Cleansing with soap and water is preferred when hands are visibly dirty or contaminated with organic materials. The Centers for Disease Control and Prevention (CDC) has published guidelines for hand hygiene in health care settings. The guidelines are available at www.cdc.gov/handhygiene.

Hand hygiene should be practiced immediately before touching a patient, performing an invasive procedure, or manipulating an invasive device; immediately after touching a patient or contaminated items or surfaces; and after removing gloves or touching items or surfaces in the immediate patient care environment, even if the patient was not touched. Clinicians should perform hand hygiene when leaving a patient's room even if they didn't touch the patient because bacteria can survive on patient care equipment and surfaces for days.

The use of sterile or nonsterile gloves also is important in preventing serious hospital infections. Important reasons for the routine use of gloves by hospital personnel include the following:

- Providing an effective barrier between contaminated material or contaminated equipment and the caregiver's hands
- Reducing the likelihood of acquiring an infectious organism from a patient who is already colonized or infected with a known pathogen
- Preventing the transmission of a skin-carried pathogenic organism from hospital staff to patients

The use of gloves does not mean that proper hand hygiene can be omitted because there can be defects or tears in gloves and skin can become contaminated when gloves are removed. Studies have demonstrated that organisms, such as methicillin-resistant *S aureus*, still can be recovered from surgeons' hands after gloves have been removed. Consequently, routine hand washing before and immediately after the use of gloves is required.

Isolation and Standard Precautions

The CDC's "Guideline for Isolation Precautions: Preventing Transmission of Infectious Agents in Healthcare Settings in 2007" includes recommendations for preventing transmission of infectious agents across all health care settings. The CDC guidelines are based on the rationale that identification of a pathogen, its source, and the mode of transmission will suggest a logical means to prevent transmission. All personnel should be educated about the use of precautions and about their responsibility for adhering to them.

The CDC recommends that standard precautions be used consistently for all patients. Because medical history and examination cannot identify reliably all patients infected with human immunodeficiency virus (HIV) or other bloodborne pathogens, the CDC recommends the use of standard precautions for all patients to protect health care workers from infectious body fluids. These recommendations incorporate the prior concept of universal precautions to prevent transmission of bloodborne pathogens and recognize the importance of all body fluids, secretions, and excretions in the transmission of health care-associated infections.

These precautions apply to the following:

- Blood
- All body fluids, secretions, and excretions except sweat, regardless of whether they contain visible blood
- Nonintact skin
- Mucous membranes

Standard precautions include the following techniques:

- Perform hand hygiene after touching blood or body fluids and contaminated items, even when gloves are worn, and between patient contacts.
- Wear gloves when touching blood, body fluids, and contaminated items, and remove them promptly after use, before touching non-contaminated surfaces.
- Wear a mask and eye and face protection during activities that may generate a splash or spray of blood or body fluids to the face.
- Wear a gown during activities that may generate a splash or spray of blood or body fluids to clothing or skin.
- Handle patient care equipment soiled with blood or body fluids so as to prevent contamination of skin, mucous membranes, clothing, and other surfaces. Single-use items should be discarded properly, and reusable equipment must be cleaned and reprocessed appropriately.

- Have written procedures for routine cleaning, care, and disinfection of frequently touched surfaces.
- Have written procedures for handling soiled linen to prevent contamination of clean surfaces.
- Take care to prevent injuries when using sharp instruments. Never recap used needles; instead, place used disposable syringes, needles, scalpel blades, and other sharps in puncture-resistant, disposable containers located as close as practical to the area where the items are normally used. Evaluate and use, as appropriate, devices to prevent exposures, such as blunt-tip suture needles, safety scalpels, self-sheathing needles, and needle-holding devices. (The U.S. Food and Drug Administration, the CDC's National Institute for Occupational Safety and Health, and the Occupational Safety and Health Administration strongly encourage health care providers in surgical settings to use blunt-tip suture needles as an alternative to standard suture needles, when clinically appropriate, to reduce the risk of needlestick injury and subsequent pathogen transmission to surgical personnel.) Use a no-touch method to pass sharp instruments between individuals.
- Have mouthpieces readily available to use as an alternative to mouth-to-mouth resuscitation.
- Follow respiratory hygiene and cough etiquette.
- Adhere to safe injection practices.
- Wear a mask for insertion of catheters or injection of material into spinal or epidural spaces via lumbar puncture procedures (eg, myelogram or spinal or epidural anesthesia).

Postexposure Testing and Prophylaxis

If one is inadvertently exposed to the blood of a patient, immediate attention is required, specifically the following: wash needlestick injuries and cuts with soap and water; flush splashes to the nose, mouth, or skin with water; and irrigate eyes with clean water, saline, or sterile irrigants. Using antiseptics or squeezing the wound has not been shown to reduce the risk of transmission of a bloodborne pathogen. Additionally, the use of caustic agents such as bleach is not recommended.

Public Health Service guidelines for the management of occupational exposures to HIV, including recommendations for postexposure prophylaxis, are available (see Resources). Postexposure HIV prophylaxis for percutaneous injuries, mucous membrane exposure, and nonintact skin exposures are based on the severity and volume of exposure as well as the infection status of the source. Prophylaxis consists of a 4-week course of two or more antiretroviral drugs, based on the level of risk of HIV transmission. Consideration of the adverse effects of the agents, as well as potential drug interactions with concomitant drugs, supplements, or over-the-counter medications, is important in the selection of the antiretroviral drug regimen.

The CDC advises that if a health care worker is exposed to blood or body fluids that might result in hepatitis B virus (HBV) transmission, the recommended postexposure management strategy depends on the health care worker's HBV vaccination status and HBV antibody levels and on the source patient's hepatitis B surface antigen status (see Bibliography). After an occupational exposure, such as a needlestick injury, the health care worker, as well as the patient, should be tested for the antibody to hepatitis C virus (HCV). Postexposure prophylaxis for HCV is not effective and is not recommended. However, early antiviral therapy may be effective in reducing the risk of progression to chronic HCV infection.

Management of Infected Health Care Workers

The risk of transmission of bloodborne infectious agents from infected health care workers to patients must be considered, although the rate is exceedingly low. Clinicians infected with a bloodborne virus must make a decision as to which procedures they can continue to perform safely. This decision will depend on the category of clinical activity and the circulating viral burden. The physician's level of expertise and his or her medical condition, including mental status, are other factors to be considered. The Society for Healthcare Epidemiology of America (SHEA) and the CDC recommend that the decision be made in consultation with an expert review panel, although the CDC indicates that oversight by an expert review panel is not needed for clinicians infected with HBV who do not perform exposure-prone procedures. The expert review panel should be a locally convened panel of experts that represents a variety of perspectives. It may include the physician's personal physician, an infectious disease specialist with expertise in the procedures performed by the physician, state or local public health official(s), and a hospital epidemiologist or other member of the infection-control committee of the hospital. If the physician works only from an office, the panel's functions should be fulfilled by the city, county, or state health department. The decision may possibly involve the chief of the department or the chief of the medical staff. If clinicians avoid procedures that place patients at risk of harm, they have no obligation to inform the patient of their infectious disease history.

The SHEA and the CDC have categorized obstetric–gynecologic procedures according to the level of risk of bloodborne pathogen transmission. Some aspects of obstetrics and gynecology do not involve measurable risk of transmission of infection. For example, routine vaginal examinations carry negligible risk of bloodborne virus transmission. Hysterectomies carry a definite risk of bloodborne virus transmission. There is some disagreement between the SHEA and CDC guidelines. The SHEA guidelines, unlike those from the CDC, include a category of intermediate risk. In the SHEA guidelines, bloodborne virus transmission is deemed theoretically possible but unlikely for minor gynecologic procedures (such as insertion and removal of contraceptive devices).

In addition to the type of procedure, the restriction of clinical practice also depends on the type of virus and the circulating viral burden. High-viral load concentrations have been associated with an increased risk of transmission, but guidelines vary as to the viral burden that would trigger the need for expert review panel oversight or practice limitation.

Cleaning and Disinfecting Patient Care Equipment

To reduce the risk of disease transmission in the health care environment, it is imperative that all facilities follow established infection-control practices in cleaning, disinfecting, and sterilizing patient care equipment. Health care workers should be aware that practices regarding the selection and use of sterilization methods and disinfectants continue to evolve, with new recommendations coming forth as new products and information become available. The CDC and the Association for Professionals in Infection Control and Epidemiology provide recommendations for the preferred methods for disinfection and sterilization of patient care equipment in the health care environment (see Bibliography). The American Institute of Ultrasound in Medicine has published guidelines for cleaning and preparing endocavitary ultrasound transducers between patients (see Box 2-2).

Environmental Infection Control

The CDC also has issued guidelines and recommendations for environmental infection control in health care facilities. These guidelines include such topics as infection control for ventilation and water systems; use of

---

Box 2-2. Guidelines for Cleaning and Preparing Endocavitary Ultrasound Transducers Between Patients

1. Remove probe cover and clean probe with running water and a mild, nonabrasive, liquid soap. A brush may be used to clean crevices. Rinse and dry.

2. Disinfect with a sterilant approved by the U.S. Food and Drug Administration* that is in accordance with the manufacturer's instructions concerning compatible disinfecting agents.

3. Cover the probe with a barrier before use. Nonlubricated, nonmedicated condoms are an excellent barrier. Nonlatex barriers should be available for latex-sensitive patients.

4. Wear gloves when performing transvaginal ultrasonographic examinations, removing the barrier, and cleaning the probe.

---

*For a list of U.S. Food and Drug Administration-approved sterilants, see http://www.fda.gov/medicaldevices/deviceregulationandguidance/reprocessingofsingle-usedevices/ucm133514.htm.

Data from American Institute of Ultrasound in Medicine. Guidelines for cleaning and preparing endocavitary ultrasound transducers between patients. Available at: http://www.aium.org/resources/viewStatement.aspx?id=27. Retrieved July 12, 2013.

dust-control procedures and barriers during construction, repair, renovation, and demolition; environmental infection control measures for special areas with patients at high risk; environmental surface cleaning and disinfection strategies with respect to antibiotic-resistant microorganisms; use of barrier protective coverings for difficult-to-clean equipment, such as computer keyboards; and infection-control procedures for health care laundry (see Resources).

Bibliography

American Institute of Ultrasound in Medicine. Guidelines for cleaning and preparing endocavitary ultrasound transducers between patients. Laurel (MD): AIUM; 2003. Available at: http://www.aium.org/resources/viewStatement.aspx?id=27. Retrieved July 16, 2013.

Association for Professionals in Infection Control and Epidemiology. APIC text of infection control and epidemiology. 3rd ed. Washington, DC: APIC; 2009.

CDC guidance for evaluating health-care personnel for hepatitis B virus protection and for administering postexposure management. National Center for HIV/AIDS, Viral Hepatitis, STD, and TB Prevention, Centers for Disease Control and Prevention. MMWR Recomm Rep 2013;62:1–19.

Food and Drug Administration. FDA-cleared sterilants and high level disinfectants with general claims for processing reusable medical and dental devices–March 2009. Silver Spring (MD): FDA; 2009. Available at: http://www.fda.gov/MedicalDevices/DeviceRegulationandGuidance/ReprocessingofSingle-UseDevices/ucm133514.htm. Retrieved January 30, 2014.

Henderson DK, Dembry L, Fishman NO, Grady C, Lundstrom T, Palmore TN, et al. SHEA guideline for management of healthcare workers who are infected with hepatitis B virus, hepatitis C virus, and/or human immunodeficiency virus. Society for Healthcare Epidemiology of America. Infect Control Hosp Epidemiol 2010;31:203–32.

Human immunodeficiency virus. ACOG Committee Opinion No. 389. American College of Obstetricians and Gynecologists. Obstet Gynecol 2007;110:1473–8.

Rutala WA, Weber DJ. Guideline for disinfection and sterilization in healthcare facilities, 2008. Healthcare Infection Control Practices Advisory Committee. Atlanta (GA): Centers for Disease Control and Prevention; 2008. Available at: http://www.cdc.gov/hicpac/pdf/guidelines/disinfection_nov_2008.pdf. Retrieved July 16, 2013.

Siegel JD, Rinehart E, Jackson M, Chiarello L. 2007 guideline for isolation precautions: preventing transmission of infectious agents in healthcare settings. Healthcare

Infection Control Practices Advisory Committee. Atlanta (GA): Centers for Disease Control and Prevention; 2007. Available at: http://www.cdc.gov/hicpac/pdf/isolation/Isolation2007.pdf. Retrieved July 16, 2013.

Updated CDC recommendations for the management of hepatitis B virus-infected health-care providers and students. Centers for Disease Control and Prevention. MMWR Recomm Rep 2012;61(RR-3):1–12.

Resources

Boyce JM, Pittet D. Guideline for hand hygiene in health-care settings. Recommendations of the Healthcare Infection Control Practices Advisory Committee and the HICPAC/SHEA/APIC/IDSA Hand Hygiene Task Force. Society for Healthcare Epidemiology of America/Association for Professionals in Infection Control/Infectious Diseases Society of America. Healthcare Infection Control Practices Advisory Committee; HICPAC/SHEA/APIC/IDSA Hand Hygiene Task Force. MMWR Recomm Rep 2002;51:1–45, quiz CE1–4.

Centers for Disease Control and Prevention. Exposure to blood: what healthcare personnel need to know. Atlanta (GA): CDC; 2003. Available at: http://www.cdc.gov/HAI/pdfs/bbp/Exp_to_Blood.pdf. Retrieved July 16, 2013.

Centers for Disease Control and Prevention. Guide to infection prevention for outpatient settings: minimum expectations for safe care. Atlanta (GA): CDC; 2011. Available at: http://www.cdc.gov/HAI/pdfs/guidelines/standatds-of-ambulatory-care-7-2011.pdf. Retrieved July 16, 2013.

Centers for Disease Control and Prevention. Hand hygiene in healthcare settings. Available at: http://www.cdc.gov/handhygiene. Retrieved July 16, 2013.

Centers for Disease Control and Prevention. Healthcare-associated infections. Available at: http://www.cdc.gov/hai. Retrieved July 16, 2013.

Centers for Disease Control and Prevention. Occupational HIV transmission and prevention among health care workers. Atlanta (GA): CDC; 2013. Available at: http://www.cdc.gov/hiv/pdf/risk_occupational_factsheet.pdf. Retrieved September 26, 2013.

Facilities Guidelines Institute. Guidelines for design and construction of health care facilities. 2014 ed. Chicago (IL): American Society for Healthcare Engineering of the American Hospital Association; 2014.

Food and Drug Administration. Reprocessing of single-use devices. Available at: http://www.fda.gov/medicaldevices/deviceregulationandguidance/reprocessingofsingle-usedevices/ucm133514.htm. Retrieved January 23, 2014.

Makulowich GS. AHRQ toolkit helps hospitals improve antibiotic selection to reduce deadly C. difficile infections. Agency for Healthcare Research and Quality.

AHRQ Res Act 2013;1, 3–5. Available at: http://www.ahrq.gov/legacy/research/feb13/0213RA.pdf. Retrieved August 14, 2013.

O'Grady NP, Alexander M, Burns LA, Dellinger EP, Garland J, Heard SO, et al. Guidelines for the prevention of intravascular catheter-related infections. Healthcare Infection Control Practices Advisory Committee (HICPAC). Clin Infect Dis 2011; 52:e162-93.

Panlilio AL, Cardo DM, Grohskopf LA, Heneine W, Ross CS. Updated U.S. Public Health Service guidelines for the management of occupational exposures to HIV and recommendations for postexposure prophylaxis. U.S. Public Health Service. MMWR Recomm Rep 2005;54:1-17.

Recommended practices for cleaning and caring for surgical instruments and powered equipment. Association of periOperative Registered Nurses. AORN J 2002;75:627–30, 633–6, 638 passim.

Recommended practices for sterilization in the perioperative practice setting. AORN Recommended Practices Committee. AORN J 2006;83:700-3, 705–8, 711–6 passim.

Rutala WA, Weber DJ. Disinfection, sterilization and control of hospital waste. In: Mandell GL, Bennett JE, Dolin R, editors. Mandell, Douglas, and Bennett's principles and practice of infectious diseases. 7th ed. Philadelphia (PA): Churchill Livingstone/Elsevier; 2010. p. 3677–95.

Sehulster L, Chinn RY. Guidelines for environmental infection control in healthcare facilities. Recommendations of CDC and the Healthcare Infection Control Practices Advisory Committee (HICPAC). MMWR Recomm Rep 2003;52:1–42.

Tablan OC, Anderson LJ, Besser R, Bridges C, Hajjeh R. Guidelines for preventing health-care-associated pneumonia, 2003: recommendations of CDC and the Healthcare Infection Control Practices Advisory Committee. MMWR Recomm Rep 2004;53:1–36.

ANCILLARY SERVICES

Ancillary services, including pharmacy, radiology, laboratory, and anesthesia, are a component of patient care. The following recommendations for ancillary services should be considered general recommendations and are not necessarily requirements or mandates. Such services, whether on site or off site, should be accredited. Physicians should check state and federal laws and regulations on self-referral prohibitions before referring a patient for health care services in which the physician or an immediate family member has a financial interest (see also the "Human Resources" section in Part 1). These laws and regulations continue to evolve, and current requirements should be reviewed. All ancillary services must meet all applicable federal and state requirements.

Pharmacy Services

An appropriate selection of medications and means for obtaining medications not onsite should be available. Prescribing, preparing, and dispensing medication should follow established procedures that are in compliance with legal regulations, licensure, and professional practice standards. Appropriate records and security are essential to maintain the safe and controlled dispensing of medications and to allow patient notification in the event of a drug recall or newly reported complications. The pharmacy must be supervised by a licensed pharmacist or physician.

When medications are dispensed, patients should be given instructions and important medication information. The quality and appropriateness of the medications used should be monitored as part of the quality improvement program. Adverse medication effects should be monitored and addressed. The U.S. Food and Drug Administration (FDA) has established MedWatch, the FDA Safety Information and Adverse Event Reporting Program, to provide safety information about prescription and over-the-counter drugs, biologics, medical devices, and dietary supplements. The American College of Obstetricians and Gynecologists, a MedWatch Partner, encourages women's health care clinicians to participate in MedWatch. More information is available on the FDA web site at www.fda.gov/Safety/MedWatch/default.htm. Reports also can be made online.

Drug samples must be stored in a secure location. Thorough documentation and records of drug samples received and dispensed should be maintained and should include information regarding drug name, lot number, date of receipt, inventory, and dispensing details. There must be complete accountability and auditing of drug sample stocks. Proper disposition of expired or recalled drug samples must be documented. The Prescription Drug Marketing Act of 1987 governs the distribution of drug samples and forbids their sale. This regulation extends to charging a dispensing fee for a prescription drug sample. When dispensing drug samples, physicians should be cognizant of the effect that free samples may have on their subsequent choice of pharmacotherapy. Physicians may choose to provide samples or vouchers; however, they should be aware that providing samples may promote patients' ongoing use of a particular medication, when other potential alternatives exist. When vouchers or samples are dispensed, consideration should be given to providing them preferentially to those patients with a true need and dispensing a supply sufficient for a full course of therapy.

State laws differ in requirements for the labeling of drug samples provided to patients. Drug samples that are dispensed should be in the required packaging and should include the name and strength of the drug, directions for use, and the expiration date of the product. Federal and state laws require a note in the patient's chart indicating that a drug sample has been dispensed.

The pharmacy compounding law includes a limited exception to the requirement that prescription drugs be approved by the FDA based on studies that demonstrate their safety and effectiveness. Because preapproval drug studies are performed on a very specific drug formula and dosage, even relatively small compounding changes can convert an approved drug into an unapproved one with different risks and effects. Most compounded products have not undergone any rigorous clinical testing for either safety or efficacy, and issues of quality assurance regarding the purity, potency, and quality of compounded products are a concern.

However, compounded drugs may be considered in some circumstances. Examples include a situation in which there is no FDA-approved drug formulation for the patient's condition or individual situation (eg, the patient cannot use the standard version of a drug because of an allergy to one of its inactive ingredients) or a situation in which it is necessary for a commercially available drug product to be compounded into a powder, liquid, lozenge, suppository, or other form to facilitate use.

The FDA's pharmacy compounding law was designed to provide protections against unsafe and ineffective compounded products. The main provisions of this law include the following:

- The compounded product must be prescribed for an identified patient.
- The drug's active ingredient can qualify for use in compounding if any of these conditions are met:
  — It is currently part of an FDA-approved drug.
  — It is recognized and listed in the book of widely used drug substances published by the U.S. Pharmacopeial Convention, an independent standard-setting organization.
  — The FDA has acknowledged it as acceptable for pharmacy compounding.
- Previously marketed drugs found to be unsafe or ineffective and removed from the market may not be compounded.
- Drug products listed in FDA regulations as difficult to compound may not be compounded.

More information on pharmacy compounding is available on the FDA's web site at www.fda.gov/Drugs/GuidanceComplianceRegulatoryInforma tion/PharmacyCompounding/default.htm.

Laboratory and Pathology Services

Laboratory and pathology services must serve patient and clinician needs and meet professional practice standards and state and federal legal requirements. Quality-control procedures should include validating test results through the use of standardized controls and appropriate documentation. A written report should be generated for all laboratory and pathology examinations performed. This report should be included in the patient's medical record, and there should be documentation of review by the clinician. A qualified physician should oversee the laboratory. Competent, appropriately trained personnel should conduct the laboratory work.

Imaging Services

Diagnostic imaging services, including but not limited to radiographic, fluoroscopic, and ultrasonographic services, must be available to meet patient and clinician needs. There should be adequate space and equipment to ensure the safe delivery of these services. Such provision should include policies for handling, storing, and disposing of potentially hazardous materials and for proper shielding where potentially hazardous energy sources are used. Performance and interpretation of imaging services should be permitted in offices or ambulatory surgical centers when these conditions are met.

A written report, signed by the interpreting physician, should be considered an integral part of the performance and interpretation of an imaging study. For optimal patient care, imaging studies should be performed and interpreted in a timely manner. Dated reports of service must be maintained and available in the patient's file. Quality assurance must be maintained by periodic review. Imaging services should be performed only on the order of a qualified clinician.

Obstetrician–gynecologists who are experienced in diagnostic imaging methods should receive privileges to perform and interpret imaging studies on the basis of their training, experience, and demonstrated current clinical competence. Obstetrician–gynecologists can perform the immediate and timely interpretation of imaging studies, correlate these studies with clinical findings, counsel the patient, and assume the responsibility for determining the treatment of the patient. Any policy that prohibits obstetrician–gynecologists from performing and interpreting imaging studies at which they are demonstrably competent interferes with the patient's access to optimal care. The American College of Obstetricians and

Gynecologists reaffirms that current certification by the American Board of Obstetrics and Gynecology, Inc., and maintenance of certification by obstetrician–gynecologists is validation of the medical, surgical, imaging, and laboratory knowledge and patient care skills relevant to the practice of the specialty. No additional certification should be required for credentialing for those procedures and care which fall within the scope of an individual's current certification by the American Board of Obstetrics and Gynecology, Inc.

Radiation monitoring devices should be provided to personnel who might be exposed to harmful energy, and personnel exposure records should be maintained in accordance with relevant regulations. Proper warning signs must be posted to alert the public and office personnel to the presence of hazardous energy fields, with particular attention given to pregnant women and patients with pacemakers.

Gynecologic ultrasonography can help in assessment of a patient's pelvic anatomy as an adjunct to physical examination and other diagnostic modalities to confirm the presence or absence of a suspected problem. In addition, gynecologic ultrasonography can be of assistance when a pelvic examination either provides insufficient information because of the difficulty of examination, or findings are abnormal and more information is desired. The clinician should use the technique that allows for optimal examination of the targeted organ. The American Institute of Ultrasound in Medicine has published standards for performance of ultrasonographic examination of the female pelvis and documentation of such examination; these standards are available at www.aium.org/resources/guidelines/pelvic.pdf.

Results from ultrasonographic examination are considered part of the medical record and should be documented and stored appropriately. The report, signed by the interpreting physician, should be placed in the patient's medical record. Vaginal probes must be covered (with a nonlatex covering for latex-allergic patients) during use, and a policy for cleaning the probe between uses must be in place (see also the "Infection Control" section earlier in Part 2).

Gynecologic ultrasonographic procedures should be explained fully to the patient in advance. Consideration should be given to the patient's privacy and sensitivity because the transvaginal ultrasonographic examination can be physically problematic, psychologically problematic, or both for some women. Because of the sensitive nature of the transvaginal examination, it may be advisable to have a chaperone present. Personnel who can serve as chaperones should be available whenever there is a request from the clinician or a patient.

Obstetrician–gynecologists with adequate training and experience are qualified to perform and interpret ultrasonographic examinations. Training in performance and interpretation of gynecologic ultrasonography may be acquired during residency training or from courses supplemented by supervised experience and follow-up. The American Institute of Ultrasound in Medicine and the American College of Radiology offer ultrasound facility accreditation. Practices, not individuals, may be accredited. Physicians must be aware that they are responsible for the quality and accuracy of ultrasound examinations performed in their names, regardless of whether or not they personally produced the images; they also are responsible for the quality of the documentation and the quality control and safety of the environment and procedures.

Anesthesia and Analgesia

When anesthesia is necessary, the level and type of anesthesia administered should be dictated by the procedure, patient's medical condition, and patient preference. Adequate space and equipment should be provided for the safe delivery of anesthesia services, and no explosive anesthetics should be used. A preanesthesia assessment should be conducted for any patient for whom anesthesia is planned. Before the administration of any sedation, staff must confirm that the patient has an escort to drive her home.

A person responsible for administration of medication and monitoring the patient must be present in the procedure room. The administration of any anesthetic must be performed or supervised by a qualified physician. Depending on the level of anesthesia, patient monitoring might be assumed by a medical assistant, nurse, certified nurse anesthetist, or anesthesiologist. In all but the last case, these individuals must work under protocols with the surgeon assuming responsibility. Physicians who administer or supervise moderate sedation or analgesia, deep sedation or analgesia, or general anesthesia should have appropriate education and training.

An adequately staffed, designated recovery area must be available. The patient must be monitored closely for depth of sedation, using all recommended monitoring equipment and procedures, regardless of the mode of delivery (oral versus intravenous); monitoring should continue during and after the procedure until the patient has adequately recovered. For more information, see the "Ambulatory Gynecologic Surgery" section in Part 4.

Follow-up Services

Discharge or transition care planning should begin the first day of hospitalization and address the patient's needs in all of the following areas: physical, emotional, social, activities of daily living, and transportation. A partial list of follow-up services includes adult foster care, case management, home health services, hospice, wound care, long-term care, ambulatory care, support groups, and rehabilitation services.

Some services are best provided in an outpatient ambulatory setting or a freestanding specialized facility, such as a nursing home. For individual care delivered to the patient at home, visiting nurses are recognized for their expertise at providing a wide range of home health and hospice care. The Visiting Nurse Associations of America are community-based, nonprofit home health and hospice providers who care for patients of all ages from infants to the elderly and offer maternal–child health programs, case-based management, infusion therapy, rehabilitation, hospice care, behavioral therapy, wound care, pain management, telemedicine, and other home health services. These services often are available regardless of ability to pay.

TRANSITION CARE

Because of the current fragmented health care system, there often exists a vacuum of care when a patient is transitioned between inpatient and outpatient care or from one location to another. Good transitional care is based on a comprehensive plan, the availability of well-trained staff who have current information about the patient's clinical status, and coordination among health care providers involved in the transition. Ineffective coordination may lead to treatment delays, medication errors, adverse events, litigation, and increased costs. Effective coordination requires a team effort, and some physicians may choose to delegate this responsibility to a health care provider on their staff, such as an advanced practice nurse or physician assistant.

It is the responsibility of the physician or his or her designee to see that practitioners who provide follow-up care receive a summary of the care previously provided, the patient's progress toward goals, and information regarding instructions and referrals provided to the patient. The patient, her family, her primary health care providers, and her ancillary practitioners should communicate clearly with one another and understand the patient assessment and plan. The use of an integrated electronic health record greatly facilitates this process. The patient and her family should receive written and verbal education regarding their responsibilities for daily care and follow-up appointments, the safe use of prescribed medications, adverse reactions or complications that must be reported to the clinician, and the name and phone number of a person to call in an emergency. The patient or family should be referred to community resources, including mental health, social services, and financial services, as needed. Tools to assist individuals and institutions in improving transitional care are provided by the Society of Hospital Medicine (www.hospitalmedicine. org/ResourceRoomRedesign/RR_CareTransitions/CT_Home.cfm) and the National Transitions of Care Coalition (www.ntocc.org/WhoWeServe/HealthCareProfessionals.aspx).

Physicians should consider carefully the agency to which they are referring patients for follow-up care. It is recommended that such agencies be accredited by a third party, such as the The Joint Commission, Community Health Accreditation Program, or Accreditation Commission for Health Care. It also is recommended that the agency hold a current state license.

ETHICS IN AFTERCARE

Physicians and other health care providers must provide and document "patient choice" in selecting aftercare. Many hospitals and some physicians are stakeholders in home health agencies or aftercare companies. A conflict of interest exists when the patient's well-being (primary interest) and the physician's financial well-being (secondary interest) are in conflict. Such a conflict of interest is not by its nature wrong, but creates an opportunity for the physician to breach a primary obligation to the patient. Such conflicts should be avoided whenever possible; if they are unavoidable and material to a patient's decision-making process, it is the physician's responsibility to disclose any such conflicts to the patient. Physicians should be aware of federal government legislation and any state "anti-kickback laws" that might be applicable.

Bibliography

American College of Obstetricians and Gynecologists. Certification and procedural credentialing. College Statement of Policy 84. Washington, DC: American College of Obstetricians and Gynecologists; 2012.

American Institute of Ultrasound in Medicine. AIUM practice guideline for the performance of pelvic ultrasound examinations. Laurel, MD: AIUM; 2009. Available at: http://www.aium.org/resources/guidelines/pelvic.pdf. Retrieved July 19, 2013.

Communication strategies for patient handoffs. Committee Opinion No. 517. American College of Obstetricians and Gynecologists. Obstet Gynecol 2012; 119:408–11.

Food and Drug Administration. Compounding Quality Act. Available at: http://www.fda.gov/Drugs/GuidanceComplianceRegulatoryInformation/PharmacyCompounding/default.htm. Retrieved July 19, 2013.

Practice guidelines for sedation and analgesia by non-anesthesiologists. American Society of Anesthesiologists Task Force on Sedation and Analgesia by Non-Anesthesiologists. Anesthesiology 2002;96:1004–17.

Professional relationships with industry. Committee Opinion No. 541. American College of Obstetricians and Gynecologists. Obstet Gynecol 2012;120:1243–9.

Resources

Accreditation Commission for Health Care. Available at: http://www.achc.org/. Retrieved July 19, 2013.

American Association of Blood Banks. Standards for blood banks and transfusion services. 27th ed. Bethesda (MD): AABB; 2011.

American College of Radiology. Accreditation. Available at: http://www.acr.org/ Quality-Safety/Accreditation. Retrieved July 19, 2013.

American College of Radiology. Practice parameters and technical standards. Available at: http://www.acr.org/Quality-Safety/Standards-Guidelines. Retrieved July 19, 2013.

American Institute of Ultrasound in Medicine. AIUM ultrasound practice accreditation. Available at: http://www.aium.org/accreditation/accreditation.aspx. Retrieved July 19, 2013.

Centers for Medicare and Medicaid Services. Home health compare. Available at: http://www.medicare.gov/homehealthcompare/search.html. Retrieved July 19, 2013.

Community Health Accreditation Program. Available at: http://www.chapinc.org/. Retrieved July 19, 2013.

Compounded bioidentical menopausal hormone therapy. Committee Opinion No. 532. American College of Obstetricians and Gynecologists and the American Society for Reproductive Medicine. Obstet Gynecol 2012;120:411–5.

Food and Drug Administration. MedWatch: the FDA safety information and adverse event reporting program. Available at: http://www.fda.gov/Safety/MedWatch/ default.htm. Retrieved July 19, 2013.

National Transitions of Care Coalition. Available at: www.ntocc.org. Retrieved July 19, 2013.

Seeking and giving consultation. ACOG Committee Opinion No. 365. American College of Obstetricians and Gynecologists. Obstet Gynecol 2007;109:1255–60.

Society of Hospital Medicine. Overview: project BOOST implementation toolkit. Available at: http://www.hospitalmedicine.org/ResourceRoomRedesign/RR_Care Transitions/CT_Home.cfm. Retrieved July 19, 2013.

The Joint Commission. Comprehensive accreditation manual for laboratory and point-of-care testing: CAMLAB. Oakbrook Terrace (IL): The Commission; 2014.

The Joint Commission. Comprehensive accreditation manual for ambulatory care: CAMAC. Oakbrook Terrace (IL): The Commission; 2014.

Visiting Nurse Associations of America. Available at: http://vnaa.org. Retrieved July 19, 2013.

INFORMATION MANAGEMENT

Because modern medical practice frequently involves several clinicians and other professionals, every health care facility needs information management systems in place to provide effective means of communication among all members of the health care team. This section provides recommendations for the maintenance of medical records and the documentation of all patient communication, including informed consent.

Medical Records

An accurate medical record must be maintained for each patient in a secure, confidential, and accessible way. A policy should be developed to verify the identity of all patients before treatment. Where feasible, a government-issued picture identification should be used. A copy of this identification can be included in the patient's record for future identification. The patient's name should appear on each page of the record, pertinent information should be firmly attached, and a problem list should be maintained. Pertinent information, including allergies, should be readily accessible. The record should be legible, concise, cogent, and complete. Every entry should have identifying data and be dated, completed promptly, and signed by the qualified health care provider. Some symbols and abbreviations can be confusing and should be avoided (see also the "Patient Safety" section in Part 1).

When surgery has been performed, the inpatient medical record should contain sufficient information and documentation to justify the preoperative diagnosis, the operative procedure, and the postoperative course. Where feasible, medical records used in an ambulatory surgical facility should be standardized and conform to the record used in the facility or backup hospital. In addition, an ambulatory surgical facility should keep registers of admissions and discharges, operations, results of follow-up contacts, and controlled substances dispensed.

The medical record should allow an easy assessment of the care provided to determine whether the patient's health care needs have been identified, diagnosed, and managed effectively. Because modern medical practice frequently involves several physicians and professionals, the medical record should serve as a vehicle for communication among all members of the health care team. Entries by all health care workers should be signed or initialed, dated, and timed. Any abbreviations should be clear to all health care workers who use the patient's medical record. A medical record should not be altered except to correct an error. Erroneous entries in a medical record should not be erased, deleted, blacked out, or written over so that they are no longer visible; rather, a single line should be drawn through the incorrect entry and the correct information, if any, should be entered and signed. Corrections to previous entries must be dated and signed and should include reasons for the corrections. Late entries should be clearly stated as such and should include the current date and time, as well as the date, time, and circumstance for which the late entry is written.

A patient may have access to copies of her written or electronic medical record. Although a written request is not required based on Health Insurance Portability and Accountability Act (HIPAA) regulations, it is nevertheless wise to obtain a written request so that all releases of records are documented. A patient also may ask for a correction of inaccurate information. The request must be made in writing, and a written answer should be provided within 60 days. If the correction request is denied, the patient's disagreement must be noted in her file. Copies or scans of the written request and the answer should be included in the patient's file, regardless of the outcome.

Medical records should be organized in a consistent manner. A system should be in place to avoid misplacing or misfiling medical records. Records should be protected against fire, theft, and other damage. Records may be kept in their original format or transferred to another medium. When disposing of records, or any documentation with patient-identifying information, physicians should ensure that the records are completely destroyed to protect confidentiality.

The medical staff should be made aware of the need for strict confidentiality of a patient's medical records (see also the "Human Resources" section in Part 1). Electronic storage and transfer of patient information requires safeguards to limit access and protect confidentiality (see also "Electronic Health Records" later in this section).

There should be an established protocol for handling requests for records by the patient, her family, an attorney, an insurance company, or another third party. A signed authorization compliant with HIPAA must be obtained from the patient before the release of any medical information contained in her medical record other than for treatment, payment, operations, or as otherwise declared in the Notice of Privacy Practices (eg, subpoenas, neglect or domestic violence reporting). Only copies should be transmitted; the original record should be retained in the office.

When feasible, patient financial records should be kept in a separate confidential file, apart from the patient's medical record. All correspondence or notation of conversations between physicians and professional liability insurance carriers or defense counsel pertaining to a patient should be kept in a confidential file separate from the patient's medical record.

Medical and legal considerations determine the length of time records are retained. When records are no longer needed for medical purposes, federal and state laws determine how long they are to be kept. Some states have specific legal requirements for retaining medical records, specific requirements for retaining business records, or both; a medical record often is considered a business record. The statute of limitations for filing medical liability actions also helps determine how long to retain medical records. Most states have different statutes of limitations for adults and minors, and these statutes vary from state to state. Frequently, statutes of limitations for medical liability actions that involve an adult provide for a 2–5-year period in which to bring a lawsuit. A minor usually has more time to file, and in some states a minor may have until she is 18 years of age or older before the statute of limitations applies. Normally, the statute of limitations begins to run when the patient—or parents or guardians in the case of a minor—should reasonably know that there is a basis for a liability claim. Some states interpret this to mean that the statute does not begin to run until the reasonable party has received legal advice that an actionable claim exists. For these reasons, physicians should consult their attorney, state medical society or professional liability insurance carrier for information on retaining medical records. The American Medical Association (AMA) provides links to all state medical society web sites at www.ama-assn.org/ama/pub/category/7630.html. Records of Medicare or Medicaid patients must be retained for at least 5 years.

The HIPAA Privacy Rule does not include medical record retention requirements but does include requirements for record-related disclosure and information protection activities. According to the privacy regulation, documents that relate to the following must be maintained for 6 years: uses and disclosures, authorization forms, business partner contracts, notices of privacy practices, responses to patients who want to amend or correct their information, patients' statements of disagreement, and complaint records. There is also a 6-year federal statute of limitations for civil penalties imposed for fraud and abuse violations related to participation in federal health care programs.

Electronic Health Records

The electronic health record (EHR) represents a fundamental change in the way health professionals approach the management of clinical information, and has the potential to improve the quality, safety, and efficiency of patient care when fully implemented. The advantages of the EHR include facilitating improved communication among health care providers; assisting with medication safety, tracking, and reporting; and promoting quality of care through optimized compliance with guidelines. Numerous vendors are offering a variety of platforms for the EHR. The use of the EHR is becoming more common, and conversion to this format is encouraged by the government through the Medicare and Medicaid EHR Incentive Programs, which provide financial incentives for the "meaningful use" of certified EHR technology to improve patient care. To receive an EHR incentive payment, health care providers have to show that they are "meaningfully using" their EHRs by meeting thresholds for a number of objectives established by the Centers for Medicare & Medicaid Services. Financial penalties take effect in 2015 for Medicare and Medicaid providers who do not transition to EHRs.

The best system for a medical practice is one that allows for efficient collection and storage of medical information. The EHR should have the capability to perform proper tracking and follow-up. The goal is improved medical care: reduction of medical errors, improved communication, and reduction of drug errors. Acceptance of EHR implementation within an institution is facilitated when a single, specific program is installed across a network of computers, along with the establishment of an information technology support department provided by the organization.

Interoperability, the transfer of data among EHR systems and various health care providers, is slowly becoming a reality but is still a work in progress. Interoperability will enhance patient safety and reduce costs by ensuring patient information is available when and where needed and by reducing the need for duplicative testing.

Protecting patients' health information is of paramount importance. Health information technology systems should be compatible with HIPAA requirements and flexible enough to accommodate state privacy laws, a particular concern for adolescent care, assisted reproductive technology, and genetic testing.

Specific administrative, physical, and technical safeguards to protect electronic information from unauthorized disclosure also are mandated under HIPAA. Although no computer system with online access is completely safe, the following interventions can be taken to help protect computer systems from unauthorized users:

- Install security patches and fixes to update the safety of the computer's operating system regularly. Make sure that antivirus security programs and operating systems are up to date and are able to respond to the continuously emerging computer and Internet threats that could threaten the system.

- Install a firewall if it is not already a feature of the operating system.

- Protect passwords. Passwords should never be words that can be found in the dictionary. Good passwords are at least eight characters long, consist of both numbers and letters, and are case sensitive.

- Change passwords at regular intervals.

- Encrypt laptops and mobile devices that access patient information in case of loss or theft.

- Use only encrypted e-mail and data storage tools for sharing of patient-sensitive information. Double-check the recipients and information included in the message before sending it.
- Keep file sharing to a minimum, and only share a single folder.
- Never open attachments from unknown people, and be wary of attachments from those who are known; viruses can be spread in an attachment without the sender realizing it.
- Use antivirus software, and run e-mail attachments through it.
- The EHR program should have an automatic logout time that closes the record after a period of inactivity to protect the contents from unauthorized viewing.
- Instruct all users not to leave e-mails open on unattended computer screens.

As with paper medical records, a copy of the patient's picture identification (preferably, government issued) or a photographic image produced onsite can be included in the patient's record for future identification. Many vendors of EHRs are including these capabilities in their products. Despite obstacles to widespread adoption and implementation, use of the EHR as a real-time, evidence-based support tool can help busy obstetrician–gynecologists improve the quality of the care they provide through improved care coordination, communication, and documentation.

Patient Communication and Follow-up

All telephone contact regarding clinical matters should be documented in the patient's medical record. A method should be established to document or log such contacts during and after office hours. An answering service for telephone calls or specific equipment to receive and transmit patient messages after normal office hours should be in place. The practitioner should be notified when a telephone message from a patient specifically requests that care be provided by that practitioner. Ideally, staff members should inform the patient of an approximate time when the call would be returned by the practitioner. All telephone prescription renewals should be verified by the practitioner.

A protocol should exist for processing pertinent clinical information that may arrive by telephone, facsimile, mail, or electronic means (see also "Electronic Communication and Patient Confidentiality" later in this section). A clear procedure should be in place to ensure that clinical information—such as laboratory, radiology, and pathology reports—and pertinent patient telephone messages are reviewed by the health care team. All such information should be initialed or signed and dated by the physician or qualified health care worker and then filed in the medical record.

TRACKING AND REMINDER SYSTEMS

As more health care providers adopt an EHR system, choosing a system that can enhance the tracking and reminder process is an important consideration. Office tracking systems should be created for results of laboratory studies, imaging studies, or consultation. The process for good patient follow-up begins with the practitioner's explaining to the patient at the initial visit any needed test, referral, or follow-up and documenting this discussion in the medical record. The next step is logging these open items into a tracking or reminder system promptly and reviewing them frequently and regularly according to the office's established procedures.

Tracking systems may be in the form of a paper medical record log or computerized. Once information is entered into the system, it should be retrieved and reviewed regularly with accompanying documentation of any actions taken or discussions with the patient.

Each office should establish priorities for tracking important information, test results, and follow-up ordered by the health care provider. Referrals to consultants should be tracked, noting whether the patient has visited with the consultant and whether the consultant's report has been filed in the medical record. Referrals of patients from other clinicians also should be tracked, with notification to the referring physician once the patient has been seen. The following are important elements to be tracked:

- Date ordered
- Patient name
- Identifying number

- Test, procedure, consultation, or referral
- Date of results
- Follow-up required
- Evaluation completed and patient notified

All printed results, including cervical cytology reports, mammography reports, consultations, and pathology reports, should be reviewed, initialed, and dated by a clinician who has been designated to perform this function. Electronic results should be signed off electronically and time stamped. Test results then should be filed permanently in the medical record, whether paper or electronic, including a notation of what follow-up testing or procedures are recommended.

The following characteristics are important for any tracking and reminder system, whether electronic or paper based:

- Policies and procedures. An office policy and procedure on tracking should be developed with input from the staff. All office members should agree to follow the same protocols. The office policy should address how to contact the patient and how to document the follow-up in the patient's medical record. Usual time frames for when to expect various types of results should be defined, and a protocol should be established for dealing with delayed or missing reports.

- HIPAA compliance. When contacting patients—whether by mail, by phone, or electronically—physicians and their staff must follow HIPAA regulations. Care also must be taken to limit the amount of information disclosed by way of voice mail or to other individuals who may answer the call without prior consent. Instead, it may be preferable to leave a name and telephone number, asking the patient to call the office. The HIPAA Privacy Rule allows covered health care providers to communicate electronically, such as through e-mail, with their patients, provided they apply reasonable safeguards when doing so (see Bibliography). If the use of unencrypted e-mail is unacceptable to a patient who requests confidential communications, other means of communicating with the patient, such as by more secure electronic methods, or by mail or telephone, should be offered and accommodated (see also "Electronic Communication and Patient Confidentiality" later in this section).

- Specificity. The reminder system should contain specific data and dates, including the dates for receipt of information and time lines for notifying the patient.

- Central location. The reminder system should be located centrally in the office and should not be kept in individual patient medical records. Reminders should be accessible to the entire staff.

- Reliability. The tracking system should not be the responsibility of a single individual. Office staff should be cross-trained so that the system is reliable and efficient. It should be updated and monitored regularly.

A protocol should be established to ensure that patients are informed of all significant abnormal test results. This notification should be documented in the patient's medical record. Computerized tracking and reminder systems, although not required, are available with custom alerts, telephone reminders, and telephone numbers to call for automated test results using individual identifying numbers. Some practices are now using secure patient portals where patients can receive their test results electronically as well as electronic reminders about when their next test should be scheduled. A method should exist for monitoring patients' adherence to recommendations that are made based on abnormal test results. The patient or her family should be given individualized instructions for continuing care after office operative procedures, and this instruction should be documented in the patient's medical record.

An established protocol also should exist for follow-up with patients who do not appear for an appointment after several appointments have been made. Missed appointments can lead to delays in diagnosis and treatment; therefore, a system of scheduling appointments and reviewing missed ones is important. The following principles can be applied to scheduling and rescheduling appointments to protect the patient and practitioner:

- Schedule appointments based on medical need.
- Indicate the follow-up interval in the medical record, and ask staff to schedule the follow-up appointment before the patient leaves the office.
- Identify and review missed appointments, because a prolonged follow-up interval may interfere with the patient receiving timely treatment.
- Instruct staff to call patients to find out their reason for missing an appointment and to reschedule. Send a letter if there is no answer, only an answering machine is reached, or the patient refuses to be seen during the recommended interval. Consider using certified mail for nonresponsive patients with potentially serious conditions. Document in the record, and include a photocopy or scanned copy of the letter in the chart, if possible.
- When patients are referred from another physician but miss or do not make an appointment, notify the referring physician (by phone and in writing) that the patient did not show up for, or cancelled, the appointment. Also, clarify with the referring physician who will follow up with the patient. This information should be documented in the medical record.
- The number of attempts to contact a patient who consistently misses appointments should be tailored to the risk involved. A clearly defined policy consistent with any state regulations must be established for the type and number of attempts that will be made to contact the patient.

The AMA states that it is ethical for physicians to charge for missed appointments or for appointments not canceled at least 24 hours in advance if patients are fully advised of the possibility of such charges. However, procedures and policies regarding missed appointments differ from state to state.

Missed appointments, nonadherence to medical advice, and refusal of a recommended test or procedure should be documented in the patient's medical record. Clinicians have the right to terminate patient–practitioner relationships. The clinician should be aware of any legal and managed care contractual requirements that apply to termination of the patient–practitioner relationship. All steps undertaken to terminate the relationship should be documented in the patient's medical record. Recommendations regarding the closing of a practice are found in the "Risk Management" section in Part 1.

ELECTRONIC COMMUNICATION AND PATIENT CONFIDENTIALITY

The use of technology for exchanging medical information among patients and health care providers is increasing. Electronic communication media, including cellular telephones, telephone answering machines, facsimile machines, electronic mail, and wireless devices all improve access among clinicians and patients but increase the possibility that a breach of patient confidentiality may occur (see also the "Human Resources" section in Part 1) and that third parties may have authorized or unauthorized access to the health care provider's or the patient's communication system. The HIPAA Privacy Rule allows covered health care providers to communicate electronically, provided they apply reasonable safeguards when doing so. Further, although the Privacy Rule does not prohibit the use of unencrypted e-mail for treatment-related communication between health care providers and patients, other safeguards should be applied to reasonably protect privacy, such as limiting the amount or type of information disclosed through unencrypted e-mail. Office computer stations should be placed to minimize unauthorized access. Unauthorized electronic access can be minimized by using procedures such as password-protected screen savers and automatic logout.

It can be useful to provide patients with written information on the privacy risks of electronic communication, guidelines for how and when the patient and practitioner may use this form of communication, and the expected turnaround time for processing each communication. Patients should understand that no clinician or institution can guarantee complete security of electronically transmitted data and that communications about highly sensitive subjects should not be e-mailed or faxed. In addition, electronic communications may not be received in a timely manner or be read at all; therefore, time-sensitive and urgent issues should not be communicated electronically. Recommendations for e-mail use have been published (see Box 2-3).

Box 2-3. Suggestions for Electronic Communications

- Obtain informed consent for use of e-mail with patients.
- Include guidelines for when e-mail may and may not be used.
- Request that patients write their full name and an identifier (eg, medical record number, birth date, address) in the text of the message.
- Establish turnaround times for messages and who will view messages.
- Establish types of appropriate communications (eg, prescription refill request, appointment reminder, results of home monitoring of blood pressure or glucose).
- Never use e-mail for highly sensitive or urgent matters.
- When replying to patient queries, include the full text of the query in the reply.
- Describe security measures that are in place.
- Indemnify against information lost because of technical failure.
- Do not forward patient-identifying information.
- Keep professional and personal e-mail accounts separate.
- Double-check all addressee fields before sending messages to ascertain that the e-mail is not going to multiple and unintended addressees.
- Back up e-mail regularly, and store a copy of each query and reply with the patient's medical record.
- Ideally, health care providers and patients will acknowledge to each other that messages have been received, read, and acted on. Use an automatic out-of-office reply feature if e-mails will not be serviced according to turnaround times previously agreed upon.
- If an e-mail is sent to a group of patients, use the blind copy feature so that the recipients' addresses are not visible.
- Health care providers should add an automatic footer to their e-mails telling patients to call or make an appointment if the e-mail reply has not been sufficient to meet their needs.
- Health care providers should not leave e-mails open on computer screens. E-mail accounts should be password protected and have automatic logout.

Data from Kane B, Sands DZ. Guidelines for the clinical use of electronic mail with patients. The AMIA Internet Working Group, Task Force on Guidelines for the Use of Clinic-Patient Electronic Mail. J Am Med Inform Assoc 1998;5:104–11.

Social media can be an effective tool to disseminate important health messages, reach out to patients, and advocate for women's health issues. But with this new territory comes new rules and risks. Protected health information should never be shared or discussed on a social media platform. Clinicians can have a successful and rewarding social media presence by educating themselves about potential liability pitfalls and being alert to possible privacy violations. Box 2-4 includes some helpful "do's and don'ts" to consider when using social media.

REMOTE CONSULTATIONS

Physicians should become familiar with their own state's regulations concerning remote consultations. Most states require that all physicians, wherever located, who provide medical advice to patients in that state have a medical license for that state. Practice web sites should carry clear disclaimers stating that the site is for informational purposes only, that the site is not intended to give medical advice, and that use of the site does not establish a patient–physician relationship.

Informed Consent

The clinician is responsible for securing the patient's informed consent. It is imperative that the patient understand all aspects of her treatment, and so informed consent is an ongoing process. The risks and benefits of each procedure as well as alternatives should be discussed (see also the "Ethical Issues" section in Part 1). Patient education information, when available, should be provided to assist in the informed consent process and in discussions that relate to specific treatments, tests, operations, and procedures. The patient should be informed of the common adverse effects of prescribed drugs and the importance of reading the patient package inserts for drugs or devices. All informed consent discussions and informational material provided should be documented appropriately in the patient's medical record.

If a patient refuses a recommended test, treatment, or procedure, this refusal also should be documented. Documentation should include the following:

- That the clinician recommended a particular test, treatment, or procedure to the patient

- That the clinician explained the need for the test, treatment, or procedure, and the benefits and risks involved
- That the clinician explained the consequences of refusing the recommendation
- That the patient refused the treatment or procedure and her reasons for the refusal

---

Box 2-4. Social Media DOs and DON'Ts

Some of the most important rules for physicians using social media include the following:

DOs	DON'Ts
Always maintain your professionalism.	Don't discuss patients online, even in general terms.
Be careful with humor and political opinions.	Don't give medical advice.
Speak in lay terms patients and consumers will understand.	Don't post photos of patients or newborns.
Ask your employer, hospital, or both if it has social media guidelines you must follow.	Don't post anything you don't want the entire world to read. Everything you do and say online is public.
Consider creating a social media policy for your practice.	Don't "friend" your patients on Facebook. If you have a personal Facebook page, consider creating a separate professional one.
Ask your professional liability carrier if it has social media coverage or guidelines.	Don't spend too much time directly promoting your practice. Social media is about having a conversation, so limit self-serving practice promotions, such as "We have 4-D fetal ultrasonography at our downtown location!"

Modified from Social media guide: how to connect with patients and spread women's health messages. ACOG Today. November 2012. American Congress of Obstetricians and Gynecologists: Washington, DC; p. 6.

When presenting medical information to a patient, whether as part of obtaining an informed consent or simply presenting educational information, the clinician must be sensitive to the patient's ability to understand and process the information presented. The health literacy of the patient may present an impediment to the informed consent process. All medical information and instructions should be presented in a manner and at a level that allows the patient to comprehend and participate in the decision-making process. The use of medical jargon should be avoided (see also the "Patient Safety" section in Part 1 for a discussion of patient–provider communication).

Practitioners also should comply with specific state and federal informed consent laws and regulations that apply to specific treatments or procedures. Doing so may include informing patients of risks and benefits specified in the laws and having patients sign an approved consent form. Specific additional requirements may apply to minors (see also the "Ethical Issues" section in Part 1 and the "Adolescents" section in Part 3).

Bibliography

American College of Obstetricians and Gynecologists. Professional liability and risk management: an essential guide for obstetrician-gynecologists. 2nd ed. Washington, DC: ACOG; 2008.

American College of Obstetricians and Gynecologists. Quality and safety in women's health care. 2nd ed. Washington, DC: American College of Obstetricians and Gynecologists; 2010.

Americans with Disabilities Act, 42 U.S.C. §12101 (2011). Available at: http://www.gpo.gov/fdsys/pkg/USCODE-2011-title42/pdf/USCODE-2011-title42-chap126.pdf. Retrieved September 20, 2013.

Centers for Medicare and Medicaid Services. EHR incentive programs. Available at: http://www.cms.gov/Regulations-and-Guidance/Legislation/EHRIncentivePrograms/index.html. Retrieved September 26, 2013.

Cultural sensitivity and awareness in the delivery of health care. Committee Opinion No. 493. American College of Obstetricians and Gynecologists. Obstet Gynecol 2011;117:1258–61.

Department of Health and Human Services, Office for Civil Rights. Does the HIPAA Privacy Rule permit health care providers to use e-mail to discuss health issues and treatment with their patients? Washington, DC: OCR; 2008. Available at: http://www.hhs.gov/ocr/privacy/hipaa/faq/health_information_technology/570.html. Retrieved October 22, 2013.

Department of Health and Human Services, Office of Minority Health. Think cultural health. Available at: https://www.thinkculturalhealth.hhs.gov. Retrieved July 19, 2013.

Effective patient–physician communication. Committee Opinion No. 587. American College of Obstetricians and Gynecologists. Obstet Gynecol 2014;123:389–93.

General administrative requirements, 45 C.F.R. part 160 (2012). Available at: http://www.gpo.gov/fdsys/pkg/CFR-2012-title45-vol1/pdf/CFR-2012-title45-vol1-part160.pdf. Retrieved September 20, 2013.

Health literacy. Committee Opinion No. 585. American College of Obstetricians and Gynecologists. Obstet Gynecol 2014;123:380–3.

Informed consent. ACOG Committee Opinion No. 439. American College of Obstetricians and Gynecologists. Obstet Gynecol 2009;114:401–8.

Modifications to the HIPAA privacy, security, enforcement, and breach notification rules under the Health Information Technology for Economic and Clinical Health Act and the Genetic Information Nondiscrimination Act; other modifications to the HIPAA rules. Fed Regist 2013;78:5565-702.

Partnering with patients to improve safety. Committee Opinion No. 490. American College of Obstetricians and Gynecologists. Obstet Gynecol 2011;117:1247–9.

Patient safety and the electronic health record. Committee Opinion No. 472. American College of Obstetricians and Gynecologists. Obstet Gynecol 2010; 116:1245-7.

Security and privacy, 45 C.F.R. part 164 (2012). Available at: http://www.gpo.gov/fdsys/pkg/CFR-2012-title45-vol1/pdf/CFR-2012-title45-vol1-part164.pdf. Retrieved September 20, 2013.

The limits of conscientious refusal in reproductive medicine. ACOG Committee Opinion No. 385. American College of Obstetricians and Gynecologists. Obstet Gynecol 2007;110:1203–8.

Tracking and reminder systems. Committee Opinion No. 546. American College of Obstetricians and Gynecologists. Obstet Gynecol 2012;120:1535–7.

Resources

Adolescent confidentiality and electronic health records. Committee Opinion No. 599. American College of Obstetricians and Gynecologists. Obstet Gynecol 2014;123:1148–50.

American Congress of Obstetricians and Gynecologists. Health information technology. Washington, DC: American Congress of Obstetricians and Gynecologists; 2013. Available at: http://www.acog.org/About_ACOG/ACOG_Departments/Health_Information_Technology. Retrieved September 30, 2013.

American Congress of Obstetricians and Gynecologists. Social media and professionalism in the medical community (DVD). Washington, DC: American Congress of Obstetricians and Gynecologists; 2013.

American Medical Association. Implementing health IT. Available at: http://www.ama-assn.org//ama/pub/physician-resources/health-information-technology/implementing-health-it.page. Retrieved July 19, 2013.

Civil money penalties, assessments and exclusions. 42 C.F.R. part 1003 (2012). Available at: http://www.gpo.gov/fdsys/pkg/CFR-2012-title42-vol5/pdf/CFR-2012-title42-vol5-part1003.pdf. Retrieved September 20, 2013.

Department of Health and Human Services. Health information privacy: the privacy rule. Available at: http://www.hhs.gov/ocr/privacy/hipaa/administrative/privacyrule/index.html. Retrieved July 19, 2013.

Integrating the Healthcare Enterprise. Available at: http://www.ihe.net. Retrieved July 22, 2013.

Kane B, Sands DZ. Guidelines for the clinical use of electronic mail with patients. The AMIA Internet Working Group, Task Force on Guidelines for the Use of Clinic-Patient Electronic Mail. J Am Med Inform Assoc 1998;5:104–11.

Sands DZ. Help for physicians contemplating use of e-mail with patients [editorial]. J Am Med Inform Assoc 2004;11:268–9.

PRACTICE MANAGEMENT

Issues to consider in the management of a successful health care practice include staffing requirements; billing systems; patient care coordination; appointments, scheduling, and patient flow; practice coverage for absent physicians; and systems for proper storage and disposal of drugs and other sensitive materials.

Staffing

STAFFING LEVELS

Staffing requirements for an office or institution will vary. Factors in setting staffing levels and types include the anticipated need for chaperoning, population served, and scope of services to be provided. State regulations may be relevant, depending on the health care providers needed and their scope of practice. In some cases, contractual arrangements may be required to assist patients with their health care needs (eg, with providers of nutrition, ultrasonography, and social services).

The efficient operation of an ambulatory surgical facility requires that the assignment of administrative and professional personnel be based on the number of patients, patient characteristics (eg, intensity of care required and types of procedures performed), the level of preparation and experience of those who provide care, and the facility design. A sufficient number of staff members with the skills needed to provide optimal care for specific procedures should be available to prevent undue delays in the provision of care. Departments in large institutions generally derive their staffing levels from institutional guidelines. Some professional organizations, such as the Association of Women's Health, Obstetric and Neonatal Nurses, have established staffing guidelines for patients in the labor and delivery suite and mother-to-newborn nursing ratios. Institutions may use these guidelines to establish their own staffing levels. There are no established national staffing guidelines regarding gynecologic care for patients. However, in 1999, California became the first state to pass a comprehensive minimum staffing bill, which requires that the state department of health services establish minimum nurse-to-patient ratios for hospitals. According to the American Nurses Association, as of 2012, 14 other states and the District of Columbia had enacted legislation, adopted regulations, or both to address nurse staffing.

TYPES OF PRACTITIONERS

A health care team may include many professionals. These professionals should be licensed and possess the credentials required by their respective professional organizations.

Obstetrician–Gynecologists

Obstetrician–gynecologists are physicians with additional education and experience in reproductive medicine and women's health care. They have completed a 4-year residency and many go on to be certified by the American Board of Obstetrics and Gynecology, Inc. Those who received their initial board certification in or after November 1986 have time-limited certificates that must be renewed every 6 years through a process of maintenance of certification (see also the "Evaluating Credentials and Granting Privileges" section in Part 1). Obstetrician–gynecologists who are board certified or active candidates may become members of the American Congress of Obstetricians and Gynecologists. Some obstetrician–gynecologists seek additional training in a subspecialty. At present, the American Board of Obstetrics and Gynecology offers subspecialty certification in four areas: 1) reproductive endocrinology and infertility, 2) maternal–fetal medicine, 3) gynecologic oncology, and 4) female pelvic medicine and reconstructive surgery.

Osteopathic obstetrician–gynecologists receive roughly 200 hours of osteopathic manipulation medicine training during the traditional 4 years of medical school. There is an optional 1-year fellowship in osteopathic manipulation medicine for physicians who desire additional training. After completion of a residency training program, osteopathic obstetrician–gynecologists can apply for board certification from the American

Osteopathic Board of Obstetrics and Gynecology. The American Osteopathic Association, Accreditation Council for Graduate Medical Education, and American Association of Colleges of Osteopathic Medicine have entered into an agreement to form a unified accreditation system beginning in July 2015.

Registered Nurses

Nursing personnel who care for gynecology patients should be familiar with the special aspects of gynecologic conditions and the equipment needed to care for these patients. Delivery of safe and effective nursing care requires appropriately qualified registered nurses in adequate numbers to meet the needs of each patient in accordance with the care setting. The number of staff members and level of skill required are influenced by the scope of nursing practice and the degree of nursing responsibilities within an institution. Nursing responsibilities in individual hospitals vary according to the level of care provided by the facility, practice procedures, number of professional registered nurses and ancillary staff, and professional nursing activities in continuing education and research.

Changing trends in medical management and technological advances influence, and may increase, the nursing workload. Each hospital should determine the scope of nursing practice for each nursing unit and specialty department. The scope of practice should be based on national nursing standards and guidelines for the specialty area of practice and should be in accordance with state law or regulations. A multidisciplinary committee comprising representatives from hospital, medical, and nursing administration should follow published professional standards and guidelines, consult state nurse practice acts and any accompanying regulations, identify the types and number of procedures performed in each unit, delineate direct and indirect nursing care activities performed, and identify activities to be performed by nonnursing personnel.

Hospitalists

The term hospitalist refers to a physician whose primary professional focus is the general medical care of hospitalized patients. Increasing numbers of physicians and physician practices use hospitalists. These doctors may or may not provide 24-hour inpatient coverage. Some hospitalists are in private practice and rotate to inpatient care days. Many more hospitals are putting hospitalists on their payrolls and giving physicians the option to use hospitalists when patients require inpatient care. Patient care is transferred back to the original clinician when the patient is discharged from the hospital.

Within the specialty of obstetrics and gynecology, the concept of the hospitalist or laborist is an evolving model of care and an alternative type of practice for some physicians. The term laborist commonly refers to an obstetrician–gynecologist who is employed by a hospital or physician group and whose primary focus is to care for laboring patients and to manage obstetric emergencies. There is no single accepted definition; however, there is general agreement that the specialist hospitalist and the laborist treat patients only in a hospital setting.

For the obstetric–gynecologic hospitalist, practicing solely in the hospital setting relieves the pressures of a private practice, such as overhead and collections, and may help with liability premiums. Among the possible benefits may be more predictable schedules, competitive compensation, paid benefits, and guaranteed time off. The benefits to the hospital include enhancement of patient safety and an increased level of nursing satisfaction because a health care provider is always present and available. In addition, improved outcomes may result from hospitalists being well rested when coming onto their shifts. For obstetrician–gynecologists in general practice in the community, having an obstetric–gynecologic hospitalist in practice at their admitting hospital affords several advantages. For example, obstetric–gynecologic hospitalists can assume the responsibilities of on-call obligations, provide coverage for patients who come to the hospital uninsured or unassigned for prenatal care, and afford office-based physicians greater autonomy over their personal and family lives.

However, critics point out that the transfer of care from the office physician to the hospitalist may increase medical errors and that patients dislike the concept of health care delivery by a physician they have never met. A key element for instituting an effective obstetric–gynecologic hospitalist program within a facility is the establishment of clear communication methods between obstetric–gynecologic hospitalists and outpatient obstetrician–gynecologists or primary women's health care providers. In addition, physicians should inform patients that hospitalists and laborists are part of the health care team that may provide their care.

The obstetric–gynecologic hospitalist model may be met with some resistance from some physicians and patients. However, this model may be appealing, particularly for younger obstetrician–gynecologists who are concerned about maintaining liability coverage, establishing an independent practice, and maintaining a balanced life style. The model of the obstetric–gynecologic hospitalist is still evolving, yet it is one potential solution to achieving increased professional and patient satisfaction while maintaining safe and effective care across delivery settings.

Certified Nurse–Midwives and Certified Midwives

Certified nurse–midwives (CNMs) and certified midwives (CMs) are primary care providers who focus on pregnancy, childbirth, the postpartum period, care of the newborn, and the family planning and gynecologic needs of women. A CNM is a registered nurse who has been educated in the two disciplines of nursing and midwifery; a CM is not a nurse but has met the same standards for midwifery education and certification as the CNM. To obtain certification, applicants must successfully complete a graduate program in midwifery from a school of midwifery accredited by the Accreditation Commission for Midwifery Education. The certification of a CNM or CM is conferred through a national examination and verified by the American Midwifery Certification Board, Inc. As of 2010, entry into clinical practice required completion of a master's or doctoral degree. A CNM or CM must be licensed by the state in which care is given. Although CNMs are licensed in all 50 states, the District of Columbia, and the U.S. territories, CMs currently are licensed only in New Jersey, New York, and Rhode Island.

Clinical Nurse Specialists

Clinical nurse specialists are registered nurses who have completed a formal educational program at the master's degree level. Clinical nurse specialists can handle a wide range of physical and mental health problems. They generally work in inpatient settings and are certified by the credentialing unit of the American Nurses Association.

Nurse Practitioners

Nurse practitioners (NPs) are licensed registered nurses with advanced-practice education, including supervised clinical instruction in health maintenance and diagnosis and treatment of illness. Completion of an NP program may lead to a certificate or a master's or doctoral degree.

Certification as an NP is required in some jurisdictions and is voluntary in others. Certification is based on completing an approved educational program, passing a national certification examination, or both. Nurse practitioners who specialize in women's health are certified by the National Certification Corporation. Requirements for certification vary according to the specialty area and are determined by the certifying organization.

Nurse practitioners are qualified to provide a wide range of primary and preventive health care services, including obtaining medical, surgical, and psychosocial histories; performing physical examinations; and diagnosing and treating common illnesses and injuries. They generally work in primary care outpatient clinics, health maintenance organizations, specialty clinics, and schools. An increasing number of NPs are employed in inpatient settings.

Women's Health Nurse Practitioners

The women's health nurse practitioner (WHNP) is an advanced-practice registered nurse who is prepared through academic and clinical study to provide health care, with an emphasis on reproductive–gynecologic and well-woman health, to women throughout the life span. Women's health nurse practitioners are licensed and regulated by boards of nursing. In many states they also are subject to regulation by state medical boards, particularly in areas of prescribing and collaboration agreements. The WHNP functions in a variety of settings and provides care that includes wellness promotion and management of gynecologic and common nongynecologic problems. The National Certification Corporation is the recognized certifying body for WHNPs. Educational programs for WHNPs are based in a college or university graduate nursing program and should include at least 200 didactic hours of content and at least 600 hours of supervised clinical practice.

Physician Assistants

Physician assistants (PAs) enter the profession from a variety of backgrounds and are educated to provide care as part of a health care team under the supervision of a physician. The Accreditation Review Commission on Education for the Physician Assistant accredits PA programs. Most of these programs have been established in, or have strong affiliations with, medical schools. Applicants generally have at least 4 years of college education, and many programs require applicants to have acquired health care experience or community experience before admission. The educational program traditionally consists of 24–32 months of didactic instruction and clinical rotations. Curriculum design for most PA programs involves basic sciences, clinical sciences, and supervised clinical instruction. Physician assistant students complete, on average, more than 2,000 hours of supervised clinical practice before graduation. Although all programs recognize the professional component of PA education with a document of completion for the professional credential (PA), 80% of the programs award a master's degree, 15% award bachelor's degrees, and 5% award associate degrees or certificates.

Physician assistants practice in virtually all specialty areas, in outpatient and inpatient settings, as first or second assistants in surgery, and in providing preoperative and postoperative care. All jurisdictions require PAs to pass a national certification examination before they can practice. The examination is given only to graduates of accredited PA programs and is developed by the independent National Commission on Certification of Physician Assistants. To maintain national certification and use the credential Physician Assistant–Certified, an individual must complete 100 hours of continuing medical education every 2 years and take a recertification examination every 6 years.

Surgical Assistants

Competent surgical assistants should be available for all major obstetric and gynecologic operations. In many cases, the complexity of the surgery or the patient's condition will require the assistance of one or more physicians or other personnel with special surgical training to provide safe, quality patient care. Often, the complexity of a given surgical procedure cannot be determined prospectively. The judgment and prerogative of the primary surgeon to determine the number and qualifications of appropriately compensated assistants should not be overruled by public or private third-party payers. Registered nurses and other personnel assisting in the provision of surgical services should be appropriately trained, be granted privileges to assist in specific procedures, and remain under the direct supervision of the surgeon.

Registered nurse first assistants are employed in hospital-based settings, ambulatory care settings, collaborative practice with physicians, and independent practice. The role of the registered nurse first assistant falls within the scope of nursing in all 50 state boards of nursing. Registered nurse first assistants must demonstrate the following:

- Competency in performing individualized surgical nursing care management before, during, and after surgery
- Competency in recognizing surgical anatomy, physiology, and operative technique
- Competency in carrying out intraoperative nursing behaviors of handling tissue, providing exposure, using surgical instruments, suturing, and controlling blood loss
- Competency in recognizing surgical hazards and initiating appropriate corrective and preventive action, including but not limited to recognizing abnormal laboratory values and diagnostic test results
- Achievement of Basic Cardiac Life Support Certification, Advanced Cardiac Life Support Certification, or both
- Achievement of national Certification in Operating Room Nursing

Other Health Care Providers

Certified professional midwives are certified through the North American Registry of Midwives. There is no single standard for education through the North American Registry of Midwives; a midwife can learn through a structured program, apprenticeship, or self-study, although certified professional midwives usually pass a written and practical examination for certification. Some states recognize the certified professional midwife credential as the basis for licensure or use the North American Registry of Midwives written examination. However, some midwives act outside of state recognition and oversight and, in fact, are not licensed by the state. Although the American College of Obstetricians and Gynecologists supports women having a choice in determining their providers of care, it does not support the provision of care by midwives who are not certified by the American College of Nurse-Midwives or the American Midwifery Certification Board. Most unlicensed midwives do not have hospital privileges, and practice and licensing requirements vary from state to state.

A naturopathic physician (ND) is the highest level of trained practitioner in the field of naturopathic medicine. At schools of naturopathic medicine, NDs are trained in medical sciences and conventional diagnostics, therapeutic nutrition, botanical medicine, homeopathy, natural childbirth, classical Chinese medicine, hydrotherapy, manipulative therapy, pharmacology, and minor surgery. Some states have licensing laws for NDs that allow them to practice as primary care general practice physicians, but most states do not license these individuals.

Billing

When scheduling an appointment, the office staff should discuss with the patient customary fees, methods of payment, billing, third-party insurance procedures, requirements for co-payments, practitioner participation, facility affiliation, and preauthorization or referrals that may be required at the visit. Verification of third-party coverage and compliance with continuing authorization requirements should occur at each visit.

The clinician should encourage the patient to review medical plan participation and identification of contractual requirements, including laboratory and imaging facility designations. A system should be in place to ensure proper participating laboratory and imaging service referrals. Appropriate referrals and approvals should be verified. A system should be established to ensure that all preprocedure requirements (laboratory tests, consents, examination records, and third-party authorizations) are met in advance of a procedure.

Staff should be aware of third-party contractual requirements for service and billing and participate in ensuring compliance with payer contracts.

The clinician is responsible for ensuring accuracy in the coding of bills. The clinician must ensure that appropriate documentation exists in the record to justify the level of service billed. Information regarding the Medicare documentation guidelines for evaluation and management services appears in the "Well-Woman Annual Health Assessment" section in Part 3. Many resources are available for reference and help with coding issues (see Box 2-5 and Resources).

Box 2-5. The American Congress of Obstetricians and Gynecologists' Coding Resources

- Workshops and webcasts—These workshops are held several times a year in different parts of the country and are designed to teach physicians the essential elements of correct coding and documentation. The American Congress of Obstetricians and Gynecologists' (ACOG) monthly webcasts cover coding, practice management, and professional liability topics from 1:00–2:30 PM Eastern Time on the second Tuesday of each month. For more information or to register, please visit ACOG's Education and Events web page at www.acog.org/Education_and_Events.

- List serv—"The Practice Management and Coding Update" is a free monthly e-mail news service that includes effective coding tips, practice management advice, information about regulatory issues, and the latest news on what ACOG is doing to help address reimbursement concerns and improve the practice environment. To subscribe to the list serv, send an e-mail message to coding-request@suse.acog.org.

- Specific questions—Physicians and their staff can submit specific coding questions to ACOG staff by fax at (202) 484-7480 or e-mail at coding@acog.org. (Per the Health Insurance Portability and Accountability Act regulations, please do not include any patient identifiable information in your fax or e-mail message.)

- Publications—A variety of coding publications may be ordered from ACOG's catalog, web site (http://sales.acog.org/), or distribution center (1-800-762-2264).

If a patient questions the customary fees, the clinician should be informed and should advise staff as to the appropriate method of addressing the patient's concerns. Ideally, a specific staff member should be assigned responsibility for handling the financial concerns or complaints of patients.

Despite the recent passage of landmark health care legislation, every practice will continue to deal with the uninsured patient. According to the Kaiser Family Foundation, in 2011, 21.68% of women of childbearing age (15–44 years of age) were uninsured, and more than 19 million women aged 18–64 years were without health insurance. It is advisable to designate someone in the office who is knowledgeable regarding Medicaid or other state-sponsored programs for the uninsured, as well as community resources such as subsidized clinics or voucher programs.

Care Coordination

The concept of the patient-centered medical home is being advanced by health professionals, administrators, and patient advocates as a cost-effective alternative to the current episodic, sometimes fragmented system of health care delivery. The principles of the medical home model are based generally on a physician who leads a team of clinicians and staff who in turn provide continuous, comprehensive, coordinated care based on a "whole person" orientation. Care is coordinated across all elements of a complex health care system and the patient's community using means such as new health systems technologies. In this care model, information exchange between medical providers and between patients and the medical home is especially important. The American Congress of Obstetricians and Gynecologists (ACOG) supports the women's medical home, which will provide targeted, continuous, coordinated, confidential, and comprehensive care to eligible individuals. The women's medical home focuses especially on women who are at risk of premature birth, the prevention of cervical cancer, care for women with breast or gynecologic cancer, and care for chronic conditions. For more information, see ACOG's Medical Home Toolkit web page, available at www.acog.org/About_ACOG/ACOG_Departments/Practice_Management_and_Managed_Care/ACOG_Medical_Home_Toolkit.

Appointments, Scheduling, and Patient Flow

AMBULATORY CARE

The most efficient method of managing patient access and flow in an office setting or clinic begins with appointment scheduling. Appointments should be booked realistically to maintain the clinician's schedules and allow sufficient time for emergency appointments. The personnel in each facility should establish a realistic goal for minimizing waiting time. The average time a practitioner spends with a patient for various procedures (eg, new patient visit, yearly checkup, and gynecologic procedure) can be analyzed easily to form a basis by which scheduling can be optimized. Such scheduling should be analyzed periodically to ensure minimal patient waiting. Procedures for the following circumstances should be established:

- Rescheduling missed or canceled appointments
- Informing patients when their appointments will be delayed substantially or when an emergency situation may prevent the clinician from keeping an appointment
- Processing patients in a timely manner
- Guiding patients to specific areas of the facility (eg, the laboratory or insurance office)

OPERATING ROOM DATA AND DATA TRACKING

Operating room data tracking is necessary for scheduling procedures and personnel and for billing. Data tracking provides a means to evaluate the operating room's utilization, efficiency, and productivity. Specific data points to be tracked depend on the needs of the institution. Data commonly collected include the following:

- Type of procedure
- Surgeon
- Length of procedure by surgeon
- Time of the
    — patient arrival in unit
    — patient in procedure room

— anesthesia induction

— incision

— patient out of room

— room cleanup start and finish

— case time (time from room setup to cleanup)

- Turnover time (time from preceding patient out of room to next patient in room)

Practice Coverage

All obstetrician–gynecologists should have appropriate coverage agreements with practitioners within their own group practice or other practitioners to care for their patients in their absence. When possible, these clinicians should be obstetrician–gynecologists. Careful consideration should be given to managed care contractual agreements and participating physician coverage. Billing policies and procedures should be established in advance and consideration given to reimbursement agreements. The clinicians should be familiar with each other's practice style and capabilities, and practitioners should have privileges at the same hospital or other facilities. An established protocol should exist to introduce the covering practitioner to hospitalized patients and patients with special problems. The institution and answering service should be advised of the dates of a clinician's absence or unavailability, as well as the names, telephone numbers, and office addresses of the covering practitioner. The covering practitioner, when feasible, should have access to patients' medical records (see also the "Risk Management" section in Part 1).

Control and Disposal of Drugs and Other Sensitive Materials

A system must be in place for maintaining the security of all controlled drugs. Ideally, a secure system also should be in place for the control of syringes, needles, and prescription pads. An established procedure should exist for monitoring the expiration date of drugs, including sample drugs and laboratory reagents, and proper disposal techniques. Also, procedures should exist for the shredding or other means of destruction of medical records and other sensitive data (see the "Information Management" section earlier in Part 2).

Bibliography

American College of Nurse–Midwives. Comparison of certified nurse-midwives, certified midwives, and certified professional midwives: clarifying the distinctions among professional midwifery credentials in the U.S. Washington, DC: ACNM; 2014. Available at: http://www.midwife.org/acnm/files/cclibraryfiles/filename/000000001031/cnm%20cm%20cpm%20comparison%20chart%20march%202011.pdf. Retrieved April 10, 2014.

American College of Obstetricians and Gynecologists, American College of Nurse-Midwives. Joint statement of practice relations between obstetricians-gynecologists and certified nurse-midwives/certified midwives. College Statement of Policy 87. Washington, DC: American College of Obstetricians and Gynecologists; 2011.

American College of Obstetricians and Gynecologists. Midwifery education and certification. College Statement of Policy 82. Washington, DC: American College of Obstetricians and Gynecologists; 2011.

American College of Obstetricians and Gynecologists. Professional liability and risk management: an essential guide for obstetrician-gynecologists. 2nd ed. Washington, DC: ACOG; 2008.

American College of Obstetricians and Gynecologists. Statement on surgical assistants. ACOG Committee Opinion 240. Washington, DC: ACOG; 2000.

American Congress of Obstetricians and Gynecologists. Midwifery legislation. Washington, DC: American Congress of Obstetricians and Gynecologists; 2013. Available at: http://www.acog.org/~/media/Departments/Members%20Only/State%20Legislative%20Activities/2013StateLegRoundtable.pdf#page=7. Retrieved March 27, 2014.

American Nurses Association. Nurse staffing plans and ratios: summary of approaches. Available at: http://www.nursingworld.org/MainMenuCategories/Policy-Advocacy/State/Legislative-Agenda-Reports/State-StaffingPlansRatios/Nurse-Staffing-Plans-and-Ratios-Summary-of-Approaches.html. Retrieved July 19, 2013.

American Osteopathic Association. Available at: http://www.osteopathic.org. Retrieved July 22, 2013.

American Osteopathic Board of Obstetrics and Gynecology. Available at: http://www.aobog.org/. Retrieved July 22, 2013.

Henry J. Kaiser Family Foundation. Health insurance coverage of women ages 18 to 64, by state, 2010–2011. Menlo Park (CA): KFF; 2012. Available at: http://kaiserfamilyfoundation.files.wordpress.com/2013/02/1613-12.pdf. Retrieved July 22, 2013.

The obstetric-gynecologic hospitalist. Committee Opinion No. 459. American College of Obstetricians and Gynecologists. Obstet Gynecol 2010;116:237–9.

U.S. Census Bureau. Table 29. Health Insurance Status by Sex and Age: 2011. Washington, DC: Census Bureau; 2012. Available at: http://www.census.gov/population/age/data/files/2011/2011gender_table29.xlsx. Retrieved July 22, 2013.

Resources

American College of Obstetricians and Gynecologists. Guidelines for implementing collaborative practice. Washington, DC: ACOG; 1995.

American College of Surgeons. Physicians as assistants at surgery: 2011 study. Chicago (IL): ACS; 2011. Available at: http://www.facs.org/ahp/pubs/2011physasstsurg.pdf. Retrieved July 22, 2013.

American Congress of Obstetricians and Gynecologists. 2014 Ob/Gyn coding manual: components of correct procedural coding. Washington, DC: American Congress of Obstetricians and Gynecologists; 2014.

American Congress of Obstetricians and Gynecologists. ACOG Medical home toolkit. Washington, DC: American Congress of Obstetricians and Gynecologists. Available at: http://www.acog.org/About_ACOG/ACOG_Departments/Practice_Management_and_Managed_Care/ACOG_Medical_Home_Toolkit. Retrieved July 17, 2013.

American Congress of Obstetricians and Gynecologists. Frequently asked questions in obstetric and gynecologic coding. 5th ed. Washington, DC: American Congress of Obstetricians and Gynecologists; 2011.

American Congress of Obstetricians and Gynecologists. ICD-9-CM to ICD-10-CM gynecologic and general medicine diagnoses crosswalk. Washington, DC: American Congress of Obstetricians and Gynecologists; 2013.

American Congress of Obstetricians and Gynecologists. Practice Management and Managed Care. Washington, DC: American Congress of Obstetricians and Gynecologists; 2013. Available at: http://www.acog.org/About_ACOG/ACOG_Departments/Practice_Management_and_Managed_Care. Retrieved July 16, 2013.

Association of periOperative Registered Nurses. Perioperative standards and recommended practices. 2013 ed. Denver, CO: AORN; 2013.

Association of Women's Health, Obstetric and Neonatal Nurses. Standards for professional nursing practice in the care of women and newborns. 7th ed. Washington, D.C.: AWHONN; 2009.

Ethical ways for physicians to market a practice. Committee Opinion No. 510. American College Obstetricians and Gynecologists. Obstet Gynecol 2011;118:1195–7.

Patient-Centered Primary Care Collaborative. Available at: http:www.pcpcc.net. Retrieved July 16, 2013.

Scroggs JL, Strunk AL. An introduction to the medical home [editorial]. Clin Rev 2010;15(3):1–7.

The Joint Commission. Comprehensive accreditation manual for ambulatory care: CAMAC. Oakbrook Terrace (IL): The Commission; 2014.

The Joint Commission. Comprehensive accreditation manual for hospitals: CAMH. Oakbrook Terrace (IL): The Commission; 2014.

WELL-WOMAN CARE

The practice of obstetrics and gynecology encompasses a broad spectrum of care directed to many aspects of a woman's health (see also Appendix J). During the reproductive years, the obstetric–gynecologic provider often serves as a woman's point of entry into the health care system, a source of continuity in her health care, and her provider of routine screening and preventive care. Routine visits are opportunities for health care providers to educate and counsel patients regarding risk factors and lifestyle issues, identified by the screening history or physical examination, that place them at risk of illness or injury.

The scope of services provided by obstetric–gynecologic providers in the ambulatory setting will vary from practice to practice (see Box 3-1). For example, a practitioner may feel comfortable in providing preventive screening for healthy asymptomatic women, but not in treating chronic diseases. Therefore, it is important to clarify with the patient whether she has a primary care physician who will be providing medical care, preventive health services, and subspecialty referrals for issues that are outside the purview of her obstetrician–gynecologist. The scope of services provided in inpatient settings also varies depending on the obstetrician–gynecologist's training and experience. For example, in some hospitals a hospitalist may provide care for inpatients, or the gynecologic surgeon may not have privileges for a procedure that the patient requires.

The following sections review the broad range of women's health care needs addressed by obstetrician–gynecologists, including reproductive, medical, surgical, psychosocial, and preventive care. Also addressed are issues that play an important role in the delivery of women's health care, including access to health care and awareness of—and responsiveness to—women with diverse needs, such as women with disabilities. The clinical recommendations presented are based on the best available evidence (see also Appendix K). Information about U.S. organizations concerned with gynecology and women's health care is provided in Appendix L.

Box 3-1. Scope of Ambulatory Women's Health Care Services

Well-Woman Care
- Age-specific routine assessment (asymptomatic women)
- Immunizations
- Health status evaluation and counseling
  - Weight
  - Nutrition
  - Exercise
- Routine detection and prevention of disease
  - Cardiovascular disorders
  - Diabetes mellitus
  - Osteoporosis
  - Sexually transmitted infections
  - Substance use and abuse
- Psychosocial issues: early detection and management
  - Sexuality and sexual dysfunction
  - Depression and mood disorders; eating disorders
  - Intimate partner violence
  - Child abuse and neglect
  - Elder abuse and neglect
- Family planning
- Preconception care
- Menopausal management

(continued)

Box 3-1. Scope of Ambulatory Women's Health Care Services *(continued)*

Obstetrics
- Obstetric care: high and low risk

Gynecologic Services
- Initial and periodic evaluation and treatment of gynecologic conditions (including breast conditions)
- Abortion-related services
- Evaluation and treatment of incontinence
- Gynecologic ultrasonography
- Evaluation and treatment of endocrine dysfunction and infertility

Part III: Use of Ambulance ... Services

ACCESS TO CARE

The American College of Obstetricians and Gynecologists (the College) supports access to quality, affordable health care for women, and since 1971 has called for universal access to maternity care. The College believes a full array of clinical services should be available throughout a woman's life, without delays or the imposition of cultural, geographic, financial, or legal barriers. The College and its members are committed to facilitating the provision of and access to high-quality women's health care. The College focuses on the following principles as essential for meeting women's lifetime health needs:

- Health coverage should be accessible and affordable to everyone, with priority given to pregnant women and infants.

- A health care system should promote preventive care, provide continuity of care, and guarantee benefits regardless of employment, income, health status, or location.

- A successful health care system can build on the strengths of the private–public financing and delivery system.

- Coverage needs to be affordable for individuals, families, and businesses.

- Discrimination based on health status, gender, and other factors must be prohibited.

- Emphasizing prevention, reducing administrative costs, and enacting tort reform can help lower health care costs.

More than one half of women report delaying or avoiding needed care because of cost. Additionally, some women experience challenges in receiving coverage for critical services, such as maternity care. The Patient Protection and Affordable Care Act (ACA), the federal health care reform law passed in 2010, has the potential to improve access to care for millions of underserved women across the nation. Medicaid coverage is granted to very low-income women in most states, and subsidies are available for other low-income women to help purchase insurance coverage through health insurance exchanges. Insurers are prohibited from denying coverage because of preexisting conditions. Women no longer face increases in premium rates because of gender or health status. Through expansion of coverage, women up to age 26 years can be covered under their parents' insurance policies. Additionally, the ACA allows direct access to obstetrician–gynecologists, which facilitates women's health care service delivery, including access to maternity care and preconception care, as well as contraceptive services.

For many, the challenges to accessing health care are due to their lack of insurance or inadequate coverage, but barriers such as health care provider shortages and educational, cultural, and logistical factors also can compromise access to care. These obstacles to health care access, as well as proposed strategies to address them, are discussed in this section.

Increasing Access to High-Quality Care

The current lack of women's health care providers in the United States, believed to be due in part to the increasing costs of liability practice insurance and changes in practice patterns, is a growing concern around the country. In 2010, the national ratio of obstetrician–gynecologists per 10,000 women was 2.1, the lowest ratio in more than 30 years (2.3 in 1978, 2.5 in 1988, and 2.7 in 1993). Approximately one half (49%) of the 3,107 U.S. counties lack obstetrician–gynecologists, and nearly 9.5 million Americans live in those predominantly rural counties. Although there are nonobstetrician–gynecologist clinicians who provide care, such as certified nurse–midwives and family physicians, this statistic speaks to the lack of access.

Under the ACA, more women have access to health care, which increases pressure for the provision of care by a wide range of trained health care providers. These changing needs will require seamless integrated health care provider relationships across specialties. Obstetrician–gynecologists provide women's health care throughout the lifespan, often functioning as primary health care providers in a collaborative team. The College has long supported collaborative practice in an integrated, patient-focused health care delivery system to help ensure high-quality care. Such high-quality care depends on appropriately trained and certified health care providers, open communication and transparency, ongoing health care provider performance evaluation, use of evidence-based guidelines, and patient education. Exemplary systems of care with these characteristics should be identified and replicated. To ensure access to high-quality programs that meet the health care needs of all women, Fellows of the College should exercise their responsibility to improve the health status of women and their offspring in the traditional patient–physician relationships and by working within their communities at the local, state, and national levels.

Health Literacy

The problem of limited health literacy is widespread. Patient health literacy includes the ability to understand instructions on prescription drug bottles, appointment slips, patient education brochures, and consent forms and the ability to negotiate complex health care systems. Whereas approximately 10% of Americans have low general literacy (skills necessary to perform simple and everyday literacy activities), 50% of adults are estimated to have marginal health literacy skills to low health literacy skills. Patients with specific educational or linguistic challenges also may have limited health literacy. Senior citizens often have low health literacy skills and, therefore, poor comprehension of information on medication labels. On a broader level, a woman's health literacy may determine how or if she attempts to access the health care setting. This alone can be a significant obstacle to access to care.

At the level of the patient–clinician interaction, it is critical that health care providers understand the broad variation in health literacy that may affect the evaluation of patients and their adherence to treatment. Health care providers need to be able to assess a woman's health literacy and provide appropriate instructions and explanations about her care. Specific strategies for making health information understandable and accessible to all patients are included in the U.S. Department of Health and Human Services' Office of Disease Prevention and Health Promotion's *Quick Guide to Health Literacy* (see Resources), as well as in the "Patient Safety" section in Part 1.

At the systems level, responsibility for recognizing and addressing the problem of limited health literacy lies with all entities in the health care profession, from the primary health care team to public health care systems. Making information understandable and accessible to all patients involves a systematic approach toward health literacy in physicians' offices, hospitals, clinics, national organizations, local health organizations, advocacy organizations, medical and allied health professional schools, residency training programs, and continuing medical education programs. Because nursing and support staff are often the ones who identify the level of health literacy among patients, it is extremely important to also provide them with the appropriate training and resources so they can help navigate these patients through the health care system. Community-based partnerships to help understand and address the needs of the local community and consumer health information organizations to focus on the issue of health literacy are needed in the effort to improve health literacy. The U.S. Department of Health and Human Services' 2010 National Action Plan to Improve Health Literacy outlines goals and strategies to improve health literacy by engaging organizations, professionals, policymakers, communities, individuals, and families in a linked, multisector effort (see Resources).

Health Care for the Uninsured

Uninsured individuals often defer obtaining preventive and medical services, thus jeopardizing the health and well-being of themselves and their families. The need for universal health care coverage is urgent, given that a considerable and increasing portion of the U.S. population does not have health insurance.

The College supports universal coverage that is designed to improve the individual and collective health of society. The College has put forward the following five necessary principles to achieve universal health care that meets women's lifetime health needs: 1) cover everyone; 2) guarantee benefits; 3) engage employers, individuals, and governments; 4) make coverage affordable; and 5) enhance quality and patient safety.

The ACA addresses many of these principles, expanding coverage options and access to minimum essential health benefits, such as preventive care. For example, as of 2014, the ACA gave states the option to expand Medicaid to include individuals younger than 65 years with incomes up to 133% of the federal poverty level but also included a provision to disregard the first 5% of income, effectively extending Medicaid to all individuals with incomes up to 138% of the federal poverty level. The expansion of Medicaid is expected to result in improved access to health care, less delay in obtaining health care, better self-reported health, and reductions in mortality. The percentage of uninsured women aged 19–64 years could decrease from 20% to 8% if all states implement the Medicaid expansion, with enormous anticipated health benefits to women. The ACA also provides subsidies for individuals with incomes between 100% and 400% of the federal poverty level to help them purchase private health insurance. Despite the promise of the ACA to improve health insurance coverage, some populations may be left out. It is estimated that with full implementation of the ACA, 23 million individuals living in the United States who are younger than 65 years will remain uninsured. Approximately 25% of these individuals will be undocumented immigrants. Up to 16.2% will be legal residents who may be exempt from the individual mandate to purchase health insurance because the cost of insurance may be found to be unaffordable, even with subsidies. Accordingly, continued efforts to expand health coverage to all Americans must remain a high priority.

Health Care for Undocumented Immigrants

Adequate provision of health care to undocumented, immigrant women remains a problem. In 2010, an estimated 11.2 million undocumented immigrants were living in the United States. Many immigrants are of Hispanic ethnicity, and approximately one third of Hispanics lack health insurance. This same group also reports linguistic and cultural barriers. There is great variation among communities and among states in policies that concern undocumented, immigrant women and access to health care providers. Health care providers can play an important role in improving access to needed health care for undocumented immigrants through implementation of the following strategies:

- Helping society understand the importance of universal health care access
- Advocating for local, state, and national policy and legislation to secure quality, affordable coverage for all
- Supporting the safety net system and provision of care in the community and office setting for the uninsured
- Providing a comfortable office atmosphere with translators and materials available in languages appropriate for the patient population
- Becoming informed and involved in the College's government relations outreach activities. (For more information go to www.acog.org/About_ACOG/ACOG_Departments/Government_Relations_and_Outreach.)

Health Care for Homeless Women

Homelessness continues to be a significant problem in the United States. Women and families represent the fastest growing segment of the homeless population. Lack of access to health care is a profound issue for the homeless population. As a result, homeless women lack preventive care, such as prenatal care, mammograms, and Pap tests, compared with women who are not homeless. In addition, they have higher rates of poor health status, mental illness, poor birth outcomes, and mortality.

The factors that contribute to homeless women being unable to obtain needed health care include the lack of health insurance, the inability to purchase or acquire medications, the lack of knowledge of where and when to obtain health care, long wait times at medical facilities, and the lack of transportation to and from medical facilities. Mental illness, substance abuse, domestic violence, and being too sick to seek care create additional obstacles in obtaining needed services. Medical providers who do not want to care for homeless individuals in their offices and the lack of available treatment facilities result in limited access to health care. Inadequate inpatient discharge planning and follow-up care and lack of referral to services available within the community for homeless individuals also act as barriers.

Health care for homeless women is a challenge but an important issue that needs to be addressed. Strategies to help health care providers address the needs of homeless individuals include the following:

- Identify patients within the practice who may be homeless or at risk of becoming homeless (ie, ask about living conditions, nutrition, mental health issues, substance abuse, and domestic violence).

- Provide health care for these homeless women without bias, including preventive care, and do not withhold treatment based on concerns about lack of adherence.

- Become familiar with and inform patients who are (or at risk of becoming) homeless about appropriate community resources, including local substance abuse programs, domestic violence services, and social service agencies.

- Simplify medical regimens and address barriers, including transportation needs, for follow-up health care visits.

- Advocate for initiatives to address homelessness, such as increased funding for housing, case management services, substance abuse treatment, mental health services, domestic violence programs, and primary and preventive care for homeless individuals.

- Volunteer to provide health care services at homeless shelters and other facilities that serve homeless individuals.

- Increase access to long-acting reversible contraceptives.

The ACA has the potential to improve the health care of homeless individuals. Although it does not directly address the homeless population, under the ACA, a portion of the homeless population will qualify for Medicaid in states that opt to expand their Medicaid programs. There are certain Medicaid benefits that can play an important role in assisting individuals who are at risk of or experience chronic homelessness, including behavioral health services (which include mental health and substance abuse services), case management, personal care and personal assistance services, and home-based and community-based services. Increased health care coverage may lead to improved access and coordination of care. Additionally, increased coverage could result in benefits such as less uncompensated care for physicians and emergency departments, thus, lowering the health care costs of caring for homeless individuals.

Health Care for Women in the Military and Women Veterans

An increasing number of women are serving in the military, and a greater proportion of United States veterans are women. Because obstetrician–gynecologists may be the primary medical providers for women in the military and women veterans, they are in a position to interact with these women and intervene early and appropriately with their unique reproductive health care needs.

Women in the military and women veterans may seek primary and reproductive health care at military treatment facilities, through the U.S. Department of Defense's TRICARE program, at the civilian sector (through Medicaid, Medicare, or private insurance), through the U.S. Department of Veterans Affairs (VA), or some combination thereof. Connecting women veterans to services available through the VA may facilitate needed comprehensive health care; VA facilities may be located by consulting a web-based directory (www2.va.gov/directory/guide/vetcenter_flsh.asp). Women who are honorably discharged from the military may qualify for a variety of benefits through the VA, including health care benefits. This eligibility is based on multiple criteria (details are available at www.va.gov/healthbenefits/apply/veterans.asp). Many mechanisms are in place to support the health needs of women veterans. Each Veterans Health Administration facility nationwide has a designated women veterans program manager who advocates for women and provides leadership in establishing, coordinating, and integrating quality health care services for women. Many VA sites have specialized women's health clinics and services available to provide care for women veterans either onsite or through referrals to non-VA health care providers.

Partnerships between academic departments of obstetrics and gynecology and local branches of the Veterans Health Administration are encouraged as a means of optimizing the provision of comprehensive health care to women veterans. This will allow all health care providers who treat women veterans to ensure that veterans in their care are aware of health care resources offered through the VA and to provide referrals as needed. Such collaboration offers unique opportunities to share best practices, foster the development and implementation of a robust research agenda regarding the reproductive health care needs of women veterans, and enhance delivery and coordination of care.

Bibliography

Allen J, Bharel M, Brammer S, Centrone W, Morrison S, Phillips C, et al. Adapting your practice: treatment and recommendations on reproductive health care for homeless patients. Nashville (TN): Health Care for the Homeless Clinicians' Network, National Health Care for the Homeless Council,Inc.; 2008. Available at: http://www.nhchc.org/wp-content/uploads/2011/09/ReproductiveHealth.pdf. Retrieved May 29, 2013.

American College of Obstetricians and Gynecologists. Health care for women, health care for all: a reform agenda. Washington, DC: ACOG; 2008. Available at: http://www.acog.org/~/media/Departments/Resource%20Center/HCFWHCFA-ReformPrinciples.pdf?dmc=1&ts=20130905T1010044353. Retrieved September 5, 2013.

American Medical Association. Physician characteristics and distribution in the U.S, 2013. Chicago (IL): AMA; 2013.

American Medical Association. The Affordable Care Act. Available at: http://www.ama-assn.org/ama/pub/advocacy/topics/affordable-care-act.page?. Retrieved August 13, 2013.

Benefits to women of Medicaid expansion through the Affordable Care Act. Committee Opinion No. 552. American College of Obstetricians and Gynecologists. Obstet Gynecol 2013;121:223–5.

Berg CJ, Harper MA, Atkinson SM, Bell EA, Brown HL, Hage ML, et al. Preventability of pregnancy-related deaths: results of a state-wide review. Obstet Gynecol 2005;106:1228–34.

Buettgens M, Hall MA. Who will be uninsured after health insurance reform? Princeton (NJ): Robert Wood Johnson Foundation; 2011. Available at: http://www.rwjf.org/content/dam/farm/reports/issue_briefs/2011/rwjf69624. Retrieved July 22, 2013.

Centers for Medicare and Medicaid Services. Affordable Care Act: eligibility. Available at: http://www.medicaid.gov/AffordableCareAct/Provisions/Eligibility. html. Retrieved July 22, 2013.

Community involvement and volunteerism. ACOG Committee Opinion No. 437. American College of Obstetricians and Gynecologists. Obstet Gynecol 2009;114: 203–4.

Gusmano MK. Undocumented immigrants in the United States: demographics and socioeconomic status. Garrison (NY): Hastings Center; 2012. Available at: http://www.undocumentedpatients.org/issuebrief/demographics-and-socioeconomic-status. Retrieved July 22, 2013.

Health care for homeless women. Committee Opinion No. 576. American College of Obstetricians and Gynecologists. Obstet Gynecol 2013;122:936–40.

Health care for undocumented immigrants. ACOG Committee Opinion No. 425. American College of Obstetricians and Gynecologists. Obstet Gynecol 2009; 113:251–4.

Health care for women in the military and women veterans. Committee Opinion No. 547. American College of Obstetricians and Gynecologists. Obstet Gynecol 2012;120:1538–42.

Health care systems for underserved women. Committee Opinion No. 516. American College of Obstetricians and Gynecologists. Obstet Gynecol 2012;119:206–9.

Health literacy. Committee Opinion No. 585. American College of Obstetricians and Gynecologists. Obstet Gynecol 2014;123:380–3.

Passel JS. The size and characteristics of the unauthorized migrant population in the U.S.: estimates based on the March 2005 Current Population Survey. Washington, DC: Pew Hispanic Center; 2006. Available at: http://www.pewhispanic.org/files/reports/61.pdf. Retrieved September 5, 2013.

Professional liability and gynecology-only practice. Committee Opinion No. 567. American College of Obstetricians and Gynecologists. Obstet Gynecol 2013; 122:186.

Rayburn WF. The obstetrician-gynecologist workforce in the United States: facts, figures, and implications 2011. Washington, DC: American Congress of Obstetricians and Gynecologists; 2011.

Sommers BD, Baicker K, Epstein AM. Mortality and access to care among adults after state Medicaid expansions. N Engl J Med 2012;367:1025–34.

The Henry J. Kaiser Family Foundation. Health reform: frequently asked questions: Who will be eligible for subsidies to make health insurance more affordable? Menlo Park (CA): KFF; 2013. Available at: http://kff.org/health-reform/faq/health-reform-frequently-asked-questions/. Retrieved September 5, 2013.

The uninsured. ACOG Committee Opinion No. 416. American College of Obstetricians and Gynecologists. Obstet Gynecol 2008;112:731–4.

Resources

American College of Obstetricians and Gynecologists. Access to women's health care. College Statement of Policy. Washington, DC: ACOG; 2013.

American Congress of Obstetricians and Gynecologists. Government relations and outreach. Washington, DC: American Congress of Obstetricians and Gynecologists; 2013. Available at: http://www.acog.org/About_ACOG/ACOG_Departments/Government_Relations_and_Outreach. Retrieved July 16, 2013.

American Congress of Obstetricians and Gynecologists. Health system reform: the law, your practice, your patients. Washington, DC: American Congress of Obstetricians and Gynecologists; 2010. Available at: http://www.acog.org/About_ACOG/ACOG_Departments/Health_Care_Reform. Retrieved July 16, 2013.

American Congress of Obstetricians and Gynecologists. Practice management and managed care. Washington, DC: American Congress of Obstetricians and Gynecologists; 2013. Available at: http://www.acog.org/About_ACOG/ACOG_Departments/Practice_Management_and_Managed_Care. Retrieved July 16, 2013.

Department of Health and Human Services, Office of Disease Prevention and Health Promotion. National action plan to improve health literacy. Washington, DC: HHS; Available at: http://www.health.gov/communication/HLActionPlan/pdf/Health_Literacy_Action_Plan.pdf. Retrieved July 22, 2013.

Department of Health and Human Services, Office of Disease Prevention and Health Promotion. Quick guide to health literacy. Available at: http://www.health.gov/communication/literacy/quickguide/Quickguide.pdf. Retrieved July 22, 2013.

Department of Veterans Affairs. Health benefits: veteran eligibility. Available at: http://www.va.gov/healthbenefits/apply/veterans.asp. Retrieved July 22, 2013.

Department of Veterans Affairs. Vet centers - locations. Available at: http://www2.va.gov/directory/guide/vetcenter_flsh.asp. Retrieved July 22, 2013.

Ethical considerations for performing gynecologic surgery in low-resource settings abroad. Committee Opinion No. 466. American College of Obstetricians and Gynecologists. Obstet Gynecol 2010;116:793–9.

World Health Organization. Sexual and reproductive health. Available at: http://www.who.int/reproductivehealth/en. Retrieved July 22, 2013.

WELL-WOMAN ANNUAL HEALTH ASSESSMENT

The annual health assessment ("annual examination") is a fundamental part of medical care and is valuable in promoting prevention practices, recognizing risk factors for disease, identifying medical problems, and establishing the patient–physician relationship. New recommendations and improving technologies continue to influence guidelines and the necessary components of the annual health assessment of women. Recommendations are based on the available evidence (Appendix L).

Recommendations for preventive services have been issued by a number of health care organizations in addition to the American College of Obstetricians and Gynecologists (the College) and differ somewhat in their specifics. The Agency for Healthcare Research and Quality acts in part as a clearinghouse for evidence-based clinical practice guidelines, thus providing a readily available means for clinicians to compare different guidelines for a specific medical condition or intervention. The National Guideline Clearinghouse can be found at www.guideline.gov.

The recommendations discussed in this section have been selected from many sources, and they describe routine assessments for women based on age group and risk factors. (Adolescent preventive services are addressed in the "Adolescents" section later in Part 3.) These assessments, yearly or as appropriate, include screening, evaluation, counseling, and immunizations. Variations to routine assessments may be required to adjust to the needs of a specific individual. For example, certain risk factors may influence additional assessments and interventions. During evaluation, the patient should be made aware of high-risk conditions that require targeted screening or treatment. The College has comprehensive recommendations and resources for the annual health assessment of women available online at www.acog.org/wellwoman.

Importance of the Annual Visit

Obstetrician–gynecologists have a tradition of providing preventive care to women. An annual visit provides an excellent opportunity to counsel patients about maintaining a healthy lifestyle and minimizing health risks. Annual visits for reproductive and well-woman care are recommended, even if individual components of that visit (eg, cervical cancer screening) may not be indicated each year. The annual health assessment should include screening, evaluation and counseling, and immunizations based on age and risk factors. The interval for specific individual services may vary for individual patients, and the scope of services provided may vary in different ambulatory care settings. The performance of a physical examination is a key part of an annual visit, and the components of that examination may vary depending on the patient's age, risk factors, and physician preference. In general, the physical examination will include obtaining standard vital signs, determining body mass index (BMI), palpating the abdomen and inguinal lymph nodes, and making an assessment of the patient's overall health. Many, but not all, women will have a pelvic examination and a clinical breast examination as a part of the physical examination. Information on these core elements of the physical examination is provided later in this section.

In particular, adolescents, the elderly, and individuals with medical, psychologic, or social issues may have needs that require more than the standard time allotted. It may not be possible to address all of the patient's concerns in one visit; the physician and patient will need to prioritize medical problems, and additional visits may need to be scheduled. In addition, if a clinician believes that a patient's health interests are jeopardized by the policies of her medical insurance plan, he or she should consider making an appeal to the plan or medical director.

The decision to perform an internal pelvic examination, breast examination, or both should be made by the physician and the patient after shared communication and decision making. Concerns, such as individual risk factors, patient expectations, or medical–legal concerns may influence the decision to perform an internal pelvic examination or clinical breast examination. In these situations, the medical record should reflect the pertinent details of the patient's medical and family history and overall condition, documentation of the physical examination, and the issues discussed between the patient and physician. The decision to perform any type of pelvic or breast examination should always be made with the consent of the patient.

Medical History

A comprehensive medical record should be kept and updated periodically, including medical history, physical examination, and laboratory and radiology results. Information from referrals and other medical services outside the purview of the obstetrician–gynecologist should be integrated into the medical record.

CONDUCTING AN INTERVIEW

The diagnostic process begins when the health care provider meets the patient. When obtaining the patient's medical history, the health care provider should greet the patient by title and name, make eye contact, shake hands, and be welcoming. The physical environment can enhance the quality of the interview. Whenever possible, the interview should take place in a quiet, private, well-lit room with comfortable and adequate space and seating, with the patient dressed. Instruments that may be intimidating should be covered.

As much as possible, allow the patient to express her story in her own words. Listen without interruption, and be aware that the presence of family members could be an impediment to an honest interview, especially in cases of intimate partner violence. If the family is present, include time in the interview for a private conversation in the absence of family members. Communication is the key to a successful medical history interview (see Box 3-2). The health care provider should make the patient comfortable enough to speak freely, and the questions should be understood easily and be tailored to the individual patient. The help of a medically trained interpreter should be sought for patients who do not easily understand or speak the language or languages in which the clinician is fluent. Use of family members as translators is discouraged because of issues of privacy, confidentiality, and bias and the sensitive nature of many issues of women's health. For those who do not speak English, efforts should be

Box 3-2. The RESPECT Communication Model

Rapport
Connect on a social level.
See the patient's point of view.
Consciously suspend judgment.
Recognize and avoid making assumptions.

Empathy
Remember that the patient has come to you for help.
Seek out and understand the patient's rationale for her behaviors or illness.
Verbally acknowledge and legitimize the patient's feelings.

Support
Ask about and understand the barriers to care and compliance.
Help the patient overcome barriers.
Involve family members, if appropriate.
Reassure the patient that you are and will be able to help.

Partnership
Be flexible with regard to control issues.
Negotiate roles, when necessary.
Stress that you are working together to address health problems.

Explanations
Check often for understanding.
Use verbal clarification techniques.

Cultural Competence
Respect the patient's cultural beliefs.
Understand that the patient's view of you may be defined by ethnic or cultural stereotypes.
Be aware of your own cultural biases and preconceptions.
Know your limitations in addressing medical issues across cultures.
Understand your personal style and recognize when it may not be working with a given patient.

Trust
Recognize that self-disclosure may be difficult for some patients.
Consciously work to establish trust.

Modified with permission from Mutha S, Allen C, Welch M. Toward culturally competent care: a toolbox for teaching communication strategies. San Francisco (CA): Center for the Health Professions, University of California; 2002.

made to provide written translations of forms and patient education materials. In some circumstances, federal and state laws and regulations impose responsibilities on health care providers to accommodate individuals with limited English proficiency.

The goal of a medical history interview is to gather pertinent and basic information about the patient's health status. A health care provider should consider all aspects of the patient's presentation and condition and prioritize areas for further evaluation. The health care provider should be aware of the influence of social, economic, and cultural factors in shaping the nature of the patient's concerns and her descriptions of health status and symptoms. Issues of cultural competency and barriers to effective communication must be examined and addressed when developing patient communication and documentation systems. Clinicians and staff members should be aware of the "culture of medicine" and their own cultural attitudes. Increased sensitivity to cultural issues can facilitate more positive interactions and help the patient feel comfortable with her health care team. Patient communication procedures should respect cultural differences in the role of the extended family in health care decision making, religious beliefs, and the role of traditional and alternative remedies. In addition, clinicians should be attuned to the possible intimidation that may be felt by patients with little exposure to the health care system. The volume of paperwork and the use of professional jargon often associated with health care information systems can be overwhelming.

Mutual trust and respect in the patient–clinician relationship helps to facilitate a complete history. This is particularly important when addressing questions and concerns about sexuality. An awareness by the clinician of his or her own biases and a nonjudgmental approach by the clinician are essential for effective counseling. Box 3-3 includes an example of a sexual history questionnaire from the College's Women's Health Record (see also the "Sexual Function and Dysfunction" section in Part 4).

Many common diseases that affect women's health can be moderated or controlled by behavioral change. However, effectively promoting changes in a patient's behavior, such as dietary and exercise habits, alcohol use, or sexual practices, can be difficult for the health care provider and the patient. The use of motivational interviewing techniques has been shown

---

Box 3-3. Sexual History Questions

- Have you ever had sex? ___
- Are you currently sexually active (vaginal, oral, anal)? ___
- Number of sexual partners (lifetime): ___
- Sexual partners are: ___men ___women ___both
- Sexual orientation and gender identity: ___heterosexual ___homosexual ___bisexual ___transgendered
- Relationship status: ___married ___living with partner ___single ___widowed ___divorced
- Number of people in household: ___
- Have you been sexually abused, threatened, or hurt by anyone? ___

Reprinted from American College of Obstetricians and Gynecologists. The women's health record. Washington, DC: American College of Obstetricians and Gynecologists; 2011.

---

to be effective in promoting behavioral change. With this technique, the physician helps the patient identify the thoughts and feelings that cause her to continue unhealthy behaviors and helps her to develop new thought patterns to aid in behavior change. This technique is implemented most effectively after the physician has established a trusting rapport with the patient. By expressing empathy, providing personalized feedback, and supporting the patient's ability to help herself, the physician creates an effective interaction for helping promote behavioral changes and better health.

CONTENT OF THE MEDICAL HISTORY

Information contained in the medical history includes discussions of the chief complaint, history of present illness, review of systems, history of past illnesses, family history, social history, and sexual history. Because many patients are reluctant to volunteer problems of urinary and fecal incontinence, substance use, sexual dysfunction, or current or past intimate partner violence, abuse, or sexual assault, women should routinely be asked about these conditions. Direct and behaviorally specific questions generally result in more accurate responses about these sensitive issues (see also the "Abuse" section later in Part 3).

In 1995 and 1997, the Health Care Financing Administration (currently known as the Centers for Medicare & Medicaid Services [CMS]) developed Medicare documentation guidelines for problem-oriented evaluation and management services (see the CMS Medicare Learning Network at www.cms.gov/MLNGenInfo). These guidelines, developed jointly by the American Medical Association and the CMS, provide physicians and claims reviewers with advice about preparing or reviewing such documentation. Physicians can use either the 1995 or 1997 guidelines, depending on which one is most appropriate for their practice. The difference between the two sets of guidelines is in the examination only. Many practices have modified their medical records to reflect the requirements specified by the CMS, and these requirements typically are included in electronic health records. These requirements are reflected in the Woman's Health Record produced by the College.

The levels of services described by the CMS are based on four types of history: 1) problem focused, 2) expanded problem focused, 3) detailed, and 4) comprehensive. Each type of history includes some or all of the following elements:

- Chief complaint
- History of present illness
- Review of systems
- Past, family, and social history

The extent of history of present illness; review of systems; and past, family, and social history that is obtained and documented depends on clinical judgment and the nature of the presenting problem.

Chief Complaint

The chief complaint is a concise statement describing the symptom, problem, condition, diagnosis, physician-recommended return, or other factor that is the reason for the encounter. It usually is stated in the patient's words.

History of Present Illness

The history of present illness is a chronologic description of the development of the patient's present illness. It describes the illness from the first sign or symptom or from the previous encounter to the present.

Review of Systems

The review of systems is an inventory of body systems that is obtained through a series of questions seeking to identify signs and symptoms that the patient may be experiencing or have experienced. For example, a history related to breast disorders would include duration, onset, and cyclicity of signs and symptoms, including any breast discharge; menstrual and reproductive history; hormone use; dietary habits; and breast surgery, including implants. The Woman's Health Record published by the College includes a review of the systems recognized by the CMS. The importance of the review of systems is highlighted in the case of ovarian cancer; a high index of suspicion for persistent and progressive symptoms, such as an increase in bloating, pelvic or abdominal pain, or difficulty eating or feeling full quickly, provides the best way to detect early ovarian cancer.

Past, Family, and Social History

The past, family, and social history consists of a review of general medical, surgical, obstetric and gynecologic history; family health history; allergies; current medications; and sexual and social history. Clinicians also should ask patients about their level of physical activity (eg, frequency, intensity, and timing), provide counseling to promote a healthy weight and lifestyle, and document this in the patient's medical record (see also the "Fitness" section later in Part 3).

Implementation of a medication reconciliation process is a National Patient Safety goal of The Joint Commission. After the patient provides and the clinician documents a list of the patient's current medications, a process is required to compare this list to a list of new medications to be provided. In addition, The Joint Commission requires that a complete list of the patient's medications be communicated to the next provider of care when a patient is referred or transferred.

Patients should be asked about their use of or exposure to substances that could be harmful to their health. Asking patients questions about their use of "medications" or "drugs" may not elicit answers related to the use of over-the-counter medications or complementary and alternative medicines. Most patients who use complementary and alternative medicines do not tell their physicians they are doing so. Thus, their medical record is incomplete, and the possibility of medical risk cannot be adequately addressed. Patients can be asked questions similar to "Have you used, or have you been considering using, other kinds of treatment or medications for relief of your symptoms or to maintain wellness?" Follow-up questions to a positive answer can include asking when the patient decided to use complementary or alternative medicines, what results she was expecting, how she chose the method, and how it has worked for her. This information then can be documented in the patient's medical record (see also the "Complementary and Alternative Medicine" section later in Part 3).

General Physical Examination

The general physical examination serves to detect abnormalities suggested by the medical history as well as unsuspected problems. Specific information the patient gives during the history should guide the practitioner to areas of physical examination that may not be surveyed in a routine screening. The extent of the examination is based on the practitioner's clinical relationship with the patient, what is being medically managed by other clinicians, and what is medically indicated. Once a problem has been identified, intervention can take the form of behavior modification, additional monitoring, treatment, or referral, as necessary. The focus of a preoperative examination will depend on the procedure (see also the "Ambulatory Gynecologic Surgery" section in Part 4).

The recommendations for periodic health assessment from the College include weight, height, and blood pressure measurements. Body mass index, which takes into account height and weight and provides the best general assessment of weight, should be calculated. (Calculations for BMI and a link to a BMI calculator are provided in the "Fitness" section later in Part 3.) Clinicians should offer patients appropriate interventions or referrals to promote a healthy weight and lifestyle (see also the "Fitness" section later in Part 3). Classification of blood pressure should be based on the average of two or more readings (see also the "Cardiovascular Disorders" section later in Part 3).

Clinical Breast Examination

For women aged 20–39 years, the performance of a clinical breast examination is recommended every 1–3 years. A clinical breast examination should be performed annually for women aged 40 years and older. Detailed recommendations for the performance of clinical breast examinations are available (see Bibliography). Currently, there is an evolution away from teaching breast self-examination and toward the concept of breast self-awareness. The College, the American Cancer Society, and the National Comprehensive Cancer Network endorse breast self-awareness, which is defined as women's awareness of the normal appearance and feel of their breasts. Breast self-awareness should be encouraged and can include breast self-examination. Breast self-examination instruction should be considered for high-risk patients. Women should report any changes in their breasts to their health care providers.

The clinical breast examination involves both visual assessment of skin changes and palpation. A visual examination should be performed while the patient is sitting or standing with her hands on her hips. The axillary and supraclavicular areas should be palpated to detect adenopathy. To assess any palpable dominant mass, the examiner should use the fingertips to palpate all of the breast tissue, including the axilla, with the patient in the upright and supine positions. The presence of nipple discharge should be ascertained by gentle pressure. A palpable mass, skin changes, breast pain, or nonlactational nipple discharge requires evaluation, which may include a follow-up examination or additional diagnostic testing (see also the "Cancer Screening and Prevention" section later in Part 3).

Patients should be encouraged to undergo screening by mammography in accordance with College guidelines (see also the "Cancer Screening and Prevention" section later in Part 3). Women should be educated about the predictive value of screening mammography and the potential for false-positive or false-negative results. Women should be informed of the potential for additional imaging or biopsies that may be recommended based on screening results.

Obstetrician–gynecologists may diagnose and manage (consistent with their training and experience) or refer for treatment those patients with a solid or cystic breast mass, a mammographic abnormality, breast pain, physiologic and abnormal nipple discharge, mastitis, or fibrocystic changes of the breast (see also the "Cancer Diagnosis and Management" section in Part 4). Institutions that grant physicians privileges to perform breast surgery should apply the same criteria for privileging to obstetrician–gynecologists as to other physicians.

When a nonpalpable mass is perceived on screening mammography, the patient should be referred to a professional experienced in the diagnosis of breast cancer. When a patient is referred to another physician for diagnostic testing or consultation, the obstetrician–gynecologist should ensure that the patient is provided with the following:

- An explanation that she needs further care
- The names of qualified physicians from whom the patient can receive care
- An opportunity to have her questions answered
- A summary of the history, physical examination, and diagnostic tests performed
- Information for the consultant if diagnostic imaging is required for a reason of clinical concern rather than merely routine screening

Documentation of these steps and a description of the clinical findings should be included in the medical record.

Pelvic Examination

The pelvic examination includes three elements: 1) inspection of the external genitalia, urethral meatus, vaginal introitus, and perianal region (external examination); 2) speculum examination of the vagina and cervix; and 3) bimanual examination of the uterus, cervix, and adnexa (the latter two elements constitute the internal examination). When indicated, a rectovaginal examination also should be performed. Annual pelvic examination of patients 21 years of age or older is recommended by the College. At this time, this recommendation is based on expert opinion, and limitations of the internal pelvic examination should be recognized. A pelvic examination always is an appropriate component of a comprehensive evaluation of any patient who reports or exhibits symptoms suggestive of female genital tract, pelvic, urologic, or rectal problems.

EXTERNAL EXAMINATION

After emptying her bladder, the patient should be assisted to the lithotomy position and properly draped. Other positions may be appropriate, depending on the age or physical limitations of the patient (see also the "Pediatric Gynecology" section and the "Women With Disabilities" section later in Part 3). Careful inspection of the vulva and perianal area with adequate lighting is performed first. The labia are then gently separated to allow visualization of the urethral meatus and introitus. The clinician should carefully note and record any pertinent findings.

SPECULUM EXAMINATION

After the external examination, a warm speculum of appropriate size should be inserted gently into the vagina, with posterior pressure against the perineal and levator muscles until the cervix can be visualized entirely. If the speculum does not pass easily, it may be moistened with water. If lubricant is used, care should be taken to avoid contaminating any sample, because lubricant can interfere with the interpretation of results of conventional cervical cytologic studies and with the growth of microorganisms if a culture is taken. After adequate inspection of the cervix and vaginal fornices has been performed, the speculum should be slowly removed so that the vaginal walls can be inspected.

If appropriate, a sample for cervical cancer screening is obtained (see also the "Cancer Screening and Prevention" section later in Part 3). If abnormal vaginal or cervical discharge is noted, or if the history indicates, appropriate sample collection and testing for sexually transmitted infections should be performed. Routine annual screening for chlamydial infection and gonorrhea is recommended for all sexually active women aged 25 years and younger and for other asymptomatic women at high risk of infection (see also the "Sexually Transmitted Infections" section later in Part 3). Nucleic acid amplification tests for gonorrhea and chlamydial infection can be performed on urine or vaginal swab specimens. If a pelvic examination is not indicated, appropriate screening for chlamydial infection and gonorrhea may still be carried out with a self-collected vaginal swab or a first-catch urine specimen.

BIMANUAL EXAMINATION

After completion of the speculum examination, a bimanual examination is carried out to evaluate the vagina and the cervix and the size, shape, and position of the uterus. The adnexa are then examined for size, shape, and tenderness.

When indicated, a rectovaginal examination should be performed as the last part of the examination to evaluate the rectovaginal septum, the posterior uterine surface, the adnexal structures, the uterosacral ligaments, and the posterior cul-de-sac. Uterosacral nodularity or posterior uterine tenderness associated with pelvic endometriosis can be assessed in this manner. In addition, this examination may identify hemorrhoids, anal fissures, sphincter tone, and possible rectal polyps or carcinoma. Taking a stool sample for fecal occult blood testing during the digital rectal examination is not recommended because it is not adequate for the detection of colorectal cancer (see also the "Cancer Screening and Prevention" section later in Part 3).

Bibliography

American College of Obstetricians and Gynecologists. Contemporary perspectives on breast health. Washington, DC: ACOG; 2005.

American College of Obstetricians and Gynecologists. The women's health record. Washington, DC: American College of Obstetricians and Gynecologists; 2011.

Breast cancer screening. Practice Bulletin No. 122. American College of Obstetricians and Gynecologists. Obstet Gynecol 2011;118:372–82.

Cultural sensitivity and awareness in the delivery of health care. Committee Opinion No. 493. American College of Obstetricians and Gynecologists. Obstet Gynecol 2011;117:1258–61.

Department of Health and Human Services, Office of Minority Health. National standards for culturally and linguistically appropriate services in health and health care: a blueprint for advancing and sustaining CLAS policy and practice. Rockville (MD): OMH; 2013. Available at: https://www.thinkculturalhealth.hhs.gov/pdfs/ EnhancedCLASStandardsBlueprint.pdf. Retrieved September 26, 2013.

Effective patient-physician communication. Committee Opinion No. 587. American College of Obstetricians and Gynecologists. Obstet Gynecol 2014;123:389–93.

Health literacy. Committee Opinion No. 585. American College of Obstetricians and Gynecologists. Obstet Gynecol 2014;123:380–3.

Motivational interviewing: a tool for behavioral change. ACOG Committee Opinion No. 423. American College of Obstetricians and Gynecologists. Obstet Gynecol 2009;113:243–6.

Mutha S, Allen C, Welch M. Toward culturally competent care: a toolbox for teaching communication strategies. San Francisco (CA): Center for the Health Professions, University of California; 2002.

Papp JR, Schachter J, Gaydos CA, Van Der Pol B. Recommendations for the laboratory-based detection of Chlamydia trachomatis and Neisseria gonorrhoeae–2014. Division of STD Prevention, National Center for HIV/AIDS, Viral Hepatitis, STD, and TB Prevention, CDC. MMWR Recomm Rep 2014;63(RR02):1–19.

The role of the obstetrician-gynecologist in the early detection of epithelial ovarian cancer. Committee Opinion No. 477. American College of Obstetricians and Gynecologists. Obstet Gynecol 2011;117:742–6.

Well-woman visit. Committee Opinion No. 534. American College of Obstetricians and Gynecologists. Obstet Gynecol 2012;120:421–4.

Resources

Agency for Healthcare Research and Quality. Guide to clinical preventive services, 2012. Recommendations of the U.S. Preventive Services Task Force. Rockville (MD): AHRQ; 2011. Available at: http://www.ahrq.gov/professionals/clinicians-providers/ guidelines-recommendations/guide/index.html. Retrieved July 22, 2013.

Agency for Healthcare Research and Quality. Prevention and chronic care. Available at: http://www.ahrq.gov/professionals/prevention-chronic-care/index.html. Retrieved July 22, 2013.

American College of Obstetricians and Gynecologists. Annual women's health care. Available at: http://www.acog.org/wellwoman. Retrieved October 1, 2013.

American College of Obstetricians and Gynecologists. Benign breast problems and conditions. Patient Education Pamphlet AP026. Washington, DC: American College of Obstetricians and Gynecologists; 2012.

American College of Obstetricians and Gynecologists. Cervical cancer screening. Patient Education Pamphlet AP085. Washington, DC: American College of Obstetricians and Gynecologists; 2013.

American College of Obstetricians and Gynecologists. Making the most of your health care visit. Patient Education Fact Sheet PFS001. Washington, DC: American College of Obstetricians and Gynecologists; 2011. Available at: http://www.acog.org/For_Patients/Search_FAQs/documents/Making_the_Most_of_Your_Health_Care_Visit. Retrieved September 4, 2013.

American College of Obstetricians and Gynecologists. Screening for breast problems. Patient Education Pamphlet AP178. Washington, DC: American College of Obstetricians and Gynecologists; 2012.

Centers for Medicare and Medicaid Services. 1997 documentation guidelines for evaluation and management services. Baltimore (MD): CMS; 1997. Available at: http://www.cms.gov/Outreach-and-Education/Medicare-Learning-Network-MLN/MLNEdWebGuide/Downloads/97Docguidelines.pdf. Retrieved July 22, 2013.

Coleman VH, Laube DW, Hale RW, Williams SB, Power ML, Schulkin J. Obstetrician-gynecologists and primary care: training during obstetrics-gynecology residency and current practice patterns. Acad Med 2007;82:602–7.

Maciosek MV, Coffield AB, Edwards NM, Flottemesch TJ, Goodman MJ, Solberg LI. Priorities among effective clinical preventive services: results of a systematic review and analysis. Am J Prev Med 2006;31:52–61.

National Heart, Lung, and Blood Institute. Available at: http://www.nhlbi.nih.gov. Retrieved September 10, 2013.

Saslow D, Hannan J, Osuch J, Alciati MH, Baines C, Barton M, et al. Clinical breast examination: practical recommendations for optimizing performance and reporting. CA Cancer J Clin 2004;54:327–44.

The Joint Commission. Comprehensive accreditation manual for ambulatory care : CAMAC. Oakbrook Terrace (IL): The Commission; 2014.

The Joint Commission. Comprehensive accreditation manual for hospitals: CAMH. Oakbrook Terrace (IL): The Commission; 2014.

Yarnall KS, Pollak KI, Ostbye T, Krause KM, Michener JL. Primary care: is there enough time for prevention? Am J Public Health 2003;93:635–41.

IMMUNIZATIONS

In the United States, vaccination programs that focus on infants and children have decreased the occurrence of many vaccine-preventable diseases. However, many adolescents and adults continue to be affected adversely by vaccine-preventable diseases, such as influenza, pertussis, varicella, hepatitis A, hepatitis B, human papillomavirus (HPV), measles, mumps, rubella, and pneumococcal pneumonia. In part, this is because vaccine programs have not focused on improving vaccination coverage. The following four factors have contributed to the low level of immunization in adults: 1) a disinterest by the general public and physicians in adult immunization because of the attitude that immunization is for children, 2) misconceptions about the safety and efficacy of vaccines compared with the consequences of the diseases, 3) concerns about liability, and 4) a poorly developed immunization system. The approval of vaccines against HPV has made the topic of immunization particularly relevant to obstetrician–gynecologists, and vaccines against HPV are discussed in some detail later in this section. For information on immunization of health care providers, see the "Human Resources" section in Part 1.

The American College of Obstetricians and Gynecologists (the College) has developed the dedicated immunization web site Immunization for Women (available at www.immunizationforwomen.org) to provide up-to-date information and resources to help obstetrician–gynecologists become routine vaccinators. The College's guide *Immunization Coding for Obstetrician–Gynecologists* addresses reimbursement and coding for vaccinations and includes coding examples and other coding resources. For additional sources of College information on immunization, see Resources at the end of this section.

Integrating Immunizations Into Practice

Given demonstrated vaccine efficacy, safety, and the large potential for prevention of many infectious diseases, obstetrician–gynecologists and other women's health care providers should embrace immunizations as an integral part of their practice. Physician recommendation has been shown to be a very effective way to ensure patients accept vaccinations. Physicians also can provide vaccinations or referrals to vaccination clinics or services, when indicated. The combination of recommending immunization and offering the vaccine at the same time has proved to be the most effective strategy for patient acceptance.

Obstetrician–gynecologists and other clinicians who provide well-woman examinations and preconception care have opportunities in which to counsel women on the need for immunizations. It is helpful to ask new patients who are scheduling well-woman examinations or preconception counseling to bring previous vaccination records. Clinicians should attempt to gather a complete immunization history from each woman, including risk factors indicating the need for immunization; they also should attempt to obtain previous records. If there are doubts about past immunizations, it is safest to assume that a woman has not been immunized and to initiate the appropriate vaccination or vaccination series.

The vaccination of adolescents poses unique challenges for obstetrician–gynecologists related to privacy, confidentiality, and informed consent. College Fellows should respect the importance of protecting adolescents' access to reproductive health care services, including HPV vaccination, while complying with local and national professional norms and applicable legal requirements.

The following are recommended key strategies for integrating immunizations into practice:

- Talk with patients directly and recommend indicated immunizations (see "Recommended Immunizations and Schedules" later in this section).

- Designate a vaccine coordinator in the office and identify a backup coordinator who is trained in the event that the designated coordinator is absent. Among other duties, the vaccine coordinator orders the vaccines, receives vaccine deliveries, and ensures that vaccines are stored properly.

- Document that recommended vaccines have been offered, that patients have been educated on indicated immunizations, and that patients accepted, refused, or obtained their vaccines at an outside facility.

- Always give a vaccine information statement (VIS) for all vaccines recommended by the Advisory Committee on Immunization Practices of the Centers for Disease Control and Prevention (CDC) before vaccine administration (see "Vaccine Information Statements" later in this section).

- When a vaccine has been administered, record the following information in the patient's permanent medical record (or a permanent office log):
  — The name, address, and title of the person who administered the vaccine
  — The date of administration
  — The vaccine manufacturer
  — The lot number of the vaccine used

- Use prompts, paper or electronic, to help remind staff and health care providers which patients are due for immunizations (see also the "Information Management" section in Part 2).

If financial or business concerns limit a physician's ability to provide vaccinations in his or her practice, the physician should provide information about alternative sources for vaccination and, when possible, refer patients to alternative community sources, such as state or local health department clinics.

Rarely, vaccine availability can be limited because of increased demand, decreased supply, or both. In cases of limited availability, allocation strategies may be developed by health care or regulatory authorities to prioritize vaccine administration to specific subsets of the population. It is critical that health care providers understand and comply with these guidelines and recommendations regarding vaccination and allocation. Health care providers should be prepared to explain to patients the importance of, and the rationale for, allocation mechanisms while continuing to address their patients' health care needs through alternative strategies other than vaccination.

RECOMMENDED IMMUNIZATIONS AND SCHEDULES

The current CDC immunization schedules, which are approved by the College, can be found online at www.cdc.gov/vaccines/schedules/hcp/adult.html. A listing of the College's recommended routine immunizations for women without risk factors by age group is available at the College's Immunization for Women web site at www.immunizationforwomen.org. Additional or earlier immunizations are recommended for women with certain high-risk factors (see also "Special Populations" at www.immunizationforwomen.org/Immunization_Facts/Special_Populations). This information also is available at the College's well-woman web site at www.acog.org/wellwoman.

Immunization recommendations can change quickly, as was seen in 2009 during the H1N1 influenza outbreak. Obstetrician–gynecologists can refer to the CDC web site (www.cdc.gov/vaccines) as well as the College's Immunization for Women web site for the most current recommendations.

VACCINE ADMINISTRATION, STORAGE, AND HANDLING

The clinician should read vaccine package inserts thoroughly. The storage temperature, body site for injection (usually the deltoid), route of injection (eg, intramuscular, subcutaneous, or intradermal), and length of needle are critical items in maximizing efficacy.

CONTRAINDICATIONS TO VACCINATION

Contraindications to vaccination are conditions under which vaccination should not be administered because of an increased likelihood of a severe reaction. The CDC notes that the only contraindication that is applicable to all vaccines is a history of a severe allergic reaction to a previous dose of a vaccine or a vaccine component. Severe hypersensitivity reactions following immunizations, including anaphylaxis, are rare. The reactions are almost always caused by hypersensitivity to one or more of the vaccine components (residual animal proteins, antibiotics, preservatives, or stabilizers). On rare occasions, an anaphylactic reaction will be caused by trace amounts of an antibiotic, such as neomycin or streptomycin (eg, neomycin in measles–mumps–rubella vaccine). Vaccination is contraindicated in women with a previous anaphylactic reaction to a vaccine or one of its components. It is important to note that none of the current licensed vaccines contain penicillin; therefore, a history of penicillin hypersensitivity is not a contraindication to vaccination. Syncope or presyncope following immunization is a potential adverse effect, especially in adolescents, and a 15-minute observation period following injection is recommended for all vaccines.

According to the CDC, the following conditions are *not* contraindications to vaccination:

- Mild acute illness with or without fever
- Mild-to-moderate local reaction (ie, swelling, redness, soreness); low-grade or moderate fever after previous dose
- Lack of previous physical examination in a well-appearing person
- Current antimicrobial therapy (Antibacterial drugs might interfere with Ty21a oral typhoid vaccine, and certain antiviral drugs might interfere with varicella vaccines and live, attenuated influenza vaccine.)
- Convalescent phase of illness
- Recent exposure to an infectious disease
- History of penicillin allergy, other nonvaccine allergies, relatives with allergies, or receiving allergen extract immunotherapy

For a complete list of contraindications for specific vaccines, see the CDC's guide to contraindications and precautions, available at www.cdc.gov/vaccines/schedules/hcp/imz/adult-contraindications.html.

VACCINE INFORMATION STATEMENTS

Federal law requires that a VIS developed by the CDC be given to all patients, regardless of age, before the administration of every dose of certain vaccines. State health departments or the CDC should be consulted to determine which vaccines are currently covered by this federal law. Vaccine information statements are available on the Internet at www.cdc.gov/ vaccines/hcp/vis/index.html. The federal requirement to provide a relevant VIS is in addition to any applicable state laws, and no state law can negate that requirement. In addition, some states may have informed consent laws regarding immunization.

REPORTING OF ADVERSE EVENTS

Health care providers are encouraged to report all vaccine-related adverse events to the Vaccine Adverse Event Reporting System, a national vaccine safety surveillance program cosponsored by the CDC and the U.S. Food and Drug Administration (FDA). It collects and analyzes information from reports of adverse events following immunization. By monitoring such events, the Vaccine Adverse Event Reporting System helps to identify any important new safety concerns and thereby assists in ensuring that the benefits of vaccines continue to be far greater than the risks. Information on the Vaccine Adverse Event Reporting System program, including reporting forms and frequently asked questions, can be found at www.vaers.hhs. gov/.

Immunization Against Human Papillomavirus

The first vaccine shown to be effective at preventing infection with some genotypes of HPV was licensed by the FDA in 2006. This quadrivalent HPV vaccine is indicated to prevent cancers and intraepithelial neoplasias of the cervix, anus, vulva, and vagina and genital warts associated with HPV genotypes 6, 11, 16, and 18. Approximately 70% of all cases of cervical cancer are caused by HPV genotypes 16 and 18, and 90% of cases of genital warts are caused by HPV genotypes 6 and 11. Indications, dosage, and storage are addressed in Box 3-4. Originally approved for nonpregnant females aged 9–26 years, the administration of this vaccine was subsequently approved for males aged 9–26 years for the prevention of genital warts.

A second, bivalent formulation of an HPV vaccine was approved by the FDA in 2009 for administration to females aged 9–25 years (see Box 3-4) for the prevention of cervical cancer, cervical intraepithelial neoplasia 2 or worse and adenocarcinoma in situ, and cervical intraepithelial neoplasia 1 caused by oncogenic HPV genotypes 16 and 18. Results of

Box 3-4. Key Information Regarding the Bivalent and Quadrivalent Human Papillomavirus Vaccines*

Dosage
Administered intramuscularly as three separate 0.5-mL doses based on the following schedule:
1. First dose: at elected date
2. Second dose: 1–2 months after the first dose
3. Third dose: 6 months after the first dose

Minimum interval between first and second dose is 4 weeks, between second and third dose is 12 weeks, and between first and third dose is 24 weeks. If the vaccine schedule is interrupted, the series does not need to be restarted, regardless of the length of time between doses. Whenever possible, the same vaccine product should be used for all doses in the series.

Recommended Age
- Target population: females and males† aged 11 years or 12 years (can be started as early as age 9 years)
- Females and males† who did not receive the vaccination at the target age can be vaccinated from age 13 years through 26 years

Contraindications
Individuals who develop symptoms indicative of hypersensitivity to the active substances or to any of the components of either vaccine after receiving a dose of vaccine should not receive further doses of the product. Safety and effectiveness of the two formulations have not been established in pregnant women. Any exposure to it during pregnancy should be reported to the manufacturer by calling 1-877-888-4231 for the quadrivalent vaccine and 1-888-452-9622 for the bivalent vaccine.

Precautions
As with any vaccine, vaccination may not protect all vaccine recipients. Neither vaccine is intended to be used for treatment of active disease (ie, genital warts, cervical cancer, cervical intraepithelial neoplasia, vulvar intraepithelial neoplasia, or vaginal intraepithelial neoplasia). Human papillomavirus (HPV) vaccines can be administered simultaneously or at any time before or after a different inactivated or live vaccine administration. Because vaccinated individuals may develop syncope, sometimes resulting in falling with injury, health care providers should consider observing patients for 15 minutes after vaccine administration.

(continued)

Box 3-4. Key Information Regarding the Bivalent and Quadrivalent Human Papillomavirus Vaccines* *(continued)*

Storage
Both formulations should be refrigerated at 2–8°C (36–46°F), should not be frozen, and should be protected from light.

Vaccine Adverse Event Reporting
To report an adverse event associated with administration, go to http://vaers.hhs.gov.

Advisory Committee on Immunization Practices Recommendations
For current recommendations by the Advisory Committee on Immunization Practices, go to http://www.cdc.gov/vaccines/recs/acip/default.htm.

Current Procedural Terminology Code‡
The American Medical Association has established a Current Procedural Terminology code of 90649 for quadrivalent HPV vaccination and 90650 for bivalent HPV vaccine.

---

*Note that the U.S. Food and Drug Administration labeling for the bivalent vaccine indicates it is for use in females aged 9–25 years. In addition, the U.S. Food and Drug Administration approved dosage intervals for the quadrivalent and bivalent vaccines to be 0 months, 2 months, and 6 months and 0 months, 1 month, and 6 months, respectively.

†The U.S. Food and Drug Administration has approved the quadrivalent vaccine for use in males aged 9–26 years for the prevention of genital warts.

‡Current Procedural Terminology (CPT) copyright 2012 American Medical Association. All rights reserved. CPT is a registered trademark of the American Medical Association.

Data from Centers for Disease Control and Prevention. FDA licensure of bivalent human papillomavirus vaccine (HPV2, Cervarix) for use in females and updated HPV vaccination recommendations from the Advisory Committee on Immunization Practices (ACIP). MMWR Morb Mortal Wkly Rep 2010;59:626–9.

studies of the bivalent vaccine indicate that it offers protection similar to the quadrivalent vaccine against HPV infections caused by genotypes 16 and 18.

The need for booster doses remains to be demonstrated but is unlikely. Both of the current three-dose HPV vaccine series are designed to maximize the primary immune response and enhance long-term protection. The durability of the immune response (ie, how long protection lasts) is being monitored in various long-term studies, and there is currently no indication for a booster vaccine.

Although obstetrician–gynecologists are not likely to care for many patients in the initial vaccination target group, they play a critical role during the catch-up vaccination period (Box 3-4). They also play an essential role in engaging mothers to vaccinate their children. During a health care visit with a patient in the age range for vaccination, an assessment of the patient's HPV vaccine status should be conducted and documented in the patient record. Testing for HPV is not required or recommended as a prerequisite for administration of the vaccine. Vaccination with either HPV vaccine is not recommended for pregnant women. The presence of immunosuppression, such as that experienced in patients with human immunodeficiency virus (HIV) infection, is not a contraindication to administration of either the quadrivalent or bivalent HPV vaccine. However, the immune response may be smaller in the immunocompromised patient than in immunocompetent patients.

The HPV vaccine is most effective if given before any exposure to HPV infection, but sexually active women can receive and benefit from vaccination. Women with previous abnormal cervical cytologic findings or genital warts also can receive the HPV vaccine. Patients should be counseled that the vaccine may be less effective in women who have been exposed to HPV before vaccination than in women who were HPV naive at the time of vaccination.

The vaccine can be given to patients with previous cervical intraepithelial neoplasia, but practitioners need to emphasize that the benefits may be limited, and cervical cancer screening and corresponding management based on College recommendations must continue. The HPV vaccines are a preventive tool and not a substitute for cancer screening. Current cervical cancer screening recommendations should be followed regardless of vaccination status (see also the "Cancer Screening and Prevention" section later in Part 3 and the "Abnormal Cervical Cytology" section in Part 4). Similarly, HPV vaccines are not intended to treat patients with cervical cytologic abnormalities or genital warts. Patients with these conditions should undergo the appropriate evaluation and treatment.

Bibliography

American College of Obstetricians and Gynecologists. Immunization for women: immunizations for ob-gyns and their patients. Washington, DC: American College of Obstetricians and Gynecologists; 2012. Available at: http://www.immunization forwomen.org/. Retrieved September 4, 2013.

American College of Obstetricians and Gynecologists. Immunization for adolescents. Guidelines for adolescent health care [CD-ROM]. 2nd ed. ed. Washington, DC: American College of Obstetricians and Gynecologists; 2011. p. 73–84.

Centers for Disease Control and Prevention. Conditions commonly misperceived as contraindications to vaccination. Available at: http://www.cdc.gov/vaccines/recs/vac-admin/contraindications-misconceptions.htm. Retrieved July 23, 2013.

Centers for Disease Control and Prevention. Vaccines and immunizations. Available at: http://www.cdc.gov/vaccines. Retrieved July 16, 2013.

Donovan B, Franklin N, Guy R, Grulich AE, Regan DG, Ali H, et al. Quadrivalent human papillomavirus vaccination and trends in genital warts in Australia: analysis of national sentinel surveillance data. Lancet Infect Dis 2011;11:39–44.

Ethical issues with vaccination for the obstetrician-gynecologist. Committee Opinion No. 564. American College of Obstetricians and Gynecologists. Obstet Gynecol 2013;121:1144–50.

General recommendations on immunization—recommendations of the Advisory Committee on Immunization Practices (ACIP). National Center for Immunization and Respiratory Diseases [published erratum appears in MMWR Recomm Rep 2011;60:993]. MMWR Recomm Rep 2011;60:1–64.

GlaxoSmithKline Biologicals. Cervarix: highlights of prescribing information. Research Triangle Park (NC): GSK; 2012. Available at: http://us.gsk.com/products/assets/us_cervarix.pdf. Retrieved November 4, 2013.

Human papillomavirus vaccination. Committee Opinion No. 588. American College of Obstetricians and Gynecologists. Obstet Gynecol 2014;123:712–8.

Integrating immunizations into practice. Committee Opinion No. 558. American College of Obstetricians and Gynecologists. Obstet Gynecol 2013;121:897–903.

Merck & Company, Inc. Gardasil: highlights of prescribing information. Whitehouse Station (NJ): Merck; 2013. Available at: http://www.merck.com/product/usa/pi_circulars/g/gardasil/gardasil_pi.pdf. Retrieved November 4, 2013.

Resources

American College of Obstetricians and Gynecologists. Annual women's health care. Available at: http://www.acog.org/wellwoman. Retrieved October 1, 2013.

American College of Obstetricians and Gynecologists. Immunization coding for obstetrician–gynecologists 2011. Washington, DC: American College of Obstetricians and Gynecologists; 2011. Available at: http://www.acog.org/~/media/ Department%20Publications/ImmunizationCoding.pdf?dmc=1&ts=2012051 1T1605167391. Retrieved August 20, 2013.

American College of Obstetricians and Gynecologists. Immunization for women: special populations for ob-gyns. Available at: http://www.immunizationforwomen. org/Immunization_Facts/Special_Populations. Retrieved October 1, 2013.

American College of Obstetricians and Gynecologists. Immunization resources for obstetrician–gynecologists: a comprehensive tool kit. Available at: http://www.acog. org/~/media/Departments/Immunization/ImmunizationToolkit.pdf?dmc=1&ts=2 0130709T1011229407. Retrieved July 9, 2013.

Atkinson W, Wolfe C, Hamborsky J, editors. Epidemiology and prevention of vaccine-preventable diseases. Centers for Disease Control and Prevention. 12th ed. Washington, DC: Public Health Foundation; 2012.

Centers for Disease Control and Prevention. Immunization schedules. Available at: http://www.cdc.gov/vaccines/schedules/hcp/index.html. Retrieved July 23, 2013.

Centers for Disease Control and Prevention. Contraindications and precautions to commonly used vaccines in adults. Atlanta (GA): CDC; 2013. Available at: http:// www.cdc.gov/vaccines/schedules/hcp/imz/adult-contraindications.html. Retrieved July 23, 2013.

Centers for Disease Control and Prevention. Travelers' health. Available at: http:// wwwnc.cdc.gov/travel. Retrieved July 23, 2013.

Centers for Disease Control and Prevention. Vaccine information statements. Available at: http://www.cdc.gov/vaccines/hcp/vis/index.html. Retrieved July 23, 2013.

Centers for Disease Control and Prevention. Vaccine storage and handling toolkit. Atlanta (GA): CDC; 2012. Available at: http://www.cdc.gov/vaccines/recs/storage/ toolkit/storage-handling-toolkit.pdf. Retrieved July 23, 2013.

Centers for Disease Control and Prevention. Vaccines and preventable diseases: HPV vaccination. Available at: http://www.cdc.gov/vaccines/vpd-vac/hpv/. Retrieved July 24, 2013.

Immunization Action Coalition. Adults only vaccination: a step-by-step guide. St. Paul (MN): IAC; 2004. Available at: http://www.immunize.org/guide/aovguide_all. pdf. Retrieved July 24, 2013.

Immunization Action Coalition. State information: state mandates on immuniza- tion and vaccine-preventable diseases. Available at: http://www.immunize.org/laws. Retrieved July 24, 2013.

Immunization of health-care personnel: recommendations of the Advisory Committee on Immunization Practices (ACIP). Centers for Disease Control and Prevention. MMWR Recomm Rep 2011;60 (RR-7):1–45.

National Foundation for Infectious Diseases. Adult vaccination: professional resources. Available at: http://adultvaccination.org/professional-resources. Retrieved July 24, 2013.

National Institute of Allergy and Infectious Diseases. Vaccines. Available at: http://www.niaid.nih.gov/topics/vaccines/Pages/Default.aspx. Retrieved July 24, 2013.

National Network for Immunization Information. Available at: http://www.immunizationinfo.org/. Retrieved July 24, 2013.

Update on immunization and pregnancy: tetanus, diphtheria, and pertussis vaccination. Committee Opinion No. 566. American College of Obstetricians and Gynecologists. Obstet Gynecol 2013;121:1411–4.

Vaccination guidelines for female infertility patients: a committee opinion. Practice Committee of American Society for Reproductive Medicine. Fertil Steril 2013;99:337–9.

Vaccine Adverse Event Reporting System. Available at: http://vaers.hhs.gov. Retrieved July 24, 2013.

▌FITNESS

General fitness assessment is an important aspect of every individual's physical examination. Obstetrician–gynecologists should evaluate each patient's fitness level and offer appropriate interventions or referrals to promote healthy living. Goals should include maintaining an appropriate weight, consuming a healthy diet, and participating in regular physical activities at appropriate intensity and duration.

Weight

WEIGHT ASSESSMENT

Body mass index (BMI) describes relative weight for height and is used as a practical marker to assess obesity. The calculation is as follows:

$$\frac{\text{Weight in kilograms}}{(\text{Height in meters})^2}$$

If pounds and inches are used to calculate BMI, multiply the division results by 703 as follows:

$$\frac{\text{Weight in pounds}}{(\text{Height in inches})^2} \times 703$$

Online resources, electronic medical records, and charts have made calculating BMI much easier. The National Heart, Lung, and Blood Institute online adult BMI calculator is available at www.nhlbi.nih.gov/guidelines/obesity/BMI/bmicalc.htm. Although the BMI value is calculated the same way for adolescents and adults, the interpretation of the BMI number varies for adolescents depending on age (see also the "Adolescents" section later in Part 3).

Obesity management guidelines issued jointly in 2013 by the American College of Cardiology, the American Heart Association, and The Obesity

Society support the following BMI classification published in 1998 by the National Heart, Lung, and Blood Institute:

- Underweight: BMI lower than 18.5
- Normal weight: BMI 18.5–24.9
- Overweight: BMI 25.0–29.9
- Obesity: BMI 30.0 or greater
    — Obesity Class I: BMI 30.0–34.9
    — Obesity Class II: BMI: 35.0–39.9
    — Obesity Class III (extreme): 40.0 or more

Measuring waist circumference, which specifically assesses abdominal fat content, is another useful tool. In women, a waist circumference greater than 35 inches is considered to be abnormal; however, more recent guidelines recommend including a measurement of 35 inches in the abnormal classification. Elevated waist circumference in the specific population of patients with a BMI between 25 and 34.9 is associated with an increased risk of type 2 diabetes mellitus, hypertension, dyslipidemia, and coronary vascular disease. This measurement is a useful adjunct to the BMI because it can provide an estimate of increased abdominal fat even in the absence of a change in BMI. Waist measurements in patients with a BMI of 35 or higher, however, are not useful because predictive power is lost. Waist measurement is performed as follows:

- The patient stands and the examiner, positioned at the right of the patient, palpates the upper hip bone to locate the right iliac crest.
- Just above the uppermost lateral border of the right iliac crest, the measuring tape is placed in a horizontal plane around the abdomen and parallel to the floor with the tape snug, but not compressing the skin.
- The measurement is made at a normal minimal respiration.

WEIGHT LOSS BENEFITS

Most Americans are aware that losing weight is beneficial to their health if they are not at their optimum weight, but physicians should relay what specific benefits may be reaped based on available evidence. Weight loss has been proved to lower elevated blood pressure in overweight and obese patients with hypertension. It also lowers elevated levels of total cholesterol, low-density lipoprotein cholesterol, and triglycerides while increasing high-density lipoproteins in overweight and obese patients with dyslipidemia. Patients with type 2 diabetes mellitus will decrease their blood glucose levels with weight loss. In addition, exercise will strengthen muscles, maintain bone health, and give more energy (see also "Exercise" later in this section).

Weight loss also can decrease the likelihood of developing morbidities associated with obesity, including heart disease, infertility, gallbladder disease, osteoarthritis, and many types of cancer, including breast, uterine, and colon cancer. For example, endometrial cancer is five times more prevalent in obese women than in nonobese women. Heart disease, the leading cause of death of women, is directly associated with obesity.

DIETARY THERAPY FOR WEIGHT LOSS

Dietary therapy for weight loss involves a diet in which fewer calories are consumed than expended. The 2010 Dietary Guidelines for Americans developed by the U.S. Department of Agriculture (USDA) includes recommendations to help individuals achieve a healthy diet. A useful adjunct to the guidelines is the ChooseMyPlate web site (www.choosemyplate.gov/), which offers an interactive web-based program to determine the number of servings needed per day in each food group and the recommended number of calories per day based on weight and height. The site also provides tables to best determine how many calories are in some of the most common food items.

Calculating caloric intake in any given day is an important tool to assist with weight loss. A 20–25% reduction in calories from the amount required for baseline maintenance will result in gradual and safe weight loss of approximately 1–2 lb/wk. Table 3-1 includes the Dietary Guidelines for Americans' recommendations for women's daily caloric needs by age and level of physical activity. If, for example, baseline caloric needs for maintenance are 2,000 kcal/d, a 25% reduction to 1,500 kcal/d would be suggested. Simply keeping a diet and calorie diary can be illuminating and

Table 3-1. Estimated Daily Caloric Needs for Nonpregnant Adolescents and Women by Level of Physical Activity*

Age (years)	Physical Activity Level		
	Sedentary[†]	Moderately Active[‡]	Active[§]
14–18	1,800[‖]	2,000[‖]	2,400[‖]
19–30	1,800–2,000	2,000–2,200	2,400
31–50	1,800	2,000	2,200
51+	1,600	1,800	2,000–2,200

*The estimated calories are rounded to the nearest 200 calories and are based on Estimated Energy Requirement equations, using reference heights (average) and reference weights (healthy) for each age group. For adolescents, reference height and weight vary. For women, the reference is height 5 ft 4 in. and weight 126 lb. An individual's caloric needs may be higher or lower than these average estimates. Estimates do not include women who are pregnant or breastfeeding. Estimated Energy Requirement equations are from the Institute of Medicine. Dietary Reference Intakes for Energy, Carbohydrate, Fiber, Fat, Fatty Acids, Cholesterol, Protein, and Amino Acids. Washington (DC): The National Academies Press; 2002.

[†]Sedentary means a lifestyle that includes only the light physical activity associated with typical day-to-day life.

[‡]Moderately active means a lifestyle that includes physical activity equivalent to walking approximately 1.5–3 miles per day at 3–4 miles per hour, in addition to the light physical activity associated with typical day-to-day life.

[§]Active means a lifestyle that includes physical activity equivalent to walking more than 3 miles per day at 3–4 miles per hour, in addition to the light physical activity associated with typical day-to-day life.

[‖]The calorie ranges shown are to accommodate needs of different ages within the group. For adolescents, more calories are needed at older ages. For women, fewer calories are needed at older ages.

Modified from Table 2-3 In: Department of Agriculture, Department of Health and Human Services. Dietary guidelines for Americans, 2010. 7th ed. Washington, DC: Government Printing Office; 2010. Available at: http://www.cnpp.usda.gov/DGAs2010-PolicyDocument.htm. Retrieved July 24, 2013.

can assist with weight loss. The USDA's SuperTracker web site (available at www.supertracker.usda.gov/default.aspx) allows individuals to create personalized nutrition and exercise plans and track their progress. Apps for smart phones and tablets also are available.

Successful weight reduction by following a low-calorie diet is more likely to occur when dietary allowances are met. Dietary education focuses on the following:

- Understanding energy values of different foods
- Understanding food composition (fats, carbohydrates, and proteins)
- Preparing foods
- Developing new food-purchasing habits
- Avoiding overeating high-calorie foods
- Maintaining adequate fluid intake
- Reducing portion sizes
- Limiting alcohol consumption

Table 3-1 provides estimated daily caloric intake requirements for women based on age group and level of physical activity.

PHARMACOTHERAPY FOR WEIGHT LOSS

The American College of Cardiology, American Heart Association, and The Obesity Society recommend that weight-loss drugs approved by the U.S. Food and Drug Administration (FDA) are only to be used as part of a comprehensive program that includes physical activity and dietary therapy. In addition, their use is recommended only in patients with a BMI greater than or equal to 30 with no concomitant obesity-related risk factors or diseases or in patients with a BMI greater than or equal to 27 with hypertension, dyslipidemia, type 2 diabetes mellitus, sleep apnea, or coronary heart disease. Because of the risks associated with the use of weight-loss drugs and the lack of long-term safety data beyond 1 year, the administration of these drugs is limited to these select patient populations. Because weight loss using phentermine and topiramate extended-release can cause fetal harm, females capable of becoming pregnant should have a negative pregnancy test result before initiation and every month while using the drug and should use effective contraception consistently while taking phentermine and topiramate extended-release.

The availability of pharmacologic therapy for weight loss continues to change at a rapid pace. The FDA provides information about currently approved weight-loss drugs on their web site, available at www.fda.gov/Drugs/DrugSafety/InformationbyDrugClass/ucm308412.htm.

WEIGHT LOSS SURGERY

Surgical options for weight loss currently include gastroplasty (including sleeve gastrectomy), adjustable gastric banding, and gastric bypass (Roux-en-Y). The primary function of each procedure is to reduce food consumption. The American College of Cardiology, American Heart Association, and The Obesity Society consider surgical candidates to be patients with a BMI greater than or equal to 40 or greater than or equal to 35 with comorbid conditions, such as cardiovascular disease, type 2 diabetes mellitus, and sleep apnea. The goal is to create enough of a caloric deficit that sufficient weight loss is achieved to decrease weight-associated risk factors or comorbidities. Beyond the risks associated with a major surgical intervention, nutritional deficiencies can occur long term. Thus, there is a need for monitoring and maintenance, and a multidisciplinary team is highly recommended for these patients. Long-term outcome studies have shown that all-cause mortality is 40% lower in patients who undergo gastric bypass surgery compared with controls. Women who have had bariatric surgery with malabsorptive procedures (eg, Roux-en-Y gastric bypass, biliopancreatic diversion) should generally avoid the use of oral contraceptives (combined estrogen and progestin and progestin-only) because failure rates may be higher because of inadequate gastrointestinal absorption. There are no contraceptive method interactions with restrictive bariatric procedures.

WEIGHT LOSS MAINTENANCE

Patients involved in a multifocused approach to weight loss, including dietary therapy, physical activity, and behavior therapy, are more successful at maintaining weight loss than others. Behavior therapy includes strategies such as self-monitoring. This involves recording what types of food are eaten, their caloric value, and their nutrient composition. Other types of therapy include stress management, stimulus control, cognitive–behavioral therapy, and the use of social supports. There also is an association between weight loss success and more frequent patient–practitioner visits, which provide encouragement and accountability.

Nutrition

Consuming a nutritious, balanced diet is essential for achieving and maintaining good health and an appropriate weight. Despite the wide variety of nutritious foods available, many Americans do not eat the array of foods that will provide all needed nutrients while staying within caloric needs. Daily intakes of nutrient-dense foods are lower than recommended, whereas consumption of nutrient-lacking foods and food components exceeds recommended levels. Box 3-5 and Box 3-6 include key recommendations from the USDA's report, *Dietary Guidelines for Americans, 2010*, which recommends food choices that should be emphasized as well as those to be limited to help close nutrient gaps and move toward healthful eating patterns. For additional information, please see the full USDA report (available at www.cnpp.usda.gov/DGAs2010-PolicyDocument.htm) as well as the dietary reference intake tables from the Institute of Medicine (IOM) (available at www.iom.edu/Activities/Nutrition/SummaryDRIs/DRI-Tables.aspx).

Box 3-5. Foods and Nutrients to Increase to Achieve a Healthy Diet

Key Recommendations

Individuals should meet the following recommendations as part of a healthy eating pattern and while staying within their caloric needs. Recommended daily amounts listed below are based on an adult diet of 2,000 calories per day.

- Fruits (2 cups)—Eat a variety of fruit. Choose whole or cut-up fruits more than fruit juice.

- Vegetables (2.5 cups)—Eat a variety of vegetables, especially dark-green, red, and orange vegetables and beans and peas.

- Grains (6 oz)*—Consume at least one half of all grains as whole grains. Increase whole-grain intake by replacing refined grains with whole grains.

- Dairy (3 cups)—Increase intake of fat-free or low-fat milk and dairy products, such as milk, yogurt, cheese, or fortified soy beverages†.

- Protein Foods (5.5 oz)—Choose a variety of protein foods, which include seafood, lean meat, poultry, eggs, beans and peas, soy products, and unsalted nuts and seeds. Increase the amount and variety of seafood consumed by choosing seafood in place of some meat and poultry. Replace protein foods that are higher in solid fats with choices that are lower in fats and calories.

- Oils (6 teaspoons)—Use oils to replace solid fats where possible.

(continued)

Box 3-5. Foods and Nutrients to Increase to Achieve a Healthy Diet *(continued)*

Key Recommendations *(continued)*
- Nutrients—Choose foods that provide more of the following nutrients, which are inadequately consumed by the general population: potassium, dietary fiber, calcium, and vitamin D.[‡]

Additional Recommendations for Specific Population Groups
Women Capable of Becoming Pregnant[§]
- Choose foods that supply heme iron (ie, iron from animal foods that originally contained hemoglobin, such as red meat, fish, and poultry), which is more readily absorbed by the body. Absorption of nonheme iron (ie, from plant sources) can be enhanced by combining intake with vitamin C-rich foods.
- Consume 0.4 mg per day of synthetic folic acid (from fortified foods, supplements, or both) in addition to food forms of folate from a varied diet.[¶]

Women Who Are Pregnant or Breastfeeding[§]
- Consume 8–12 oz of seafood per week from a variety of seafood types. Because of their methyl mercury content, limit white (albacore) tuna to 6 oz per week and do not eat the following four types of fish: tilefish, shark, swordfish, and king mackerel.
- If pregnant, take an iron supplement as recommended by an obstetrician or other health care provider.

Individuals Aged 50 Years and Older
- Consume foods fortified with vitamin B_{12}, such as fortified cereals, or dietary supplements.

---

[*]Examples of 1-oz equivalents of grain include 1 oz slice bread; 1 oz uncooked pasta or rice; 1/2 cup cooked rice, pasta, or cereal; 1 tortilla (6" diameter); 1 pancake (5" diameter); 1 oz ready-to-eat cereal (approximately 1 cup cereal flakes).

[†]Fortified soy beverages have been marketed as "soymilk," a product name consumers could see in supermarkets and consumer materials. However, the U.S. Food and Drug Administration's regulations do not contain provisions for the use of the term soymilk. Therefore, in this document, the term "fortified soy beverage" includes products that may be marketed as soymilk.

(continued)

Box 3-5. Foods and Nutrients to Increase to Achieve a Healthy Diet *(continued)*

‡See the Institute of Medicine Dietary Reference Intake tables for recommended daily allowances and adequate intake levels of these nutrients: http://www.iom.edu/Activities/Nutrition/SummaryDRIs/DRI-Tables.aspx.

§Includes adolescent girls.

¶"Folic acid" is the synthetic form of the nutrient, whereas "folate" is the form found naturally in foods.

Modified from Chapter 4: Foods and nutrients to increase. In: Department of Agriculture, Department of Health and Human Services. Dietary guidelines for Americans, 2010. 7th ed. Washington, DC: Government Printing Office; 2010. Available at: http://www.cnpp.usda.gov/DGAs2010-PolicyDocument.htm. Retrieved July 24, 2013.

FOODS AND NUTRIENTS TO INCREASE

Greater consumption of nutrient-dense foods is advised to provide recommended levels of vitamins and minerals while controlling caloric intake and reducing the risk of chronic health conditions, such as obesity, cardiovascular disease, and type 2 diabetes mellitus. Nutrient-dense foods include vegetables, fruits, whole grains, fat-free or low-fat dairy products, and lean protein that are prepared without added solid fats, sugars, starches, and sodium. In the United States, inadequate consumption of these foods has led to lower than recommended intake of dietary fiber and other essential nutrients (Box 3-5), several of which are particularly important for women's health, including calcium, vitamin D, folic acid, and iron.

Dietary Fiber

Dietary fiber is the nondigestible form of carbohydrates and lignin. Dietary fiber naturally occurs in plants and is important in promoting bowel regularity. Because foods that contain fiber are digested slowly, they help provide a greater feeling of fullness and are helpful in maintaining a healthy weight and controlling blood glucose levels. The IOM recommends that individuals intake 14 g of fiber per 1,000 calories consumed. Some of the best sources of dietary fiber are beans and peas, such as navy beans, split

Box 3-6. Foods and Food Components to Reduce

- Reduce daily sodium intake to less than 2,300 mg and further reduce intake to 1,500 mg among individuals who are 51 years and older and those of any age who are African American or have hypertension, diabetes, or chronic kidney disease. The 1,500-mg recommendation applies to approximately one half of the U.S. population, including children and most adults.*

- Consume less than 10% of calories from saturated fatty acids by replacing them with monounsaturated and polyunsaturated fatty acids.

- Consume less than 300 mg per day of dietary cholesterol. Consuming less than 300 mg/d of cholesterol can help maintain normal blood cholesterol levels, and intake of less than 200 mg/d can further help individuals at high risk of cardiovascular disease.

- Keep trans-fatty acid consumption as low as possible, especially by limiting foods that contain synthetic sources of trans-fats, such as partially hydrogenated oils, and by limiting other solid fats.

- Reduce the intake of calories from solid fats and added sugars.

- Limit the consumption of foods that contain refined grains, especially refined grain foods that contain solid fats, added sugars, and sodium.

- If alcohol is consumed, it should be consumed in moderation—up to one drink per day† for women—and only by adults of legal drinking age.

---

*Because a recommended dietary allowance for sodium could not be determined, the Institute of Medicine set adequate intake (AI) levels for this nutrient. The AI value is the recommended daily average intake level of a nutrient, and usual intakes at or above the AI have a low probability of inadequacy. The sodium AI for individuals aged 9–50 years is 1,500 mg per day. Because older individuals consume fewer calories than their younger counterparts, their recommended daily AI values are lower: 1,300 mg for those aged 51–70 years, and 1,200 mg for individuals aged 71 years and older. For individuals aged 14 years and older, the Institute of Medicine set the tolerable upper intake level at 2,300 mg per day. The tolerable upper intake level is the highest daily nutrient intake level that is likely to pose no risk of adverse health effects (eg, for sodium, increased blood pressure) to almost all individuals in the general population.

†One drink is defined as 12 fluid oz of regular beer (5% alcohol), 5 fluid oz of wine (12% alcohol), or 1.5 fluid oz of 80 proof (40% alcohol) distilled spirits. One drink contains 0.6 fluid oz of alcohol.

Reprinted from Chapter 3: Foods and food components to reduce. In: Department of Agriculture, Department of Health and Human Services. Dietary guidelines for Americans, 2010. 7th ed. Washington, DC: Government Printing Office; 2010. Available at: http://www.cnpp.usda.gov/DGAs2010-PolicyDocument.htm. Retrieved July 24, 2013.

peas, lentils, pinto beans, and black beans. Additional sources of dietary fiber include other vegetables, fruits, whole grains, and nuts.

Calcium and Vitamin D

To help promote good bone health and reduce fracture risk, the IOM's recommended dietary allowance of calcium is 1,000 mg/d for women aged 19–50 years and 1,200 mg/d for women 51 years and older. This is the necessary amount of calcium that should be consumed through food sources to achieve peak bone mass and maintain bone health. Vitamin D has a role in calcium absorption, muscle performance, and balance. The most common sources are fortified milk, cereals, egg yolks, salt-water fish, and liver. The recommended dietary allowance is 600 international units/day for most of life and 800 international units/day for adults older than 70 years.

Folic Acid

Daily intake of 0.4 mg/d of folic acid is recommended for all women capable of becoming pregnant because the preconception ingestion of folic acid has been shown to reduce the risk of neural tube defects. Daily supplementation with a multivitamin is recommended for all women in this group because most women are unable to attain this level of folic acid through dietary sources alone, and approximately 50% of pregnancies are unplanned. A higher folic acid dosage of 4 mg/d is recommended for women who take anticonvulsant medication, have a history of neural tube defects, or have already given birth to a child affected by a neural tube defect. This higher dosage of folic acid should be prescribed by a health care provider. Although folic acid is relatively nontoxic, increasing the doses of multivitamin preparations to reach the higher level is not advised because of the potential for ingesting excessive amounts of other vitamins that may be harmful.

Iron

Many women of reproductive age are deficient in iron. The IOM's recommended dietary allowance of iron is 18 mg/d for women aged 19–50 years. Women can improve their iron status by choosing foods that supply heme iron, which is readily absorbed by the body, as well as foods that enhance iron absorption such as those rich in vitamin C. Sources of heme iron include lean meat, poultry, and seafood. Additional sources of iron include most breads and cereals, which are enriched with iron. Plant sources of nonheme iron—the less bioavailable form of iron—include white beans, lentils, and spinach.

FOODS AND FOOD COMPONENTS TO REDUCE

Decreased consumption of nutrient-lacking foods and food components is advised. Sodium, solid fats, added sugars, and refined grains should be consumed in moderation (Box 3-6).

Sodium

Sodium is an essential nutrient but is needed by the body in relatively small quantities, provided that substantial sweating does not occur. On average, the higher an individual's sodium intake, the higher the individual's blood pressure. Sodium is found in a wide variety of foods, some expected—such as deli meats and canned soups—and others more surprising—such as breakfast cereals and baked goods. Caloric intake is associated with sodium intake; therefore, reducing caloric intake can help reduce sodium intake, thereby contributing to the health benefits that occur with lowering sodium intake. Recommended daily sodium intake levels are listed in Box 3-6. Individuals can reduce their consumption of sodium in a variety of ways, including consuming more fresh foods, choosing low-sodium processed foods, and limiting the use of salt when cooking or dining out.

Solid Fats and Added Sugar

Fats should provide no more than 20–35% of the total calories in an adult diet, with most fats coming from sources of polyunsaturated fatty acids and monounsaturated fats. It is also important to include sources of omega-3 fatty acids, which may be beneficial for disease prevention and maintenance of overall health. Intake of saturated fatty acids, trans-fatty acids, and cholesterol should be limited.

Reducing dietary fat alone without reducing overall calories is not sufficient for weight loss. Added sugar is another major source of excess empty calories. Most sugars in typical American diets are sugars added to foods during processing or preparation or at the table. Reducing the consumption of solid fats and added sugars allows for increased intake of nutrient-dense foods without exceeding overall caloric needs. Individuals can reduce their consumption of solid fat and added sugar by focusing on eating the most nutrient-dense forms of foods from all food groups; limiting the amount of solid fats and added sugars when cooking or eating; and consuming fewer and smaller portions of foods and beverages that contain solid fats, added sugars, or both, such as grain-based desserts, sodas, and other sugar-sweetened beverages.

Refined Grains

The refining of whole grains involves a process that results in the loss of dietary fiber, vitamins, and minerals. Most refined grains are enriched with iron, thiamin, riboflavin, niacin, and folic acid before being further used as ingredients in foods; however, dietary fiber and some vitamins and minerals that are present in whole grains are not routinely added back to refined grains. In addition, because many refined grain products are high in solid fats and added sugars, they commonly provide excess calories when consumed beyond recommended levels. For individuals maintaining a 2,000-calorie daily diet, the USDA recommends consumption of no more than 3 ounce-equivalents per day. Consumption of refined grain products that also are high in solid fats, added sugars, or both—such as cakes, cookies, donuts, and other desserts—should be reduced. Refined grains should be replaced with whole grains, such that at least half of all grains eaten are whole grains.

SPECIAL DIETS

Special diets abound for a variety of reasons and conditions. Some are based on clinical evidence, whereas others are merely popular fads or trends based on testimonials.

The vegetarian diet continues to grow in popularity, with the increasing number of vegetarian products available in supermarkets, vegetarian menu options at restaurants, and vegetarian cookbooks and web sites as evidence of the considerable interest in this dietary way of life. Although there are many variations, the Academy of Nutrition and Dietetics (formerly, the American Dietetic Association) defines a vegetarian diet as one that excludes meat (or fowl), seafood, or products containing these foods. A vegan diet differs from a vegetarian diet in that it excludes eggs, dairy, and other animal products. According to the Academy, vegetarian diets (including total vegetarian or vegan diets) support good health when appropriately planned to meet nutrient and energy needs and may help in the prevention and treatment of certain diseases.

The gluten-free diet has gained recent popularity, although it has been in existence for decades as the treatment for celiac disease. More recently, it has been suggested that the avoidance of dietary gluten, a protein found in wheat, rye, and barley, can lead to better sleep, increased energy, weight loss, and feelings of health and well-being. At this time, scientific evidence does not support the benefits of a gluten-free diet for individuals without a known diagnosis of celiac disease or gluten sensitivity.

For individuals with lactose intolerance, a dairy-free diet might seem to be the only option for symptom management. However, most people with lactose intolerance can tolerate small volumes of milk and lactose from dairy foods other than milk, such as cheese and yogurt. Because milk and milk products are a significant source of calcium and other important nutrients, complete dietary avoidance is not recommended, especially for women who may be at risk of osteoporosis. Instead, strategies such as limiting the consumption of dairy products, choosing dairy products with added lactase, and using lactase enzyme supplements when eating foods containing lactose are generally recommended to help individuals manage the symptoms of lactose intolerance.

Exercise

All adults should engage in regular physical activity. Women should be counseled about various medical limitations, such as arthritis, that may limit their activities, or be referred to a fitness instructor for safety guidelines. There are two general types of exercise: 1) aerobic and 2) muscle strengthening. Inactive adults should work gradually toward the aerobic exercise and muscle-strengthening goals listed in the following discussions. To avoid injury risks, it is important to exercise for shorter periods of time at a light or moderate intensity with more frequent sessions spread throughout the week. For example, walking sessions could begin at 5 minutes three times a day for 5–6 days of the week. The length of time could then gradually be lengthened and the walking speed slowly increased.

Aerobic Exercise

Aerobic exercises, by definition, are physical activities that move large muscles in a rhythmic manner for a sustained period. These include running, brisk walking, bicycling, dancing, and swimming. These activities increase the heart rate to meet the increased oxygen demands of the body during exercise. Aerobic exercise guidelines for adults are as follows:

- For substantial health benefits, the recommendation is for moderate-intensity aerobic activity (eg, brisk walking) for 150 minutes (2 hours, 30 minutes) per week or vigorous-intensity aerobic activity (eg, jogging or running) for 75 minutes (1 hour and 15 minutes) per week, spread throughout the week in episodes of at least 10 minutes each.

- For additional and more extensive health benefits, increasing this time span to 300 minutes (5 hours) of moderate-intensity aerobic physical activity or 2 hours and 30 minutes of vigorous-intensity physical activity per week will lower the risk of colon and breast cancer, prevent unhealthy weight gain, and lower risk of heart disease and diabetes.

- Activities spread over at least 3 days of the week produce health benefits and may help reduce the risk of injury and avoid fatigue.

Older adults should follow these aerobic exercises guidelines. If chronic conditions limit their activities, older adults should be as physically active as their abilities allow. They should avoid inactivity. Older adults should do exercises that maintain or improve balance if they are at risk of falling.

Measurement of heart rate during exercise is an excellent method by which to evaluate cardiovascular fitness. The heart rate at which conditioning will develop is called the target heart rate. As conditioning improves, the heart rate stabilizes at a fixed level. The following formula is used to calculate the target heart rate:

220 – (patient's age) = maximum heart rate

60–80% of the maximum heart rate = target heart rate

It is recommended that individuals know their heart rate while exercising and aim for being within the target heart rate range for 20–30 minutes. Exceeding the target heart rate range may be dangerous and should be done only under supervision.

MUSCLE STRENGTHENING

Muscle-strengthening exercises are activities that overload the muscles to increase bone strength and maintain muscle mass. These exercises work the major muscle groups of the body: legs, hips, back, chest, abdomen, shoulders, and arms. Weight training, calisthenics, working with resistance bands, carrying heavy loads, and heavy gardening activities (including digging, raking, shoveling, and sweeping) are all examples. Muscle-strengthening activity recommendations for adults are as follows:

- No specific amount of time per day is recommended, but 2 days per week is the minimum.
- Sets of 8–12 repetitions of each exercise are effective, but 2–3 sets of these repetitions are even more effective. Increasing the amount of weight or the number of days per week will result in stronger muscles.

Bibliography

Adams TD, Gress RE, Smith SC, Halverson RC, Simper SC, Rosamond WD, et al. Long-term mortality after gastric bypass surgery. N Engl J Med 2007;357:753–61.

American College of Obstetricians and Gynecologists. Obesity in adolescents. Guidelines for adolescent health care [CD-ROM]. 2nd ed. ed. Washington, DC: American College of Obstetricians and Gynecologists; 2011. p. 148–63.

Craig WJ, Mangels AR. Position of the American Dietetic Association: vegetarian diets. American Dietetic Association. J Am Diet Assoc 2009;109:1266–82.

Department of Agriculture, Department of Health and Human Services. Dietary guidelines for Americans, 2010. 7th ed. Washington, DC: Government Printing Office; 2010. Available at: http://www.cnpp.usda.gov/DGAs2010-PolicyDocument.htm. Retrieved July 24, 2013.

Department of Health and Human Services. Physical activity guidelines for Americans at-a-glance: a fact sheet for professionals. Available at: http://www.health.gov/paguidelines/factsheetprof.aspx. Retrieved July 24, 2013.

Gaesser GA, Angadi SS. Gluten-free diet: imprudent dietary advice for the general population? J Acad Nutr Diet 2012;112:1330–3.

Institute of Medicine. Dietary reference intakes tables and application. Available at: http://www.iom.edu/Activities/Nutrition/SummaryDRIs/DRI-Tables.aspx. Retrieved July 24, 2013.

Jensen MD, Ryan DH, Apovian CM, Ard JD, Comuzzie AG, Donato KA, et al. 2013 AHA/ACC/TOS guideline for the management of overweight and obesity in adults: a report of the American College of Cardiology/American Heart Association Task Force on Practice Guidelines and The Obesity Society. Circulation 2013; DOI: 10.1161/01.cir.0000437739.71477.ee. J Am Coll Cardiol 2013; DOI: 10.1016/j.jacc.2013.11.004. Obesity (Silver Spring). 2013 Nov 12. DOI: 10.1002/oby.20660.

Moyer VA. Behavioral counseling interventions to promote a healthful diet and physical activity for cardiovascular disease prevention in adults: U.S. Preventive Services Task Force recommendation statement. U.S. Preventive Services Task Force. Ann Intern Med 2012;157:367–72.

Moyer VA. Screening for and management of obesity in adults: U.S. Preventive Services Task Force recommendation statement. U.S. Preventive Services Task Force. Ann Intern Med 2012;157:373–8.

National Heart, Lung, and Blood Institute. Clinical guidelines on the identification, evaluation, and treatment of overweight and obesity in adults: the evidence report. NIH Publication No. 98-4083. Bethesda (MD): NHLBI; 1998. Available at: http://www.nhlbi.nih.gov/guidelines/obesity/ob_gdlns.pdf. Retrieved July 24, 2013.

National Institute of Diabetes and Digestive and Kidney Diseases. Lactose intolerance. Available at: http://digestive.niddk.nih.gov/ddiseases/pubs/lactoseintolerance. Retrieved July 24, 2013.

Understanding and using the U.S. Medical Eligibility Criteria For Contraceptive Use, 2010. Committee Opinion No. 505. American College of Obstetricians and Gynecologists. Obstet Gynecol 2011;118:754–60.

Resources

American College of Obstetricians and Gynecologists. Annual women's health care. Washington, DC: American College of Obstetricians and Gynecologists; 2011. Available at: http://www.acog.org/wellwoman. Retrieved July 19, 2013.

American College of Obstetricians and Gynecologists. Exercise and fitness: a guide for women. Patient Education Pamphlet AP045. Washington, DC: American College of Obstetricians and Gynecologists; 2010.

American College of Obstetricians and Gynecologists. Healthy eating. Patient Education Pamphlet AP130. Washington, DC: American College of Obstetricians and Gynecologists; 2013.

American College of Obstetricians and Gynecologists. Weight control: eating right and keeping fit. Patient Education Pamphlet AP064. Washington, DC: American College of Obstetricians and Gynecologists; 2013.

Department of Agriculture. ChooseMyPlate. Available at: http://www.choosemy plate.gov/. Retrieved July 24, 2013.

Department of Agriculture. ChooseMyPlate: information for health care professionals. Available at: http://www.choosemyplate.gov/information-healthcare-profes sionals.html. Retrieved July 24, 2013.

Department of Agriculture. Dietary guidelines for Americans. Available at: http://www.cnpp.usda.gov/dietaryguidelines.htm. Retrieved July 24, 2013.

Department of Agriculture. SuperTracker. Available at: https://www.supertracker. usda.gov/default.aspx. Retrieved July 24, 2013.

Food and Drug Administration. Weight loss drugs. Available at: http://www.fda. gov/Drugs/DrugSafety/InformationbyDrugClass/ucm308412.htm. Retrieved July 24, 2013.

Hall KD. What is the required energy deficit per unit weight loss? Int J Obes (Lond) 2008;32:573-6.

Haskell WL, Lee IM, Pate RR, Powell KE, Blair SN, Franklin BA, et al. Physical activity and public health: updated recommendation for adults from the American College of Sports Medicine and the American Heart Association. American College of Sports Medicine and American Heart Association. Circulation 2007;116:1081–93.

Kushi LH, Byers T, Doyle C, Bandera EV, McCullough M, McTiernan A, et al. American Cancer Society Guidelines on Nutrition and Physical Activity for cancer prevention: reducing the risk of cancer with healthy food choices and physical activity. American Cancer Society 2006 Nutrition and Physical Activity Guidelines Advisory Committee. CA Cancer J Clin 2006;56:254,81; quiz 313–4.

National Foundation for Celiac Awareness. Celiac disease and women's health. Available at: http://www.celiaccentral.org/education/Women-s-Health/438. Retrieved August 20, 2013.

National Heart, Lung, and Blood Institute. Aim for a healthy weight. Available at: http://www.nhlbi.nih.gov/health/public/heart/obesity/lose_wt/index.htm. Retrieved July 24, 2013.

National Heart, Lung, and Blood Institute. Calculate your body mass index. Available at: http://www.nhlbi.nih.gov/guidelines/obesity/BMI/bmicalc.htm. Retrieved July 24, 2013.

National Institute of Diabetes and Digestive and Kidney Diseases. Digestive disorders. Available at: http://www.nutrition.gov/nutrition-and-health-issues/digestive-disorders. Retrieved July 24, 2013.

Osteoporosis. Practice Bulletin No. 129. American College of Obstetricians and Gynecologists. Obstet Gynecol 2012;120:718–34.

Ross AC, Manson JE, Abrams SA, Aloia JF, Brannon PM, Clinton SK, et al. The 2011 report on dietary reference intakes for calcium and vitamin D from the Institute of Medicine: what clinicians need to know. J Clin Endocrinol Metab 2011;96:53–8.

COMPLEMENTARY AND ALTERNATIVE MEDICINE

Complementary and alternative medicine (CAM) can be defined as those systems, practices, interventions, modalities, professions, therapies, applications, theories, or claims that are currently not an integral part of the dominant or conventional medical system (known as allopathy in North America). Importantly, over time some of the individual modalities do overlap with, or become integrated into, Western medicine.

In 2007, 38.3% of Americans used some form of CAM over the previous 12 months, spending $33.9 billion out of pocket. This trend of increased CAM use will continue as it is reinforced and supported by continuing media attention; intense commercial efforts by providers of CAM products and services, including proprietary pharmaceutical companies; third-party reimbursement for some CAM practices and products; and the increasing over-the-counter access to CAM products in drugstores and supermarkets.

Types of Therapy

The spectrum of CAM encompasses more than 350 different techniques and treatments. These can be classified into the following major categories, with some overlap.

MIND–BODY PRACTICES

Mind–body practices typically focus on intervention strategies that are believed to promote health and well-being and include yoga, relaxation-response techniques, meditation, tai chi, hypnotherapy, spirituality, support groups, visual imagery, and biofeedback. This field views illness as an opportunity for growth and transformation.

WHOLE MEDICAL SYSTEMS

Whole medical systems use multiple modalities when promoting health and treating illness and are exemplified by traditional Chinese medicine.

Other approaches in this category include homeopathy, Ayurveda, natu-ropathy, chiropractic medicine, Native-American medicine, and the various forms of acupuncture.

BIOLOGICALLY BASED PRACTICES

Biologically based practices include, but are not limited to, the use of botanicals, animal-derived extracts, vitamins, minerals, fatty acids, amino acids, proteins, whole diets, functional foods, and probiotics. A large num-ber of these substances have historically formed the basis of the Western pharmacopeia.

Nutrition-based and diet-based practices encompass the use of vitamins, minerals, and nutritional supplements, in general, and cancer and cardio-vascular disease diets, in particular. Dietary supplements that have gained popularity in Western culture include the use of glucosamine for arthritis, of echinacea for upper respiratory infections, and of fish oil for cardio-vascular disease. Other diet-based and nutrition-based treatments include megadosing, elimination of or excessive intake of certain foods, vegetarian and macrobiotic diets, and diets associated with various physicians (see also the "Fitness" section earlier in Part 3).

Functional foods are components of the usual diet that may have bio-logically active components (eg, fish oils and polyphenols). Specific examples include dark chocolate, soy, and nuts. Sales of functional foods are explod-ing, thanks in part to the ability of manufacturers to advertise directly to consumers.

Probiotics are defined by the World Health Organization and the Food and Agriculture Organization of the United Nations as "live microorgan-isms, which, when administered in adequate amounts, confer a health benefit on the host." Probiotics are enjoying increasing popularity, par-ticularly among women. These bacteria, often used to promote digestion, are similar to bacteria found normally in the gut, either *lactobacillus* or *bifidobacterium* species. Of interest to the obstetrician–gynecologist are women who use probiotics to treat irritable bowel syndrome or infections of the female urinary or genital tract. Probiotics are available in foods and dietary supplements and in some other forms as well. In probiotic foods and supplements, the bacteria may have been present originally or added during preparation. Examples of foods that contain probiotics include yogurt, fermented and unfermented milk, miso, tempeh, and some juices and soy beverages.

MANIPULATIVE AND BODY-BASED PRACTICES

Manipulative and body-based practices focus mainly on the structures and systems of the body, including the bones and joints, the soft tissues, and the circulatory and lymphatic systems. These are among the most widely accepted and commonly used CAM therapies. Examples include massage and chiropractic and osteopathic manipulation.

ENERGY MEDICINE

Energy medicine describes a domain of CAM that uses two types of energy to affect health: 1) veritable, which is of specific measurable wavelengths or frequencies, and 2) putative (or biofield), which has so far eluded measurement. Veritable energy medicine includes the use of magnets to treat musculoskeletal and neurologic pain; of low-frequency thermal waves for deep tissue heat treatment (or diathermy); of pulsed electromagnetic waves to treat bone fractures; of transcutaneous electrical nerve stimulation for pain relief; and of light to treat conditions such as seasonal affective disorder. Putative energy medicine is based on the concept that humans are infused with subtle forms of energy. Examples include the use of qi in acupuncture, Reiki, therapeutic touch, Ayurveda, and distant healing.

Safety Concerns

Safety is the critical issue when a patient asks about the merit of using a CAM product or intervention. The potential can exist for direct and indirect risks. These risks can include patient delay in or avoidance of seeking appropriate conventional treatment, a misdiagnosis, toxic reactions from ingested substances, and interference with the mechanism of action of a prescribed drug or treatment.

Over-the-counter herbal preparations and dietary supplements, such as those marketed to relieve menopausal symptoms, may be of particular concern to the obstetrician–gynecologist. There can be uncertainty as to the identity of the active ingredient and its potency. Also, the chemical composition may vary from manufacturer to manufacturer and by lot number, and there may be adulteration without this being identified on the label. In 2007, the U.S. Food and Drug Administration was given the authority to oversee the manufacture of domestic and foreign-made dietary supplements, including herbal supplements. The regulations require supplement manufacturers to evaluate the identity, purity, strength, and composition of their dietary supplements to ensure that they contain what their labels claim and are free of contaminants. It is also important to note that these regulations do not change the fact that dietary supplements are regulated as foods, not as medications and, therefore, do not have to provide evidence to the U.S. Food and Drug Administration of effectiveness or safety.

Concerns about safety can be tempered for some CAM modalities. For instance, it is unlikely that homeopathic preparations, acupuncture, biofeedback, or prayer will be associated with direct adverse effects. In contrast, intravenous hydrogen peroxide, chelation therapy, and megadosing of supplements can be toxic and dangerous. Accordingly, when informed that a patient is using CAM, her clinician can advise her if there is supporting published research, warn her about real or potential dangers, ascertain whether the CAM method can be continued in conjunction with conventional treatment, and monitor her treatment for positive and negative effects over time.

Addressing Patient Use and Interest

Most patients who use CAM are self-referred and do not tell their physicians about their use of CAM treatments. Thus, their medical record is incomplete, and the possibility of medical risk cannot be addressed. Inquiring about the patient's interest in, or use of, CAM and providing information on safety and effectiveness can be integral to the physician's role as a patient advocate. Patients can be asked questions such as, "Have you used or have you been considering other kinds of treatment or medications for relief of your symptoms or to maintain wellness?" Follow-up questions to a positive answer can include asking when she decided to use CAM, what results she was expecting, how she chose the method, and how it has worked for her. This information can then be documented in the patient's medical record.

Some patients will request a referral to a local alternative care provider. Any such referral should be made only to a state-licensed provider. All states license chiropractors, but not all license other CAM providers, such as naturopathic physicians, acupuncturists, or massage therapists. Physicians should be aware of possible liability consequences of such referrals. If the referral itself is negligent because it is inconsistent with generally accepted standards of medical practice, the referring physician may be exposed to liability if the patient is injured by the subsequent treatment. Also, liability may arise if the referring physician supervises the CAM care, jointly treats the patient, or knows (or should have known) that the CAM provider is unlicensed.

It can be anticipated that patients will continue to use CAM with or without physician referral. Accompanying this use is the public's expectation that health insurance plans will reimburse for CAM treatment. A growing number of third-party payers have responded by doing so under a variety of clinical guidelines. This willingness can result in conflict between physicians and CAM providers if important operational issues are not addressed. These issues include the creation of protocols and plans of care for specific diagnoses, procedures for monitoring and follow-up with finite clinical endpoints, evidence for safety and effectiveness, and identified criteria for referral to conventional care.

Health Care Provider Education

Each physician can determine to what extent he or she wishes to learn more about various aspects of CAM. There are a number of ways to obtain information. Clinical studies in peer-reviewed, conventional medical journals now appear on a regular basis. In addition to continuing medical education courses, there are peer-reviewed medical journals, textbooks, and newsletters devoted to the subject. Computer databases and web pages specifically oriented to CAM now are accessible by physicians and patients (see Bibliography and Resources).

In the coming years, it is likely that there will be a continued blending of conventional medicine with various CAM therapies as evidence-based research data support clinical decision making in patient care. This comprehensive approach is known as integrated medical care.

Bibliography

Barnes J, Anderson LA, Phillipson JD. Herbal medicines. 3rd ed. London: Pharmaceutical Press; 2007.

Blumenthal M, editor. The complete German Commission E monographs: Therapeutic guide to herbal medicines. Austin (TX): American Botanical Council; 1998.

Blumenthal M. Herbal medicine: expanded Commission E monographs. 1st ed. Newton (MA): Integrative Medicine Communications; 2000.

Jonas WB, Levin JS, editors. Essentials of complementary and alternative medicine. Philadelphia (PA): Lippincott Williams & Wilkins; 1999.

Mayo Clinic. Herbal supplements: what to know before you buy. Available at: http://www.mayoclinic.com/health/herbal-supplements/SA00044. Retrieved July 24, 2013.

Nahin RL, Barnes PM, Stussman BJ, Bloom B. Costs of complementary and alternative medicine (CAM) and frequency of visits to CAM practitioners: United States, 2007. Natl Health Stat Report 2009;(18):1–14.

National Center for Complementary and Alternative Medicine. National Institutes of Health. Available at: http://nccam.nih.gov. Retrieved July 24, 2013.

National Institutes of Health. Alternative medicine: expanding medical horizons: a report to the National Institutes of Health on alternative medical systems and practices in the United States. Bethesda (MD): NIH; 1995.

PDR for herbal medicines. 4th ed. Montvale (NJ): Medical Economics Co.; 2007.

Segen JC. Dictionary of alternative medicine. Stamford (CT): Appleton & Lange; 1998.

Resources

American Botanical Council. Available at: http://abc.herbalgram.org. Retrieved July 24, 2013.

Center for Complementary and Integrative Medicine. Weill Cornell Medical College. Available at: http://weill.cornell.edu/ccim. Retrieved July 24, 2013.

National Cancer Institute. Complementary and alternative medicine. Available at: http://www.cancer.gov/cancertopics/cam. Retrieved July 24, 2013.

National Center for Complementary and Alternative Medicine. Herbs at a glance. Available at: http://nccam.nih.gov/health/herbsataglance.htm. Retrieved July 24, 2013.

National Center for Complementary and Alternative Medicine. Resources for health care providers. Available at: http://nccam.nih.gov/health/providers. Retrieved August 20, 2013.

National Library of Medicine. Available at: http://www.nlm.nih.gov. Retrieved July 24, 2013.

Office of Dietary Supplements. National Institutes of Health. Available at: http://ods.od.nih.gov. Retrieved July 24, 2013.

CARDIOVASCULAR DISORDERS

Cardiovascular disease (CVD) is the leading cause of death in U.S. women. Cardiovascular disease often presents differently and has a higher mortality rate in women than in men. The obstetrician–gynecologist can educate, screen, monitor, and treat women to reduce their risk of morbidity and mortality from CVD, such as from myocardial infarction and stroke. For women of reproductive age who have CVD or related disorders, it is particularly important to avoid unintended pregnancy until the disorder is under control, given the risks of pregnancy to the woman and her fetus. The U.S. Medical Eligibility Criteria for Contraceptive Use (www.cdc.gov/reproductivehealth/unintendedpregnancy/usmec.htm) is an excellent resource that can help guide practitioners in regard to contraception for patients with cardiovascular disorders as well as other coexisting medical conditions (see also the "Family Planning" section later in Part 3).

Patients should be counseled about factors that increase their risk of CVD: family history of CVD, dyslipidemia, hypertension, obesity, lack of exercise, and smoking. Individuals with polycystic ovary syndrome may be at increased risk of coronary heart disease (CHD) because of underlying chronic anovulation and hyperandrogenism (see also the "Polycystic Ovary Syndrome" section in Part 4). Other conditions unique to women that also can increase a woman's risk of CVD include pregnancy-induced hypertension, preeclampsia, and gestational diabetes. Nonmodifiable risk factors for CVD include age older than 55 years, a family history of premature CHD (defined as myocardial infarction or sudden death in a first-degree male relative before age 55 years or a first-degree female relative before age 65 years), and a personal history of peripheral arterial disease. Risk factors that can be modified include cigarette smoking; physical inactivity; obesity; a poor diet; and medical conditions such as diabetes, hypertension, and hyperlipidemia.

Patients with major medical risk factors, life habit risk factors, and emerging risk factors are characterized by a condition called metabolic syndrome. The National Heart, Lung, and Blood Institute and the American Heart Association define metabolic syndrome in women as the presence of three or more of the following components:

- Waist circumference equal to or greater than 35 inches
- Triglyceride level 150 mg/dL or higher
- High-density lipoprotein (HDL) cholesterol less than 50 mg/dL
- Blood pressure 130/85 mm Hg or higher
- Fasting glucose level 100 mg/dL or higher

Pharmaceutical treatment for elevated triglyceride levels, reduced HDL cholesterol levels, elevated blood pressure, or elevated fasting glucose are alternative indicators for those measures.

The clinician should address the following issues with patients as indicated, depending on age, risk factors, and medical history:

- Educate patients regarding risk factors for, and symptoms of, CVD.
- Educate patients regarding heart attack symptoms: sudden, intense pressure or pain in the chest; shortness of breath; chest pain that spreads to the shoulders, neck, or arms; and feelings of lightheadedness, fainting, sweating, or nausea. Although many women do experience these symptoms, women are more likely than men to have atypical symptoms, such as "heartburn," or pain only in their shoulders, neck, or arms.
- Counsel patients regarding lifestyle modifications.
  — Diet low in saturated fat, trans-fatty acids, and sodium
  — Moderate exercise (see also the "Fitness" section earlier in Part 3)
  — Smoking cessation
  — Weight control (maintain body mass index [calculated as weight in kilograms divided by height in meters squared] between 18.5 and 24.9)
  — Limiting alcohol consumption
- Counsel patients regarding safe and effective contraceptive methods.

- Screen for hypertension.
- Screen for cholesterol.
- Screen for other conditions that can affect CVD (see "Hypertension" and "Dyslipidemia" in this section and the "Diabetes Mellitus" section later in Part 3).
- Counsel patients with diabetes on the need to maintain normoglycemia.
- Treat or refer when risk factors are identified.
- In women aged 55–79 years, the U.S. Preventive Services Task Force recommends low-dose aspirin therapy if the benefit for prevention of ischemic stroke is likely to outweigh the risk of gastrointestinal bleeding. The optimum dose of aspirin for preventing CVD events is not known, but a dosage of approximately 75 mg/d seems as effective as higher dosages. The decision about the exact stroke risk level at which the potential benefits outweigh harms is an individual one. Some women may decide that avoiding a stroke is of great value but experiencing a gastrointestinal bleeding event is not a major problem. These women would probably decide to take low-dose aspirin at a lower stroke risk level than those who are more concerned about having a bleeding event. Women younger than 55 years should be discouraged from taking aspirin for CVD prevention.

Guidelines on the assessment of CVD risk and on lifestyle management to reduce risk have been published jointly by the American College of Cardiology (ACC) and the American Heart Association (AHA) (see Resources).

Hypertension

Hypertension, generally defined as blood pressure higher than 140/90 mm Hg, affects 68 million adults in the United States. The incidence of hypertension increases with each decade of life. Approximately one half of U.S. women in their 50s are hypertensive, and the prevalence continues to increase thereafter. At every age, African-American women have a higher prevalence of hypertension than white women. Hypertension increases the risk of CVD events, including CHD, congestive heart failure, stroke, peripheral vascular disease, and renal failure. Untreated hypertension is a major cause of mortality, with risk directly proportional to the degree of hypertension.

CLASSIFICATION

In 2004, the National Heart, Lung, and Blood Institute published its *Seventh Report of the Joint National Committee on Prevention, Detection, Evaluation, and Treatment of High Blood Pressure* (JNC 7), which classifies blood pressure levels as normal, prehypertension, stage 1 hypertension, or stage 2 hypertension (Table 3-2). Guidelines for the management of hypertension released subsequently do not address classification of blood pressure levels, so it is reasonable to continue to follow the classification schema in JNC 7. Most patients with hypertension have primary hypertension (elevated blood pressure with no demonstrable cause), and perhaps 5% of affected patients have secondary hypertension (hypertension associated with other diseases) or malignant hypertension (severe hypertensive state, with diastolic pressure as high as 130 mm Hg or more and a poor prognosis). High-risk groups for hypertension include African-American women, older women, women with prehypertension, women with a family history of hypertension, and women with lifestyle factors associated with hypertension (eg, obesity and excessive alcohol use).

Table 3-2. Classification of Blood Pressure for Adults 18 Years and Older

BP Classification	Systolic BP (mm Hg)		Diastolic BP (mm Hg)
Normal	Less than 120	and	Less than 80
Prehypertension	120–139	or	80–89
Stage 1 hypertension	140–159	or	90–99
Stage 2 hypertension	160 or more	or	100 or more

Abbreviation: BP, blood pressure.

Reprinted from National Heart, Lung, and Blood Institute. The seventh report of the Joint National Committee on Prevention, Detection, Evaluation, and Treatment of High Blood Pressure. NIH Publication No. 04-5230. Bethesda (MD): NHLBI; 2004. Available at: http://www.nhlbi.nih.gov/guidelines/hypertension/jnc7full.pdf. Retrieved September 10, 2013.

IDENTIFICATION AND EVALUATION

Obstetrician–gynecologists can assume a pivotal role in the prevention of hypertension-related morbidity and mortality. Suggestions for modifying lifestyle can be incorporated into patient counseling to prevent the development of chronic hypertension. Identification and management of women with prehypertension or stage 1 hypertension are within the capabilities of the obstetrician–gynecologist (see Table 3-2). More advanced stages should be referred for specialist consultation.

Blood pressure readings higher than 120/80 mm Hg should alert the physician to begin counseling for lifestyle modifications to prevent the development of chronic hypertension. However, a single blood pressure measurement is insufficient for diagnosis. At least two measurements should be made and the average recorded. Proper technique is crucial to measuring blood pressure accurately. The method recommended by JNC 7 is shown in Box 3-7. Particularly important is proper assessment of Korotkoff heart sounds.

Laboratory assessments in women with hypertension include urinalysis, complete blood count, serum chemistries (eg, potassium, sodium, creatinine, and fasting glucose measurements), and lipid profile. Electrocardiography should be performed, and if ventricular hypertrophy is indicated, echocardiography should be considered.

MANAGEMENT

The goal of managing hypertension is to achieve a systolic blood pressure below 140 mm Hg and a diastolic blood pressure less than 90 mm Hg. Whether individuals 60 years of age or older should have a higher systolic blood pressure goal is controversial. Panel members appointed to the Eighth Joint National Committee on the Prevention, Detection, Evaluation, and Treatment of High Blood Pressure (JNC 8) recommend a systolic blood pressure treatment goal of less than 150 mm Hg for this population; during the development of these guidelines, the National, Heart, Lung, and Blood Institute decided to discontinue developing guidelines, so these recommendations do not reflect the views of the Institute. However, a science advisory from the ACC, AHA, and the Centers for Disease Control

Box 3-7. Recommended Techniques of Blood Pressure Measurement

- A properly calibrated and validated instrument should be used for blood pressure measurement.
- Patients should be seated in a chair with their feet on the floor, their backs supported, and their arms bared and supported at the level of their hearts. Patients should refrain from smoking or ingesting caffeine for at least 30 minutes before the blood pressure measurement.
- Blood pressure measurement should be taken after 5 minutes of rest.
- The appropriate-sized cuff should be used to ensure accuracy. The bladder of the blood pressure cuff should encircle at least 80% of the arm.
- Systolic and diastolic blood pressures should be recorded. Systolic blood pressure is defined by the first appearance of Korotkoff heart sounds (phase I), and diastolic blood pressure is defined by the disappearance of Korotkoff heart sounds (phase V).

Data from National Heart, Lung, and Blood Institute. The seventh report of the Joint National Committee on Prevention, Detection, Evaluation, and Treatment of High Blood Pressure. NIH Publication No. 04-5230. Bethesda (MD): NHLBI; 2004. Available at: http://www.nhlbi.nih.gov/guidelines/hypertension/jnc7full.pdf. Retrieved September 10, 2013.

and Prevention retains the systolic blood pressure goal of less than 140 mm Hg set by JNC 7. Lifestyle modifications for prevention and management of hypertension include the following:

- Quitting smoking
- Weight loss (in overweight patients)
- Limiting alcohol intake for women who consume two or more alcoholic beverages daily
- Increasing aerobic physical activity (see also the "Fitness" section earlier in Part 3)
- Reducing sodium intake to less than 2,300 mg/d for the general population and to 1,500 mg/d for people at risk (individuals 51 years or older; African Americans; and those with hypertension, diabetes, or chronic kidney disease)

- Reducing dietary intake of saturated fat and cholesterol
- Ensuring adequate dietary intake of potassium, calcium, and magnesium

A variety of pharmacologic therapies are available for managing hypertension, including thiazide diuretics, adrenergic blockers, angiotensin-converting enzyme inhibitors, angiotensin II receptor blockers, and calcium channel blockers. Note that angiotensin-converting enzyme inhibitors should be used with caution in women who may become pregnant.

Dyslipidemia

Coronary heart disease is the leading cause of death for men and women in the United States and accounts for approximately 500,000 deaths each year. Clinical trials have shown that a 1% reduction in serum cholesterol levels results in a 2% reduction in CHD rates. Approximately one quarter to one third of individuals who have a first coronary event will die as a result. Although cholesterol level reduction is anticipated to result in a short-term benefit in patients at risk of future CHD, the near-term benefit of decreasing cholesterol levels is greater among patients with established CHD. Thus, primary prevention (ie, prevention for patients without established CHD) and secondary prevention (ie, prevention for patients with established CHD) are both important goals.

IDENTIFICATION AND EVALUATION

Abnormal cholesterol levels have been firmly linked to atherosclerosis and cardiovascular and cerebrovascular disease. However, standards that apply to the identification of candidates for testing and frequency of testing differ among organizations. Furthermore, the value of lipid screening in women without definite risk factors (eg, tobacco use, hypertension, diabetes, or a family history of CVD) remains disputed. Current guidelines from the American College of Obstetricians and Gynecologists recommend that women without risk factors have a lipid profile assessment (measurement of total cholesterol, low-density lipoprotein [LDL] cholesterol, HDL cholesterol, and triglyceride levels) every 5 years, beginning at age 45 years. Earlier screening may be appropriate in women with risk factors (see www.acog.org/About_ACOG/ACOG_Departments/Annual_Womens_ Health_Care/High-Risk_Factors).

The 2013 ACC and AHA guideline for the management of high blood cholesterol levels is based on assessment of atherosclerotic cardiovascular disease risk to determine individuals who would most benefit from cholesterol-lowering therapy. In addition to evaluation of blood cholesterol levels with a fasting lipid profile (Box 3-8), the 2013 ACC and AHA guidelines recommend calculation of 10-year cardiovascular disease risk with a risk calculator developed for the guidelines (see Resources). The well-known Framingham risk score, which incorporates various risk factors to derive an estimated risk of developing CHD within 10 years, was rejected by the 2013 ACC and AHA guideline developers because it was developed with solely a white population and provided risk estimates only for CHD. The new calculator includes levels of total cholesterol and HDL cholesterol (Box 3-8), but the guidelines indicate that evidence is insufficient to establish treatment targets for LDL cholesterol or other non-HDL cholesterol. These guidelines and the risk calculator on which they rely have been criticized.

MANAGEMENT

Research indicates that elevated LDL cholesterol is a major cause of CHD. In addition, recent clinical trials show that LDL cholesterol–lowering therapy reduces the risk of CHD. Treatment for high LDL cholesterol levels can include therapeutic lifestyle changes, drug therapy, or both depending on the risk category of the patient. Therapeutic lifestyle changes include dietary changes to reduce intake of saturated fats and cholesterol and enhance intake of plant stanols, sterols, and soluble fiber; weight reduction; and increased physical activity. Drug therapy options include statins, bile acid sequestrants, and nicotinic acids. However, 2013 guidelines on the management of high blood cholesterol levels issued jointly by the ACC and the AHA recommend primary drug therapy with statins based on evidence that nonstatins do not provide acceptable risk reduction compared with the potential for adverse events.

Thromboembolic Disease

Venous thromboembolic disease represents a spectrum of conditions that range from peripheral thrombosis to pulmonary embolism and stroke.

Box 3-8. Fasting Lipoprotein Profile

Low-Density Lipoprotein Cholesterol (mg/dL)

Less than 100	Optimal
100–129	Near optimal or above optimal
130–159	Borderline high
160–189	High
190 or more	Very high

High-Density Lipoprotein Cholesterol (mg/dL)

Less than 40	Low
50 or more	Optimal

Total Cholesterol (mg/dL)

Less than 180	Optimal
180–199	Nonoptimal
200–239	Elevated risk factor
240 or more	Major risk factor

Serum Triglycerides (mg/dL)

Less than 150	Normal
150–199	Borderline high
200–499	High
500 or more	Very high

Data from National Heart, Lung, and Blood Institute. Third report of the Expert Panel on Detection, Evaluation, and Treatment of High Blood Cholesterol in Adults (Adult Treatment Panel III). Bethesda (MD): NHLBI; Available at: http://www.nhlbi.nih.gov/guidelines/cholesterol/index.htm. Retrieved July 25, 2013 *and* Eckel RH, Jakicic JM, Ard JD, Hubbard VS, de Jesus JM, Lee IM, et al. 2013 AHA/ACC guideline on lifestyle management to reduce cardiovascular risk: a report of the American College of Cardiology/American Heart Association Task Force on Practice Guidelines. Circulation 2013; DOI: 10.1161/01.cir.0000437740.48606.d1. J Am Coll Cardiol 2013; DOI: 10.1016/j.jacc.2013.11.003.

Risk factors for venous thromboembolic disease include age, prolonged immobility (eg, due to stroke or paralysis), surgery, trauma, malignancy, pregnancy, use of estrogenic medications (eg, hormonal contraceptives, hormone therapy, raloxifene, and tamoxifen), congestive heart failure, hyperhomocystinemia, diseases that increase blood viscosity (eg, polycythemia, sickle cell disease, and multiple myeloma), and inherited thrombophilia. Patients with inheritable causes of thrombosis usually do not have spontaneous venous thrombosis until they have been exposed to another environmental risk factor, such as pregnancy, trauma, surgery, or immobilization.

Venous thromboembolism is a leading cause of morbidity and mortality in hospitalized patients in the United States. The presence of an asymptomatic deep vein thromboembolism is strongly linked to the development of a clinically significant pulmonary embolism. Most patients who die from a pulmonary embolism do so within 30 minutes of the event, leaving little time for therapeutic interventions. Thus, it is important to assess patient risk and adopt appropriate preventive measures before surgery or hospitalization. Evidence-based risk assessment classifications and recommended prophylaxis strategies based on risk have been published by the American College of Chest Physicians (see Resources).

Bibliography

Aspirin for the prevention of cardiovascular disease: U.S. Preventive Services Task Force recommendation statement. US Preventive Services Task Force. Ann Intern Med 2009;150:396–404.

Department of Agriculture, Department of Health and Human Services. Dietary guidelines for Americans, 2010. 7th ed. Washington, DC: Government Printing Office; 2010. Available at: http://www.cnpp.usda.gov/DGAs2010-PolicyDocument. htm. Retrieved July 24, 2013.

Department of Health and Human Services. The Heart Truth: lecture materials and PowerPoint slides. Available at: http://www.womenshealth.gov/heart-truth/clinical-education/lecture-materials.php. Retrieved July 25, 2013.

Eckel RH, Jakicic JM, Ard JD, Hubbard VS, de Jesus JM, Lee IM, et al. 2013 AHA/ACC guideline on lifestyle management to reduce cardiovascular risk: a report of the American College of Cardiology/American Heart Association Task Force on Practice Guidelines. Circulation 2013; DOI: 10.1161/01.cir.0000437740.48606.d1. J Am Coll Cardiol 2013; DOI: 10.1016/j.jacc.2013.11.003.

Go AS, Bauman MA, Coleman King SM, Fonarow GC, Lawrence W, Williams KA, et al. An effective approach to high blood pressure control: a science advisory from the American Heart Association, the American College of Cardiology, and the Centers for Disease Control and Prevention. J Am Coll Cardiol 2014;63:1230–8 and Hypertension 2014;63:878–85.

Goff DC Jr, Lloyd-Jones DM, Bennett G, Coady S, D'Agostino RB S, Gibbons R, et al. 2013 ACC/AHA guideline on the assessment of cardiovascular risk: a report of the American College of Cardiology/American Heart Association Task Force on Practice Guidelines. Circulation 2013; DOI: 10.1161/01.cir.0000437741.48606.98. J Am Coll Cardiol 2013; DOI: 10.1016/j.jacc.2013.11.005.

Grundy SM, Cleeman JI, Daniels SR, Donato KA, Eckel RH, Franklin BA, et al. Diagnosis and management of the metabolic syndrome: an American Heart Association/National Heart, Lung, and Blood Institute Scientific Statement. American Heart Association and National Heart, Lung, and Blood Institute [published errata appear in Circulation 2005;112:e297. Circulation 2005;112:e298]. Circulation 2005;112:2735–52.

James PA, Oparil S, Carter BL, Cushman WC, Dennison-Himmelfarb C, Handler J, et al. 2014 evidence-based guideline for the management of high blood pressure in adults: report from the Panel Members Appointed to the Eighth Joint National Committee (JNC 8). JAMA 2013; DOI: 10.1001/jama.2013.284427.

Moyer VA. Behavioral counseling interventions to promote a healthful diet and physical activity for cardiovascular disease prevention in adults: U.S. Preventive Services Task Force recommendation statement. U.S. Preventive Services Task Force. Ann Intern Med 2012;157:367–72.

National Cholesterol Education Program. Third report of the Expert Panel on Detection, Evaluation, and Treatment of High Blood Cholesterol in Adults (Adult Treatment Panel III). National Heart, Lung, and Blood Institute. Bethesda (MD): NHLBI; Available at: http://www.nhlbi.nih.gov/guidelines/cholesterol/index.htm. Retrieved July 25, 2013.

National Heart, Lung, and Blood Institute. The seventh report of the Joint National Committee on Prevention, Detection, Evaluation, and Treatment of High Blood Pressure. NIH Publication No. 04-5230. Bethesda (MD): NHLBI; 2004. Available at: http://www.nhlbi.nih.gov/guidelines/hypertension/jnc7full.pdf. Retrieved September 10, 2013.

Polycystic ovary syndrome. ACOG Practice Bulletin No. 108. American College of Obstetricians and Gynecologists. Obstet Gynecol 2009;114:936–49.

Prevention of deep vein thrombosis and pulmonary embolism. ACOG Practice Bulletin No. 84. American College of Obstetricians and Gynecologists. Obstet Gynecol 2007;110:429–40.

Stone NJ, Robinson J, Lichtenstein AH, Bairey Merz CN, Lloyd-Jones DM, Blum CB, et al. 2013 ACC/AHA guideline on the treatment of blood cholesterol to reduce atherosclerotic cardiovascular risk in adults: a report of the American College of Cardiology/American Heart Association Task Force on Practice Guidelines. J Am Coll Cardiol 2013; DOI: 10.1016/j.jacc.2013.11.002. Circulation 2013; DOI: 10.1161/01.cir.0000437738.63853.7a.

Yoon PW, Gillespie CD, George MG, Wall HK. Control of hypertension among adults–National Health and Nutrition Examination Survey, United States, 2005–2008. Centers for Disease Control and Prevention. MMWR Morb Mortal Wkly Rep 2012;61(suppl):19–25.

Resources

American College of Cardiology. Guidelines and quality standards. Available at: http://www.cardiosource.org/Science-And-Quality/Practice-Guidelines-and-Quality-Standards.aspx. Retrieved January 30, 2014.

American College of Cardiology, American Heart Association. 2013 prevention guideline tools and risk calculator. Available at: http://www.cardiosource.org/science-and-quality/practice-guidelines-and-quality-standards/2013-prevention-guideline-tools.aspx. Retrieved January 30, 2014.

American College of Cardiology, American Heart Association. CV risk calculator. Available at: http://my.americanheart.org/professional/StatementsGuidelines/PreventionGuidelines/Prevention-Guidelines_UCM_457698_SubHomePage.jsp. Retrieved January 30, 2014.

American College of Obstetricians and Gynecologists. Annual women's health care: high risk factors. Available at: http://www.acog.org/About_ACOG/ACOG_Depart ments/Annual_Womens_Health_Care/High-Risk_Factors. Retrieved October 1, 2013.

American College of Obstetricians and Gynecologists. Cholesterol and your health. Patient Education Pamphlet AP101. Washington, DC: American College of Obstetricians and Gynecologists; 2013.

American College of Obstetricians and Gynecologists. Keeping your heart healthy. Patient Education Pamphlet AP122. Washington, DC: American College of Obstetricians and Gynecologists; 2004.

American College of Obstetricians and Gynecologists. Managing high blood pressure. Patient Education Pamphlet AP123. Washington, DC: American College of Obstetricians and Gynecologists; 2010.

Gould MK, Garcia DA, Wren SM, Karanicolas PJ, Arcelus JI, Heit JA, et al. Prevention of VTE in nonorthopedic surgical patients: Antithrombotic therapy and prevention of thrombosis, 9th ed: American College of Chest Physicians evidence-based clinical practice guidelines. American College of Chest Physicians [published erratum appears in Chest 2012;141:1369]. Chest 2012;141:e227S–77S.

Mosca L, Benjamin EJ, Berra K, Bezanson JL, Dolor RJ, Lloyd-Jones DM, et al. Effectiveness-based guidelines for the prevention of cardiovascular disease in women—2011 update: a guideline from the American Heart Association. Circulation 2011;123:1243–62.

National Heart, Lung, and Blood Institute. Information for health professionals: cholesterol. Available at: http://www.nhlbi.nih.gov/health/prof/heart/index. htm#chol. Retrieved January 30, 2014.

National Heart, Lung, and Blood Institute. Information for professionals: other heart and vascular diseases. Available at: http://www.nhlbi.nih.gov/health/prof/heart/index.htm#hd. Retrieved January 30, 2014.

Ozaki A, Bartholomew JR. Venous thromboembolism (deep venous thrombosis & pulmonary embolism). Cleveland (OH): Cleveland Clinic Foundation; 2012. Available at: http://www.clevelandclinicmeded.com/medicalpubs/diseasemanagement/cardiology/venous-thromboembolism. Retrieved July 25, 2013.

Screening for high blood pressure: U.S. Preventive Services Task Force reaffirmation recommendation statement. U.S. Preventive Services Task Force. Ann Intern Med 2007;147:783–6.

U.S. Medical Eligibility Criteria for Contraceptive Use, 2010. Centers for Disease Control and Prevention. MMWR Recomm Rep 2010;59(RR-4):1-86. Available at: http://www.cdc.gov/mmwr/pdf/rr/rr5904.pdf. September 26, 2013.

U.S. Preventive Services Task Force. Screening for Lipid Disorders in Adults: U.S. Preventive Services Task Force Recommendation Statement. AHRQ Publication No. 08-05114-EF-2, June 2008 Agency for Healthcare Research and Quality, Rockville, MD. Available at: http://www.uspreventiveservicestaskforce.org/clinic/uspstf08/lipid/lipidrs.htm. Retrieved July 25, 2013.

Vandvik PO, Lincoff AM, Gore JM, Gutterman DD, Sonnenberg FA, Alonso-Coello P, et al. Primary and secondary prevention of cardiovascular disease: antithrombotic therapy and prevention of thrombosis, 9th ed: American College of Chest Physicians evidence-based clinical practice guidelines. American College of Chest Physicians [published erratum appears in Chest 2012;141:1129]. Chest 2012; 141:e637S–e668S.

DIABETES MELLITUS

Diabetes mellitus is a group of disorders that share hyperglycemia as a common feature. Diabetes results from a combination of insulin resistance, increased hepatic output of glucose, and pancreatic insufficiency. Type 2 diabetes mellitus, which is characterized by insulin resistance, is the most common form of diabetes. Other forms include type 1 diabetes mellitus (characterized by absent or insufficient insulin production), gestational diabetes mellitus (or GDM, defined as carbohydrate intolerance that begins or is first recognized in pregnancy), and diabetes that is due to other causes (eg, genetic defects in beta-cell function or in insulin action). Approximately 30% of people with diabetes in the United States, or 6.2 million people, are undiagnosed. Even when symptoms are not present, the disease can cause long-term complications. As many as 25% of people with a new diagnosis of diabetes already have established diabetic retinopathy or microalbuminuria, which has been interpreted to mean that there is, on average, a 7-year gap between actual onset and clinical recognition. Diabetes that is due to obesity may be preventable or reversible with weight loss. Exercise increases insulin sensitivity and may forestall or prevent the development of diabetes. Management of diabetes often requires a multidisciplinary team approach and needs to take into account the goals of treatment in the multiple organ systems affected.

Prevention

There is good evidence that structured programs that emphasize lifestyle changes with moderate weight loss (7% of body weight), regular physical activity (150 min/wk), and a diet of reduced calories and reduced fat intake can decrease the risk of developing type 2 diabetes in high-risk patients (Box 3-9). The oral hypoglycemic drugs metformin and acarbose are less effective than lifestyle measures in the prevention of diabetes. Nutrition

Box 3-9. American Diabetes Association Criteria for Testing for Diabetes in Asymptomatic Adults

1. Testing should be considered in all adults who are overweight (BMI greater than or equal to 25 kg/m^2*) and have additional risk factors:
   - Physical inactivity
   - First-degree relative with diabetes
   - High-risk race/ethnicity (eg, African American, Latino, Native American, Asian American, Pacific Islander)
   - Women who gave birth to a newborn weighing more than 9 lb or were diagnosed with GDM
   - Hypertension (blood pressure greater than or equal to 140/90 mm Hg or on therapy for hypertension)
   - HDL cholesterol level less than 35 mg/dL (0.90 mmol/L) and/or a triglyceride level greater than 250 mg/dL (2.82 mmol/L)
   - Women with polycystic ovary syndrome
   - Hemoglobin A$_{1c}$ greater than or equal to 5.7%, IGT, or IFG on previous testing
   - Other clinical conditions associated with insulin resistance (eg, severe obesity, acanthosis nigricans)
   - History of cardiovascular disease
2. In the absence of the above criteria, testing for diabetes should begin at age 45 years.
3. If results are normal, testing should be repeated at least at 3-year intervals, with consideration of more frequent testing depending on initial results (eg, those with prediabetes should be tested yearly) and risk status.

Abbreviations: BMI, body mass index; GDM, gestational diabetes mellitus; HDL, high-density lipoprotein; IFG, impaired fasting glucose; IGT, impaired glucose tolerance.

*At-risk BMI may be lower in some ethnic groups.

Modified with permission from Standards of medical care in diabetes–2014. American Diabetes Association. Diabetes Care 2014;37 Suppl 1:S14-80. Copyright 2014 American Diabetes Association.

control is an integral component of preventive care for women with prediabetes (ie, individuals with impaired glucose tolerance, impaired fasting glucose, or both [see Table 3-3]). These women need thorough dietary counseling and may need the services of a dietitian to help with planning their diet. Health care providers should recommend and facilitate lifestyle interventions to help prevent or delay the onset of diabetes in patients at increased risk. However, when counseling patients, clinicians should be realistic about what behavioral modifications are possible and take into consideration the patient's readiness to change and any significant environmental factors that might impede change.

Screening and Diagnosis

It is best to identify and treat diabetes early in the disease process. The American Diabetes Association and the American College of Obstetricians and Gynecologists recommend that individuals at average risk be screened every 3 years beginning at age 45 years. Screening should begin

Table 3-3. Screening and Diagnostic Criteria for Diabetes Mellitus

Test	Prediabetes Screening*	Diabetes Diagnosis[†]
Fasting plasma glucose	100–125 mg/dL (impaired fasting glucose)	Greater than or equal to 126 mg/dL
2-h, 75-g oral glucose tolerance test	140–199 mg/dL (impaired glucose tolerance)	Greater than or equal to 200 mg/dL
Hemoglobin A_{1c}	5.7–6.4%	Greater than or equal to 6.5%
Random plasma glucose	N/A	Greater than or equal to 200 mg/dL in a patient with classic symptoms of hyperglycemia or hyperglycemic crisis

*If screening results are negative, screen again in 3 years; if screening results are positive, repeat screening using the same method, if possible.

[†]If the results of two different tests are both above diagnostic thresholds, the diagnosis of diabetes is confirmed.

Data from Standards of medical care in diabetes–2014. American Diabetes Association. Diabetes Care 2014;37 Suppl 1:S14–80.

at a younger age and be performed more frequently in individuals with risk factors (see Box 3-9).

There has been some controversy regarding how to screen, diagnose, and treat diabetes. According to the American Diabetes Association, appropriate tests for prediabetes or diabetes include the fasting plasma glucose test; hemoglobin A_{1c} test; or the 2-hour, 75-g oral glucose tolerance test (Table 3-3). The hemoglobin A_{1c} test has several advantages compared with the fasting plasma glucose test and the glucose tolerance test: it does not require patients to fast; it assesses blood glucose control over the past 2–3 months; it has standardized and reliable laboratory methods; and it results in infrequent errors caused by nonglycemic factors. However, these advantages must be balanced against the hemoglobin A_{1c} test's greater cost and its inaccurate assessment of glycemia in certain individuals (eg, those with certain anemias and hemoglobinopathies).

Management

Women's health care providers who wish to implement a treatment plan for women with diabetes can refer to the American Diabetes Association's *Standards of Medical Care in Diabetes* (see Bibliography), which provides annually updated guidelines for management of diabetes. Ongoing treatment, however, usually requires management by a health care provider with expertise in diabetes care.

The goal of management is to ensure adequate glucose control. In asymptomatic patients, lifestyle changes (ie, dietary control, weight loss, and active exercise programs) should be instituted, and the patient should be educated about her disease. If symptoms are present, immediate drug therapy may be necessary. The patient's condition should be assessed to detect complications of the disease, such as organ damage from vascular changes. Considerations for the use of pharmacologic agents include efficacy, cost, adverse effects, comorbidities, and patient preference. If not contraindicated and if tolerated, metformin is the recommended initial pharmacologic agent for the treatment of type 2 diabetes. Common adverse effects of metformin, such as bloating and diarrhea, may be decreased by initiating therapy at low doses and gradually increasing the amounts until therapeutic levels are attained. Metformin administration should be discontinued before radiologic procedures that use iodinated contrast material, such as intravenous pyelography. Insulin therapy often is indicated at some point for many patients with type 2 diabetes.

The American Diabetes Association recommends that nonpregnant women with diabetes lower hemoglobin A_{1c} levels to less than 7.0% to help reduce the risk of microvascular disease. However, a more aggressive goal (such as less than 6.5%) might be considered in patients who are relatively young, such as women of reproductive age; who have short duration of disease; and who have no cardiovascular disease. Less stringent targets (such as less than 8%) might be reasonable in patients with short life expectancy or a history of hypoglycemic episodes, multiple complications, or comorbid conditions or when stricter goals are too difficult to reach.

Because of the greater risk of coronary problems in patients with diabetes, their target blood pressure (less than 140/80 mm Hg) is lower than it is for patients with uncomplicated hypertension. An even lower target level of less than 130/80 mm Hg may be appropriate if this goal can be achieved without undue treatment burden. Based on the clear synergistic risks of hypertension and diabetes, the American Diabetes Association recommends lifestyle changes for patients with diabetes with a blood pressure of more than 120/80 mm Hg and prompt pharmacologic therapy plus lifestyle changes for those with a confirmed blood pressure of more than 140/80 mm Hg.

Another consideration in the care of women with diabetes is contraceptive use. Avoidance of unintended pregnancy is particularly important until diabetes is under control, given the risks of pregnancy to the woman and her fetus. The American Diabetes Association recommends that women with diabetes achieve hemoglobin A_{1c} levels as close to normal (less than 7%) as possible before attempting to conceive. Combined hormonal contraceptives and depot medroxyprogesterone acetate are not recommended in women with type 1 or type 2 diabetes mellitus and nephropathy, retinopathy, other vascular disease, or a history of diabetes for more than 20 years. The risks and benefits of progesterone-only contraceptives should be weighed in this population before use is recommended. Health care providers should reference the Centers for Disease Control and Prevention's

U.S. Medical Eligibility Criteria for Contraceptive Use, 2010 (available at www.cdc.gov/mmwr/pdf/rr/rr5904.pdf) for more detailed information on the use of contraception in women with diabetes and other comorbidities (see also the "Family Planning" section later in Part 3).

Gestational Diabetes Mellitus

Gestational diabetes mellitus (GDM) affects 2–10% of pregnancies in the United States, depending on the characteristics of the population studied. Pregnancy itself impairs insulin action. Although the carbohydrate intolerance of GDM frequently resolves after delivery, up to one third of women who develop GDM will have diabetes or impaired glucose metabolism at postpartum screening and up to 50% will eventually develop diabetes. Women who develop GDM should be screened postpartum with a fasting plasma glucose test or oral glucose tolerance test. Women with normal values should be screened every 3 years thereafter (see also the "Preconception and Interconception Care" section later in Part 3).

Bibliography

Colberg SR, Sigal RJ, Fernhall B, Regensteiner JG, Blissmer BJ, Rubin RR, et al. Exercise and type 2 diabetes: the American College of Sports Medicine and the American Diabetes Association: joint position statement. American College of Sports Medicine and American Diabetes Association. Diabetes Care 2010;33: e147–67.

Ganda OP. Refining lipoprotein assessment in diabetes: apolipoprotein B makes sense. Endocr Pract 2009;15:370–6.

Gestational Diabetes Mellitus. Practice Bulletin No. 137. American College of Obstetricians and Gynecologists. Obstet Gynecol 2013;122:406–16.

Saudek CD, Herman WH, Sacks DB, Bergenstal RM, Edelman D, Davidson MB. A new look at screening and diagnosing diabetes mellitus. J Clin Endocrinol Metab 2008;93:2447–53.

Screening for type 2 diabetes mellitus in adults: U.S. Preventive Services Task Force recommendation statement. U.S. Preventive Services Task Force [published erratum appears in Ann Intern Med 2008;149:147]. Ann Intern Med 2008;148:846–54.

Standards of medical care in diabetes–2014. American Diabetes Association. Diabetes Care 2014;37 Suppl 1:S14–80.

Understanding and using the U.S. Medical Eligibility Criteria For Contraceptive Use, 2010. Committee Opinion No. 505. American College of Obstetricians and Gynecologists. Obstet Gynecol 2011;118:754–60.

U.S. Medical Eligibility Criteria for Contraceptive Use, 2010. Centers for Disease Control and Prevention. MMWR Recomm Rep 2010;59 (RR-4):1–86.

Xiang AH, Kawakubo M, Kjos SL, Buchanan TA. Long-acting injectable progestin contraception and risk of type 2 diabetes in Latino women with prior gestational diabetes mellitus. Diabetes Care 2006;29:613–7.

Resources

Agency for Healthcare Research and Quality. Women at high risk for diabetes: access and quality of health care, 2003–2006. Rockville (MD); 2011. Available at: http://www.ahrq.gov/research/findings/final-reports/women-and-diabetes-2003-2006/index.html. Retrieved September 3, 2013.

American College of Obstetricians and Gynecologists. Diabetes and women. Patient Education Pamphlet AP142. Washington, DC: American College of Obstetricians and Gynecologists; 2011.

American Diabetes Association. Women and diabetes. Available at: http://www.diabetes.org/living-with-diabetes/treatment-and-care/women. Retrieved March 28, 2014.

Department of Health and Human Services. National agenda for public health action: the national public health initiative on diabetes and women's health. Atlanta (GA): USDHHS, Centers for Disease Control and Prevention; 2003. Available at: http://stacks.cdc.gov/view/cdc/6488. Retrieved September 3, 2013.

Umpierrez GE, Hellman R, Korytkowski MT, Kosiborod M, Maynard GA, Montori VM, et al. Management of hyperglycemia in hospitalized patients in non-critical care setting: an endocrine society clinical practice guideline. Endocrine Society. J Clin Endocrinol Metab 2012;97:16–38.

OSTEOPOROSIS

Osteoporosis is a skeletal disorder characterized by loss of bone mass, deterioration of microarchitecture, and a decline in bone quality, all of which lead to an increased vulnerability to fracture. The time of most rapid bone loss in women coincides with the marked decline in estrogen levels associated with menopause. Approximately 9% of U.S. women aged 50 years and older have osteoporosis at the femur neck or lumbar spine, and another 49% of women older than 50 years have low bone mass at the femur neck or lumbar spine, according to the most recent data from the National Health and Nutrition Examination Survey (2005–2008).

Bone mass decreases with age, and bone fragility increases with age. At any bone density, the likelihood of fracture is greater in older women (and men) because of the increase in bone fragility. Although there are many factors that contribute to the likelihood of a fracture, low bone mass is a key determinant and one that is potentially modifiable. Although morbidity and mortality are especially high with hip fractures, the more common thoracic compression spine fracture also is a source of marked morbidity, including pain, deformity, loss of independence, and reduced cardiovascular, respiratory, and even digestive function.

The risk of postmenopausal osteoporosis is a function of the peak bone mass acquired during adolescent growth and the rate of bone loss in adulthood. A decline in adult estrogen levels has been associated with the loss of bone mineral density (BMD) in a number of conditions: anorexia nervosa, lactation, menopause, hypogonadism, and prolonged use of medications such as progestin-only contraceptives (eg, depot medroxyprogesterone acetate [DMPA]), gonadotropin-releasing hormone agonists, and aromatase inhibitors. Certain other drugs and certain diseases or medical conditions also are known to be associated with bone loss (see Box 3-10).

Osteoporosis is a treatable complication of aging. Preventive measures, screening strategies, and pharmacologic interventions for women at high

Box 3-10. Conditions, Diseases, and Medications That Cause or Contribute to Osteoporosis and Fractures

- Lifestyle factors: low calcium intake, vitamin D insufficiency, excess vitamin A, high caffeine intake, high salt intake, aluminum intake (in antacids), alcohol intake (three or more drinks per day), inadequate physical activity, immobilization, smoking (active or passive), falling, thinness
- Genetic factors: cystic fibrosis, homocystinuria, osteogenesis imperfecta, Ehlers-Danlos syndrome, hypophosphatasia, parental history of hip fracture, Gaucher disease, idiopathic hypercalciuria, porphyria, glycogen storage diseases, Marfan syndrome, Riley-Day syndrome, hemochromatosis, Menkes (steely hair) syndrome
- Hypogonadal states: androgen insensitivity, hyperprolactinemia, Turner and Klinefelter syndromes, anorexia nervosa and bulimia, panhypopituitarism, athletic amenorrhea, premature ovarian failure
- Endocrine disorders: adrenal insufficiency, diabetes mellitus, thyrotoxicosis, Cushing's syndrome, hyperparathyroidism
- Gastrointestinal disorders: celiac disease, inflammatory bowel disease, primary biliary cirrhosis, gastric bypass, malabsorption, gastrointestinal surgery, pancreatic disease
- Hematologic disorders: hemophilia, multiple myeloma, systemic mastocytosis, leukemia and lymphomas, sickle cell disease, thalassemia
- Rheumatic and autoimmune diseases: ankylosing spondylitis, lupus, rheumatoid arthritis
- Miscellaneous conditions and diseases: alcoholism, emphysema, muscular dystrophy, amyloidosis, end-stage renal disease, parenteral nutrition, chronic metabolic acidosis, epilepsy, posttransplant bone disease, congestive heart failure, idiopathic scoliosis, prior fracture as an adult, depression, multiple sclerosis, sarcoidosis
- Medications: anticoagulants (heparin), cancer chemotherapeutic drugs, gonadotropin-releasing hormone agonists, anticonvulsants, cyclosporine A and tacrolimus, lithium, aromatase inhibitors, depot medroxyprogesterone, barbiturates, corticosteroids (5 or more mg/d of prednisone or equivalent for 3 or more months)

risk are available to reduce the risk of osteoporosis and reduce the incidence of fracture.

Prevention Counseling

Physical activity, adequate nutrition, and good health are necessary for bone health. The effect of lifestyle and nutrition on bone health should be considered for girls and women of all ages, and patients should be counseled accordingly as part of the annual gynecologic examination. Counseling should include recommending the following preventive measures:

- Adequate calcium and vitamin D consumption—In its 2011 report, the Institute of Medicine (IOM) recommended a dietary allowance for calcium of 1,000 mg/d for adults aged 19–50 years and 1,200 mg/d for adults aged 51 years and older. The IOM's recommendations for vitamin D are 600 international units/d for most of life and 800 international units/d for individuals older than 70 years. Routine screening for vitamin D levels is not recommended in the absence of risk factors for vitamin D deficiency. Whether to recommend supplementation, as opposed to dietary sources, is uncertain. Health care providers are advised to refer to the U.S. Preventive Services Task Force for up-to-date, evidence-based vitamin D supplementation recommendations.

- A minimum of 30 minutes three times per week of weight-bearing exercise on an ongoing basis is recommended to reduce falls and prevent fractures and help to "pad" the bones and provide protection if there is a fall (see also the "Fitness" section earlier in Part 3).

- Smoking cessation (see also the "Substance Use and Abuse" section later in Part 3)

- Moderation of alcohol intake

- Fall prevention strategies, including removal of throw rugs and use of hip protectors, for women prone to falling

Bone Mineral Density Screening

Bone mineral density screening recommendations from the American College of Obstetricians and Gynecologists are shown in Fig. 3-1. Several

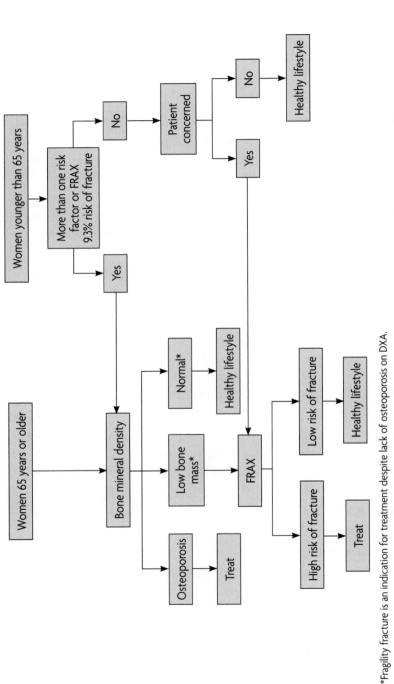

*Fragility fracture is an indication for treatment despite lack of osteoporosis on DXA.

Fig. 3-1. Screening and treating postmenopausal women for fracture prevention. (Screening and treating premenopausal women is generally restricted to women who have diseases, condition, or medication use known to increase risk of fractures.) Abbreviations: FRAX, fracture risk assessment tool; DXA, dual-energy X-ray absorptiometry. (Reprinted from Osteoporosis. Practice Bulletin No. 129. American College of Obstetricians and Gynecologists. Obstet Gynecol 2012;120:718–34.)

tests measure BMD. Dual energy X-ray absorptiometry (DXA) is the preferred method because it is reliable and highly precise, is widely available and relatively inexpensive, and exposes the patient to minimal radiation. Most of the recent large, randomized, controlled clinical trials have used DXA of the hip and spine to monitor response to interventions. The BMD measurement of the patient (preferably the femoral neck, total hip, and lumbar spine) is compared with the mean BMD of a young, healthy cohort of females to produce a T-score. The T-score categories are normal, low bone mass (formerly called osteopenia), and osteoporosis (Table 3-4).

Bone mineral density screening with DXA should begin at age 65 years for women, and DXA screening can be used selectively for women younger than 65 years if they are postmenopausal and have other risk factors for fracture (Box 3-11). Alternatively, the fracture risk assessment tool (FRAX) can be used in women younger than 65 years to determine which women should have a DXA scan (see "Fracture Risk Assessment Tool" later in this section). Routine screening of newly menopausal women is not recommended nor is a "baseline" screen recommended. In addition, practitioners should not perform BMD monitoring solely in response to DMPA use because any observed short-term loss in BMD associated with DMPA use may be recovered and is unlikely to place an adolescent or adult woman at risk of fracture during use or in later years.

In the absence of new risk factors, DXA screening should not be performed more frequently than every 2 years. For women without a high risk of fracture, data from the Study of Osteoporotic Fractures suggest a screening interval of 15 years for those older than 65 years with a normal BMD or mild bone loss (T-score greater than or equal to -1.5), a 5-year screening interval for a T-score from -1.5 to -1.99, and a 1-year screening interval for a T-score between -2.0 and -2.49. The FRAX fracture risk assessment tool, a description of which immediately follows, should continue to be used on an annual basis to monitor the important effect of age on fracture risk.

Fracture Risk Assessment Tool

In 2008, the World Health Organization introduced FRAX to allow clinicians to estimate the 10-year probability of hip and major osteoporotic fractures (forearm, hip, shoulder, or spine) for patients aged 40–90 years

Table 3-4. Diagnosing Osteoporosis Using Bone Densitometry Criteria Developed by the World Health Organization

Category	T-Score*
Normal	Greater than or equal to –1.0
Low Bone Mass (formerly osteopenia)	Less than –1 to greater than –2.5
Osteoporosis	Less than or equal to –2.5

*T-score is the number of standard deviations above or below the mean average bone density value for young adult women.

Reprinted from Osteoporosis. Practice Bulletin No. 129. American College of Obstetricians and Gynecologists. Obstet Gynecol 2012;120:718–34.

Box 3-11. When to Screen for Bone Density Before Age 65 Years

Bone density should be screened in postmenopausal women younger than 65 years if any of the following risk factors are noted:
- Medical history of a fragility fracture
- Body weight less than 127 lb
- Medical causes of bone loss (medications or diseases)
- Parental medical history of hip fracture
- Current smoker
- Alcoholism
- Rheumatoid arthritis

Reprinted from Osteoporosis. Practice Bulletin No. 129. American College of Obstetricians and Gynecologists. Obstet Gynecol 2012;120:718–34.

---

based on sex, ethnicity, and region of the world (available at www.shef.ac.uk/FRAX). This tool incorporates BMD and clinical risk factors. The clinical risk factors used in FRAX include, age, sex, body mass index, previous fragility fracture, parental hip fracture, current smoking status, corticosteroid use (greater than or equal to 5 mg prednisolone per day for 3 months), alcohol intake greater than or equal to 3 units per day (approximately three drinks), rheumatoid arthritis, and other secondary causes of osteoporosis.

The National Osteoporosis Foundation recommends FRAX be used in women who are postmenopausal, are not receiving osteoporosis treatment, have a T-score indicating low bone mass, and have no prior hip or vertebral fracture. In the United States, FRAX has been most widely used as an aid in decision making regarding treatment initiation when the patient's BMD score is in the low bone mass range. The fracture risk assessment tool also can be used in women younger than 65 years to determine which women should have a DXA scan. Those women with a FRAX 10-year risk of major osteoporotic fracture of 9.3% or greater could justifiably be referred for DXA because that is the risk of fracture found in a 65-year-old Caucasian woman with no risk factors.

Pharmacologic Interventions

Medical treatment should be recommended for women who have a BMD T-score of less than or equal to −2.5. For women with a BMD T-score between −1 and −2.5, the FRAX calculator can be used to make an informed decision about the need for treatment (Fig. 3-1). Women who are found to have a 10-year risk of major osteoporotic fracture greater than or equal to 20% or a risk of hip fracture greater than or equal to 3% using the FRAX calculator are candidates for medical pharmacologic therapy. Women who have had a low-trauma fracture (especially of the vertebra or hip) also are candidates for treatment even in the absence of osteoporosis on the DXA report (Fig. 3-1).

There are now several pharmacologic options available for osteoporosis prevention, treatment, or both. All of these agents are antiresorptive (slow bone loss) with the exception of parathyroid hormone, which is an anabolic agent (builds new bone).

- Bisphosphonates—These drugs, which can be used for the prevention and treatment of osteoporosis, inhibit resorption of bone by osteoclasts, ultimately leading to an increase in BMD and a decrease in bone turnover. Products are available that can be taken orally (daily, weekly, monthly) or intravenously (quarterly or yearly).

- Selective estrogen receptor modulators—This class of partial estrogen agonists/antagonists reduces the risk of vertebral fractures and is available in daily oral formulation. Raloxifene is approved for osteoporosis prevention and treatment.

- Hormone therapy—Estrogen therapy and combined estrogen and progestogen therapy are approved for the prevention of osteoporosis in women at an increased risk of osteoporosis and fracture (see also the "Menopause" section later in Part 3).

- Parathyroid hormone – Recombinant human parathyroid hormone is an anabolic bone treatment agent that increases trabecular size and connectivity and is administered by subcutaneous injection daily.

- Calcitonin—A naturally occurring hormone, calcitonin reduces fractures but appears to be less effective than other treatment agents. It can be administered by injection (subcutaneous or intramuscular) or nasal spray. In 2013, a U.S. Food and Drug Administration advisory panel reviewed evidence that indicated a potential risk of cancer may outweigh the benefit of fracture prevention. Updated labeling indicates that calcitonin-salmon treatment should be used only in patients for whom alternative treatments are not suitable, and use should be reevaluated on a periodic basis.

- RANK ligand inhibitor—This human monoclonal antibody to the receptor activator of nuclear factor-$\kappa\beta$ ligand decreases bone resorption and increases BMD. This medication is administered subcutaneously every 6 months.

Clinicians should take into account patient symptoms and medical history and should weigh the potential benefits and risks when selecting medication for the prevention or treatment of osteoporosis. Pharmacologic treatment should be used in conjunction with dietary modifications and supplements, weight-bearing exercises, and modification of risk factors for falling (see "Prevention Counseling" earlier in this section).

Testing with DXA to assess the effect of treatment generally should not be undertaken before 2 years after initiation of treatment because it often takes 18–24 months to document a clinically meaningful change. If the BMD is improved or stable (no significant change), the DXA does not usually need to be repeated in the absence of new risk factors.

Bibliography

Chen WY, Manson JE, Hankinson SE, Rosner B, Holmes MD, Willett WC, et al. Unopposed estrogen therapy and the risk of invasive breast cancer. Arch Intern Med 2006;166:1027–32.

Chlebowski RT, Hendrix SL, Langer RD, Stefanick ML, Gass M, Lane D, et al. Influence of estrogen plus progestin on breast cancer and mammography in healthy postmenopausal women: the Women's Health Initiative Randomized Trial. WHI Investigators. JAMA 2003;289:3243–53.

Depot medroxyprogesterone acetate and bone effects. Committee Opinion No. 602. American College of Obstetricians and Gynecologists. Obstet Gynecol 2014;123:1398–402.

Food and Drug Administration. Questions and answers: changes to the indicated population for miacalcin (calcitonin-salmon). Available at: http://www.fda.gov/Drugs/DrugSafety/PostmarketDrugSafetyInformationforPatientsandProviders/ucm388641.htm. Retrieved April 10, 2014.

Gourlay ML, Fine JP, Preisser JS, May RC, Li C, Lui LY, et al. Bone-density testing interval and transition to osteoporosis in older women. N Engl J Med 2012;366:225–33.

Hormone therapy. American College of Obstetricians and Gynecologists. Obstet Gynecol 2004;104 (suppl):1S–129S.

Kanis JA, Johnell O, Oden A, Johansson H, McCloskey E. FRAX and the assessment of fracture probability in men and women from the UK. Osteoporos Int 2008;19:385–97.

Looker AC, Borrud LG, Dawson-Hughes B, Shepherd JA, Wright NC. Osteoporosis or low bone mass at the femur neck or lumbar spine in older adults: United States, 2005–2008. NCHS Data Brief 2012;(93):1–8.

Management of osteoporosis in postmenopausal women: 2010 position statement of The North American Menopause Society. Menopause 2010;17:25–54; quiz 55–6.

Moyer VA. Prevention of falls in community-dwelling older adults: U.S. Preventive Services Task Force recommendation statement. U.S. Preventive Services Task Force. Ann Intern Med 2012;157:197–204.

Moyer VA. Vitamin D and calcium supplementation to prevent fractures in adults: U.S. Preventive Services Task Force recommendation statement. U.S. Preventive Services Task Force. Ann Intern Med 2013;158:691–6.

National Osteoporosis Foundation. Clinician's guide to prevention and treatment of osteoporosis. Washington, DC: NOF; 2013. Available at: http://www.nof.org/files/nof/public/content/file/2237/upload/878.pdf. Retrieved August 29, 2013.

Osteoporosis prevention, diagnosis, and therapy. NIH Consensus Development Panel on Osteoporosis Prevention, Diagnosis, and Therapy. JAMA 2001;285: 785–95.

Osteoporosis. Practice Bulletin No. 129. American College of Obstetricians and Gynecologists. Obstet Gynecol 2012;120:718–34.

Ross AC, Manson JE, Abrams SA, Aloia JF, Brannon PM, Clinton SK, et al. The 2011 report on dietary reference intakes for calcium and vitamin D from the Institute of Medicine: what clinicians need to know. J Clin Endocrinol Metab 2011;96:53–8.

Screening for osteoporosis: U.S. preventive services task force recommendation statement. U.S. Preventive Services Task Force. Ann Intern Med 2011;154:356–64.

The 2012 hormone therapy position statement of the North American Menopause Society. North American Menopause Society. Menopause 2012;19:257–71.

Resources

American College of Obstetricians and Gynecologists. Osteoporosis. Patient Education Pamphlet AP048. Washington, DC: American College of Obstetricians and Gynecologists; 2013.

American College of Obstetricians and Gynecologists. The menopause years. Patient Education Pamphlet AP047. Washington, DC: American College of Obstetricians and Gynecologists; 2013.

World Health Organization Collaborating Centre for Metabolic Bone Diseases. WHO Fracture Risk Assessment Tool (FRAX). Sheffield, United Kingdom: University of Sheffield; 2013. Available at: http://www.shef.ac.uk/FRAX/. Retrieved September 30, 2013.

GENETIC RISK ASSESSMENT

Genetic testing is poised to play a greater role in the practice of obstetrics and gynecology. With the success of the Human Genome Project, a growing number of diseases are now known to have a genetic contribution. In addition to conditions widely understood as having a genetic contribution, such as fragile X syndrome, neural tube defects, and hemoglobinopathies, other conditions commonly seen in gynecologic practice—for example, diabetes mellitus, hypertension, cancer (breast, endometrial, ovarian, and colon), and cancer syndromes (such as hereditary breast and ovarian cancer syndrome and Lynch syndrome)—are also known to have a genetic contribution. Identification and management of genetic risk factors have the potential to affect the quality and length of a woman's life. Genetic risk factors that may be identified in a particular patient include the relatively common ones associated with cancer and heart disease, as well as more specific ones that may be discovered through the patient's family or medical history (Box 3-12).

The list of medical conditions that have, or are suspected to have, a genetic contribution continues to grow as new genetic risks are discovered, and additional tests for these conditions are continually developed. The National Center for Biotechnology Information of the National Institutes of Health provides a resource for reviewing these conditions and tests (available at www.ncbi.nlm.nih.gov/gtr/). Clinicians need to maintain competence in the face of this evolving science, including the ability to identify patients within their practices who are candidates for genetic counseling, genetic testing, or both.

Genetic risk assessment has an especially important role in preconception and prenatal screening. The testing may affect a patient's decisions regarding her reproductive choices. Genetic risk assessment not related to reproductive care has the potential for identifying factors that will affect the patient's health and possible longevity. The purpose of testing in this case is

---

Box 3-12. Red Flags for Genetic Conditions

- Family history of a known or suspected genetic condition
- Ethnic predisposition to certain genetic disorders
- Consanguinity
- Multiple affected family members with the same or related disorders
- Earlier than expected age of onset of disease
- Diagnosis in less-often-affected sex
- Multifocal or bilateral occurrence of disease (often cancer) in paired organs
- Disease in the absence of risk factors or after application of preventive measures
- One or more major malformations
- Developmental delays or mental retardation
- Abnormalities in growth (growth restriction, asymmetric growth, or excessive growth)
- Recurrent pregnancy losses (two or more)

Data from National Coalition for Health Professional Education in Genetics. Genetic red flags. Available at: http://www.nchpeg.org/index.php?option=com_content&view=article&id=59&Itemid=75. Retrieved on September 26, 2013.

---

to identify risks that may be modified by changes in lifestyle or therapeutic interventions (see also the "Cancer Screening and Prevention" section later in Part 3 and the "Cancer Diagnosis and Management" section in Part 4).

Family History

A family history that may identify genetic risks should be gathered. Women should be informed of genetic risks and offered appropriate counseling and testing. Specific counseling is needed for testing that may have medical or psychosocial consequences. Counseling includes outlining the risks, benefits, and alternatives to genetic testing and should be neutral. Pretest and posttest counseling facilitate women's access to appropriate health care. Most obstetrician–gynecologists are capable of basic genetic risk identification and counseling, but referral may be needed for comprehensive counseling. Personnel with more advanced training, such as genetic counselors and medical geneticists, are appropriate for patients with common and more unusual abnormalities.

Assisted Reproductive Technology

Genetic services also may play a role in assisted reproductive technology. Gamete donors should be screened for heritable disorders through evaluation of pedigree, counseling, and—when appropriate—testing procedures. In some circumstances it is possible to identify embryos affected by certain diseases before implantation, in which case the affected embryos are not transferred. Preimplantation genetic testing often is used in instances when the potential disease might have a significant effect on the health of the future child. Consideration of such screening can raise ethical issues that the health care provider, genetic counselor, and patient should openly discuss before implementation.

Ethical Issues

Ethical issues related to the use of information gathered as a result of all genetic risk assessments need to be anticipated and discussed with the patient at the first genetic counseling session. Concerns about the effect of information about genetic conditions on such factors as employability and insurability have been raised. The Genetic Information Nondiscrimination Act of 2008 is designed to prohibit discrimination in health insurance coverage and employment based on genetic information. Patients should be encouraged to consider the importance of relatives being made aware of genetic disorders in the family, and confidentiality issues must be considered carefully (see also the "Human Resources" section in Part 1). The patient should be informed prospectively about policies regarding the use of information and legal requirements. Ordinarily, information may not be revealed without the patient's express consent. However, there may be situations in which the information may not be protected. The health care provider should be familiar with state or federal requirements regarding genetic screening, reporting, disclosure, breach of confidentiality, and discrimination based on genetic information.

Bibliography

2008 Guidelines for gamete and embryo donation: a Practice Committee report. American Society for Reproductive Medicine and Society for Assisted Reproductive Technology. Fertil Steril 2008;90:S30–44.

Ethical issues in genetic testing. ACOG Committee Opinion No. 410. American College of Obstetricians and Gynecologists. Obstet Gynecol 2008;111:1495–502.

Family history as a risk assessment tool. Committee Opinion No. 478. American College of Obstetricians and Gynecologists. Obstet Gynecol 2011;117:747–50.

National Coalition for Health Professional Education in Genetics. Genetic red flags. Available at: http://www.nchpeg.org/index.php?option=com_content&view=article &id=59&Itemid=75. Retrieved on September 26, 2013.

Patient testing: ethical issues in selection and counseling. ACOG Committee Opinion No. 363. American College of Obstetricians and Gynecologists. Obstet Gynecol 2007;109:1021–3.

The importance of preconception care in the continuum of women's health care. ACOG Committee Opinion No. 313. American College of Obstetricians and Gynecologists. Obstet Gynecol 2005;106:665-6.

Resources

American College of Obstetricians and Gynecologists. Cystic fibrosis: prenatal screening and diagnosis. ACOG Patient Education Pamphlet AP171. Washington, DC: American College of Obstetricians and Gynecologists; 2009.

American Medical Association. Family medical history. Available at: http://www. ama-assn.org/ama/pub/physician-resources/medical-science/genetics-molecular- medicine/family-history.page. Retrieved July 25, 2013.

Breast cancer screening. Practice Bulletin No. 122. American College of Obstetricians and Gynecologists. Obstet Gynecol 2011;118:372–82.

Carrier screening for fragile X syndrome. Committee Opinion No. 469. American College of Obstetricians and Gynecologists. Obstet Gynecol 2010;116:1008–10.

Department of Health and Human Services. Surgeon general's family health history initiative. Available at: http://www.hhs.gov/familyhistory. Retrieved April 16, 2013.

Direct-to-consumer marketing of genetic testing. ACOG Committee Opinion No. 409. American College of Obstetricians and Gynecologists. Obstet Gynecol 2008;111:1493–4.

Elective and risk-reducing salpingo-oophorectomy. ACOG Practice Bulletin No. 89. American College of Obstetricians and Gynecologists. Obstet Gynecol 2008;111: 231–41.

Genetic Alliance, Genetics and Public Policy Center at the Johns Hopkins University. National Coalition for Health Professional Education in Genetics. GINA: Genetic Information Nondiscrimination Act. Available at: http://www.ginahelp.org. Retrieved July 25, 2013.

Genetics and molecular diagnostic testing. Technology Assessment in Obstetrics and Gynecology No. 11. American College of Obstetricians and Gynecologists. Obstet Gynecol 2014;123:394–413.

Genetics and Public Policy Center. Genetic Information Nondiscrimination Act (GINA). Available at: http://www.dnapolicy.org/gina. Retrieved April 10, 2014.

Hemoglobinopathies in pregnancy. ACOG Practice Bulletin No. 78. American College of Obstetricians and Gynecologists. Obstet Gynecol 2007;109:229–37.

Hereditary breast and ovarian cancer syndrome. ACOG Practice Bulletin No. 103. American College of Obstetricians and Gynecologists and Society of Gynecologic Oncologists. Obstet Gynecol 2009;113:957–66.

March of Dimes. Your family health history. Available at: http://www.marchofdimes. com/pregnancy/your-family-health-history.aspx. Retrieved July 25, 2013.

National Cancer Institute. Cancer genetics risk assessment and counseling (PDQ®). Available at: http://www.cancer.gov/cancertopics/pdq/genetics/risk-assessment-and-counseling/HealthProfessional. Retrieved July 25, 2013.

National Center for Biotechnology Information, National Library of Medicine. Genetic testing registry. Available at: http://www.ncbi.nlm.nih.gov/gtr. Retrieved July 25, 2013.

National Coalition for Health Professional Education in Genetics. Available at: http://www.nchpeg.org/. Retrieved September 26, 2013.

National Library of Medicine. Why is it important to know my family medical history? Genetics home reference. Available at: http://ghr.nlm.nih.gov/handbook/inheritance/familyhistory. Retrieved July 26, 2013.

National Society of Genetic Counselors. Your genetic health: patient information. Understanding and collecting your family history. Available at: http://nsgc.org/p/cm/ld/fid=52. Retrieved April 10, 2014.

Preconception and prenatal carrier screening for genetic diseases in individuals of Eastern European Jewish descent. ACOG Committee Opinion No. 442. American College of Obstetricians and Gynecologists. Obstet Gynecol 2009;114:950–3.

Screening for Tay-Sachs disease. ACOG Committee Opinion No. 318. American College of Obstetricians and Gynecologists. Obstet Gynecol 2005;106:893–4.

Spinal muscular atrophy. ACOG Committee Opinion No. 432. American College of Obstetricians and Gynecologists. Obstet Gynecol 2009;113:1194–6.

Update on carrier screening for cystic fibrosis. Committee Opinion No. 486. American College of Obstetricians and Gynecologists. Obstet Gynecol 2011;117:1028–31.

▌CANCER SCREENING AND PREVENTION

Cancer is currently the second leading cause of death in women, after cardiovascular disease. Many treatments are available, but early detection significantly improves treatment outcomes and reduces mortality. Because the obstetrician–gynecologist may be the only physician providing routine care, every obstetrician–gynecologist should be able to recommend immunizations against viruses known to cause cancer, routine cancer screenings for gynecologic cancers and nongynecologic cancers, and risk-reducing options for those women at high risk of cancer. The obstetrician–gynecologist should discuss both the benefits and limitations of screening tests with the patient. Evaluation of the risk of cancer includes assessment of high-risk behaviors and family history (see also the "Genetic Risk Assessment" section earlier in Part 3).

The estimated number of women in the United States who would develop various malignancies and the number expected to die of these types of cancer in 2014 is shown in Table 3-5. Although breast cancer is the most frequent cancer in women, with approximately 232,670 new cases expected in 2014, the American Cancer Society reports that lung and bronchus cancer is the most common cause of cancer-related deaths in women in the United States, with approximately 72,330 deaths estimated in 2014.

According to currently available information, the most important factors in the development of cancer appear to be tobacco use, diet, infectious agents, alcohol consumption, and geographic location. The most well understood of these factors is tobacco use, which is thought to cause approximately 30% of cancer-related deaths in developed countries. Another major cause of cancer is the more complex factor of diet and nutrition, with 35% of cancer-related deaths associated with dietary practices. Recent research has identified clear associations between cancer risk and certain infectious agents, such as the association of some types of human papillomavirus with cervical, vulvar, vaginal, penile, anal, and

Table 3-5. Estimated Number and Lifetime Risk of U.S. Women Who Will Develop or Die From Various Types of Cancer in 2014

Type of Cancer	Number of New Cases	Lifetime Risk of Developing Cancer	Number of Deaths	Lifetime Risk of Dying from Cancer
Breast	232,670	1 in 8	40,000	1 in 36
Lung and bronchus	108,210	1 in 16	72,330	1 in 20
Colorectal	65,000	1 in 22	24,040	1 in 53
Endometrial	52,630	1 in 37	8,590	1 in 182
Melanoma	32,210	1 in 63	3,240	1 in 476
Ovarian	21,980	1 in 73	14,270	1 in 101
Cervical	12,360	1 in 152	4,020	1 in 435

Data from Siegel R, Ma J, Zou Z, Jemal A. Cancer Statistics, 2014. CA Cancer J Clin 2014;64:9–29 *and* American Cancer Society. Lifetime risk of developing or dying from cancer. Available at: http://www.cancer.org/cancer/cancerbasics/lifetime-probability-of-developing-or-dying-from-cancer. Retrieved January 14, 2014.

oropharyngeal cancer. In addition, striking associations exist between hepatitis viruses and liver cancer and between Epstein-Barr virus and nasopharyngeal cancer. Current estimates suggest that at least 10% of cases of human cancer may be the result of infection, and it is expected that further research in this area will increase this estimate significantly. Most of the other proposed causes of cancer, including alcohol consumption, industrial by-products, food additives, and other constitutional and geographic factors, account for much smaller proportions of cancer-related deaths.

Breast Cancer

Breast cancer is the most commonly diagnosed noncutaneous cancer in women in the United States, and the second leading cause of death from cancer in American women—second only to lung cancer (Table 3-5). The incidence of breast cancer increases with age. Breast cancer mortality can be effectively reduced through screening. Factors that increase the risk of breast cancer are outlined in Table 3-6, and the American College of Obstetrians and Gynecologists (the College) recommendations on individuals who warrant earlier or more frequent testing are available at www.acog.org/About_ACOG/ACOG_Departments/Annual_Womens_Health_Care/High-Risk_Factors.

Table 3-6. Factors That Increase the Relative Risk of Breast Cancer in Women

Relative Risk	Factor
>4.0	Female
	Age (65+ years vs <65 years, although risk increases across all ages until age 80)
	Certain inherited genetic mutations for breast cancer (*BRCA1*, *BRCA2*, or both)
	Two or more first-degree relatives with breast cancer diagnosed at an early age
	Personal history of breast cancer
	High breast tissue density
	Biopsy-confirmed atypical hyperplasia
2.1–4.0	One first-degree relative with breast cancer
	High-dose radiation to chest
	High bone density (postmenopausal)
1.1–2.0 Factors that affect circulating hormones	Late age at first full-term pregnancy (>30 years)
	Early menarche (<12 years)
	Late menopause (>55 years)
	No full-term pregnancies
	Never breastfed a child
	Recent oral contraceptive use
	Recent and long-term use of estrogen and progestin
	Obesity (postmenopausal)
Other factors	Personal history of endometrial or ovarian cancer
	Alcohol consumption
	Height (tall)
	High socioeconomic status
	Ashkenazi Jewish heritage

Modified with permission from Hulka BS, Moorman PG. Breast cancer: hormones and other risk factors. Maturitas 2001;38:103–13; discussion 113–6. Copyright 2001, with permission from Elsevier.

Screening

Breast cancer screening has traditionally included three elements: 1) breast imaging (primarily mammography), 2) clinical breast examination, and 3) patient self-screening (breast self-examination or breast self-awareness). The College continues to endorse inclusion of all three strategies in breast cancer screening.

Mammography

At present, mammography is the recommended screening method in most women to detect subclinical or occult breast cancer, the stage least likely to have spread to regional lymph nodes and beyond. Based on the incidence of breast cancer, the sojourn time for breast cancer growth, and the potential reduction in breast cancer mortality, the College recommends that women aged 40 years and older be offered screening mammography annually. Women should be educated on the predictive value of screening mammography and the potential for false-positive results and false-negative results. Women should be informed of the potential for additional imaging or biopsies that may be recommended based on screening results.

Digital mammography detects some cases of cancer that are not identified by film mammography, but overall detection is similar for many women. However, for women younger than 50 years or women who have dense breast tissue, overall detection is somewhat higher with digital mammography. Digital mammography may detect cases of breast carcinoma that are obscured or "hidden" by dense breast tissue or detect the low contrast of the tumor in comparison with the surrounding breast tissue. Dense breast tissue can mask tumors by lying directly above and below a tumor in a two-dimensional view. Image processing of digital data allows the degree of contrast in the image to be manipulated so that contrast can be increased in the dense areas of the breast with the lowest contrast.

The American College of Radiology's Breast Imaging Reporting and Data System (also known as BI-RADS) classifies abnormalities identified by mammography with a standardized reporting system (see Bibliography). Mammography results are classified as Categories 0–6 based on likelihood of malignancy. A Category 3 result indicates a 0–2% chance of malignancy.

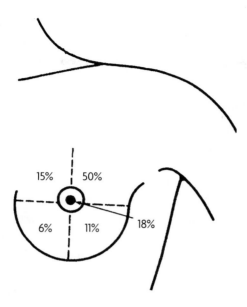

Fig. 3-2. Relative location of malignant lesions of the breast. (Reprinted with permission from DiSaia PJ, Creasman WT. Clinical gynecologic oncology. 6th ed. St. Louis [MO]: Elsevier/Mosby; Copyright 2002.)

A Category 5 classification is used for findings with an approximate 95% or higher chance of malignancy. Findings that fall between these two categories are designated Category 4. The American College of Radiology has recommended an optional division of Category 4 into three subgroups to provide more concrete evaluation for treatment and outcome studies. Obstetrician–gynecologists who provide mammography services should be in compliance with the Mammography Quality Standards Act and its regulations (see also the "Compliance With Government Regulations" section in Part 1).

Clinical Breast Examination

The clinical breast examination involves visual assessment of skin changes and palpation. Malignant lesions of the breast are more common in the upper outer quarter (Fig. 3-2). For women aged 20–39 years, clinical breast examinations are recommended every 1–3 years. Clinical breast examination should be performed annually for women aged 40 years and older (see also the "Well-Woman Annual Health Assessment" section earlier in Part 3).

Patient Self-Screening

Breast self-examination is the performance of an examination of the breasts in a consistent, systematic way by the individual on a regular basis, typically monthly. Currently, there is an evolution away from teaching breast self-examination toward educating patients about the concept of breast self-awareness, which is defined as women's awareness of the normal appearance and feel of their breasts. Breast self-awareness should be encouraged and can include breast self-examination. Women who desire to perform self-examination as a part of this breast self-awareness strategy may be instructed in the appropriate technique, although emphasis is not on examination techniques. Women should report any changes in their breasts to their health care providers.

Enhanced Screening

Women who are estimated to have a lifetime risk of breast cancer of 20% or greater, based on risk models that rely largely on family history (such as BRCAPRO, BODACEA, or Claus), but who are either untested or test negative for *BRCA* gene mutations, can be offered enhanced screening. For women who test positive for *BRCA1* and *BRCA2* mutations, enhanced screening should be recommended and risk-reduction methods discussed. Enhanced screening for these women includes twice-yearly clinical breast examinations, annual mammography, annual breast magnetic resonance imaging, and instruction in breast self-examination.

Other Imaging Techniques

Mammography has been the primary screening test for early breast cancer for more than five decades, but conventional mammography imaging continues to have limitations in sensitivity and specificity. Alternative breast imaging modalities that have been developed to improve cancer detection include ultrasonography, magnetic resonance imaging (MRI), and three-dimensional digital breast tomosynthesis. These imaging tests may be indicated for women at increased risk of developing breast cancer, such as those with a *BRCA1* or *BRCA2* mutation, a strong family history of breast cancer or ovarian cancer, or prior chest radiation therapy. Women with dense breasts have a modestly increased risk of breast cancer and experience reduced sensitivity of mammography to detect breast cancer. However, current published evidence does not demonstrate meaningful outcome benefits (eg, reduction in breast cancer mortality) with supplemental tests (eg, ultrasonography and magnetic resonance imaging) to screening mammography or with alternative screening modalities (eg, breast tomosynthesis) in women with dense breasts who do not have additional risk factors. Thus, the American College of Obstetricians and Gynecologists does not recommend routine use of alternative or adjunctive tests in these cases. However, it recommends that health care providers comply with state laws that may require disclosure to women of their breast density as recorded in a mammogram report.

Ultrasonography is an established adjunct to mammography in the imaging evaluation. It is useful in evaluating inconclusive mammographic findings, in evaluating young patients and other women with dense breast tissue and other risk factors for breast cancer, in guiding tissue core-needle biopsy and other biopsy techniques, and in differentiating a cyst from a solid mass. It is not recommended as a screening modality for women at average risk of developing breast cancer. Ultrasonography may be an option for additional screening in women at high risk who are candidates for MRI screening but cannot receive MRI because of gadolinium contrast allergy, claustrophobia, or other barriers.

A three-dimensional modality used for breast cancer screening is MRI. Studies that use MRI for breast cancer screening indicate greater sensitivity but less specificity than mammography for detection of breast cancer in high-risk women. The American Cancer Society recommends annual screening using MRI in addition to mammography beginning at age 30 years for women at high risk of breast cancer (greater than 20–25% lifetime risk).

Digital breast tomosynthesis is another three-dimensional imaging technology that involves acquiring images of a stationary compressed breast at multiple angles during a short scan. The individual images are reconstructed into a series of thin high-resolution slices that can be displayed individually or in a dynamic cine mode. Digital breast tomosynthesis offers the potential to overcome one of the primary limitations of mammography, which is the inability to image overlapping dense normal breast tissue. This common clinical finding can reduce the accuracy of conventional mammography and digital mammography in distinguishing benign and malignant lesions. Digital breast tomosynthesis creates multiple projections that are imaged across a range of viewing angles to produce a series of section images. This procedure results in a reduction in the amount of superimposed breast tissue in each tomosynthesis section with presumed improved sensitivity for small tumors compared with mammography. Clinical data suggest that digital mammography with tomosynthesis produces a better image, improved accuracy, and lower recall rates compared with digital mammography alone. Further study will be necessary to confirm whether digital mammography with tomosynthesis is a cost-effective approach that is capable of replacing digital mammography alone as the first-line screening modality of choice for breast cancer screening.

DIAGNOSTIC MAMMOGRAPHY

Mammography may be used as either a screening device or an adjunct in the diagnosis of a palpable mass. A palpable mass, in the presence of normal findings on mammography, requires further evaluation. Malignant lesions of the breast are more common in the upper outer quarter (Fig. 3-2). Normal diagnostic mammography alone is not always sufficient to rule out malignancy in a patient with a palpable breast mass. Ultrasonography may be useful to define a cystic lesion. If a cyst is aspirated and the fluid is clear (transparent and not bloody), there is no need for cytologic evaluation. If the cyst does not disappear after aspiration or recurs within 6 weeks, surgical follow-up should be considered. In adult women, a solid, dominant, persistent mass requires tissue diagnosis by core-needle biopsy or other biopsy techniques. Physical examination, imaging, and cytologic evaluations all contribute information but are not definitive (see also the "Cancer Diagnosis and Management" section in Part 4).

RISK ASSESSMENT AND REDUCTION

The clinician should be knowledgeable regarding the indications and options for reducing the incidence of breast cancer, including prophylactic mastectomy and chemoprevention. A key factor to be considered is the woman's risk of breast cancer. It is important that clinicians take a thorough history to assess the risk adequately. Researchers from the National Cancer Institute and the National Surgical Adjuvant Breast and Bowel Project have developed a computer-based tool to allow clinicians to project a woman's individualized estimate of breast cancer risk. The Breast Cancer Risk Assessment Tool is a computer program that a woman and her health care provider can use to estimate her chances of developing breast cancer based on several established risk factors. The program is available at no charge in PC-compatible and Macintosh computer formats or online (see Resources).

Consideration should be given to tamoxifen or raloxifene chemopreventive therapy for women at high risk of developing breast cancer. Individualized risk assessment should be performed to determine whether a patient is a candidate for breast cancer risk reduction by chemoprevention unless she has ductal carcinoma in situ or lobular carcinoma in situ, in which case the benefit of chemoprevention already has been documented.

Cervical Cancer

The American Cancer Society estimates that there are more than 12,000 new cases of cervical cancer in the United States each year, with more than 4,000 deaths from the disease (Table 3-5). Estimates suggest that 50% of the women in whom cervical cancer is diagnosed never had cervical cytology testing, and another 10% have not been screened within the 5 years before diagnosis. Thus, approximately 60% of diagnoses of cervical cancer are a result of inadequate screening. Although rates of cervical cancer are decreasing in women born in the United States with access to screening, women who are immigrants to the United States, those lacking a regular source of health care, and the uninsured are at especially high risk.

Cervical cancer screening should begin at age 21 years. Women younger than 21 years should not be screened regardless of the age of sexual initiation or the presence of other behavior-related risk factors. Women aged 21–29 years should be tested with cervical cytology alone, and screening should be performed every 3 years. Co-testing with cytology and human papillomavirus (HPV) testing should not be performed in women younger than 30 years. For women aged 30–65 years, co-testing every 5 years is preferred, and screening with cytology alone every 3 years is acceptable. Annual screening should not be performed in women at average risk. Women who have received the HPV vaccine should be screened according to the same guidelines as women who have not been vaccinated.

Screening should be discontinued after age 65 years in women with evidence of adequate negative prior screening results and no history of cervical intraepithelial neoplasia (CIN) 2 or higher. Adequate negative prior screening results are defined as three consecutive negative cytology results or two consecutive negative co-test results within the previous 10 years, with the most recent test performed within the past 5 years. Women with a history of CIN 2, CIN 3, or adenocarcinoma in situ should continue to undergo routine age-based screening for 20 years after the initial post-treatment surveillance period, even if it requires that screening continue past age 65 years. In women who have had a total hysterectomy for benign indications and no history of CIN 2 or higher, routine cytology screening and HPV testing should be discontinued and not restarted for any reason. Women who have a history of cervical cancer, have human immunodeficiency virus (HIV) infection, are immunocompromised, or were exposed to diethylstilbestrol in utero may require more frequent cervical cytology screening and should not follow routine screening guidelines (see also the "Abnormal Cervical Cytology" section in Part 4).

Liquid-based and conventional methods of collecting samples for cervical cancer screening are acceptable. A cellular sample from the endocervical canal obtained with an endocervical brush and a scraping of the portio, to include the entire transformation zone, provides a reliable sample for cervical cancer screening. An endocervical brush should be used to obtain the endocervical cell sampling because it is more reliable in terms of identifying CIN, providing adequate cytology specimens, and limiting false-negative test results than other tools for collection.

Certain measures can be taken to help ensure an adequate sample is obtained. Cells should be collected before the bimanual examination. Care should be taken to avoid contaminating the sample with lubricant. Ideally, the entire portio of the cervix should be visible when the sample is obtained. If a conventional Pap test is being done, the specimen should be transferred and fixed as quickly as possible in an effort to reduce air-drying artifact. Routine swabbing of the discharge from the cervix may result in cytologic samples of scant cellularity.

When conventional Pap tests are performed, a single slide (combining the endocervical sample and ectocervical sample) or two separate slides can be used. The most important consideration is rapid fixation. If liquid-based preparations are used, rapid immersion in liquid media is equally important.

Endometrial Cancer

Endometrial cancer is the most common gynecologic malignancy. The American Cancer Society estimates that there are more than 52,000 new cases diagnosed in the United States each year (Table 3-5). The most common cause is an excess of endogenous or exogenous estrogen unopposed by progestin that leads to endometrial hyperplasia followed by cancer. This cause allows for prevention and early detection of the most common and most indolent form of endometrial cancer (type I or estrogen dependent). Type I endometrial cancer typically has a good prognosis. The more lethal variety of endometrial cancer, type II, accounts for approximately 10% of cases. There is no clear epidemiologic profile for type II endometrial cancer. Modifiable risk factors for type II endometrial cancer include obesity, cigarette smoking, postmenopausal unopposed estrogen therapy, and high cumulative doses of tamoxifen. Carcinosarcoma of the endometrium is the most aggressive form of endometrial cancer.

Routine screening of asymptomatic women for endometrial cancer and its precursors is not cost-effective. Obtaining a family history may alert the gynecologist to women at increased risk of genetically linked cancers, such as Lynch syndrome (also known as hereditary nonpolyposis colorectal cancer), in which young age at presentation of colon cancer is important. The most common manifestation of Lynch syndrome in women is endometrial cancer. Women with a history or evidence of abnormal vaginal bleeding are at increased risk of endometrial cancer and should be evaluated. It is important to identify women at risk in order to provide them with appropriate evaluation, prophylactic surgery, and counseling.

Ovarian Cancer

Ovarian cancer is the leading cause of death from gynecologic pelvic malignancies. More women die from ovarian cancer than from cervical cancer and endometrial cancer combined (Table 3-5). Currently, there are no techniques that have proved to be effective in the routine screening of asymptomatic low-risk women for ovarian cancer. The use of transvaginal ultrasonography and tumor markers (such as CA 125) as potential screening strategies has been evaluated. These methods, however, have proved to be ineffective for screening low-risk asymptomatic women because their sensitivity, specificity, positive predictive value, and negative predictive value all have been modest at best. It appears that the best way to detect early ovarian cancer is for the patient and her clinician to have a high index of suspicion for the diagnosis in the symptomatic woman. This strategy requires education of physicians and patients about the symptoms commonly associated with ovarian cancer. Factors that are most significantly associated with ovarian cancer, if they occur more than 12 days per month and for less than 1 year, are pelvic or abdominal pain, increase in abdominal size or bloating, and difficulty eating or feeling full.

Inherited susceptibility to ovarian cancer has the greatest effect of all ovarian cancer risk factors. Women with the highest risk of ovarian carcinoma are those with hereditary breast and ovarian cancer syndrome, followed by women with Lynch syndrome. Suggestive family histories of hereditary cancer risk include cancer occurring at young ages; cancer in first–degree relatives; cancer in multiple generations; bilateral, metachronous, or synchronous cancer in one individual; and clustering of cancer on one side of the family. Evaluating a patient's risk of a hereditary cancer syndrome should be a routine part of obstetric and gynecologic practice. Initial screening should involve asking specific questions about personal and family history of breast cancer and ovarian cancer as well as cancer types associated with Lynch syndrome. A hereditary cancer risk assessment is conducted by a health care provider with expertise in cancer genetics and includes gathering of family history information, risk assessment, education, and counseling. This assessment may include genetic testing if desired, after appropriate counseling and consent is obtained. Genetic testing can clarify ovarian carcinoma risk as well as risk of cancer to other organs. More information on genetic risk assessment can be found in the "Genetic Risk Assessment" section earlier in Part 3.

Women with an increased risk of ovarian carcinoma secondary to hereditary breast and ovarian cancer syndrome or Lynch syndrome are at risk of cancer in other organs and qualify for more intensive surveillance or prevention measures. Women with hereditary breast and ovarian cancer syndrome should be offered surveillance for breast cancer with breast magnetic resonance imaging in addition to mammography and should be counseled about the option of prophylactic mastectomy. Women with Lynch syndrome should have annual colonoscopies with removal of any polyps. Ovarian cancer risk should not be addressed in isolation without consideration of other cancer risks.

Given the limitations of current ovarian cancer screening approaches, women at high risk of ovarian cancer (women with *BRCA1* or *BRCA2* mutations) should be offered risk-reducing salpingo-oophorectomy by age 40 years or after the conclusion of childbearing. Risk-reducing salpingo-oophorectomy for these women should include careful inspection of the peritoneal cavity, pelvic washings, removal of the fallopian tubes, and ligation of the ovarian vessels at the pelvic brim. If hysterectomy is not performed, care must be taken to completely remove the fallopian tubes to the level of the cornu. Complete, serial sectioning of the ovaries and fallopian tubes is necessary, with microscopic examination for occult cancer. Carriers of the *BRCA1* and *BRCA2* mutations who undergo salpingo–oophorectomy achieve an 80–90% ovarian cancer risk reduction, as well as an approximate 50–60% decrease in breast cancer risk if surgery is performed before menopause. There are no established guidelines for age of risk-reducing surgery in women with Lynch syndrome mutations. In women with Lynch syndrome, the average age of ovarian cancer diagnosis is 42 years and the average age of endometrial cancer diagnosis is 50 years. Thus, it is also reasonable to consider prophylactic surgery in women aged 35–40 years with Lynch syndrome if childbearing is no longer desired.

Colon Cancer

Colon cancer causes nearly as many deaths among women as all gynecologic pelvic malignancies combined (Table 3-5). In most cases, it is preceded by adenomatous polyps. The College recommends colorectal cancer screening with colonoscopy every 10 years beginning at age 50 years for average-risk women and at age 45 years for African American women. The College supports stopping routine screening at age 75 years. An earlier starting age for screening is recommended in African American women because of increased incidence and earlier age of onset of colorectal cancer in this population. The College's recommendations on individuals who warrant earlier or more frequent testing are available at www.acog.org/About_ACOG/ACOG_Departments/Annual_Womens_Health_Care/High-Risk_Factors.

The advantages and limitations of other appropriate colorectal cancer screening methods also should be discussed so that women may choose to be tested by whichever method they are most likely to accept and complete. Annual testing of stool for blood using methods with high sensitivity can aid in early detection. High-sensitivity guaiac fecal occult blood testing and fecal immunochemical testing require two or three samples of stool collected by the patient at home and returned for analysis. A single stool sample for fecal occult blood testing or fecal immunochemical testing obtained by digital rectal examination is not adequate for the detection of colorectal cancer. Other acceptable screening methods include flexible sigmoidoscopy every 5 years, computed tomography colonography every 5 years, and fecal DNA testing (interval undetermined). However, the U.S. Preventive Services Task Force currently considers computed tomography colonography and fecal DNA testing to be evolving technologies with insufficient evidence of benefits or risks to make a recommendation. In addition, there currently is no fecal DNA test approved by the U.S. Food and Drug Administration. Abnormalities found with any screening method other than colonoscopy necessitate referral for diagnostic colonoscopy.

Lung Cancer

Lung cancer is the leading cause of death from malignancy for women, estimated to account for 72,330 deaths—surpassing breast cancer—in 2014. Available screening techniques are not cost-effective and have not been shown to reduce mortality from lung cancer in the general population. Accordingly, routine lung cancer screening is not recommended for women at average risk. However, the National Cancer Institute recommends consideration of lung cancer screening with low-dose helical computed tomography for patients aged 55–74 years who have at least a 30-pack-year smoking history and who currently smoke or have quit within the past 15 years. The U.S. Preventive Services Task Force has issued similar guidance that extends the age range for screening to 80 years. The only effective way to reduce mortality is to promote smoking cessation. Health care providers can make a major contribution to the long-term health of women who smoke by identifying all women who smoke and counseling them to stop (see also the "Substance Use and Abuse" section later in Part 3). A smoking-cessation plan—coupled with the use of pharmacotherapy aids when indicated—as well as proper follow-up care can help women quit smoking and avoid relapse. Legislative and voluntary measures to reduce the risk of secondary exposure to smoke also are important current efforts to reduce the incidence of lung cancer. In June 2009, the Family Smoking Prevention and Tobacco Control Act was passed. This Act provides the U.S. Food and Drug Administration with some power to regulate the tobacco industry, including a ban on most flavored cigarettes and more stringent requirements for labeling.

Bibliography

ACR BI-RADS®–mammography: assessment categories. In: ACR breast imaging reporting and data system, breast imaging atlas. 5th ed. Reston (VA): American College of Radiology; 2014. p. 135–8.

Breast cancer screening. Practice Bulletin No. 122. American College of Obstetricians and Gynecologists. Obstet Gynecol 2011;118:372–82.

Centers for Disease Control and Prevention. Cervical cancer. Available at: http://www.cdc.gov/cancer/cervical. Retrieved July 26, 2013.

Chemoprevention of breast cancer: recommendations and rationale. U.S. Preventive Services Task Force. Ann Intern Med 2002;137:56–8.

DiSaia PJ, Creasman WT. Clinical gynecologic oncology. 6th ed. St. Louis (MO): Elsevier/Mosby; 2002.

Digital breast tomosynthesis. Technology Assessment in Obstetrics and Gynecology No. 9. American College of Obstetricians and Gynecologists. Obstet Gynecol 2013;121:1415–7.

Elective and risk-reducing salpingo-oophorectomy. ACOG Practice Bulletin No. 89. American College of Obstetricians and Gynecologists. Obstet Gynecol 2008;111:231–41.

Freeman HP, Wingrove BK. Excess cervical cancer mortality: a marker for low access to health care in poor communities. NIH Pub. No. 05-5282. Rockville (MD): National Cancer Institute, Center to Reduce Cancer Health Disparities; 2005. Available at: http://crchd.cancer.gov/attachments/excess-cervcanmort.pdf. Retrieved July 26, 2013.

Hereditary breast and ovarian cancer syndrome. ACOG Practice Bulletin No. 103. American College of Obstetricians and Gynecologists and Society of Gynecologic Oncologists. Obstet Gynecol 2009;113:957-66.

Hulka BS, Moorman PG. Breast cancer: hormones and other risk factors. Maturitas 2001;38:103-13; discussion 113-6.

Induced abortion and breast cancer risk. ACOG Committee Opinion No. 434. American College of Obstetricians and Gynecologists. Obstet Gynecol 2009; 113:1417-8.

Levin B, Lieberman DA, McFarland B, Andrews KS, Brooks D, Bond J, et al. Screening and surveillance for the early detection of colorectal cancer and adenomatous polyps, 2008: a joint guideline from the American Cancer Society, the U.S. Multi-Society Task Force on Colorectal Cancer, and the American College of Radiology. Gastroenterology 2008;134:1570-95.

Lifetime risk of developing or dying from cancer. Available at: http://www.cancer.org/cancer/cancerbasics/lifetime-probability-of-developing-or-dying-from-cancer. Retrieved January 14, 2014.

Management of endometrial cancer. ACOG Practice Bulletin No. 65. American College of Obstetricians and Gynecologists. Obstet Gynecol 2005;106:413-25.

Moyer VA. Screening for lung cancer: U.S. Preventive Services Task Force recommendation statement. U.S. Preventive Services Task Force. Ann Intern Med 2014;160:330-8.

National Cancer Institute. Lung cancer screening (PDQ®). Bethesda (MD): NCI; 2013. Available at: http://www.cancer.gov/cancertopics/pdq/screening/lung/HealthProfessional. Retrieved September 26, 2013.

Saslow D, Boetes C, Burke W, Harms S, Leach MO, Lehman CD, et al. American Cancer Society guidelines for breast screening with MRI as an adjunct to mammography. American Cancer Society Breast Cancer Advisory Group [published erratum appears in CA Cancer J Clin 2007;57:185]. CA Cancer J Clin 2007;57:75-89.

Schiffman M, Wentzensen N. From human papillomavirus to cervical cancer. Obstet Gynecol 2010;116:177-85.

Schiller JS, Lucas JW, Ward BW, Peregoy JA. Summary health statistics for U.S. adults: National Health Interview Survey, 2010. Vital Health Stat 10 2012;(252):1-207.

Screening for cervical cancer. Practice Bulletin No. 131. American College of Obstetricians and Gynecologists. Obstet Gynecol 2012;120:1222-38.

Siegel R, Ma J, Zou Z, Jemal A. Cancer statistics, 2014. CA Cancer J Clin 2014;64: 9–29.

Smith RA, Manassaram-Baptiste D, Brooks D, Cokkinides V, Doroshenk M, Saslow D, et al. Cancer screening in the United States, 2014: a review of current American Cancer Society guidelines and current issues in cancer screening. CA Cancer J Clin 2014;64:30–51.

Spence AR, Goggin P, Franco EL. Process of care failures in invasive cervical cancer: systematic review and meta-analysis. Prev Med 2007;45:93–106.

The role of the obstetrician-gynecologist in the early detection of epithelial ovarian cancer. Committee Opinion No. 477. American College of Obstetricians and Gynecologists. Obstet Gynecol 2011;117:742–6.

Warner E, Messersmith H, Causer P, Eisen A, Shumak R, Plewes D. Systematic review: using magnetic resonance imaging to screen women at high risk for breast cancer. Ann Intern Med 2008;148:671–9.

Resources

Agrawal S, Bhupinderjit A, Bhutani MS, Boardman L, Nguyen C, Romero Y, et al. Colorectal cancer in African Americans. Committee of Minority Affairs and Cultural Diversity, American College of Gastroenterology [published erratum appears in Am J Gastroenterol 2005;100:1432]. Am J Gastroenterol 2005;100:515–23; discussion 514.

American College of Obstetricians and Gynecologists. Annual women's health care: high risk factors. Available at: http://www.acog.org/About_ACOG/ACOG_Departments/Annual_Womens_Health_Care/High-Risk_Factors. Retrieved October 1, 2013.

American College of Obstetricians and Gynecologists. Cancer of the cervix. Patient Education Pamphlet AP163. Washington, DC: American College of Obstetricians and Gynecologists; 2013.

American College of Obstetricians and Gynecologists. Cancer of the ovary. Patient Education Pamphlet AP096. Washington, DC: American College of Obstetricians and Gynecologists; 2011.

American College of Obstetricians and Gynecologists. Cancer of the uterus. ACOG Patient Education Pamphlet AP097. Washington, DC: American College of Obstetricians and Gynecologists; 2008.

American College of Obstetricians and Gynecologists. Cervical cancer prevention in low-resources settings. College Statement of Policy 79. Washington, DC: American College of Obstetricians and Gynecologists; 2011.

American College of Obstetricians and Gynecologists. Cervical cancer screening. Patient Education Pamphlet AP085. Washington, DC: American College of Obstetricians and Gynecologists; 2013.

American College of Obstetricians and Gynecologists. It's time to quit smoking. Patient Education Pamphlet AP065. Washington, DC: American College of Obstetricians and Gynecologists; 2012.

American College of Obstetricians and Gynecologists. Reducing your risk of cancer. Patient Education Pamphlet AP007. Washington, DC: American College of Obstetricians and Gynecologists; 2013.

American College of Obstetricians and Gynecologists. Smoking and women's health. In: Special issues in women's health. Washington, DC: ACOG; 2005. p. 151–67.

Aromatase inhibitors in gynecologic practice. ACOG Committee Opinion No. 412. American College of Obstetricians and Gynecologists. Obstet Gynecol 2008; 112:405–7.

Genetics and Public Policy Center. Johns Hopkins University. Available at: http://www.dnapolicy.org. Retrieved April 10, 2014.

Moyer VA. Screening for cervical cancer: U.S. Preventive Services Task Force recommendation statement. U.S. Preventive Services Task Force [published erratum appears in Ann Intern Med 2013;158:852]. Ann Intern Med 2012;156:880–91, W312.

National Cancer Institute. Breast cancer risk assessment tool. Available at: http://www.cancer.gov/bcrisktool/. Retrieved September 20, 2013.

Sarfaty M. How to increase colorectal cancer screening rates in practice: a primary care clinician's evidence-based toolbox and guide. Atlanta (GA): American Cancer Society; 2008. Available at: http://www.cancer.org/acs/groups/content/documents/document/acspc-024588.pdf. Retrieved July 26, 2013.

Saslow D, Solomon D, Lawson HW, Killackey M, Kulasingam SL, Cain J, et al. American Cancer Society, American Society for Colposcopy and Cervical Pathology, and American Society for Clinical Pathology screening guidelines for the prevention and early detection of cervical cancer. ACS-ASCCP-ASCP Cervical Cancer Guideline Committee. CA Cancer J Clin 2012;62:147–72.

Screening for breast cancer: U.S. Preventive Services Task Force recommendation statement. US Preventive Services Task Force [published errata appear in Ann Intern Med 2010;152:688. Ann Intern Med 2010;152:199–200]. Ann Intern Med 2009;151:716–26, W-236.

Screening for colorectal cancer: U.S. Preventive Services Task Force recommendation statement. U.S. Preventive Services Task Force. Ann Intern Med 2008;149:627–37.

Screening for ovarian cancer: recommendation statement. U.S. Preventive Services Task Force. Ann Fam Med 2004;2:260–2.

SUBSTANCE USE AND ABUSE

The use of tobacco, alcohol, and illegal drugs constitutes a substantial national health problem. In the United States, an estimated 21% of all women use tobacco products, 15.8% of women aged 12 years and older are binge drinkers, and 10.8% of nonpregnant women aged 15–44 years reported illicit drug use in the past month. Frequent use or dependency that involves more than one substance is common. Although the prevalence of tobacco, alcohol, and illegal drug use varies, it is present in all socioeconomic, cultural, and ethnic groups. Abuse of prescription drugs is a growing problem.

Evaluation of a patient for tobacco, alcohol, or other substance abuse requires appreciation of the high prevalence and wide distribution among the population of such behavior, along with the ability to take a thorough history. Traditionally, physicians have had low rates of detection and referrals in nonpregnant women. Obstetrician–gynecologists have an ethical obligation to learn and use a protocol for universal screening by questioning for illicit drug and at-risk drinking on all patients. Universal screening is the key: screening only patients who may be perceived to be at risk leads to the low rates of detection. Direct questioning of patients about their use of tobacco, alcohol, and other drugs is preferable to vague inquiry. When there is evidence of substance abuse, obstetrician–gynecologists should be able to perform a brief intervention and refer patients to appropriate treatment.

Addiction is a chronic, relapsing behavioral disorder that affects the functioning of the brain and other major organs. It is not a moral problem, an indication of bad character, a sign of weakness, or a failure of the will. Because substance abuse and dependence are medical conditions, health care providers have a key role to play in their prevention and treatment. This role includes screening patients by use of validated questionnaires; providing education, brief intervention, and referral; guiding and referring high-risk patients; advising patients about social and support groups; and practicing safe prescription writing. This section first addresses smoking, followed by alcohol and other drug use and abuse.

Smoking

Cigarette smoking is the largest preventable cause of premature death and avoidable illness among women in the United States. Physicians and office staff can encourage smoking cessation by ensuring that all smokers are identified, monitored, and counseled appropriately at every office visit.

SCREENING AND ASSESSMENT

The Agency for Healthcare Research and Quality recommends a brief smoking cessation intervention known as the "5 A's" for screening and treating tobacco dependence (see Box 3-13). The 5 A's are applicable to outpatient office visits. Meta-analysis has shown that this intervention is not only clinically effective but also extremely cost-effective relative to other commonly used disease prevention interventions and medical treatments. Smoking

---

Box 3-13. The Five A's Brief Smoking Cessation Intervention

Ask about tobacco use. Identify and document tobacco use status for every patient at every visit.

Advise to quit. In a clear, strong, and personalized manner, urge every tobacco user to quit.

Assess willingness to make a quit attempt. Is the tobacco user willing to make a quit attempt at this time?

Assist in quit attempt. For patients unwilling to make a quit attempt at the time, address tobacco dependence and willingness to quit at next clinic visit.

Arrange follow-up. Schedule follow-up contact, preferably within the first week after the quit date.

Data from Counseling and interventions to prevent tobacco use and tobacco-caused disease in adults and pregnant women: U.S. Preventive Services Task Force reaffirmation recommendation statement. U.S. Preventive Services Task Force. Ann Intern Med 2009;150:551–5.

cessation interventions delivered by health and social care providers (eg, physicians, dentists, nurses, psychologists, and social workers) markedly increase cessation rates compared with interventions with no health care provider involvement (eg, self-administered interventions).

Clinicians can enhance the motivation of individuals to quit by reviewing the many health risks associated with smoking and the numerous benefits of living smoke free. Smoking contributes to deaths from cancer, cardiovascular disease, and respiratory diseases. Women who smoke increase their risk of osteoporosis, secondary amenorrhea, and menstrual irregularity. Women often do not appreciate that smoking also is associated with early menopause and infertility. Counseling of adolescents should focus on associations that are important to them, such as body image issues. For example, in the "Advise" portion of the 5 A's approach for adolescents, personalize the message to include the fact that smoking may be associated with bad breath, clothing odors, skin changes, and limp, dull hair.

Utilizing motivational interviewing, which is discussed in more detail in the "Well-Woman Annual Health Assessment" section earlier in Part 3, has been shown to be effective in eliciting behavior change. Follow-up that reinforces the health risks of smoking and provides appropriate referrals for additional cessation counseling and medical therapy is an important component of smoking cessation intervention.

For the patient willing to make a quit attempt, use counseling and pharmacotherapy (unless contraindicated) to help her quit. Adolescents, smokeless tobacco users, and light smokers should not routinely use pharmacotherapy. For patients unwilling to make a quit attempt at first, address tobacco dependence and willingness to quit at the next clinic visit. The following systematic approach to patients is helpful:

1. Suggest and encourage the use of problem-solving methods and skills for smoking cessation (eg, identify "trigger" situations).

2. Provide social support as part of the treatment (eg, "We can help you quit").

3. Arrange social support in the smoker's environment (eg, identify a "quit buddy" and smoke-free space).

4. Provide self-help smoking cessation materials.

Every state offers free smoking cessation telephone counseling that smokers can access through a toll-free number, 800-QUIT-NOW. Quit lines offer counseling and information on local resources, and they have been proved to increase smoking cessation rates and decrease relapse. This multifaceted counseling approach has been found in meta-analysis studies to be extremely helpful in helping patients to quit. New Current Procedural Terminology codes have been developed for patient counseling.

Women experience more difficulty with smoking cessation than do men, especially in the initial cessation period, and women are more prone to relapse. Clinicians can provide brief, effective relapse prevention treatment by reinforcing the patient's decision to quit, reviewing the benefits of quitting, and assisting the patient in resolving any residual problems encountered from quitting.

Many women are deterred from quitting smoking because of the fear of weight gain. Approximately one half of those who stop smoking gain weight and most will gain fewer than 10 lb. Weight gain is not caused by a change in chronic resting metabolic rates after smoking cessation; tobacco smoke is not an anorectic or a thermogenic agent. Weight gain with smoking cessation seems to be caused by a transient increase in oral intake without any change in physical activity. Following a nutritious diet of low-caloric foods, drinking large amounts of noncaloric or low-caloric liquids, and engaging in regular exercise can help smokers cope with withdrawal symptoms and minimize weight gain. Several medications prescribed for smoking cessation (particularly nicotine replacement) may help delay weight gain; however, once the medications are discontinued, most women experience weight gain.

PHARMACOTHERAPY AND OTHER EVIDENCE-BASED SMOKING CESSATION AIDS

Pharmacologic treatment for smoking cessation (including nicotine replacement therapy and sustained-release bupropion and varenicline) should be offered to all women attempting smoking cessation unless it is contraindicated (see Table 3-7). These products may be used in combination for patients who are experiencing difficulty quitting. The clinician needs to be aware of the black box label warning on bupropion (which also is used to treat depression) and varenicline in regard to suicide ideation.

Table 3-7. Smoking Cessation Aids

Method	6-Month Abstinence Rate (%)	Cost*	Where Available
Patient desire	8	–	–
Physician advice	10.2	–	–
Group or individual counseling	14–17	Low to very high cost depending on provider	Health centers Public health programs Private counselor
Telephone counseling (Smokers' Quitline)	16	Free	1-800-QUIT NOW
Nicotine gum, patch, or lozenge	19–26	$150–$300 for 6–14 weeks	Over-the-counter
Nicotine inhaler or nasal spray	25–27	$150–$300 for up to 6 months	Requires prescription
Combined nicotine replacement therapies	24–36	$150–$400 for up to 6 months	Over-the-counter Requires prescription
Bupropion	24	$150–$300 for up to 14 weeks	Requires prescription
Varenicline	33	$250–$400 for up to 14 weeks	Requires prescription
Clonidine	25	Less than $150 for up to 12 weeks	Requires prescription
Nortriptyline	22.5	Less than $150 for up to 12 weeks	Requires prescription
Combined counseling and medication	28–32	$150 and up	Health centers Public health programs Private counselor Medication requires prescription
Hypnosis	Insufficient evidence	Greater than $300	Not covered by insurance
Acupuncture	9	Greater than $300	Not covered by insurance

*Cost of a course of treatment. This may be covered by insurance unless otherwise indicated in the patient's health insurance policy.

Data from Fiore MC, Jaen CR, Baker TB, Bailey WC, Benowitz NL, Curry SJ, et al. Treating tobacco use and dependence: 2008 update. Clinical Practice Guideline. Rockville (MD): Department of Health and Human Services; 2008.

Patients should be counseled and monitored for abrupt mood changes. The U.S. Food and Drug Administration has issued a warning concerning an increase in cardiovascular events for those individuals with cardiovascular disease who use varenicline. A downloadable, comprehensive, and patient-centered chart of evidence-based smoking cessation interventions with effectiveness ratings can be found at www.whatworkstoquit.tobaccocessation.org/NTCCguide.pdf. Hypnotherapy and the use of herbal remedies have not proved to be effective for achieving smoking cessation.

Alcohol and Other Drug Use and Abuse

Excessive alcohol consumption contributes to more than 100,000 deaths in the United States each year. In addition to motor vehicle accidents, suicide, and homicide, heavy drinking contributes to deaths from heart disease, cancer, and stroke. Half of all cirrhosis deaths are linked with alcohol. Menstrual disorders, early menopause, and osteoporosis are among the gynecologic consequences of alcohol abuse. Condom use is inversely correlated with alcohol use.

Substance use, abuse, and dependence can have serious implications for women's health. Among these implications are adverse effects on reproductive function and pregnancy. Liver disease, stroke and other cerebrovascular diseases, an increase in certain malignancies, and behavior that results in malnutrition or the acquisition of serious infections, such as human immunodeficiency virus (HIV) and hepatitis, are some of the consequences noted in women who abuse alcohol or other substances.

Deaths from prescription painkiller overdoses increased more than 400% between 1999 and 2010, with nearly 48,000 women dying of prescription painkiller overdoses during that period. The nonmedical use of prescription drugs, particularly opioids, sedatives, and stimulants, has been cited as an epidemic in the United States, accounting for increasing numbers of emergency department visits and deaths from reactions and overdoses. Those who abuse prescription drugs most often obtain them from friends and family, either through sharing or theft.

The role of the obstetrician–gynecologist or primary health care provider includes appropriate prescribing, universal screening by questionnaire, brief intervention, and referral. Prompt intervention that goes beyond screening may help the patient come to terms with her substance abuse problem. The obstetrician–gynecologist also can be effective in encouraging a patient's participation in the engagement and maintenance of her treatment and in planning for relapse prevention. Potentially addictive medications should be prescribed with caution in patients with a substance abuse history (see also "Preventing Prescription Drug Abuse" later in this section).

SCREENING AND ASSESSMENT

All women should be screened annually for alcohol and substance abuse, including prescription drug abuse, using a validated questionnaire. Box 3-14 includes examples of validated alcohol screening questionnaires. The "Drug Use Screening Tool" created by the National Institute on Drug Abuse is a brief web-based interactive assessment that guides clinicians through a series of questions to identify risky substance use in adult patients. The accompanying resources assist clinicians in providing patient feedback and arranging for specialty care, where necessary, using the 5 A's of intervention (see www.drugabuse.gov/nmassist/).

Women may not disclose tobacco, alcohol, or other substance use for a variety of reasons. Fears regarding disclosure can include the fear of intervention by government agencies, when reporting can result in punishment, incarceration, or loss of child custody. Clinicians should be aware of the variety of adverse effects and examination findings related to substances that are commonly abused and follow up on these findings as appropriate.

DRUG TESTING

If drug testing is performed, it is incumbent on the medical practitioner, as part of the procedure in obtaining consent for testing, to provide information about the nature and purpose of the test to the patient and how the results will guide management. Clinicians should be familiar with state statutes that require illicit drug use reporting. Where there are laws that require disclosure, patients should be informed in advance about specific items for which disclosure is mandated.

When indicated, and when used appropriately and with informed consent, laboratory drug tests can help identify or confirm a substance abuse problem overlooked by other detection methods. Although drug testing can be done on blood, hair, sweat, saliva, and nails, urine testing generally is the most practical option for the clinician's office. Urine testing is easy

---

Box 3-14. Alcohol Use Screening Tools

T-ACE
- T—Tolerance
  How many drinks does it take to make you feel high?
  (More than two drinks = 2 points)
- A—Annoyed
  Have people annoyed you by criticizing your drinking?
  (Yes = 1 point)
- C—Cut down
  Have you ever felt you ought to cut down on your drinking?
  (Yes = 1 point)
- E—Eye-opener
  Have you ever had a drink first thing in the morning to steady your nerves or get rid of a hangover?
  (Yes = 1 point)

A total score of 2 points or more indicates a positive screening for at-risk drinking

Alcohol Quantity and Drinking Frequency Questions
- In a typical week, how many drinks do you have that contain alcohol? (Positive for at-risk drinking if more than seven drinks)
- In the past 90 days, how many times have you had more than three drinks on any one occasion? (Positive for at-risk drinking if more than one time)

Data from Sokol RJ, Martier SS, Ager JW. The T-ACE questions: practical prenatal detection of risk-drinking. Am J Obstet Gynecol 1989;160:863–8, discussion 868–70 *and* National Institute on Alcohol Abuse and Alcoholism. Helping patients who drink too much: a clinician's guide. Bethesda (MD): NIAAA; 2005. Available at: http://pubs.niaaa.nih.gov/publications/practitioner/CliniciansGuide2005/Guide_Slideshow.htm. Retrieved July 26, 2013.

and inexpensive, and it provides a reasonable testing window for commonly used drugs (a few days in most cases). Mass-produced kits generate immediate results that can be discussed with the patient. A standard urine testing panel does not detect synthetic opioids and does not detect some stimulants and benzodiazepines, and testing alone cannot confirm intoxication, abuse, or dependence. However, when combined with a thorough medical history, physical examination, and screening questionnaire, biophysical drug testing can help the clinician provide appropriate interventions to the patient.

INTERVENTION

If alcohol, illicit drug, or prescription drug abuse is identified, the health care provider should perform a brief motivational intervention as described in the American College of Obstetricians and Gynecologists' Committee Opinion Number 423, *Motivational Interviewing: A Tool for Behavior Change* (see Bibliography). Given the potential consequences of alcohol abuse, illicit drug use, and prescription drug misuse during pregnancy, counseling on the use of effective contraception methods should be included in the intervention (see also the "Family Planning" section later in Part 3).

REFERRAL FOR TREATMENT

If alcohol or drug dependence is revealed, the patient should be referred to a substance abuse treatment specialist. No single treatment is appropriate for all individuals with substance abuse problems. Recovery from substance abuse is a long-term process. Better outcome is seen in individualized programs that provide a greater range, frequency, and intensity of services. Treatment programs for women should look beyond simple abstinence from further substance use and take into account the total health of the individual. Support services (eg, transportation and child-care services) can affect the success of substance abuse treatment. Social service departments in many hospitals are an invaluable source of assistance and referral of patients with substance abuse problems. Many additional community and clinical resources are available (see Resources).

PREVENTING PRESCRIPTION DRUG ABUSE

Patient education is central in preventing intentional and unintentional drug diversion. When prescribing medications that may be misused, physicians should educate their patients on proper use, storage, and disposal of medications.

Patients who are prescribed opioid medications for legitimate pain control are unlikely to abuse them. However, physicians should be aware of patients who try to exploit practitioner sensitivity to patient pain. Use of patient pain contracts and drug testing may help to reduce this exploitation. The U.S. Food and Drug Administration now requires manufacturers of extended-release or long-acting opioid analgesics to offer continuing education on safe prescribing of these drugs, and these programs will be helpful resources to physicians and other prescribers. Prescribers should also be aware of state laws that address the prescribing of opioids and other potential drugs of addiction (see also the "Acute and Chronic Pain Management" section in Part 4).

Patients should be instructed to take the medication only as it is prescribed to them. They should be cautioned to not share the medication with anyone else, including friends and relatives who may feel that taking the patient's medication may help them. Medication that may be abused should be stored in secure places to prevent misuse by others, particularly youth who may obtain them without anyone knowing. Unused medications should be taken to a pharmacy for proper disposal or thrown away mixed in coffee grounds or cat litter to discourage recovery of the medications by someone intending to misuse the drug. In addition, women's health care providers should consider referral to a pain management specialist for women with chronic pain.

Bibliography

At-risk drinking and alcohol dependence: obstetric and gynecologic implications. Committee Opinion No. 496. American College of Obstetricians and Gynecologists. Obstet Gynecol 2011;118:383–8.

Centers for Disease Control and Prevention. Prescription painkiller overdoses. CDC Vital Signs. Atlanta (GA): CDC; 2013. Available at: http://www.cdc.gov/vitalsigns/PrescriptionPainkillerOverdoses/. Retrieved September 27, 2013.

Counseling and interventions to prevent tobacco use and tobacco-caused disease in adults and pregnant women: U.S. Preventive Services Task Force reaffirmation recommendation statement. U.S. Preventive Services Task Force. Ann Intern Med 2009;150:551–5.

Fiore MC, Jaen CR, Baker TB, Bailey WC, Benowitz NL, Curry SJ, et al. Treating tobacco use and dependence: 2008 update. Clinical Practice Guideline. Rockville (MD): U.S. Department of Health and Human Services; 2008.

Food and Drug Administration. Risk Evaluation and Mitigation Strategy (REMS) for extended-release and long-acting opioids. Available at: http://www.fda.gov/Drugs/DrugSafety/InformationbyDrugClass/ucm163647.htm. Retrieved July 26, 2013.

Methamphetamine abuse in women of reproductive age. Committee Opinion No. 479. American College of Obstetricians and Gynecologists. Obstet Gynecol 2011;117:751–5.

Motivational interviewing: a tool for behavioral change. ACOG Committee Opinion No. 423. American College of Obstetricians and Gynecologists. Obstet Gynecol 2009;113:243–6.

National Institute on Alcohol Abuse and Alcoholism. Helping patients who drink too much: a clinician's guide. Bethesda (MD): NIAAA; 2005. Available at: http://pubs.niaaa.nih.gov/publications/practitioner/CliniciansGuide2005/Guide_Slideshow.htm. Retrieved July 26, 2013.

National Institute on Drug Abuse. NIDA drug screening tool. Available at: http://www.drugabuse.gov/nmassist. Retrieved September 27, 2013.

Nonmedical use of prescription drugs. Committee Opinion No. 538. American College of Obstetricians and Gynecologists. Obstet Gynecol 2012;120:977–82.

Sokol RJ, Martier SS, Ager JW. The T-ACE questions: practical prenatal detection of risk-drinking. Am J Obstet Gynecol 1989;160:863-8; discussion 868–70.

Tenore PL. Advanced urine toxicology testing. J Addict Dis 2010;29:436–48.

Tobacco use and women's health. Committee Opinion No. 503. American College of Obstetricians and Gynecologists. Obstet Gynecol 2011;118:746–50.

Resources

Alcoholics Anonymous. Available at: http://www.alcoholics-anonymous.org. Retrieved July 26, 2013.

American Cancer Society. The Great American Smokeout. Available at: http://www.cancer.org/healthy/stayawayfromtobacco/greatamericansmokeout/index. Retrieved July 26, 2013.

American College of Obstetricians and Gynecologists, Physician Leadership on National Drug Policy. Illicit drug abuse and dependence in women—a slide lecture presentation. Available at: http://www.acog.org/~/media/Departments/Health%20 Care%20for%20Underserved%20Women/DependenceinWoment.ashx. Retrieved September 11, 2013.

American College of Obstetricians and Gynecologists. Alcohol and women. Patient Education Pamphlet AP068. Washington, DC: American College of Obstetricians and Gynecologists; 2011.

American College of Obstetricians and Gynecologists. It's time to quit smoking. Patient Education Pamphlet AP065. Washington, DC: American College of Obstetricians and Gynecologists; 2012.

American Lung Association. Available at: http://www.lung.org/. Retrieved July 26, 2013.

American Society of Addiction Medicine. Available at: http://www.asam.org. Retrieved July 26, 2013.

Center for Substance Abuse Treatment. Substance Abuse and Mental Health Services Administration. Available at: http://www.samhsa.gov/about/csat.aspx. Retrieved July 26, 2013.

Centers for Disease Control and Prevention. The health consequences of smoking: a report of the Surgeon General. Atlanta (GA): CDC; 2004. Available at: http://www.cdc.gov/tobacco/data_statistics/sgr/2004/complete_report/index.htm. Retrieved July 26, 2013.

Centers for Disease Control and Prevention. The health consequences of involuntary exposure to tobacco smoke: a report of the Surgeon General. Atlanta (GA): CDC; 2006. Available at: http://www.surgeongeneral.gov/library/reports/second hand-smoke-consumer.pdf. Retrieved July 26, 2013.

Department of Justice, Office of Juvenile Justice and Delinquency Prevention. Substance abuse: the nation's number one health problem. OJJDP Fact Sheet No. 17. Washington, DC: DOJ; 2001. Available at: https://www.ncjrs.gov/pdffiles1/ojjdp/fs200117.pdf. Retrieved July 26, 2013.

Narcotics Anonymous. Available at: http://www.na.org. Retrieved July 26, 2013.

National Council on Alcoholism and Drug Dependence. Available at: http://www.ncadd.org. Retrieved July 26, 2013.

National Institute on Alcohol Abuse and Alcoholism. Alcohol: a women's health issue. Bethesda (MD): NIAAA; 2008. Available at: http://pubs.niaaa.nih.gov/publications/brochurewomen/Woman_English.pdf. Retrieved July 26, 2013.

National Institute on Alcohol Abuse and Alcoholism. Rethinking drinking: alcohol and your health. Bethesda (MD): NIAAA; 2010. Available at: http://pubs.niaaa.nih.gov/publications/RethinkingDrinking/Rethinking_Drinking.pdf. Retrieved July 26, 2013.

National Tobacco Cessation Collaborative. A guide to quit smoking methods. Available at: http://tobacco-cessation.org/whatworkstoquit/NTCCguide.pdf. Retrieved July 26, 2013.

Nonmedical use of prescription drugs. Committee Opinion No. 538. American College of Obstetricians and Gynecologists. Obstet Gynecol 2012;120:977–82.

Results from the 2012 National Survey on Drug Use and Health: summary of national findings. Substance Abuse and Mental Health Services Administration. Rockville (MD): Substance Abuse and Mental Health Services Administration; 2013. Available at: http://www.samhsa.gov/data/NSDUH/2012SummNatFindDetTables/NationalFindings/NSDUHresults2012.pdf. Retrieved September 4, 2013.

SMART Recovery. Available at: http://www.smartrecovery.org. Retrieved July 26, 2013.

Substance Abuse and Mental Health Services Administration. Available at: http://www.samhsa.gov. Retrieved July 26, 2013.

Women for Sobriety. Available at: http://www.womenforsobriety.org. Retrieved July 26, 2013.

FAMILY PLANNING

The United States has the highest rate of unintended pregnancy in the developed world; approximately one half of all pregnancies are unintended. Although the percentage of unintended pregnancies is highest in adolescents and women older than 40 years, approximately one third of pregnancies in the middle reproductive years also are unintended. Couples using no contraceptive method account for approximately one half of unintended pregnancies, and the other half are the result of contraceptive failures.

Methods of contraception that require the couple to take little or no action after the placement or procedure, "non–user-dependent methods," are the most effective methods of contraception. These include implants and intrauterine devices. Methods that require contraception linked to the coital act are among the less effective methods of contraception (see Table 3-8). Because one half of unintended pregnancies occur as the result of contraceptive failures, encouraging appropriate couples to consider using methods that are more effective has the potential to decrease unintended pregnancies.

Unintended pregnancies result in tremendous individual and societal consequences, which include family upheaval, nonattainment of educational goals, and financial burdens. Two thirds of American women of reproductive age wish to avoid or postpone pregnancy. When discussing contraception with these women, clinicians should tailor counseling to the individual patient's lifestyle and needs, in addition to outlining the benefits and risks of different types of contraceptive methods. Counseling also should focus on information that may help decrease contraceptive failures for the method the patient chooses.

Initial Evaluation

The initial visit for family planning, which can be combined with a general preventive care visit, provides an opportunity to assess the health status of

Table 3-8. Percentage of U.S. Women Who Experience an Unintended Pregnancy During the First Year of Typical Use and the First Year of Perfect Use of Contraception and the Percentage of Women Who Continue Use at the End of 1 Year

Method	% of Women Who Experience an Unintended Pregnancy Within the First Year of Use		% of Women Who Continue Use at 1 Year*
	Typical Use[†]	Perfect Use[‡]	
No method[§]	85	85	
Spermicides[‖]	28	18	42
Fertility awareness-based methods	24		47
Standard Days method[¶]		5	
TwoDay method[¶]		4	
Ovulation method[¶]		3	
Symptothermal method[¶]		0.4	
Withdrawal	22	4	46
Sponge			36
Parous women	24	20	
Nulliparous women	12	9	
Condom[#]			
Female	21	5	41
Male	18	2	43
Diaphragm**	12	6	57
Combined pill and progestin-only pill[††]	9	0.3	67
Patch	9	0.3	67
Ring	9	0.3	67
Medroxyprogesterone	6	0.2	56
Intrauterine contraceptive devices			
Copper	0.8	0.6	78
Levonorgestrel	0.2	0.2	80
Etonogestrel	0.05	0.05	84
Female sterilization	0.5	0.5	100
Male sterilization	0.15	0.10	

(continued)

Table 3-8. Percentage of U.S. Women Who Experience an Unintended Pregnancy During the First Year of Typical Use and the First Year of Perfect Use of Contraception and the Percentage of Women Who Continue Use at the End of 1 Year *(continued)*

*Among typical couples who initiate use of a method (not necessarily for the first time), the percentage who experience an accidental pregnancy during the first year if they do not stop use for any reason other than pregnancy. Estimates of the probability of pregnancy during the first year of typical use for spermicides and the diaphragm are taken from the 1995 National Survey of Family Growth corrected for underreporting of abortion; estimates for fertility awareness-based methods, withdrawal, the male condom, the pill, and medroxyprogesterone are taken from the 1995 and 2002 National Survey of Family Growth corrected for underreporting of abortion.

†Among couples who initiate use of a method (not necessarily for the first time) and who use it perfectly (ie, consistently and correctly), the percentage who experience an accidental pregnancy during the first year if they do not stop use for any other reason.

‡Among couples attempting to avoid pregnancy, the percentage who continue to use a method for 1 year.

§The percentage of women who become pregnant in the typical use and perfect use columns are based on data from populations where contraception is not used and from women who cease using contraception in order to become pregnant. Among such populations, approximately 89% become pregnant within 1 year. This estimate was lowered slightly (to 85%) to represent the percentage who would become pregnant within 1 year among women now relying on reversible methods of contraception if they abandoned contraception altogether.

‖Foams, creams, gels, vaginal suppositories, and vaginal film.

¶The Ovulation and TwoDay methods are based on evaluation of cervical mucus. The Standard Days method avoids intercourse on cycle days 8 through 19. The Symptothermal method is a double-check method based on evaluation of cervical mucus to determine the first fertile day and evaluation of cervical mucus and temperature to determine the last fertile day.

#Without spermicides.

**With spermicidal cream or jelly.

††These are weighted averages of estimates derived from the 1995 and 2002 National Surveys of Family Growth. The National Survey of Family Growth does not ask for brand of pill; thus, combined and progestin-only pills cannot be distinguished. However, because use of the combined pill is far more common than use of the progestin-only pill, the results from the National Survey of Family Growth overwhelmingly reflect typical use of combined pills. The efficacy of progestin-only pills may be lower than that for combined pills because progestin-only pills are probably less forgiving of nonadherence to the dosing schedule. Whether the progestin-only pill also is less effective during perfect use is unknown.

Modified with permission from Trussell J. Contraceptive efficacy. In: Hatcher RA, Trussell J, Nelson AL, Cates WJ, Kowal D,Policar MS, editors. Contraceptive technology. 20th revised ed. New York (NY): Ardent Media; 2011. p. 779–863.

the woman and to enlist her involvement in overall health maintenance. Clinicians should encourage women to formulate a reproductive health plan and should discuss it in a nondirective way at each subsequent visit.

Such a plan would address the individual's or couple's desire for a child or children (or desire not to have children); the optimal number, spacing, and timing of children in the family; and age-related changes in fertility. Because a patient's plans may change over time, creating a reproductive health plan requires an ongoing, conscientious assessment of the desirability of a future pregnancy; determination of steps that need to be taken either to prevent or to plan for and optimize a pregnancy; and evaluation of current health status.

CONTRACEPTIVE AND SEXUAL HISTORY

For all women of reproductive age, a contraceptive and sexual history should be obtained to assess the need for contraceptive services. The clinician should obtain a general medical and gynecologic history for women who request contraception. The Centers for Disease Control and Prevention (CDC) have published the *U.S. Medical Eligibility Criteria for Contraceptive Use, 2010* (U.S. MEC), which is extremely helpful in identifying contraindications to various methods. The full recommendations are available at www.cdc.gov/mmwr/pdf/rr/rr5904.pdf, and a summary chart can be accessed at www.cdc.gov/reproductivehealth/ UnintendedPregnancy/Docs/USMEC-Color-62012.docx. Updates and supporting information for clinicians are available at www.cdc.gov/reproduc tivehealth/UnintendedPregnancy/USMEC.htm.

SCREENING FOR REPRODUCTIVE AND SEXUAL COERCION AND INTIMATE PARTNER VIOLENCE

Reproductive coercion involves behavior that interferes with contraceptive use or pregnancy. The most common forms of reproductive coercion include sabotage of contraceptive methods, pregnancy coercion, and pregnancy pressure. Sexual coercion includes a range of behavior that a partner may use to pressure or coerce a person to have sex without using physical force. Examples include repeatedly pressuring a partner to have sex, threatening to end a relationship if the person does not have sex, forcing sex without a condom or not allowing other prophylaxis use, intentionally exposing a partner to a sexually transmitted infection (STI), including human immunodeficiency virus (HIV), or threatening retaliation if notified of a positive STI test result.

Because of the known link between reproductive health and violence, women's health care providers should screen women and adolescent girls for intimate partner violence and reproductive and sexual coercion at periodic intervals and include reproductive and sexual coercion and intimate partner violence as part of the differential diagnosis when patients are seen for pregnancy or STI testing, emergency contraception, or with unintended pregnancies. Some examples of screening questions include the following:

- Has your partner ever forced you to do something sexually that you did not want to do or refused your request to use condoms?

- Has your partner ever tried to get you pregnant when you did not want to be pregnant?

- Are you worried your partner will hurt you if you do not do what he wants with the pregnancy?

If a patient responds affirmatively to screening questions, the health care provider should validate her experience and commend her for discussing and evaluating her health and relationships. She should be reassured that the situation is not her fault and further assessment of her safety should be elicited and discreet contraceptive options reviewed. Interventions include education on the effect of reproductive and sexual coercion and intimate partner violence on patients' health and choices, counseling on harm-reduction strategies, and prevention of unintended pregnancies by providing discreet and confidential methods of contraception, such as intrauterine devices (IUDs), emergency contraception, depot medroxy-progesterone acetate injections, and etonogestrel implants. For additional support, patients may be offered hotline numbers, use of the office phone to access suggested care, and referral to a domestic violence advocate for additional resources (see also the "Abuse" section later in Part 3).

PHYSICAL EXAMINATION AND LABORATORY TESTS

As a companion document to the U.S. MEC, the CDC has published the *U.S. Selected Practice Recommendations for Contraceptive Use, 2013* (U.S. SPR). According to the U.S. SPR, with few exceptions, examinations and tests are not needed before initiating contraceptive methods in women who are presumed to be healthy because these assessments do not contribute substantially to safe and effective use of contraceptive methods. Examinations or tests that are not deemed necessary for safe and effective contraceptive use might be appropriate for good preventive health care or for diagnosing or assessing suspected medical conditions. For example, weight measurement or body mass index calculations are not needed to determine medical eligibility for any methods of contraception. Measuring weight and calculating body mass index at baseline might be helpful, however, for monitoring any changes and counseling women using hormonal methods or IUDs who might be concerned about weight change perceived to be associated with their contraceptive method. See "Methods" later in this section for specific examinations or tests that are recommended before initiating certain types of contraception.

COUNSELING ON METHODS

In the absence of contraindications, patient choice should be the principal factor in prescribing one method of contraception over another. To help the patient make this choice, the health care provider should do the following:

- Fully explain potential adverse effects and risks for all methods; in a healthy woman, death rates from pregnancy are higher than from any contraceptive method.
- Discuss efficacy and failure rates (see Table 3-8). Couples deciding among methods should be encouraged to choose a method they are likely to use effectively. Methods that are less user-dependent often fit this description.
- Describe ease of use and noncontraceptive benefits.
- Explain the use of barrier methods to reduce the risk of STI transmission when nonbarrier contraceptive methods are used (see also the "Sexually Transmitted Infections" section later in Part 3).

A special warning regarding the use of condoms and diaphragms should be given to patients with latex sensitivity. Women, especially, are at high risk of reaction because of mucous membrane contact with these devices.

Nonlatex male condoms and diaphragms are available. The second-generation female condom is nonlatex, being made of nitrile; this condom has the same instructions and has shown similar safety and efficacy to previously marketed polyurethane products. Provide information on when and how to use emergency contraception. To maximize the effectiveness of treatment, women should be able to obtain emergency contraception quickly when the need arises (see also "Emergency Contraception" later in this section).

Periodic Reassessment

The U.S. SPR recommendations address when routine follow-up is recommended for safe and effective continued use of contraception for healthy women. The recommendations refer to general situations and might vary for different users and different situations. Specific populations that might benefit from more frequent follow-up visits include adolescents, those with certain medical conditions or characteristics, and those with multiple medical conditions.

With the exception of hysteroscopic sterilization and vasectomy, routine follow-up visits are not needed for any contraceptive method. Clinicians should advise a woman to return at any time to discuss side effects or other problems, if she wants to change the method being used, and when it is time to remove or replace the method. At other routine visits, health care providers who see contraceptive users should assess the woman's satisfaction with her contraceptive method and whether she has any concerns about method use. The health care provider should assess any changes in health status, including medications that would change the appropriateness of the method for safe and effective use on the basis of the U.S. MEC (eg, category 3 and 4 conditions and characteristics). Specific recommendations for users of IUDs and combined hormonal contraceptives are included later in this section.

Rates of pregnancy and discontinuation are highest in the first few months after the initiation of a contraceptive method. A visit in the first few months to troubleshoot problems can be considered to help avoid discontinuation or facilitate transfer to another method. Similarly, a phone call from an office nurse after contraception initiation also may be appropriate. High rates of discontinuation may be reduced with good follow-up and the provision of a convenient opportunity to have the patient's questions about the contraceptive method answered. Once the patient has become comfortable with her method of contraception, annual follow-up examinations should be conducted in accordance with age-specific recommendations for asymptomatic women.

Special Populations

OLDER CONTRACEPTIVE USERS

Prevention of unintended pregnancy assumes increasing importance for many women during the perimenopausal years. Pregnancies in women over 40 years of age are often unintended. It may be difficult to know when it is safe to change from hormonal contraception to postmenopausal hormone treatment. Assessment of follicle-stimulating hormone levels to determine when older contraceptive users have become menopausal is expensive and may be misleading. Until a well-validated tool to confirm menopause is available, it is appropriate for healthy, nonsmoking women doing well on a combined hormonal contraceptive to continue contraceptive use until age 50–55 years. The likelihood that a woman has reached menopausal status by age 55 years is 85%.

WOMEN WITH COEXISTING MEDICAL CONDITIONS

Clinicians must balance benefits and risks when contemplating appropriate contraception in women with coexisting medical conditions. Avoidance of unintended pregnancy is particularly important, given the risks of pregnancy to the woman and her fetus, for some medical conditions. Some conditions or medications may alter contraceptive effectiveness. The U.S. MEC (www.cdc.gov/reproductivehealth/unintendedpregnancy/usmec. htm) is an excellent resource that can help guide practitioners in regard to contraception for patients with coexisting medical conditions. The U.S. MEC uses four categories to aid clinicians in their decisions regarding the use of each contraceptive method for a patient with a given characteristic or medical condition (see Box 3-15).

Box 3-15. Categories of Medical Eligibility Criteria for Contraceptive Use

1 = A condition for which there is no restriction for the use of the contraceptive method.
2 = A condition for which the advantages of using the method generally outweigh the theoretical or proven risks.
3 = A condition for which the theoretical or proven risks usually outweigh the advantages of using the method.
4 = A condition that represents an unacceptable health risk if the contraceptive method is used.

Reprinted from U.S. Medical Eligibility Criteria for Contraceptive Use, 2010. Centers for Disease Control and Prevention. MMWR Recomm Rep 2010;59(RR-4):1–86: adapted from the World Health Organization. Medical eligibility criteria for contraceptive use. 4th ed. Geneva: WHO; 2009. Available at: http://whqlibdoc.who.int/publications/2010/9789241563888_eng.pdf. Retrieved June 7, 2013.

Methods

STERILIZATION

A woman who feels that her family is complete should be informed about male and female sterilization options as well as IUDs and contraceptive implants. Intrauterine devices should be strongly considered because their efficacy is similar to that of surgical sterilization with substantially lower risks associated with insertion as compared with surgery for sterilization. The advantages of vasectomy include the fact that it is a less invasive and less expensive procedure than tubal sterilization. Vasectomy also can be performed with local anesthesia.

Female sterilization can be performed at any time when a woman is not pregnant (interval sterilization) or after pregnancy (postpartum sterilization). The choice and timing of sterilization are affected by individual patient preference, medical assessment of acute risk, access to services, and insurance coverage. The timing of the procedure influences the surgical approach and the method of tubal occlusion or ligation. Hysteroscopic techniques are not indicated for postpartum sterilization or sterilization after an abortion.

The laparoscopic approach is used for interval and postabortal tubal ligation procedures. In the United States, minilaparotomy generally is reserved for postpartum procedures and rarely considered for patients at high risk of complications associated with laparoscopic procedures.

If a patient is considering surgical sterilization, she should be told that the procedure is intended to be permanent, that there is a small chance of failure, and that the success of any subsequent attempts at surgical restoration of fertility is uncertain. Although most women do not regret their decision to have tubal sterilization, women aged 30 years or younger at the time of sterilization and those who have had a break-up or divorce are more likely to express sterilization regret. Patients who undergo hysteroscopic sterilization should have hysterosalpingography performed at 3 months to ensure tubal occlusion. They should be instructed to use another method of contraception until hysterosalpingography confirms bilateral tubal occlusion. Similarly, men who undergo vasectomy need to return for a semen analysis 8–16 weeks after the procedure to ensure it was successful. Men (and their female partners) should be advised to use additional contraceptive protection or abstain from intercourse until after the postvasectomy semen analysis confirms the success of the procedure.

Physicians need to be aware of applicable federal and state requirements that relate to consent, age restrictions, and reimbursement for surgical sterilization (see also the "Ethical Issues" section in Part 1). If the physician has any question about the patient's capacity to authorize the procedure, he or she should seek consultation to ensure that legal requirements are met.

INTRAUTERINE DEVICES

Intrauterine devices are used at lower rates by U.S. women compared with women in other nations. The National Center for Health Statistics reports that from 2006 to 2010, only 5.6% of U.S. women used an IUD as contraception. The effectiveness of IUDs is similar to that of female sterilization.

According to the U.S. MEC, the only absolute contraindications (ie, U.S. MEC 4 rating) to IUD use are as follows:

* Distorted uterine cavity
* Persistent or malignant gestational trophoblastic disease

- Current breast cancer (levonorgestrel-releasing intrauterine system [levonorgestrel IUD] only)
- Immediately after septic abortion
- Puerperal sepsis

In addition, whereas continuation of IUD use may be acceptable, IUD use should not be initiated in women with the following:

- Current pelvic inflammatory disease
- Current purulent cervicitis, chlamydial infection, or gonorrhea
- Pelvic tuberculosis
- Cervical or endometrial cancer awaiting treatment

Nulliparous and multiparous women who desire long-term reversible contraception are good candidates for IUD use. The first levonorgestrel IUD that was approved by the U.S. Food and Drug Administration is recommended for women who have had at least one child and should be replaced in 5 years. Although the 5-year levonorgestrel IUD is not approved for nulliparous women, it has a U.S. MEC 2 rating in nulliparous women because the advantages generally outweigh the risks. The recently approved 3-year levonorgestrel IUD, which postdates the publication of the U.S. MEC, is not restricted to use in parous women. The copper IUD is labeled for 10 years of use. Data support the safety of IUD use in adolescents.

Previous ectopic pregnancy is not a contraindication to IUD use. Pelvic inflammatory disease (PID) complicating IUD insertion is uncommon, and the risk of PID decreases to the baseline risk after the first 20 days following insertion. Progestin-containing IUDs have noncontraceptive benefits, including decreased menstrual flow. However, only the 5-year levonorgestrel IUD is labeled as an appropriate treatment for heavy menstrual bleeding in women who choose an IUD for contraception.

According to the U.S. SPR, few examinations or tests are needed before initiation of an IUD by healthy women. Bimanual examination and cervical inspection are necessary before IUD insertion. Recommendations should be followed for routine screening for chlamydial infection and gonorrhea (see also the "Sexually Transmitted Infections" section later in Part 3). Women who have not received indicated screening can be screened at the time of IUD insertion; the insertion should not be delayed while awaiting results. Women who have a very high likelihood of STI exposure (eg, those with a currently infected partner) generally should not undergo IUD insertion until appropriate testing and treatment occur.

For new contraceptive users and those switching from another method, either the copper IUD or levonorgestrel IUD can be inserted at any time if it is reasonably certain that the woman is not pregnant (see Box 3-16). Waiting for the next menstrual period is unnecessary. A back-up method of contraception is not needed if the levonorgestrel IUD is inserted within the first 7 days of the start of menstrual bleeding or at the time of a surgical abortion. Otherwise, the patient needs to abstain from sexual intercourse or use additional contraceptive protection for the next 7 days. Guidance on switching from the copper IUD to the levonorgestrel IUD is available in the U.S. SPR (see Bibliography). No additional contraceptive protection is needed after insertion of the copper IUD.

The copper IUD may be inserted immediately (up to 7 days) after a first-trimester or second-trimester spontaneous abortion or induced abortion. Labeling states that the 5-year and 3-year levonorgestrel IUDs may be inserted immediately after a first-trimester abortion, but insertion after a second-trimester abortion should be delayed until uterine involution is complete (for the 5-year IUD) or for a minimum of 6 weeks or until the uterus is fully involuted (for the 3-year IUD). Immediate insertion of the 5-year levonorgestrel IUD is classified as U.S. MEC 1 after a first-trimester abortion and as U.S. MEC 2 after a second-trimester abortion because of a higher risk of expulsion after a second-trimester abortion. Although there may be a higher risk of expulsions with postabortion IUD placements, studies have shown that many patients do not return for IUD placement at later times.

The U.S. SPR indicates that no routine follow-up visit is required after IUD insertion. General considerations for ongoing contraceptive management are addressed earlier in this section (see "Periodic Reassessment"). At other routine visits, health care providers who treat IUD users should consider performing an examination to check for the presence of the IUD strings. Management of common problems that may occur with IUD use (eg, bleeding irregularities, amenorrhea, PID management in an IUD user) is found in the U.S. SPR (see Bibliography).

Box 3-16. How to Be Reasonably Certain That a Woman Is Not Pregnant

A health care provider can be reasonably certain that a woman is not pregnant if she has no symptoms or signs of pregnancy and meets any one of the following criteria:

- Has started her normal menses within the past 7 days
- Has not had sexual intercourse since the start of her last normal menses
- Has been correctly and consistently using a reliable method of contraception
- Has had a spontaneous abortion or induced abortion within the past 7 days
- Has given birth within the past 4 weeks
- Is fully or nearly fully breastfeeding (exclusively breastfeeding or the vast majority [85% or more] of feeds are breastfeeds)*, amenorrheic, and less than 6 months postpartum

*Data from Labbok MH, Perez A, Valdes V, Sevilla F, Wade K, Laukaran VH, et al. The lactational amenorrhea method (LAM): a postpartum introductory family planning method with policy and program implications. Adv Contracept 1994;10:93–109.

Modified from U.S. Selected Practice Recommendations for Contraceptive Use, 2013: adapted from the World Health Organization selected practice recommendations for contraceptive use, 2nd edition. Division of Reproductive Health, National Center for Chronic Disease Prevention and Health Promotion, Centers for Disease Control and Prevention. MMWR Recomm Rep 2013;62:1–60.

CONTRACEPTIVE IMPLANTS

The contraceptive implant is a single 4-cm by 2-mm rod containing etonogestrel that provides 3 years of contraception and consistently suppresses ovulation. The efficacy of the contraceptive implant is excellent, with failure rates similar to that of sterilization. The main disadvantage to the contraceptive implant is unpredictable bleeding, which is particularly problematic in the first 3 months after insertion. Before insertion, patients should be strongly counseled about this adverse effect and assured that the bleeding is not a sign of pathology. The contraceptive implant should not be used in women with current breast cancer (U.S. MEC 4).

For new contraceptive users and those switching from another method, the contraceptive implant can be inserted at any time if it is reasonably certain that the woman is not pregnant (see Box 3-16). Waiting for the next menstrual period is unnecessary. Contraceptive implant insertion immediately (up to 7 days) after a first-trimester or second-trimester spontaneous abortion or induced abortion is classified as U.S. MEC 1, but this recommendation is based on studies of a levonorgestrel implant system no longer marketed in the United States. If the implant is placed within 5 days of the start of menstrual bleeding or at the time of a surgical abortion, no additional contraceptive protection is needed. Otherwise, the woman needs to abstain from sexual intercourse or use additional contraceptive protection for the next 7 days. Guidance on switching from an IUD to the contraceptive implant is provided in the U.S. SPR (see Bibliography).

The U.S. SPR indicates that no routine follow-up visit is required after contraceptive implant insertion. General considerations for ongoing contraceptive management are addressed earlier in this section (see "Periodic Reassessment"). Management of common problems that may occur with implant use (eg, bleeding irregularities, amenorrhea) is found in the U.S. SPR.

INJECTABLE CONTRACEPTION

There are two injectable contraceptive formulations currently available in the United States: 1) depot medroxyprogesterone acetate (DMPA) 150 mg/mL, which is given every 13 weeks intramuscularly and is by far the most common formulation, and 2) DMPA 104 mg/0.65 mL, which is given subcutaneously every 13 weeks. Repeat injections can be given early when necessary. According to the U.S. SPR, repeat injections can be given up to 15 weeks after the last injection without requiring additional contraceptive protection. The typical-use failure rate over 1 year of use is approximately 6%, which is lower than the typical-use failure rate of approximately 9% for combined oral contraceptives, the progestin-only pill, or the contraceptive patch or contraceptive ring (Table 3-8). Because injectable contraception requires minimal patient action, it is often favored by women for whom adherence to other methods is a problem. Injectable contraception use is contraindicated in women with current breast cancer (U.S. MEC 4).

For new contraceptive users and those switching from another method, the first DMPA injection can be given at any time if it is reasonably certain that the woman is not pregnant (see Box 3-16). Waiting for the next menstrual period is unnecessary. The first DMPA injection can be given immediately (up to 7 days) after a spontaneous or induced abortion. If the first DMPA injection is given within 7 days of the start of menstrual bleeding or at the time of a surgical abortion, no additional contraceptive protection is needed. Otherwise, the woman needs to abstain from sexual intercourse or use additional contraceptive protection for the next 7 days. Guidance on switching from an IUD to combined hormonal contraception injection is available in the U.S. SPR (see Bibliography).

The U.S. SPR indicates that no routine follow-up visit is required after DMPA injection. General considerations for ongoing contraceptive management are addressed earlier in this section (see "Periodic Reassessment"). Management of common problems that may occur with the injection (eg, bleeding irregularities, amenorrhea) is found in the U.S. SPR.

The use of contraceptive dosages of DMPA suppresses ovarian production of estradiol. Although DMPA is associated with bone mineral density (BMD) loss during use, current evidence suggests that partial or full recovery occurs after discontinuation of use. Concerns regarding the effect of DMPA on bone mineral density should neither prevent practitioners from prescribing nor cause them to limit its use to 2 consecutive years, despite the "black box" package labeling cautioning against prolonged use. Practitioners should not perform BMD monitoring solely in response to DMPA use, because any observed short-term loss of BMD associated with DMPA use may be recovered and is unlikely to place a woman at risk of fracture either during use or in later years. Caution is advised in the use of DMPA for women with mobility disorders who are not weight bearing.

Weight gain is a problem that may be seen in women using DMPA, although it is critical to note that it is not consistent in all women and may vary by age, ethnicity, and perhaps baseline dietary practices. A systematic review of a limited body of evidence suggests that early weight gain may predict future weight gain. Therefore, measuring weight and calculating body mass index at baseline might be helpful for monitoring any changes and counseling women receiving DMPA injections who might be concerned about weight change perceived to be associated with their contraceptive method. According to the U.S. MEC, obesity is not a contraindication for DMPA use.

COMBINED HORMONAL CONTRACEPTIVES: ORAL, PATCHES, AND RINGS

Combined hormonal contraceptives that contain an estrogen and a progestin are available in oral contraceptive pills, the contraceptive patch, and the contraceptive ring. Because all have an estrogen component, a contraindication to estrogen use precludes the use of any of these methods. Combined hormonal contraceptives should be prescribed with caution, if ever, to women who are older than 35 years and are smokers (ie, U.S. MEC 3 rating for those who smoke fewer than 15 cigarettes a day and a U.S. MEC 4 rating for those who smoke more than 15 cigarettes a day).

According to the U.S. SPR, few examinations or tests are needed before initiation of combined hormonal contraceptives by healthy women. Blood pressure should be measured before initiation of combined hormonal contraceptives. In cases in which access to health care might be limited, the blood pressure measurement can be obtained by the woman in a nonclinical setting (eg, pharmacy or fire station) and self-reported to the clinician.

According to the U.S. SPR, for new contraceptive users and those switching from another method, combination hormonal contraceptives (pills, patch, and ring) can be initiated at any time if it is reasonably certain that a woman is not pregnant (see Box 3-16). Waiting for the next menstrual period is unnecessary. Combined hormonal contraceptives can be started immediately (up to 7 days) after a first-trimester or second-trimester spontaneous abortion or induced abortion. If combined hormonal contraceptives are started within 5 days of the start of menstrual bleeding or at the time of a surgical abortion, no additional contraceptive protection is needed. Otherwise, the woman needs to abstain from sexual intercourse or use additional contraceptive protection for the next 7 days. Guidance on switching from an IUD to combined hormonal contraception is provided in the U.S. SPR (see Bibliography).

The U.S. SPR indicates that no routine follow-up visit is required after initiation of combined hormonal contraception. General considerations for ongoing contraceptive management are addressed earlier in this section (see "Periodic Reassessment"). At other routine visits, health care providers who treat users of combined hormonal contraception should assess blood pressure or, if access to health care is limited, request self-reports of blood pressure readings from patients. Management recommendations for common problems that may occur with use of combined hormonal contraceptives (eg, unscheduled bleeding, vomiting, or severe diarrhea while using the method) are found in the U.S. SPR (see Bibliography).

Oral Contraceptives

The U.S. Food and Drug Administration considers generic and brand name oral contraceptive products to be clinically equivalent and interchangeable. The College supports patient or clinician requests for branded oral contraceptives or continuation of the same generic or branded oral contraceptives if the request is based on clinical experience or concerns regarding packaging or adherence, or if the branded product is considered a better choice for that individual patient.

Although some data have suggested that use of drospirenone-containing pills has a higher risk of venous thromboembolism, this risk is still very low and is much lower than the risk of venous thromboembolism during pregnancy and the immediate postpartum period. Decisions regarding choice of oral contraceptive should be left to clinicians and their patients, taking into account the possible minimally increased risk of venous thromboembolism, patient preference, and the available alternatives. When prescribing any oral contraceptive, clinicians should consider a woman's risk factors for venous thromboembolism and refer to the U.S. MEC.

Product labeling and protocols developed by various organizations may differ in the information they provide on how to handle a missed dose of a contraceptive pill. Often, patients missing several doses will have unscheduled or breakthrough bleeding, which may serve as an adherence reminder and an opportunity to reevaluate contraceptive method choice. The protocol for missed or late pills developed for the U.S. SPR is detailed in Box 3-17. Package labeling also makes recommendations depending on the package week and number of doses missed.

Missed doses are very common for any prescription product. Practitioners can help patients with daily adherence by linking the taking of

Box 3-17. Recommended Actions After Late or Missed Combined Oral Contraceptives

If one hormonal pill is taken late (less than 24 hours since a pill should have been taken) or missed (24 hours to less than 48 hours since a pill should have been taken):

- Take the late or missed pill as soon as possible.
- Continue taking the remaining pills at the usual time (even if it means taking two pills on the same day).
- No additional contraceptive protection is needed.
- Emergency contraception is not usually needed but can be considered if hormonal pills were missed earlier in the cycle or in the last week of the previous cycle.

If two or more consecutive hormonal pills have been missed (48 hours or longer since a pill should have been taken):

- Take the most recent missed pill as soon as possible. (Any other missed pills should be discarded.)
- Continue taking the remaining pills at the usual time (even if it means taking two pills on the same day).
- Use back-up contraception (eg, condoms) or avoid sexual intercourse until hormonal pills have been taken for 7 consecutive days.
- If the pills were missed in the last week of hormonal pills (eg, days 15–21 for 28-day pill packs):
  — Omit the hormone-free interval by finishing the hormonal pills in the current pack and starting a new pack the next day.
  — If unable to start a new pack immediately, use back-up contraception (eg, condoms) or avoid sexual intercourse until hormonal pills from a new pack have been taken for 7 consecutive days.
- Emergency contraception should be considered if hormonal pills were missed during the first week and unprotected sexual intercourse occurred in the previous 5 days.
- Emergency contraception may also be considered at other times as appropriate.

Reprinted from U.S. Selected Practice Recommendations for Contraceptive Use, 2013: adapted from the World Health Organization selected practice recommendations for contraceptive use, 2nd edition. Division of Reproductive Health, National Center for Chronic Disease Prevention and Health Promotion, Centers for Disease Control and Prevention. MMWR Recomm Rep 2013;62:1–60.

the product to a daily activity, such as tooth brushing or the morning cup of coffee, and the pills can be stored next to the toothbrush or coffee products as a memory cue. Similar lifestyle reminders can be used for weekly products, for example, setting a weekly confidential reminder on a cellphone to remind oneself that the contraceptive patch needs to be changed. Programs are available that allow patients to set various computer-generated reminders including e-mails, text messages, phone applications, and pop-up cues.

Access and cost issues are common reasons why women either do not use contraception or have gaps in use. Although oral contraceptives are the most widely used reversible method of family planning in the United States, oral contraceptive use is subject to problems with adherence and continuation, often because of logistics or practical issues. The American College of Obstetricians and Gynecologists supports over-the-counter access to oral contraceptives and access to multiple pill packs at one time as potential ways to improve contraceptive access and use and possibly decrease the unintended pregnancy rate. The U.S. SPR recommends that up to a 1-year supply of combined hormonal contraception be prescribed or provided at initial and return visits. The more pill packs given up to 13 cycles, the higher the continuation rates.

Contraceptive Patch and Ring

The contraceptive patch is changed weekly for 3 weeks, followed by 1 week without the patch. It is less effective in women who weigh more than 198 lb. The vaginal contraceptive ring is initially inserted on a day between cycle days 1 and 5 and left in place for 3 weeks, followed by 1 week of no ring use. Management of delayed application or detached contraceptive patches and delayed insertion or reinsertion of the vaginal ring is addressed in Box 3-18.

Currently, only one brand of contraceptive patch and one brand of vaginal contraceptive ring are available in the United States. Both products have informational web sites sponsored by the pharmaceutical makers, which provide patients and clinicians with answers to frequently asked questions. Various scenarios, such as detached patches and what to do if the ring falls out, also are addressed in the patient package insert.

Box 3-18. Recommended Actions After Delayed Application of a Combined Hormonal Patch or Insertion of a Combined Vaginal Ring

The following is recommended if patch application or detachment* or ring insertion or reinsertion† is delayed for less than 48 hours:

- Apply patch or insert ring as soon as possible. (If detachment of a patch occurred less than 24 hours since the patch was applied, try to reapply the patch or replace with a new patch.)
- Keep the same patch change day, or keep the ring in until the scheduled removal day.
- No additional contraceptive protection is needed.
- Emergency contraception is not usually needed but can be considered if delayed patch application or detachment or ring insertion or reinsertion occurred earlier in the cycle or in the last week of the previous cycle.

The following is recommended if patch application or detachment* or ring insertion or reinsertion† is delayed for 48 hours or longer:

- Apply a new patch or insert a new ring as soon as possible.
- Keep the same patch change day or keep the ring in until the scheduled ring removal day.
- Use back-up contraception (eg, condoms) or avoid sexual intercourse until a patch or ring has been worn for 7 consecutive days.
- If the delayed patch application or detachment or ring removal occurred in the third week of use
  —omit the hormone-free week by finishing the third week of use (keeping the same patch change day) and starting a new patch or ring immediately.
  — if unable to start a new patch or ring immediately, use back-up contraception (eg, condoms) or avoid sexual intercourse until a new patch or ring has been worn for 7 consecutive days.
  — emergency contraception should be considered if the delayed patch application or detachment of the patch or ring insertion or reinsertion occurred within the first week of use and unprotected sexual intercourse occurred in the previous 5 days.

(continued)

> **Box 3-18.** Recommended Actions After Delayed Application of
> a Combined Hormonal Patch or Insertion of a Combined
> Vaginal Ring *(continued)*
>
> — emergency contraception also may be considered at other times as
> appropriate.
>
> ---
>
> *If detachment of the patch takes place but the woman is unsure when it occurred,
> consider the patch to have been detached for at least 48 hours since a patch should
> have been applied or reattached.
> †If removal of the ring takes place but the woman is unsure of how long the ring has
> been removed, consider the ring to have been removed for at least 48 hours since a ring
> should have been inserted or reinserted.
> Modified from U.S. Selected Practice Recommendations for Contraceptive Use, 2013:
> adapted from the World Health Organization selected practice recommendations for
> contraceptive use, 2nd edition. Division of Reproductive Health, National Center for
> Chronic Disease Prevention and Health Promotion, Centers for Disease Control and
> Prevention. MMWR Recomm Rep 2013;62:1–60.

PROGESTIN-ONLY PILLS

There are several progestin-only methods available in the United States, including progestin-only oral contraceptives (sometimes referred to as "minipills"). Progestin-only pills are safe for many women for whom there are strong contraindications against the use of estrogen.

For new contraceptive users and those switching from another method, progestin-only pills can be initiated at any time if it is reasonably certain that a woman is not pregnant (see Box 3-16). Waiting for the next menstrual period is unnecessary. The U.S. SPR recommends that up to a 1-year supply of progestin-only pills be prescribed or provided at initial and return visits. The more pill packs given up to 13 cycles, the higher the continuation rates. Progestin-only pills can be started immediately (up to 7 days) after a spontaneous or induced abortion. If progestin-only pills are started within 5 days of the start of menstrual bleeding or at the time of a surgical abortion, no additional contraceptive protection is needed. Otherwise, the woman needs to abstain from sexual intercourse or use additional contraceptive protection for the next 2 days. Guidance on switching from an IUD to progestin-only pills is provided in the U.S. SPR (see Bibliography).

The U.S. SPR indicates that no routine follow-up visit is required after initiation of progestin-only pills. General considerations for ongoing contraceptive management are addressed earlier in this section (see "Periodic Reassessment"). Progestin-only pills require careful attention to consistent pill-taking at the same time of day (within a 3-hour window) to help ensure contraceptive efficacy. If a pill is taken more than 3 hours late, the pill should be taken as soon as possible, and pills should be taken daily, one each day at the same time each day, even if it means taking two pills on the same day. Back-up contraception or avoidance of sexual intercourse is recommended until pills have been taken correctly, on time, for 2 consecutive days. Emergency contraception should be considered if the woman has had unprotected sexual intercourse. Vomiting and severe diarrhea that occur within 3 hours of taking a progestin-only pill is managed similarly to late pills. Irregular bleeding is seen significantly more in progestin-only pill users than in women who take combined oral contraceptives and is the major reason for discontinuation.

OVER-THE-COUNTER PRODUCTS, BARRIER METHODS, AND RARELY USED PRESCRIPTION PRODUCTS

Although over-the-counter methods are less effective than prescription methods, they may be preferred by many couples (see Table 3-8). Contraceptive sponges and spermicides are available without prescription. It is important that the patient understands that the sponge does not protect against STIs. The sponge is effective for contraception immediately after insertion for up to 24 hours after coitus. The sponge must be left in the vagina for at least 6 hours after coitus and must not be left for longer than 30 hours.

Condoms are an excellent choice as a barrier method because they prevent STIs and pregnancy. No examinations or tests are needed before initiating use of condoms or spermicides. However, patients should be aware that although condoms offer the best protection against STIs, they are not the most effective contraceptive method. Diaphragms are similar to condoms in contraceptive effectiveness and have the advantage of being female controlled but the disadvantages of not providing STI protection and requiring a health care provider visit with bimanual examination and a prescription.

Less commonly used nonhormonal prescription methods include a reusable one-size shield that is held by the vaginal wall and a cervical cap that is available in several sizes to allow for coverage of the cervix. Both devices are labeled for use with a spermicide. A bimanual examination and cervical inspection are needed for cervical cap fitting.

FERTILITY AWARENESS-BASED METHODS AND WITHDRAWAL

Fertility awareness-based methods of family planning help women to either plan or prevent pregnancy by helping them identify the days when pregnancy is likely. Identifying the fertile days involves tracking the menstrual cycle or monitoring a woman's fertility signs. The woman prevents pregnancy by avoiding unprotected intercourse on fertile days. Fertility awareness-based methods provide options for women who want to use a natural method for medical or personal reasons. They are used by approximately 1.3% of U.S. women at risk of pregnancy. The "TwoDay method" and the "Ovulation method" use cervical mucus as a marker of ovulation. In the "Standard days method," unprotected intercourse is avoided from cycle days 8 through 19. Approximately 47% of women using fertility awareness-based methods discontinue the method at 1 year, with typical use failure rates similar to those of the withdrawal method. Perfect-use failure rates with fertility awareness methods are in the 3–5% range for most methods, with the symptothermal method—which provides a cross-check—much lower at 0.4% (Table 3-8).

Withdrawal is a method that has been practiced by more than one half of all U.S. couples during their lifetimes and is widely practiced in the adolescent population. Although its typical use failure rate of 22% places it in the next-to-lowest tier of contraceptive effectiveness, withdrawal still is much more effective than use of no contraceptive method. Sperm are present in the preejaculatory fluid of some men, which is one cause of withdrawal method failure. The withdrawal method does not eliminate the transmission of STIs. Preejaculatory fluid, for example, can contain cells infected with HIV.

EMERGENCY CONTRACEPTION

Emergency contraception may be used to prevent pregnancy after an unprotected or inadequately protected act of sexual intercourse. Emergency contraception should be taken as soon as possible within 5 days of unprotected sexual intercourse. It is most effective if used within the first 24 hours. The most common emergency contraceptive method is oral progestin-only pills (levonorgestrel), but other effective methods include antiprogestin ulipristal acetate and combined regimens (high doses of ethinyl estradiol and a progestin). A copper IUD is the most effective form of emergency contraception for medically eligible women, may prevent pregnancy if inserted within 5 days of unprotected intercourse, and has the additional benefit of providing long-term, effective contraception.

Progestin-only emergency contraception is better tolerated and more efficacious than the combined regimen. In the United States, the two levonorgestrel-only regimens include a single-dose regimen (1.5 mg levonorgestrel) and a two-dose regimen (two tablets of 0.75 mg of levonorgestrel taken 12 hours apart).

The antiprogestin ulipristal acetate is at least as effective as levonorgestrel in preventing pregnancy up to 72 hours after unprotected intercourse and appears to be more effective than levonorgestrel in preventing pregnancy when used between 72 hours and 120 hours after unprotected intercourse. Ulipristal acetate may reduce the efficacy of combined hormonal contraceptive methods, such as oral contraceptives, patches, and rings. According to the U.S. SPR, any regular contraceptive method may be started immediately after using ulipristal acetate, but it is recommended that the woman abstain or use barrier contraception for 14 days or until her next menses and that she have a pregnancy test if she does not have a withdrawal bleed within 3 weeks. Guidance for the use of emergency contraception that contains levonorgestrel or combined hormonal contraceptives is similar except that abstinence or back-up methods are needed for only 7 days.

Emergency contraception should be offered or made available to women who experience unprotected or inadequately protected sexual intercourse and who do not desire pregnancy. Treatment with emergency contraception should be initiated as soon as possible to maximize efficacy, and it should be made available to patients who request it up to 120 hours after unprotected intercourse. No clinical examination or pregnancy testing is necessary before the provision or prescription of emergency contraception. Prescription or provision of emergency contraception in advance of need, particularly for adolescents younger than 17 years, can increase availability and may increase use. In 2013, the Plan B One-Step (Teva Women's Health, Inc.) single-dose levonorgestrel regimen was made available over-the-counter without age restriction. The other levonorgestrel-only regimens also are available without a prescription but only to women aged 17 years or older with government-issued photo identification. A 30-mg tablet of ulipristal acetate requires a prescription.

Access to emergency contraception can be limited by pharmacist refusal and pharmacy stocking issues. Not all pharmacies stock these dedicated products, and pharmacist refusal may occur. Access to emergency contraception remains difficult for some populations, including adolescents, immigrants, non-English speaking women, survivors of sexual assault, those living in areas with few pharmacy choices, and poor women.

Some patients may have oral contraceptives in their household that can be used for emergency contraception. Table 3-9 describes appropriate formulations from a variety of combined oral contraceptives available in the United States. To reduce the chances of nausea with the combination estrogen–progestin regimen, an antiemetic agent (such as dimenhydrinate) is recommended and may be taken 1 hour before the first emergency contraception dose.

Emergency contraception is effective only before a pregnancy is established. The major, if not sole, mechanism of emergency contraception appears to be inhibition or delay of ovulation. Emergency contraception does not disrupt a pregnancy after nidation, or implantation, has occurred. No studies have specifically investigated adverse effects of exposure to emergency contraception during early pregnancy. However, numerous studies of the teratogenic risk of conception during daily use of oral contraceptives (including older, higher-dose preparations) have found no increase in risk to either the pregnant woman or the developing fetus.

Emergency contraception may be used even if the woman has used it before, even within the same menstrual cycle. The U.S. MEC includes no conditions in which the risks of emergency contraception outweigh the

Table 3-9. Oral Contraceptives That Can Be Used for Emergency Contraception in the United States*

Brand	Company	First Dose†	Second Dose† (12 hours later)	Ulipristal Acetate per Dose (mg)	Ethinyl Estradiol per Dose (microgram)	Levon-orgestrel per Dose (mg)‡
Ulipristal acetate pills						
ella	Watson	1 white pill	None†	30	–	–
Progestin-only pills						
Plan B One-Step	Teva	1 white pill	None	–	–	1.5
Next Choice One Dose	Watson	1 peach pill	None	–	–	1.5
My Way	Gavis	1 white pill	None	–	–	1.5
Levon-orgestrel Tablets	Perrigo	2 white pills	None†	–	–	1.5
Combined progestin and estrogen pills						
Altavera	Sandoz	4 peach pills	4 peach pills	–	120	0.60
Amethia	Watson	4 white pills	4 white pills	–	120	0.60
Amethia Lo	Watson	5 white pills	5 white pills	–	100	0.50
Amethyst	Watson	6 white pills	6 white pills	–	120	0.54
Aviane	Teva	5 orange pills	5 orange pills	–	100	0.50
Camrese	Teva	4 light blue-green pills	4 light blue-green pills	–	120	0.60
CamreseLo	Teva	5 orange pills	5 orange pills	–	100	0.50
Cryselle	Teva	4 white pills	4 white pills	–	120	0.60

(continued)

Table 3-9. Oral Contraceptives That Can Be Used for Emergency Contraception in the United States* *(continued)*

Brand	Company	First Dose†	Second Dose† (12 hours later)	Ulipristal Acetate per Dose (mg)	Ethinyl Estradiol per Dose (microgram)	Levon-orgestrel per Dose (mg)‡
Combined progestin and estrogen pills						
Enpresse	Teva	4 orange pills	4 orange pills	–	120	0.50
Introvale	Sandoz	4 peach pills	4 peach pills	–	120	0.60
Jolessa	Teva	4 pink pills	4 pink pills	–	120	0.60
Lessina	Teva	5 pink pills	5 pink pills	–	100	0.50
Levora	Watson	4 white pills	4 white pills	–	120	0.60
Lo/Ovral	Akrimax	4 white pills	4 white pills	–	120	0.60
LoSeasonique	Teva	5 orange pills	5 orange pills	–	100	0.50
Low-Ogestrel	Watson	4 white pills	4 white pills	–	120	0.60
Lutera	Watson	5 white pills	5 white pills	–	100	0.50
Lybrel	Wyeth	6 yellow pills	6 yellow pills	–	120	0.54
Nordette	Teva	4 light-orange pills	4 light-orange pills	–	120	0.60
Ogestrel	Watson	2 white pills	2 white pills	–	100	0.50
Portia	Teva	4 pink pills	4 pink pills	–	120	0.60
Quasense	Watson	4 white pills	4 white pills	–	120	0.60
Seasonale	Teva	4 pink pills	4 pink pills	–	120	0.60

(continued)

Table 3-9. Oral Contraceptives That Can Be Used for Emergency Contraception in the United States* *(continued)*

Brand	Company	First Dose[†]	Second Dose[†] (12 hours later)	Ulipristal Acetate per Dose (mg)	Ethinyl Estradiol per Dose (microgram)	Levon-orgestrel per Dose (mg)[‡]
Combined progestin and estrogen pills						
Seasonique	Teva	4 light-blue-green pills	4 light-blue-green pills	–	120	0.60
Sronyx	Watson	5 white pills	5 white pills	–	100	0.50
Trivora	Watson	4 pink pills	4 pink pills	–	120	0.50

*ella, Plan B One-Step, Next Choice One Dose, My Way, and Levonorgestrel Tablets are the only dedicated products specifically marketed for emergency contraception. The regular oral contraceptives listed have been declared safe and effective for use as emergency contraceptive pills by the U.S. Food and Drug Administration. Outside the United States, approximately 100 emergency contraceptive products are specifically packaged, labeled, and marketed. Levonorgestrel-only emergency contraceptive pills are available either over-the-counter or from a pharmacist without having to see a clinician in 60 countries. In the United States, Plan B One-Step is available on the shelf with no restrictions. The one-pill generic products Next Choice One Dose and My Way will soon be available on the shelf, but will be available only to those aged 17 or older. The one-pill generic product Levonorgestrel Tablets is available at the pharmacy counter to women and men aged 17 and older, or by prescription to younger individuals. ella is available by prescription only.

†The label for Levonorgestrel Tablets says to take one pill within 72 hours after unprotected intercourse, and another pill 12 hours later. However, research has found that both pills can be taken at the same time. All of the brands listed here may be effective when used within 120 hours after unprotected sex, but should be taken as soon as possible.

‡The progestin in Cryselle, Lo/Ovral, Low-Ogestrel, and Ogestrel is norgestrel, which contains two isomers, only one of which (levonorgestrel) is bioactive; the amount of norgestrel in each tablet is twice the amount of levonorgestrel.

Reprinted with permission from Association of Reproductive Health Professionals, Office of Population Research at Princeton University. Emergency contraception website. Oral contraceptives that can be used for emergency contraception in the United States. Available at: http://ec.princeton.edu/questions/dose.html#dose. Retrieved July 29, 2013.

This information is updated on a regular basis. For the most up to date information, see The Emergency Contraception web site at http://ec.princeton.edu/questions/dose.html#dose.

benefits. These criteria note that women with previous ectopic pregnancy, cardiovascular disease, migraines, or liver disease and women who are breastfeeding may use emergency contraception. Therefore, emergency contraception may be made available to women with contraindications to the use of conventional oral contraceptive preparations.

Information regarding effective contraceptive methods should be made available either at the time that emergency contraception is prescribed or at some convenient time thereafter. Use of highly effective long-acting reversible methods should be strongly encouraged. Repetitive use of emergency contraception is not as effective as other contraceptive methods such as IUDs, implants, injections, oral contraceptives, contraceptive rings, and patches. Clinical evaluation is indicated for women who have used emergency contraception if menses are delayed by 1 week or more after the expected time or if abdominal pain or persistent irregular bleeding develops.

Postpartum Contraception

Ovulation returns quickly after delivery, with an average time to ovulation of 45 days, so contraception initiation must occur quickly in women who are not using the lactational amenorrhea method. Because approximately two thirds of couples are sexually active in the first postpartum month and more than three fourths in the second postpartum month, contraception planning during the antenatal period is ideal. If initiation of a prescription-only method is delayed, the use of condoms is an excellent option. Withdrawal also provides some protection if couples choose not to use condoms. Timing of postpartum visits may depend on and affect the method and timing of postpartum contraception.

BREASTFEEDING AND CHOICE OF CONTRACEPTIVE METHOD

Breastfeeding has multiple benefits to the mother and infant, including the potential benefit of contraception. The lactational amenorrhea method is an excellent method of contraception as long as three conditions are met: 1) menses have not returned, 2) the mother is fully or nearly fully breastfeeding (exclusively breastfeeding or the vast majority [85% or more] of feeds are breastfeeds), and 3) the infant is 6 months of age or younger.

It should especially be noted that pumping milk appears not to have the same antiovulatory effect as suckling from breastfeeding.

Traditionally, combined oral contraceptives have not been recommended as the first choice for breastfeeding women because of concerns that the estrogenic component of combined oral contraceptives can reduce the volume of milk production and the caloric and mineral content of breast milk. However, use of combined oral contraceptives by well-nourished breastfeeding women does not appear to result in infant development problems. A systematic review of randomized controlled trials concluded that existing data are of poor quality, report inconsistent findings, and are insufficient to establish an effect of hormonal contraception on lactation. Use of combined hormonal contraceptives can be considered once milk flow is well established. Overall, progestin-only methods (progestin-only pills, DMPA, levonorgestrel IUD, and etonogestrel single-rod contraceptive implant) appear to have little effect on either breastfeeding success or infant growth and health, and some obstetricians routinely initiate these methods in many women before hospital discharge, including those who choose to breastfeed.

Timing of Initiation

Postpartum women remain in a hypercoagulable state for weeks after childbirth, but ovulation can occur as early as 25 days postpartum in women who are not breastfeeding, making timely initiation of contraception important. Before initiation of contraception, the health care provider should confirm that the woman meets medical eligibility criteria for the chosen method (see U.S. MEC) and be reasonably certain that she is not pregnant (Box 3-16). Timing of initiation varies based on the contraceptive method and whether the mother is breastfeeding (Table 3-10).

Need for Back-up Contraception

A postpartum woman's need for back-up contraception depends on the method of primary contraception initiated, whether she is breastfeeding, and whether her menstrual cycle has resumed. Women who are using the copper IUD require no additional contraceptive protection, regardless of breast-feeding or menstruation status. For women who are less than 6 months postpartum, amenorrheic, and fully or nearly fully breastfeeding (exclusively breastfeeding or the vast majority [85% or more] of feeds are breastfeeds), no additional contraceptive protection is needed. Otherwise, a woman who is 21 days or more postpartum and has not experienced return of her menstrual cycle needs to abstain from sexual intercourse or use additional contraceptive protection for the next 7 days (for combined oral contraceptives users) or the next 2 days (for progestin-only pill users). If a woman's menstrual cycle has resumed and it has been more than 5 days since the start of menstrual bleeding (or more than 7 days in the case of levonorgestrel IUD or DMPA injection users), additional contraceptive protection is needed for the next 7 days (or the next 2 days for progestin-pill users).

Table 3-10. U.S. Medical Eligibility Criteria for Postpartum Initiation of Contraception*

| Contraceptive Type | Timing of Initiation (U.S. MEC Category Rating) | |
	Breastfeeding	Not Breastfeeding
Combined oral contraceptives	Less than 21 days postpartum (4)	Less than 21 days postpartum (4)
	21–29 days postpartum, regardless of venous thromboembolism risk (3)	21–42 days postpartum, with other risk factors for venous thromboembolism (3)
	30–42 days postpartum, with other risk factors for venous thromboembolism (3)	21–42 days postpartum, without other risk factors for venous thromboembolism (2)
	30–42 days postpartum, without other risk factors for venous thromboembolism (2)	
Progestin-only pills	Less than 1 month postpartum (2)[†]	Any time, including immediately postpartum (1)
	At least 1 month postpartum (1)[†]	
Injectable contraception	Any time, including immediately postpartum (1 or 2)[‡]	Any time, including immediately postpartum (1)

(continued)

Table 3-10. U.S. Medical Eligibility Criteria for Postpartum Initiation of Contraception* *(continued)*

Contraceptive Type	Timing of Initiation (U.S. MEC Category Rating)	
	Breastfeeding	Not Breastfeeding
Contraceptive implant	Less than 1 month postpartum (2)§	Any time, including immediately postpartum (1)
	More than 11 months postpartum (1)	
Intrauterine devices‖ (copper and 5-year levonorgestrel)	Any time, including immediately postpartum (after vaginal or cesarean delivery), unless contraindications exist¶ (1 or 2)	

Abbreviations: IUD, intrauterine device; U.S. MEC, U.S. Medical Eligibility Criteria for Contraceptive Use, 2010.

*Before initiation of contraception, the health care provider should confirm that the woman meets medical eligibility criteria for the chosen method (see U.S. Medical Eligibility Criteria for Contraceptive Use) and be reasonably certain that she is not pregnant.

†In nursing women who use progestin-only oral contraceptives, very small amounts of progestin are passed into the breast milk, and no adverse effects on infant growth have been observed.

‡When initiated immediately postpartum, use of depot medroxyprogesterone acetate does not adversely affect lactation or infant development.

§A category 2 rating is given because of theoretical concerns regarding milk production and infant growth and development.

‖This does not include the 3-year IUD. For information on prescribing, see Bayer HealthCare Pharmaceuticals Inc. Skyla (levonorgestrel-releasing intrauterine system): highlights of prescribing information. Wayne (NJ): Bayer; 2013. Available at: http://labeling.bayerhealthcare.com/html/products/pi/Skyla_PI.pdf. Retrieved July 26, 2013.

¶Immediate postpartum insertion of an IUD is contraindicated in cases of puerperal sepsis or septic abortion.

Data from U.S. Selected Practice Recommendations for Contraceptive Use, 2013: adapted from the World Health Organization selected practice recommendations for contraceptive use, 2nd edition. Division of Reproductive Health, National Center for Chronic Disease Prevention and Health Promotion, Centers for Disease Control and Prevention. MMWR Recomm Rep 2013;62:1–60.

Contraceptive Failure

If a pregnancy occurs while a hormonal method of contraception is being used, the method should be discontinued, although there is no substantive evidence that the use of any method of contraception during early pregnancy is associated with fetal anomalies. If a patient becomes pregnant while using an IUD, the U.S. SPR recommends an evaluation for ectopic pregnancy, counseling regarding the increased risk of spontaneous abortion (including septic abortion) and preterm delivery if the IUD is left in place, and removal of the IUD as soon as possible if the strings are visible or the device can be removed safely. If the IUD strings are not visible or the IUD cannot be removed safely, consider performing or referring for ultrasound examination to determine the location of the IUD. If ultrasonography is not available or fails to locate the device, advise the woman to seek care promptly if she has heavy bleeding, cramping, pain, abnormal vaginal discharge, or fever.

Bibliography

Access to emergency contraception. Committee Opinion No. 542. American College of Obstetricians and Gynecologists. Obstet Gynecol 2012;120:1250–3.

Access to postpartum sterilization. Committee Opinion No. 530. American College of Obstetricians and Gynecologists. Obstet Gynecol 2012;120:212–15.

Adolescents and long-acting reversible contraception: implants and intrauterine devices. Committee Opinion No. 539. American College of Obstetricians and Gynecologists. Obstet Gynecol 2012;120:983–8.

American College of Obstetricians and Gynecologists. Guidelines for adolescent health care [CD-ROM]. 2nd ed. ed. Washington, DC: American College of Obstetricians and Gynecologists; 2011.

American College of Obstetricians and Gynecologists. Reproductive health care for adolescents with disabilities: supplement to Guidelines for adolescent health care. 2nd ed. ed. Washington, DC: American College of Obstetricians and Gynecologists; 2012. Available at: http://www.acog.org/Resources_And_Publications/Guidelines_for_Adolescent_Health_Care/Reproductive_Health_Care_for_Adolescents_With_Disabilities. Retrieved July 23, 2013.

Bartz D, Greenberg JA. Sterilization in the United States. Rev Obstet Gynecol 2008; 1:23–32.

Bayer HealthCare Pharmaceuticals Inc. Mirena (levonorgestrel-releasing intrauterine system): highlights of prescribing information. Wayne (NJ): Bayer; 2013. Available at: http://labeling.bayerhealthcare.com/html/products/pi/Mirena_PI.pdf. Retrieved July 26, 2013.

Bayer HealthCare Pharmaceuticals Inc. Skyla (levonorgestrel-releasing intrauterine system): highlights of prescribing information. Wayne (NJ): Bayer; 2013. Available at: http://labeling.bayerhealthcare.com/html/products/pi/Skyla_PI.pdf. Retrieved July 26, 2013.

Benefits and risks of sterilization. Practice Bulletin No. 133. American College of Obstetricians and Gynecologists. Obstet Gynecol 2013;121:392–404.

Brand versus generic oral contraceptives. ACOG Committee Opinion No. 375. American College of Obstetricians and Gynecologists. Obstet Gynecol 2007;110: 447–8.

Depot medroxyprogesterone acetate and bone effects. Committee Opinion No. 602. American College of Obstetricians and Gynecologists. Obstet Gynecol 2014;123:1398–402.

Emergency contraception. Practice Bulletin No. 112. American College of Obstetricians and Gynecologists. Obstet Gynecol 2010;115:1100–9.

Hatcher RA, Trussell J, Nelson AL, Cates WJ, Kowal D, Policar MS, editors. Contraceptive technology. 20th revised ed. New York (NY): Ardent Media; 2011.

Increasing use of contraceptive implants and intrauterine devices to reduce unintended pregnancy. ACOG Committee Opinion No. 450. American College of Obstetricians and Gynecologists. Obstet Gynecol 2009;114:1434–8.

Institute for Reproductive Health. Fertility awareness. Available at: http://irh.org/focus-areas/fertility_awareness. Retrieved July 29, 2013.

Janssen Pharmaceuticals Inc. Ortho Evra (norelgestromin/ethinyl estradiol transdermal system): highlights of prescribing information. Titusville (NJ): Janssen; 2013. Available at: http://www.orthoevra.com/sites/default/files/assets/OrthoEvraPI.pdf. Retrieved July 29, 2013.

Jones J, Mosher W, Daniels K. Current contraceptive use in the United States, 2006–2010, and changes in patterns of use since 1995. Natl Health Stat Report 2012;(60):1–25.

Labbok MH, Perez A, Valdes V, Sevilla F, Wade K, Laukaran VH, et al. The lactational amenorrhea method (LAM): a postpartum introductory family planning method with policy and program implications. Adv Contracept 1994;10:93-109.

Long-acting reversible contraception: implants and intrauterine devices. Practice bulletin No. 121. American College of Obstetricians and Gynecologists. Obstet Gynecol 2011;118:184–96.

Lyus R, Lohr P, Prager S, Board of the Society of Family Planning. Use of the Mirena LNG-IUS and Paragard CuT380A intrauterine devices in nulliparous women. Contraception 2010;81:367–71.

Merck & Company Inc. NuvaRing® (etonogestrel/ethinyl estradiol vaginal ring). Whitehouse Station (NJ): Merck; 2012. Available at: http://www.merck.com/product/usa/pi_circulars/n/nuvaring/nuvaring_pi.pdf. Retrieved July 29, 2013.

Multifetal pregnancy reduction. Committee Opinion No. 553. American College of Obstetricians and Gynecologists. Obstet Gynecol 2013;121:405–10.

Over-the-counter access to oral contraceptives. Committee Opinion No 544. American College of Obstetricians and Gynecologists. Obstet Gynecol 2012;120: 1527–31.

Reproductive and sexual coercion. Committee Opinion No. 554. American College of Obstetricians and Gynecologists. Obstet Gynecol 2013;121:411–5.

Risk of venous thromboembolism among users of drospirenone-containing oral contraceptive pills. Committee Opinion No. 540. American College of Obstetricians and Gynecologists; Obstet Gynecol 2012;120:1239–42.

Steenland MW, Zapata LB, Brahmi D, Marchbanks PA, Curtis KM. Appropriate follow up to detect potential adverse events after initiation of select contraceptive methods: a systematic review. Contraception 2013;87:611–24.

Trussell J. Contraceptive efficacy. In: Hatcher RA, Trussell J, Nelson AL, Cates WJ, Kowal D,Policar MS, editors. Contraceptive technology. 20th revised ed. New York (NY): Ardent Media; 2011. p. 779–863.

U.S. Medical Eligibility Criteria for Contraceptive Use, 2010. Centers for Disease Control and Prevention. MMWR Recomm Rep 2010;59(RR-4):1–86. Available at: http://www.cdc.gov/mmwr/pdf/rr/rr5904.pdf. Retrieved September 11, 2013.

U.S. Selected Practice Recommendations for Contraceptive Use, 2013: adapted from the World Health Organization selected practice recommendations for contraceptive use, 2nd edition. Division of Reproductive Health, National Center for Chronic Disease Prevention and Health Promotion, Centers for Disease Control and Prevention. MMWR Recomm Rep 2013;62:1–60.

Understanding and using the U.S. Medical Eligibility Criteria For Contraceptive Use, 2010. Committee Opinion No. 505. American College of Obstetricians and Gynecologists. Obstet Gynecol 2011;118:754–60.

Understanding and using the U.S. Selected Practice Recommendations for Contraceptive Use, 2013. Committee Opinion No. 577. American College of Obstetricians and Gynecologists. Obstet Gynecol 2013;122:1132–3.

Update to CDC's U.S. Medical Eligibility Criteria for Contraceptive Use, 2010: revised recommendations for the use of contraceptive methods during the postpartum period. Centers for Disease Control and Prevention. MMWR Morb Mortal Wkly Rep 2011;60:878–83.

Watson Pharma Inc. ELLA-ulipristal acetate tablet. Parsippany (NJ): Watson; 2012. Available at: http://pi.actavis.com/data_stream.asp?product_group=1699&p =pi&language=E. Retrieved July 29, 2013.

Resources

American College of Obstetricians and Gynecologists. Barrier methods of contraception. Patient Education Pamphlet AP022. Washington, DC: American College of Obstetricians and Gynecologists; 2011.

American College of Obstetricians and Gynecologists. Birth control. Patient Education Booklet AB020. Washington, DC: American College of Obstetricians and Gynecologists; 2011.

American College of Obstetricians and Gynecologists. Combined hormonal birth control methods: pills, patches, and rings. Patient Education Pamphlet AP185. Washington, DC: American College of Obstetricians and Gynecologists; 2014.

American College of Obstetricians and Gynecologists. Emergency contraception. Patient Education Pamphlet AP114. Washington, DC: American College of Obstetricians and Gynecologists; 2013.

American College of Obstetricians and Gynecologists. Long-acting reversible contraception Patient Education Pamphlet AP184. Washington, DC: American College of Obstetricians and Gynecologists; 2014.

American College of Obstetricians and Gynecologists. Natural family planning. Patient Education Pamphlet AP024. Washington, DC: American College of Obstetricians and Gynecologists; 2012.

American College of Obstetricians and Gynecologists. Postpartum sterilization. Patient Education Pamphlet AP052. Washington DC: American College of Obstetricians and Gynecologists; 2013.

American College of Obstetricians and Gynecologists. Progestin-only hormonal birth control methods: pills and injections. Patient Education Pamphlet AP186. Washington, DC: American College of Obstetricians and Gynecologists; 2014.

American College of Obstetricians and Gynecologists. Sterilization by laparoscopy. Patient Education Pamphlet AP035. Washington, DC: American College of Obstetricians and Gynecologists; 2013.

American College of Obstetricians and Gynecologists. Sterilization for women and men. Patient Education Pamphlet AP011. Washington, DC: American College of Obstetricians and Gynecologists; 2014.

American College of Obstetricians and Gynecologists. Long-Acting Reversible Contraception. Available at http://www.acog.org/About_ACOG/ACOG_Depart ments/Long_Acting_Reversible_Contraception. Retrieved July 29, 2013.

Association of Reproductive Health Professionals, Office of Population Research at Princeton University. Emergency contraception hotline. 1-888-NOT-2-LATE.

Association of Reproductive Health Professionals, Office of Population Research at Princeton University. Emergency contraception website. Oral contraceptives that can be used for emergency contraception in the United States. Available at: http://ec.princeton.edu/questions/dose.html#dose. Retrieved July 29, 2013.

Association of Reproductive Health Professionals. A quick reference guide for clinicians: choosing a birth control method. Washington, DC: ARHP; 2011. Available at: http://wwww.arhp.org/uploadDocs/choosingqrg.pdf. Retrieved July 29, 2013.

Association of Reproductive Health Professionals. Health matters: facts about emergency contraception pills. Washington, DC: ARHP; 2012. Available at: http://wwww.arhp.org/uploadDocs/EC_healthmatters.pdf. Retrieved July 29, 2013.

Association of Reproductive Health Professionals. Method match. Available at: http://wwww.arhp.org/MethodMatch. Retrieved July 29, 2013.

Bedsider. The National Campaign to Prevent Teen and Unplanned Pregnancy. Available at: http://bedsider.org. Retrieved July 29, 2013.

Cromer BA, Scholes D, Berenson A, Cundy T, Clark MK, Kaunitz AM. Depot medroxyprogesterone acetate and bone mineral density in adolescents—the Black Box Warning: a Position Paper of the Society for Adolescent Medicine. Society for Adolescent Medicine. J Adolesc Health 2006;39:296–301.

Jaccard J. Careful, current, and consistent: tips to improve contraceptive use. Washington, DC: National Campaign to Prevent Teen and Unplanned Pregnancy; 2010. Available at: https://thenationalcampaign.org/sites/default/files/resource-primary-download/carefulcurrentconsistent.pdf. Retrieved March 28, 2014.

Jaccard J. Unlocking the contraception conundrum: reducing unplanned pregnancies in emerging adulthood. Washington, DC: National Campaign to Prevent Teen and Unplanned Pregnancy; 2009. Available at: http://thenationalcampaign.org/sites/default/files/resource-primary-download/unlocking_contraceptive.pdf. Retrieved March 28, 2014.

Johns Hopkins Bloomberg School of Public Health, Center for Communication Programs, Information and Knowledge for Optimal Health (INFO), World Health Organization. Decision-making tool for family planning clients and providers. Baltimore (MD); INFO; Geneva: WHO; 2005. Available at: http://whqlibdoc.who.int/publications/2005/9241593229_eng.pdf. Retrieved July 29, 2013.

Johns Hopkins Bloomberg School of Public Health, United States Agency for International Development, World Health Organization. Family planning: a global handbook for providers. Baltimore (MD): JHBSPH; Washington, DC: USAID; Geneva: WHO; 2011. Available at: http://whqlibdoc.who.int/publications/2011/9780978856373_eng.pdf. Retrieved July 29, 2013.

Kapp N, Curtis KM. Combined oral contraceptive use among breastfeeding women: a systematic review. Contraception 2010;82:10–6.

Planned Parenthood Federation of America. Birth control. Available at: http://www.plannedparenthood.org/health-topics/birth-control-4211.htm. Retrieved July 29, 2013.

Planned Parenthood Federation of America. My method. Available at: http://www. plannedparenthood.org/all-access/my-method-26542.htm. Retrieved July 29, 2013.

Society of Family Planning, Clinical guidelines. Available at: http://societyfp.org/ resources/guidelines.asp. Retrieved September 27, 2013.

Sterilization of women, including those with mental disabilities. ACOG Committee Opinion No. 371. American College of Obstetricians and Gynecologists. Obstet Gynecol 2007;110:217–20.

Vasquez P, Schreiber CA. The missing IUD. Contraception 2010;82:126–8.

World Health Organization. Medical eligibility criteria for contraceptive use. 4th ed. Geneva: WHO; 2009. Available at: http://whqlibdoc.who.int/publications/2010/ 9789241563888_eng.pdf. Retrieved June 7, 2013.

PRECONCEPTION AND INTERCONCEPTION CARE

Every encounter with the health care system should be viewed as an opportunity to improve reproductive health in women capable of becoming pregnant. A woman's awareness of reproductive risks, health-enhancing behaviors, and family planning options is essential to improving her own health and the outcomes of pregnancy. Nearly one half of all pregnancies in the United States are unplanned. Because women do not always seek medical care and consultation in anticipation of a planned pregnancy, it is imperative that clinicians provide ongoing education and screening to all women capable of becoming pregnant to optimize their health and identify potential maternal and fetal risks and hazards before and between pregnancies. Addressing these issues may produce benefits to the woman's health that extend beyond reproductive concerns.

Reproductive health hazards—including the use of alcohol, tobacco, and other drugs—exist across all socioeconomic and age groups; therefore, all women capable of becoming pregnant should develop a reproductive health plan and should discuss it in a nondirective way at each subsequent visit. The discussion should include assessment of the desirability of a future pregnancy; determination of steps that need to be taken either to prevent, or to plan for and optimize, a pregnancy; and evaluation of current health status (see also the "Family Planning" section earlier in Part 3). Adolescents and women in their 40s require a special approach and focus because reproductive health risks and the rates of unintended pregnancy are highest in these groups. Reproductive messages and strategies to deliver them should be developed for men as well.

Women of advanced reproductive age are more likely to have infertility issues caused by oocyte abnormalities and decreased ovarian reserve as well as an increased risk of pregnancy loss. Fecundity rates begin to decrease gradually around age 32 years and then decrease more rapidly after age

37 years. The risk of spontaneous abortion and pregnancy complications also increase with age. Women should be educated about this issue so that they can formulate a reproductive health plan that is most appropriate for them.

Reproductive health screening, contraceptive counseling, and preconception considerations should not be limited to obstetrician–gynecologists and other providers of women's health care. Because reproductive health can significantly affect the development of chronic health conditions and the management of those conditions can affect pregnancy outcomes, it is crucial that reproductive health be considered by all health care providers serving women in their reproductive years.

Preconception Care

As it is with well-woman care, contraceptive planning is a key part of preconception care. Women who do not wish to become pregnant should be encouraged to use effective methods of contraception (see also the "Family Planning" section earlier in Part 3). Women who are contemplating pregnancy should be encouraged to undergo a comprehensive preconception evaluation and counseling and to formulate a reproductive health plan that addresses the optimal number, spacing, and timing of children in the family; real and perceived barriers to achieving these goals; and age-related changes in fertility. Because unintended pregnancy is so common, elements of this visit also should be incorporated into the well-woman visit for women capable of becoming pregnant (see also the "Family Planning" section earlier in Part 3).

Although most pregnancies result in good maternal and fetal outcomes, some pregnancies result in adverse health effects for the woman, fetus, or newborn. Even though some adverse outcomes cannot be prevented, optimizing a woman's health and knowledge before she plans and conceives a pregnancy may eliminate or reduce the risk. For example, initiation of folic acid supplementation at least 1 month before pregnancy reduces the incidence of neural tube defects. Similarly, adequate blood glucose control in a woman with diabetes mellitus before and throughout pregnancy can decrease maternal morbidity, spontaneous abortion, fetal malformation, fetal macrosomia, intrauterine fetal death, and neonatal morbidity. It is important for women to be aware that the measures they take to optimize their preconceptional health in the months preceding a planned pregnancy will result in maternal and fetal benefits.

At the preconception visit, information that may have a bearing on a future pregnancy should be obtained through patient history, physical assessment, and screening and testing, as appropriate. After this information has been obtained, the clinician may provide patient counseling and make recommendations for interventions to help the patient achieve optimal physical and psychologic health before pregnancy, as well as provide information about what to expect during pregnancy. This visit also is an opportunity to identify fertility issues, with referral to a fertility specialist as appropriate.

HISTORY

A comprehensive history should be taken. Attention should be focused on how a future pregnancy might affect the woman's own health and be affected by her medical, reproductive, immunization, and family histories; use of medications or substances; nutritional status; and environmental exposures.

Medical History

Conditions that may have an effect on pregnancy should be covered in the medical history. Information should be obtained about chronic conditions, such as diabetes mellitus; phenylketonuria; thyroid disease; hypertension; epilepsy; anemia and disorders of coagulation; autoimmune disorders; herpes and other sexually transmitted infections, including human immunodeficiency virus (HIV); heart disease; kidney disease; endocrine disease; and reactive airway disease. Because some women are not aware they were ever diagnosed with phenylketonuria, they should be asked whether they were placed on a special diet during childhood. Examples of conditions that are associated with an increased risk of adverse health events as a result of unintended pregnancy are shown in Box 3-19. The history also should include menstrual history, surgical history, contraceptive methods previously used and any complications, past accidents, allergies, and childhood

Box 3-19. Conditions Associated With Increased Risk of Adverse Health Events as a Result of Unintended Pregnancy

- Breast cancer
- Complicated valvular heart disease
- Diabetes: type 1 diabetes mellitus; with nephropathy, retinopathy, neuropathy, or other vascular disease; or of more than 20 years' duration
- Endometrial or ovarian cancer
- Epilepsy
- Hypertension (systolic greater than 160 mm Hg or diastolic greater than 100 mm Hg)
- History of bariatric surgery within the past 2 years
- Human immunodeficiency virus or acquired immune deficiency syndrome
- Ischemic heart disease
- Malignant gestational trophoblastic disease
- Malignant liver tumors (hepatoma) and hepatocellular carcinoma of the liver
- Peripartum cardiomyopathy
- Schistosomiasis with fibrosis of the liver
- Severe (decompensated) cirrhosis
- Sickle cell disease
- Solid organ transplantation within the past 2 years
- Stroke
- Systemic lupus erythematosus
- Thrombogenic mutations
- Tuberculosis

Reprinted from U.S. Medical Eligibility Criteria for Contraceptive Use, 2010. Centers for Disease Control and Prevention. MMWR Recomm Rep 2010;59 (RR-4):1–86.

disease history. A psychiatric history also should be obtained to identify women who have a history of, or are currently being treated for, depression or other psychiatric disorders.

Reproductive History

Patients should be asked about conditions that may affect future pregnancy. These conditions include a history of therapy or surgery on the cervix, ovaries, uterus, or fallopian tubes; in utero exposure to diethylstilbestrol; and prior adverse pregnancy outcomes.

Immunization History

An immunization history should be obtained, and vaccination(s) should be offered to women found to be at risk (see also "Counseling" later in this section).

Family History

The patient should be questioned about specific conditions related to ethnic background and family history suggestive of genetic disorders, such as muscular dystrophy, hemophilia, Tay–Sachs disease, sickle cell disease, cystic fibrosis, thalassemia, consanguinity, mental retardation, anatomic birth defects, Down syndrome, and other chromosomal abnormalities. It is reasonable to offer cystic fibrosis carrier screening to all patients. Further genetic screening and testing may be recommended based on family history or ethnic background (see also "Counseling" later in this section).

Medication and Substance Use and Abuse

Prescription medication used to treat various medical conditions may pose an increased risk for the fetus. Patients should be asked about prescription and over-the-counter medications that they take regularly or as needed. They should be asked specifically about medications that they may be reluctant to mention (or may not consider to be medications), such as sedatives or tranquilizers, herbal supplements, or appetite suppressants. Use of tobacco, alcohol, and illegal drugs should be determined. Patients should be reassured of the confidentiality of this information in an attempt to ensure a candid response (see also "Counseling" later in this section and the "Substance Use and Abuse" section earlier in Part 3).

Nutritional Status

The patient's height and weight and a general assessment of her dietary habits should be recorded. Information about her use of dietary supplements (including folic acid and other vitamins), efforts to control weight, any history of eating disorders, such as bulimia or anorexia, and prior obesity should be obtained in the inquiry.

Environmental Factors

Patient exposure to toxic environmental chemicals and other stressors is ubiquitous, and preconception exposure to toxic environmental agents can have a profound and lasting effect on reproductive health across the life course. Obtaining a patient history during a preconception visit to identify specific types of exposure that may be harmful to a developing fetus is a key step and also should include queries of the maternal and paternal workplaces, the patient's home environment, exercise habits, and hobbies. Examples of an exposure history are available from the University of California, San Francisco, Program on Reproductive Health and the Environment (www.prhe.ucsf.edu/prhe/clinical_resources.html). A list of key chemical categories, sources of exposure, and clinical implications are provided online at www.acog.org/About_ACOG/ACOG_Departments/Health_Care_for_Underserved_Women. Additional information regarding potential teratogens may be obtained from toxicology web sites or hotlines if toxic hazards may be an issue (see Box 3-20).

PHYSICAL ASSESSMENT

After a history is obtained, a complete physical assessment of the patient should be performed, with emphasis on conditions that might affect pregnancy adversely (see Box 3-19). Body mass index (BMI) should be calculated. A pelvic examination should be conducted to detect possible reproductive anomalies that may influence conception and pregnancy.

SCREENING AND TESTING

Cervical cytologic testing and screening for sexually transmitted infections should be performed when appropriate (see also the "Cancer Screening and Prevention" section and the "Sexually Transmitted Infections" section in Part 3). Testing for HIV is recommended for women seeking preconception care. Where legal, opt-out HIV screening should be performed, in which the patient is notified that HIV testing will be performed as a routine part of gynecologic and obstetric care, unless the patient declines testing. Physicians should be aware of state laws related to HIV testing. If a patient declines HIV testing, this should be noted in the medical record.

Box 3-20. Sources of Current Teratogen Information

Several sources of useful current information regarding potential teratogens are available, including numerous teratogen information services available throughout the United States that serve specific geographic areas. For information on the teratogen service in a particular area, contact the following:
Organization of Teratology Information Specialists
5034A Thoroughbred Lane
Brentwood, TN 37027
(615) 649-3082
www.mothertobaby.org

The following web site provides a variety of resources and links:
Teratology Society
1821 Michael Faraday Drive, Suite 300
Reston, VA 20190
(703) 438-3104
www.teratology.org

The following computerized teratology and reproductive risk database offers up-to-date summaries of electronic resources that provide teratology information at no cost:
TOXNET – Toxicology Data Network
National Library of Medicine
Two Democracy Plaza, Suite 440 and Suite 510
6707 Democracy Blvd., MSC 5467
Bethesda, MD 20892
(301) 496-1131
1-888-FINDNLM
www.toxnet.nlm.nih.gov

COUNSELING

After the history and physical assessment are completed, the patient should be counseled regarding risk factors and lifestyle changes that may increase her chance of having a successful pregnancy and a healthy infant. Measures should be taken to modify behavior that may be detrimental, such as smoking, alcohol consumption, or poor nutrition. It should be stressed to the patient that a healthy lifestyle not only will improve her chances of having a healthy pregnancy but also will have long-term benefits for herself and her family; however, patients should be informed that ideal physical health before pregnancy does not prevent all complications of pregnancy. Pregnancy complications or discomforts may necessitate changes in lifestyle, such as interruption of work, that are not predictable before pregnancy or even in early pregnancy.

Immunizations

Vaccination(s) should be offered to women found to be at risk of, or susceptible to the following: measles, mumps, rubella, varicella, hepatitis A, hepatitis B, meningococcus, and pneumococcus. The Advisory Committee on Immunization Practices of the Centers for Disease Control and Prevention recommends vaccination with the inactivated influenza vaccine for all women who will be pregnant through the influenza season (October through May in the United States). In addition, women who have not been immunized with the tetanus toxoid, reduced diphtheria toxoid, and acellular pertussis (Tdap) vaccine or women whose vaccine status is unknown should be offered immunization with the Tdap vaccine. The human papillomavirus (HPV) vaccination can be offered to appropriate nonpregnant women. However, because the vaccine is not recommended during pregnancy, completion of the vaccine series may need to be delayed until the postpartum period.

Nutrition and Weight

Patients should be counseled on appropriate weight for height, recommendation for folic acid supplementation, and avoidance of excessive vitamin supplementation or food fads, with referral for in-depth counseling, if appropriate. Counseling should include the provision of specific information concerning the maternal and fetal risks of obesity in pregnancy and encouragement to undertake a weight-reduction program, if appropriate (see also the "Fitness" section earlier in Part 3).

Women should be advised to achieve a near-normal BMI before attempting conception because infertility as well as maternal and fetal complications are associated with abnormal BMI. All women should be encouraged to exercise at least 30 minutes on most days of the week (see also the "Fitness" section earlier in Part 3). Obese women should be advised regarding their increased risk of adverse perinatal outcomes, including difficulty becoming pregnant, conception of a fetus with a variety of birth defects, preterm delivery, diabetes, cesarean delivery, and hypertensive disease (see also the "Fitness" section earlier in Part 3).

The preconception ingestion of folic acid has been shown to reduce the risk of neural tube defects. The U.S. Public Health Service has advocated that all women who are capable of becoming pregnant take 0.4 mg of folic acid daily to prevent neural tube defects. For this reason, the recommended dietary allowance for folic acid has been increased to 0.4 mg as well. Although many grains now are fortified with folic acid, it is unlikely that a daily intake of 0.4 mg can be achieved through diet alone. Therefore, daily supplementation with a multivitamin is recommended for all women who are capable of becoming pregnant. Patients at high risk of neural tube defects (eg, those who have a history of neural tube defects, have had an affected infant, or are taking anticonvulsant medication) should begin ingesting 4 mg of folic acid daily at least 1 month before the time they plan to become pregnant and continue through the first 3 months of pregnancy. This higher dosage of folic acid should be prescribed by a health care provider. Although folic acid is relatively nontoxic, increasing the doses of multivitamin preparations to reach the higher level is not advised because of the potential for ingesting excessive amounts of other vitamins that may be harmful.

Chronic Medical Conditions

Patients should be counseled about the possible effects of pregnancy on existing medical conditions for the woman and the possible effects of the woman's existing medical conditions on the fetus, and interventions should be introduced. Women with metabolic diseases, such as phenylketonuria and diabetes mellitus, should be counseled regarding the importance of appropriate diet and metabolic control before, during, and after pregnancy. Dietary restrictions that result in lower maternal phenylalanine levels appear to reduce the risk of fetal abnormalities. Good glycemic control reduces the risk of miscarriage, fetal anomalies, and other adverse pregnancy outcomes in women with diabetes mellitus. To be most effective, appropriate dietary modifications should begin before pregnancy.

Medication Use

In general, using the lowest effective dose of only necessary medications is recommended. The use of known or potential teratogenic medications should be addressed. Some common teratogenic medications include the oral anticoagulant warfarin, the antiseizure drugs valproic acid and carbamazepine, isotretinoin, and angiotensin-converting enzyme inhibitors (see also "Depression and Psychiatric Illness" later in this section).

Environmental Factors

Once an environmental toxin exposure inventory has been completed, information should be given regarding the avoidance of exposure to toxic agents at home, in the community, and at work with possible referrals to occupational medicine programs or United States Pediatric Environmental Health Specialty Units if a serious exposure is found. Intervention as early as possible during the preconception period is advised to alert patients regarding avoidance of toxic exposure and to ensure beneficial environmental exposure, eg, fresh fruit and vegetables, unprocessed food, outdoor activities, and a safe and nurturing physical and social environment. Also, women in the preconception period should be advised to avoid eating some large fish, such as shark, swordfish, king mackerel, and tilefish, which are known to contain high levels of methylmercury, a known teratogen.

Physicians in the United States are required to report illnesses or injuries that may be work related, and reporting requirements vary by state. Illnesses include acute and chronic conditions, such as a skin disease (eg, contact dermatitis), respiratory disorder (eg, occupational asthma), or poisoning (eg, lead poisoning or pesticide intoxication). Resources for information about how to report occupational and environmental illnesses include local and state health agencies and the Association of Occupational and Environmental Clinics (www.aoec.org/about.htm).

Maternal Age

Women should be educated regarding pregnancy risks with advancing maternal age. Complications of pregnancy that are more common in pregnant women older than 35 years include gestational diabetes, hypertensive disorders, cesarean delivery, maternal mortality, and possibly perinatal mortality and neural tube defects. Although any woman may give birth to a child with Down syndrome or other trisomy, the risk of autosomal trisomy increases with advancing maternal age.

Genetic Counseling

Couples with identifiable risks of having a child with heritable abnormalities and couples with genetic concerns should be counseled appropriately or referred to genetic counseling services. Genetic counseling includes in-depth assessment of risks and discussion of availability and limitations of prenatal diagnosis and options. Recognizing positive carrier status before pregnancy allows couples to understand the risks outside the emotional context of pregnancy; allows time for thorough family evaluation, when indicated; and prepares the couple for prenatal diagnostic testing during pregnancy, if desired (see also the "Genetic Risk Assessment" section earlier in Part 3).

Substance Use and Abuse

The preconception interview allows for timely education about medication and substance use and abuse in pregnancy, informed decision making about the risks to the fetus, and the introduction of interventions for patients who abuse substances. Behavioral counseling for substance use and abuse issues can be particularly effective during the preconception period. Women who smoke cigarettes or use any other form of tobacco product should be encouraged and supported in an effort to quit. This is a good opportunity to offer referral to smoking cessation programs. Other important behavioral issues to address include alcohol use and misuse and the abuse of prescription and nonprescription recreational drugs. Women who are trying to become pregnant should be counseled to completely refrain from all alcohol use and from misuse and abuse of prescription and nonprescription recreational drugs. Referral relationships with appropriate resources should be established and used as needed to assist women with these issues. Women who are counseled about substance use and abuse should be monitored to assess adherence to recommendations. (For information on interventions, see also the "Substance Use and Abuse" section earlier in Part 3.)

Depression and Psychiatric Illness

Patients should be counseled regarding the possibility of postpartum depression. This condition is more common in women with a history of depression before pregnancy, previous postpartum depression, or other psychiatric disorders. Women who have been receiving treatment for depression should receive counseling concerning the management options during pregnancy. Consultation with the prescribing psychiatrist is recommended regarding antidepressant medication dosing and safety (see also the "Depression" section later in Part 3).

Intimate Partner and Domestic Violence

Aspects of an individual's home environment may be of concern. Fear and abuse are problems for many women. It is important to determine if the woman feels safe and what options she may have if she does not feel safe. In reproductive coercion, a woman's partner interferes with her reproductive choices, such as whether to become pregnant or continue a pregnancy (see also the "Abuse" section later in Part 3).

Interconception Care

Interconception care refers to care that is delivered between a woman's pregnancies. Because certain adverse outcomes in pregnancy have implications for well-woman care and the health of future pregnancies, interconception care offers a valuable opportunity to improve a woman's health and the health of any children she may have in the future. Women with preeclampsia are almost four times more likely to develop diabetes and almost 12 times more likely to develop hypertension that requires drug treatment. Up to 70% of women with gestational diabetes mellitus develop type 2 diabetes mellitus within 5 years of the pregnancy. Excessive pregnancy weight gain and failure to lose weight after delivery can adversely affect a woman's immediate and future health.

The key element in interconception care is the postpartum visit. This is a critical opportunity to gather information related to the pregnancy; perform a physical evaluation and any needed screening and testing; counsel the patient on recommended lifestyle changes and health care interventions; and transition the patient back to well-woman care for surveillance and management of any identified medical conditions.

History

At the postpartum visit, an interval history should be obtained to supplement the obstetric history. Obstetric complications should be noted, especially hypertensive disorders (such as pregnancy-induced hypertension, preeclampsia, and eclampsia), gestational diabetes, and preterm delivery. Specific inquiries should be made regarding breastfeeding and contraceptive use.

Physical Assessment

The examination should include an evaluation of weight, blood pressure, breasts, and abdomen as well as a pelvic examination. Although many contraceptive methods can be initiated immediately after delivery (see also the "Family Planning" section earlier in part 3), the postpartum visit is also an opportunity to insert long-acting reversible contraceptive methods if this was not done after delivery.

Screening and Testing

All women with gestational diabetes mellitus should be screened at 6–12 weeks postpartum. Either a fasting plasma glucose test or the 75-g, 2-hour oral glucose tolerance test is appropriate for diagnosing diabetes. According to the American Diabetes Association, the hemoglobin A_{1c} test is also appropriate for diabetes screening and diagnosis in adults. Although the fasting plasma glucose test is easier to perform, it lacks sensitivity for detecting other forms of abnormal glucose metabolism; results of the oral glucose tolerance test can confirm an impaired fasting glucose level and impaired glucose tolerance. If the results of the postpartum screen are normal, the American Diabetes Association recommends repeat testing at least every 3 years. Women should be encouraged to discuss their gestational diabetes mellitus history and need for screening with all of their health care providers (see also the "Diabetes Mellitus" section earlier in Part 3).

The postpartum visit is an opportune time to review adult immunizations, such as rubella and varicella vaccination for women who are susceptible and did not receive the vaccine immediately postpartum. Women who did not receive the Tdap vaccine during the current pregnancy or immediately after delivery should receive a dose to ensure pertussis immunity and reduce the risk of transmission to the newborn. Other testing and laboratory data should be obtained as indicated.

Depression is very common during the postpartum period, but at this time there is insufficient evidence to support a firm recommendation for postpartum screening. There are also insufficient data to recommend how often screening should be done. However, screening for depression has the potential to benefit a woman and her family and should be strongly considered. Women with a positive assessment require follow-up evaluation and treatment if indicated (see also the "Depression" section later in Part 3).

COUNSELING

The postpartum visit is an excellent time to begin preconception counseling for the woman who may wish to have children in the future (see also "Preconception Care" earlier in this section). This counseling includes review of the patient's reproductive health plan for the planning, spacing, and timing of the next pregnancy; discussion of health-promotion measures; and timely intervention to reduce medical and psychosocial risks. A woman who plans to have another child can be counseled that in its *Healthy People 2020* initiative, the U.S. Department of Health and Human Services recommends that women avoid conceiving within 18 months of a previous birth to help optimize maternal and fetal outcomes. Discussion about health promotion may include counseling regarding hazardous behaviors, such as those related to sexually transmitted infections, tobacco, alcohol, and other substance use, as well as positive recommendations regarding folic acid use, breastfeeding, and contraceptive use. Other interventions may include treatment of infections; nutrition counseling, supplementation, and guidance on postpartum weight loss; and appropriate referrals for follow-up care. Depending on the outcome of the patient's pregnancy, it may be advantageous to discuss the implications of diabetes mellitus, fetal growth restriction, preterm birth, hypertension, fetal anomalies, and other conditions that may recur in a future pregnancy.

Women with a history of substance abuse should receive supportive guidance during the postpartum visit to prevent relapse to prepregnancy behaviors. If the mother used opioid drugs before or during pregnancy, she is at high risk of an overdose during the postpartum period and should be immediately referred to an addiction medicine specialist.

Many women experience some degree of emotional lability in the post-partum period. If this persists or develops into clinically significant depression, intervention may be necessary. The emotional status of a woman whose pregnancy had an abnormal outcome also should be assessed, with referrals for counseling and treatment as appropriate.

TRANSITION TO WELL-WOMAN CARE

At the postpartum visit, the obstetrician or other obstetric care provider should identify interval care recommendations for general health promotion and for reproductive health promotion. Regardless of whether the woman's subsequent well-woman care will be provided by the obstetric care provider who attended the delivery, an internist, a family physician, or another health care provider, it is important to clearly identify needed follow-up care, such as repeat glucose screening. Patient handoffs are a necessary component of current medical care. Accurate communication of information about a patient from one member of the health care team to another is a critical element of patient care and safety. In order to be effective, communication should be complete, clear, concise, and timely.

Bibliography

American Academy of Pediatrics, American College of Obstetricians and Gynecologists. Guidelines for perinatal care. 7th ed. Elk Grove Village (IL): AAP; Washington, DC: American College of Obstetricians and Gynecologists; 2012.

American Heart Association. 2011 AHA guidelines for cardiovascular disease prevention in women: for obstetrician-gynecologists and other reproductive health professionals. Dallas (TX): AHA; 2011. Available at: http://www.womens health.gov/heart-truth/heart-truth-docs/OBGYN/508%20OBGYN%20100311.pdf. Retrieved July 29, 2013.

Carrier screening for fragile X syndrome. Committee Opinion No. 469. American College of Obstetricians and Gynecologists. Obstet Gynecol 2010;116:1008-10.

Communication strategies for patient handoffs. Committee Opinion No. 517. American College of Obstetricians and Gynecologists. Obstet Gynecol 2012;119: 408-11.

Department of Health and Human Services. Healthy People 2020 topics and objectives: family planning. Available at: http://www.healthypeople.gov/2020/topics objectives2020/overview.aspx?topicId=13. Retrieved September 27, 2013.

Exposure to toxic environmental agents. Committee Opinion No. 575. American College of Obstetricians and Gynecologists. Obstet Gynecol 2013;122:931–5.

Female age-related fertility decline. Committee Opinion No. 589. American College of Obstetricians and Gynecologists. Obstet Gynecol 2014;123:719–21.

Gestational Diabetes Mellitus. Practice Bulletin No. 137. American College of Obstetricians and Gynecologists. Obstet Gynecol 2013;122:406–16.

Maternal decision making, ethics, and the law. ACOG Committee Opinion No. 321. American College of Obstetricians and Gynecologists. Obstet Gynecol 2005;106: 1127–37.

Maternal phenylketonuria. ACOG Committee Opinion No. 449. American College of Obstetricians and Gynecologists. Obstet Gynecol 2009;114:1432–3.

Neural tube defects. ACOG Practice Bulletin No. 44. American College of Obstetricians and Gynecologists. Obstet Gynecol 2003;102:203–13.

Nonmedical use of prescription drugs. Committee Opinion No. 538. American College of Obstetricians and Gynecologists. Obstet Gynecol 2012;120:977–82.

Preconception and prenatal carrier screening for genetic diseases in individuals of Eastern European Jewish descent. ACOG Committee Opinion No. 442. American College of Obstetricians and Gynecologists. Obstet Gynecol 2009;114:950–3.

Pregestational diabetes mellitus. ACOG Practice Bulletin No. 60. American College of Obstetricians and Gynecologists. Obstet Gynecol 2005;105:675–85.

Screening for fetal chromosomal abnormalities. ACOG Practice Bulletin No. 77. American College of Obstetricians and Gynecologists. Obstet Gynecol 2007;109: 217–27.

Screening for Tay-Sachs disease. ACOG Committee Opinion No. 318. American College of Obstetricians and Gynecologists. Obstet Gynecol 2005;106:893–4.

The importance of preconception care in the continuum of women's health care. ACOG Committee Opinion No. 313. American College of Obstetricians and Gynecologists. Obstet Gynecol 2005;106:665–6.

Tobacco use and women's health. Committee Opinion No. 503. American College of Obstetricians and Gynecologists. Obstet Gynecol 2011;118:746–50.

U.S. Medical Eligibility Criteria for Contraceptive Use, 2010. Centers for Disease Control and Prevention. MMWR Recomm Rep 2010;59 (RR-4):1–86.

Update on carrier screening for cystic fibrosis. Committee Opinion No. 486. American College of Obstetricians and Gynecologists. Obstet Gynecol 2011;117:1028–31.

Update on immunization and pregnancy: tetanus, diphtheria, and pertussis vaccination. Committee Opinion No. 566. American College of Obstetricians and Gynecologists. Obstet Gynecol 2013;121:1411–4.

Resources

American College of Obstetricians and Gynecologists. Good health before pregnancy: preconception care. Patient Education Pamphlet AP056. Washington, DC: American College of Obstetricians and Gynecologists; 2012.

American College of Obstetricians and Gynecologists. Immunization for women. Washington, DC: American College of Obstetricians and Gynecologists; 2012. Available at: http://www.immunizationforwomen.org/. Retrieved September 4, 2013.

American College of Obstetricians and Gynecologists. Immunization resources for obstetrician-gynecologists: a comprehensive tool kit. Washington, DC: American College of Obstetricians and Gynecologists; 2013. Available at: http://www.acog. org/~/media/Departments/Immunization/ImmunizationToolkit.pdf?dmc=1&ts-20130709T1011229407. Retrieved September 27, 2013.

American College of Obstetricians and Gynecologists. Later childbearing. Patient Education Pamphlet AP060. Washington, DC: American College of Obstetricians and Gynecologists; 2012.

American College of Obstetricians and Gynecologists. Your pregnancy and childbirth: month to month. 5th ed. Washington, DC: American College of Obstetricians and Gynecologists; 2010.

American College of Obstetricians and Gynecologists, American Society for Reproductive Medicine. Exposure to toxic environmental agents. Washington, DC; Birmingham (AL): American College of Obstetricians and Gynecologists; ASRM; 2013. Available at: http://www.acog.org/About_ACOG/ACOG_Departments/ Health_Care_for_Underserved_Women/~/media/Committee%20Opinions/ Committee%20on%20Health%20Care%20for%20Underserved%20Women/ ExposuretoToxic.pdf. Retrieved September 27, 2013.

Association of Occupational and Environmental Clinics. Available at: http://www. aoec.org. Retrieved September 27, 2013.

Association of Reproductive Health Professionals. Fish consumption to promote good health and minimize contaminants. A quick reference guide for clinicians. Washington, DC: ARHP; 2008. Available at: http://www.arhp.org/uploadDocs/ QRGfishandhealth.pdf. Retrieved July 29, 2013.

Bombard JM, Robbins CL, Dietz PM, Valderrama AL. Preconception care: the perfect opportunity for health care providers to advise lifestyle changes for hypertensive women. Am J Health Promot 2013;27:S43–9.

Jack BW, Atrash H, Coonrod DV, Moos MK, O'Donnell J, Johnson K. The clinical content of preconception care: an overview and preparation of this supplement. Am J Obstet Gynecol 2008;199:S266–79.

Johnson K, Posner SF, Biermann J, Cordero JF, Atrash HK, Parker CS, et al. Recommendations to improve preconception health and health care–United States. A report of the CDC/ATSDR Preconception Care Work Group and the Select Panel on Preconception Care. CDC/ATSDR Preconception Care Work Group, Select Panel on Preconception Care. MMWR Recomm Rep 2006;55:1–23.

Kaye K, Suellentrop K, Sloup C. The fog zone: how misperceptions, magical thinking, and ambivalence put young adults at risk for unplanned pregnancy. Washington, DC: The National Campaign to Prevent Teen and Unplanned Pregnancy; 2009. Available at: http://thenationalcampaign.org/sites/default/files/resource-primary-download/FogZone.pdf. Retrieved March 28, 2014.

Lead screening during pregnancy and lactation. Committee Opinion No. 533. American College of Obstetricians and Gynecologists. Obstet Gynecol 2012;120: 416–20.

Mitchell EW, Verbiest S. Effective strategies for promoting preconception health—from research to practice. Am J Health Promot 2013;27:S1–3.

Mosca L, Benjamin EJ, Berra K, Bezanson JL, Dolor RJ, Lloyd-Jones DM, et al. Effectiveness-based guidelines for the prevention of cardiovascular disease in women—2011 update: a guideline from the American Heart Association. Circulation 2011;123:1243–62.

Organization of Teratology Information Specialists. Available at: http://www.mothertobaby.org. Retrieved July 30, 2013.

Preconception Health Council of California. Interconception care project of California. Available at: http://www.everywomancalifornia.org/content_display.cfm?categoriesID=121&contentID=359. Retrieved July 30, 2013.

Teratology Society. Available at: http://www.teratology.org. Retrieved July 30, 2013.

Toriello HV. Policy statement on folic acid and neural tube defects. Policy and Practice Guideline Committee of the American College of Medical Genetics. Genet Med 2011;13:593–6.

TOXNET—Toxicology Data Network. Available at: http://toxnet.nlm.nih.gov. Retrieved July 30, 2013.

University of California, San Francisco. Clinical practice: resources for health care professionals to promote environmental health. Program on Reproductive Health and the Environment. Available at: http://prhe.ucsf.edu/prhe/clinical_resources.html. Retrieved September 27, 2013.

SEXUALLY TRANSMITTED INFECTIONS*

Sexually transmitted infections (STIs) can be acquired through contact during oral, vaginal, or anal sex. The transmission of an STI may result in myriad consequences, including infertility, chronic pelvic pain, cancer, and even death; in addition to its physical effects, it can cause psychologic distress and be a strain on personal relationships. Sexually transmitted infections are the number one cause of preventable infertility and are strongly associated with ectopic pregnancy. They may increase the risk of human immunodeficiency virus (HIV) acquisition threefold to fivefold, and their management is a critical strategy in the prevention of HIV infection. The Institute of Medicine has highlighted that U.S. STI rates are the highest in the industrialized world, and in some communities they are comparable to infection rates in many developing countries.

Prevention

Prevention of STIs includes strategies to decrease exposure through delaying the onset of sexual activity, limiting the number of sexual partners, limiting exposure to high-risk partners, limiting risky sexual practices, encouraging immunization, and increasing the use of condoms. Preventing the spread of STIs in a population also can include partner notification and treatment

---

*This section includes information based on the *2010 Sexually Transmitted Diseases Treatment Guidelines* from the Centers for Disease Control and Prevention. A revision of these guidelines was underway during the production of the fourth edition of *Guidelines for Women's Health Care*. For the most up-to-date guidance on the diagnosis and management of sexually transmitted infections, please refer to the current Centers for Disease Control and Prevention guidelines (available at www.cdc.gov/std/) as well as the American College of Obstetricians and Gynecologists' guidance on the annual health assessment of women (available at www.acog.org/wellwoman).

and reporting of diseases when required. Gonorrhea, syphilis, chlamydial infection, and HIV and acquired immunodeficiency syndrome (AIDS) are reportable diseases in every U.S. state. Clinicians should be familiar with any federal, state, or local requirements for the screening, follow-up, and reporting of STIs.

Abstinence from sexual activity is the most effective way to avoid STIs, including human papillomavirus (HPV) infection. However, an abstinence-only counseling strategy is not an effective first-line strategy. Clinicians should not condemn or chastise young patients regarding sexual activity. Instead, they should provide information and counsel patients regarding the risks of STIs and unintended pregnancy. Some patients may not consider themselves to be sexually active or at risk of acquiring STIs if engaged in oral or anal sex, and this perception should be considered when taking a sexual history. Limiting the number of sexual partners may decrease one's risk of STIs, including HPV infection.

Recommended immunizations for preventable STIs, such as hepatitis and HPV infection, for various age groups are available at www.acog.org/wellwoman. A quadrivalent vaccine against HPV types 6, 11, 16, and 18 and a bivalent vaccine against HPV types 16 and 18 are now available. The Advisory Committee on Immunization Practices of the Centers for Disease Control and Prevention (CDC) has recommended the initial vaccination target of females aged 11 years or 12 years with either the bivalent or quadrivalent vaccine. In addition, the Advisory Committee on Immunization Practices recommends routine vaccination of males aged 11 years or 12 years with the quadrivalent vaccine. Although obstetrician–gynecologists are not likely to care for many girls in this initial vaccination target group, these clinicians are critical to the widespread use of the vaccine for females aged 13–26 years (see also the "Immunizations" section earlier in Part 3). The HPV vaccine is not intended to treat patients with cervical cytologic abnormalities or genital warts. Patients with these conditions should undergo the appropriate evaluation and treatment (see also the "Abnormal Cervical Cytology" section in Part 4). It is important to note that many early cytologic abnormalities can be detected and managed conservatively, given the significant rate of regression. This is especially true in adolescents and young women.

If used consistently and correctly, latex condoms reduce the likelihood of HPV acquisition and HPV-related cervical dysplasia. Clinician counseling on condoms should include educating patients on the proper use of male condoms. This education is particularly important in young populations, who have significantly higher rates of breakage and slippage. The following question may guide counseling in noncondom users who are at risk of STIs: "The last time you did not use a condom, what were the reasons?" Answers might include nonavailability, lack of time or knowledge, or partner objection. The CDC recommendations for proper use of male condoms are provided in Box 3-21.

Three types of male condoms are available in the United States: 1) natural membrane (sometimes referred to as lambskin), 2) polyurethane, and 3) latex. Natural membrane condoms are not recommended for STI prophylaxis and should be used only for pregnancy prevention, because

---

Box 3-21. Centers for Disease Control and Prevention Recommendations for Proper Use of Male Condoms

- Use a new condom with each sex act (eg, oral, vaginal, and anal).
- Carefully handle the condom to avoid damaging it with fingernails, teeth, or other sharp objects.
- Put the condom on after the penis is erect and before any genital, oral, or anal contact with the partner.
- Use only water-based lubricants (eg, glycerin) with latex condoms. Oil-based lubricants (eg, petroleum jelly, shortening, mineral oil, massage oils, body lotions, and cooking oil) can weaken latex and should not be used.
- Ensure adequate lubrication during vaginal and anal sex, which might require the use of exogenous water-based lubricants.
- To prevent the condom from slipping off, hold the condom firmly against the base of the penis during withdrawal, and withdraw while the penis is still erect.

Reprinted from Workowski KA, Berman S. Sexually transmitted diseases treatment guidelines, 2010. Centers for Disease Control and Prevention [published erratum appears in MMWR Morb Mortal Wkly Rep 2011;60:18]. MMWR Recomm Rep 2010;59:1–110.

they may allow pathogens to pass through their pores. Latex condoms are the optimal choice for most individuals. Polyurethane condoms, which are approximately double the cost of latex condoms but provide similar protection against STIs and pregnancy, are recommended if either sexual partner has a history of latex allergy. Slippage and breakage rates are significantly higher for polyurethane condoms. The CDC does not recommend condoms lubricated with spermicides for STI and HIV prevention. Condoms lubricated with spermicides are no more effective than other lubricated condoms for STI and HIV prevention. In addition, condoms lubricated with spermicide have been associated with urinary tract infection in young women, and frequent use of spermicides that contain nonoxynol-9 has been associated with a possible higher risk of HIV transmission through disruption of the genital epithelium.

Laboratory studies indicate that the female condom, which now consists of a lubricated nitrile sheath with a ring on each end that is inserted into the vagina, is an effective mechanical barrier to viruses, including HIV, and to semen. A limited number of clinical studies have evaluated the efficacy of female condoms in providing protection from STIs, including HIV. Just as the male condom, the female condom substantially reduces the risk of STI acquisition if used consistently and correctly. When a male condom cannot be used properly, sex partners should consider using a female condom. Female condoms are more costly compared with male condoms. The female condom also can be used for STI and HIV protection during receptive anal intercourse. Its efficacy in prevention of STI transmission in this setting is undefined.

Clinicians can arrange directly for partner notification or treatment of STIs or use local or state health departments as referral sites. Treatment of male sexual partners is important in the prevention of transmission and reinfection with certain STIs. Clinicians may be asked to provide a prescription for the patient's partner without having performed an examination of the individual, an approach known as expedited partner therapy. A CDC review of the evidence has found expedited partner therapy to be a useful option, especially for treatment of male partners of women with gonorrhea or chlamydial infection (see Bibliography). However, state law and liability standards may prohibit expedited partner therapy in some areas. Clinicians are encouraged to become familiar with local regulations and resources. In addition, the recent changes to CDC treatment recommendations to require an intramuscular cephalosporin as part of the first-line treatment for gonorrhea will be an impediment to expedited partner therapy. In most cases, such a prescription will result in treatment without complication. An adverse reaction to the medication is uncommon but may result in a significant health hazard to the partner. Each clinician must decide whether providing such prescriptions is appropriate. Male partners who receive expedited partner therapy should be encouraged to seek medical evaluation.

Screening

Appropriate STI screening in nonpregnant women depends on the age of the patient and assessment of risk factors elicited during the medical and sexual history. Box 3-22 details guidelines on routine screening and screening based on risk factors. Optimal rescreening intervals are ill defined but should take into account any change in sexual partners. The CDC advises that urine or swab specimens from the endocervix or vagina can be used for screening and diagnosis, and that nucleic acid amplification tests are the most sensitive tests for these specimens. Recent studies indicate that self-collected vaginal swabs combined with nucleic acid amplification tests testing are highly acceptable to patients and may result in increased screening rates. An endocervical swab is appropriate when another indication for a pelvic examination is present.

The CDC and the American College of Obstetricians and Gynecologists (the College) recommend that females aged 13–64 years be screened for HIV at least once in their lifetime and then annually thereafter based on factors related to risk (see Box 3-22). In addition, obstetrician–gynecologists should annually review patients' risk factors for HIV and assess the need for retesting. Screening after age 64 years is indicated if there is ongoing risk for HIV infection, as indicated by risk assessment (eg, new sexual partners). Ideally, opt-out HIV screening should be performed, in which the patient is notified that HIV testing will be performed as a routine part of gynecologic and obstetric care unless the patient declines testing. However, state and local laws on HIV testing may not be consistent with such an approach;

Box 3-22. The American College of Obstetricians and Gynecologists' Sexually Transmitted Infection Screening Recommendations*

Routine Screening:

- Sexually active women aged 25 years and younger should be screened annually for chlamydial infection and gonorrhea. Screening also is recommended for women older than 25 years with risk factors (see "Screening Based on Risk Factors" later in this box). Note that urine-based sexually transmitted infection (STI) screening is an efficient means for accomplishing this without a speculum examination.

- Women with developmental disabilities should be screened for STIs.

- Human immunodeficiency virus (HIV) screening is recommended for females aged 13–64 years. Obstetrician–gynecologists should annually review patients' risk factors for HIV and assess the need for retesting. Ideally, opt-out HIV screening should be performed, in which the patient is notified that HIV testing will be performed as a routine part of gynecologic and obstetric care unless the patient declines testing.[†]

- One-time hepatitis C virus testing is recommended for individuals born from 1945 through 1965 and unaware of their infection status.

Screening Based on Risk Factors:

- Women should be regularly screened for STIs if they have a history of multiple sexual partners or a sexual partner with multiple contacts; sexual contact with individuals with culture-proven STIs; repeated episodes of STIs; or attendance at clinics for STIs. Other women who should be screened regularly include asymptomatic women older than 25 years with risk factors for chlamydial infection (eg, new or multiple sexual partners) or for gonorrhea (those who live in a high-prevalence area, have had a previous gonococcal infection, have other STIs, have new or multiple sex partners, use condoms inconsistently, participate in sex work, and use drugs).

- Syphilis testing is recommended for sexually active adolescents who exchange sex for drugs or money, use intravenous drugs, are entering a detention facility, or live in a high-prevalence area.

- Human immunodeficiency virus screening should be offered at least annually to women who are injection drug users; are sex partners of injection-drug users; exchange sex for money or drugs; are sex partners

(continued)

Box 3-22. The American College of Obstetricians and Gynecologists' Sexually Transmitted Infection Screening Recommendations* *(continued)*

of HIV-infected persons; have had sex with men who have sex with men since their most recent HIV test; or have had more than one sex partner since their most recent HIV test. Human immunodeficiency virus testing should be recommended to all women seeking preconception care.

• Hepatitis C virus testing is recommended for all individuals with HIV infection, history of injecting illegal drugs, recipients of clotting factor concentrates before 1987, chronic (long-term) hemodialysis, persistently abnormal alanine aminotransferase levels, recipients of blood from donors who later tested positive for hepatitis C virus infection, recipients of blood or blood-component transfusion or organ transplant before July 1992, or occupational percutaneous or mucosal exposure to hepatitis C virus-positive blood.

*These recommendations are based on the *2010 Sexually Transmitted Diseases Treatment Guidelines* from the Centers for Disease Control and Prevention. A revision of these guidelines was underway during the production of the fourth edition of *Guidelines for Women's Health Care*. For the most up-to-date guidance on the diagnosis and management of sexually transmitted infections, please refer to the current Centers for Disease Control and Prevention guidelines (available at www.cdc.gov/std/) as well as the American College of Obstetricians and Gynecologists' guidance on the annual health assessment of women (available at www.acog.org/wellwoman).

†Although the American College of Obstetricians and Gynecologists recommends opt-out screening where legally possible, state and local laws may have specific requirements for HIV testing that are not consistent with such an approach. Physicians should be aware of, and follow, the HIV screening requirements in their jurisdiction.

Data from Routine human immunodeficiency virus screening. Committee Opinion No. 596. American College of Obstetricians and Gynecologists. Obstet Gynecol 2014;123:1137–9 *and* Workowski KA, Berman S. Sexually transmitted diseases treatment guidelines, 2010. Centers for Disease Control and Prevention [published erratum appears in MMWR Morb Mortal Wkly Rep 2011;60:18]. MMWR Recomm Rep 2010;59:1–110.

therefore, physicians should be aware of, and follow, the HIV screening requirements in their jurisdiction.

Diagnosis and Management

Many infections are asymptomatic, and presenting history and examination findings vary. Table 3-11, Table 3-12, and the following discussion provide a brief overview of the diagnosis and management of some of the most common STIs. Information on bacterial vaginosis and trichomoniasis is provided in the "Vaginitis" section in Part 4. Detailed information on the management of STIs is provided in the most recent STI treatment guidelines published by the CDC (see www.cdc.gov/std).

PELVIC INFLAMMATORY DISEASE

Pelvic inflammatory disease, a leading cause of infertility, is associated with STIs. No specific finding or test is sensitive and specific for the diagnosis of PID. Many cases go unrecognized and may present with mild, nonspecific symptoms, such as abnormal bleeding or vaginal discharge. The CDC recommends that practitioners have a low threshold for diagnosing PID, given the potential for infertility in what appears to be mild or atypical PID. The CDC advises empiric treatment for PID in sexually active young women and other women at risk of STIs if no other cause of the illness can be identified and any one of the following is present on pelvic examination: uterine tenderness, adnexal tenderness, or cervical motion tenderness. The CDC also recommends that all women with diagnosed acute PID be tested for chlamydial infection, gonorrhea, and HIV infection. Most, but not all, women with PID will have white blood cells in their vagina or a mucopurulent cervical discharge. In patients without these findings, the diagnosis of PID is unlikely, and thorough evaluation should investigate other possible sources of pain.

The routine use of laparoscopy to diagnose PID is not indicated because of cost and operative risk. However, if the diagnosis is uncertain, the patient fails to respond to therapy, or symptoms recur soon after adequate therapy, diagnostic laparoscopy may be indicated to rule out other conditions causing pain, such as endometriosis, ruptured ovarian cyst, or adnexal torsion.

The CDC recommends that therapy with recommended treatment regimens be initiated as soon as the presumptive diagnosis of PID has been

Table 3-11. Diseases Characterized by Genital Ulcers*

- Differential diagnosis: genital herpes, syphilis, chancroid, and nonsexually transmitted infections
- Diagnosis: history and physical examination frequently inaccurate; all patients should be tested for syphilis and herpes; consideration given to chancroid

Herpes	Syphilis	Chancroid
Prevalence:	Prevalence:	Prevalence:
• At least 50 million individuals in the United States have HSV infection	• Decreasing; more prevalent in metropolitan areas	• Decreasing in the United States • Usually in discrete outbreaks—high rates of HIV coinfection
Presentation:	Common presentations:	Presentation:
• Classic presentation of vesicles/ulcers absent in many cases • Many women with either HSV-1 or HSV-2 infection are asymptomatic. • Recurrences much less common with HSV-1; important fact for counseling	• Primary: ulcer or chancre • Secondary: skin rash, lymphadenopathy, mucocutaneous lesions • Tertiary: cardiac or ophthalmic manifestations, auditory abnormalities, gummatous lesions • Latent: no symptoms, diagnosed by serology	• Combination of a painful genital ulcer and tender suppurative inguinal adenopathy
Diagnostic tests:	Diagnostic tests:	Diagnosis:
• Clinical diagnosis should be confirmed by laboratory testing. • Isolation of HSV in cell culture or PCR are the preferred virologic tests. • Viral culture isolates should be typed to determine if HSV-1 or HSV-2 is the cause of the infection.	• Dark-field examinations and direct fluorescent antibody tests of lesion exudate or tissue are the definitive methods for diagnosing early syphilis. • Presumptive diagnosis is possible with nontreponemal tests (VDRL and RPR) and treponemal tests (eg, FTA-ABS and TP-PA).	• Culture media • No FDA-approved test is available • Probable diagnosis: patient with painful ulcers, no evidence of syphilis, typical chancroid presentation, and diagnostic tests negative for herpes

(continued)

Table 3-11. Diseases Characterized by Genital Ulcers* *(continued)*

Herpes	Syphilis	Chancroid
Diagnostic tests:	Diagnostic tests:	
• The serologic type-specific glycoprotein G-based assays should be specifically requested when serology is performed.	• The use of only one type of serologic test is insufficient; false-positive nontreponemal test results are sometimes associated with medical conditions unrelated to syphilis.	

*The information in this table is from the *2010 Sexually Transmitted Diseases Treatment Guidelines* from the Centers for Disease Control and Prevention. A revision of these guidelines was underway during the production of the fourth edition of *Guidelines for Women's Health Care*. For the most up-to-date guidance, please refer to the current Centers for Disease Control and Prevention guidelines, available at www.cdc.gov/std/.

Abbreviations: FDA, U.S. Food and Drug Administration; FTA-ABS, fluorescent treponemal antibody absorbed; HIV, human immunodeficiency virus; HSV, herpes simplex virus; PCR, polymerase chain reaction; RPR, rapid plasma reagin; TP-PA, T pallidum particle agglutination; VDRL, Venereal Disease Research Laboratory.

Data from Workowski KA, Berman S. Sexually transmitted diseases treatment guidelines, 2010. Centers for Disease Control and Prevention [published erratum appears in MMWR Morb Mortal Wkly Rep 2011;60:18]. MMWR Recomm Rep 2010;59:1–110.

Table 3-12. Diseases Characterized by Cervicitis or Urethritis*

Chlamydial Infection	Gonorrhea
Prevalence:	Prevalence:
• Most frequently reported infectious disease in the United States • Highest prevalence in individuals 25 years and younger	• Second most commonly reported notifiable infection; it has been estimated that 700,000 new infections occur each year in the United States • Prevalence varies widely among communities and populations. • Women younger than 25 years are at highest risk.

(continued)

Table 3-12. Diseases Characterized by Cervicitis or Urethritis* *(continued)*

Chlamydial Infection	Gonorrhea
Presentation: • Asymptomatic infection common • Other presentations: mucopurulent cervicitis, abnormal vaginal discharge, irregular intermenstrual vaginal bleeding	Presentation: • Frequently asymptomatic
Evaluation: • All sexually active women 25 years and younger should be screened annually. • Urogenital infection in women can be diagnosed by testing urine or swab specimens collected from the endocervix or vagina. • Culture, direct immunofluorescence, EIA, nucleic acid hybridization tests, and NAATs are available for the detection of *Chlamydia trachomatis* on endocervical swab specimens. • NAATs are the most sensitive tests and are the recommended testing method. They are cleared by the FDA for use with endocervical swab, vaginal swab, and urine specimens. • A clinician-collected or self-collected vaginal swab is the recommended sample type. A self-collected swab is an option for screening women when a pelvic examination is not otherwise indicated. • Consider first-catch urine screening for adolescents and others reluctant to have pelvic examination or when pelvic examination is not feasible. However, testing of urine specimens may miss up to 10% of infections compared with testing of vaginal or endocervical swab specimens.	Evaluation: • Testing is appropriate in patients at high risk of STIs. • All sexually active women younger than 25 years should be screened annually because they are at highest risk of infection. • Pharyngeal and anorectal infections should be considered based on sexual practices elicited during the sexual history. • Culture and NAATs are available for the detection of genitourinary infection with *Neisseria gonorrhoeae*. • NAATs are the most sensitive tests and are the recommended testing method. They are cleared by the FDA for use with endocervical swab, vaginal swab, and urine specimens. • Consider first-catch urine screening for adolescents and others reluctant to have pelvic examination or when pelvic examination is not feasible. However, testing of urine specimens may miss up to 10% of infections compared with testing of vaginal or endocervical swab specimens.

(continued)

Table 3-12. Diseases Characterized by Cervicitis or Urethritis* *(continued)*

Chlamydial Infection	Gonorrhea
• Certain NAATs have been FDA-approved for use on liquid-based cytology specimens. Special considerations: • Individuals treated for chlamydial infection should be instructed to abstain from sexual intercourse for 7 days after single-dose therapy or until completion of a 7-day regimen and be instructed to abstain from sexual intercourse until all of their sex partners are treated. • Test-of-cure (repeated testing 3–4 weeks after completing therapy) is not recommended for individuals treated with the recommended or alternative regimens, unless therapeutic adherence is in question, symptoms persist, or reinfection is suspected. • Because of high rates of reinfection, consider advising all women with chlamydial infection to be retested approximately 3 months after treatment and encourage retesting for all women treated for chlamydial infection whenever they next seek medical care within the following 3–12 months.	Special considerations: • Patients with gonorrhea should be treated routinely for chlamydial infection as well. • If a heterosexual partner of a patient cannot be treated within a timely fashion with the CDC-recommended treatment, expedited partner therapy using the alternative oral combination antimicrobial therapy should be considered. — If alternative oral combination therapy is given, encourage test-of-cure 7 days after treatment. • Consider advising all patients with gonorrhea to be retested 3 months after treatment. If patients do not seek retesting in 3 months, encourage retesting whenever these patients seek medical care within the following 12 months.

*The information in this table is from the *2010 Sexually Transmitted Diseases Treatment Guidelines* from the Centers for Disease Control and Prevention. A revision of these guidelines was underway during the production of the fourth edition of *Guidelines for Women's Health Care*. For the most up-to-date guidance, please refer to the current Centers for Disease Control and Prevention guidelines, available at www.cdc.gov/std/.

Abbreviations: CDC, Centers for Disease Control and Prevention; EIA, enzyme immunoassay; FDA, U.S. Food and Drug Administration; NAAT, nucleic acid amplification test; STI, sexually transmitted infection; The College, American College of Obstetricians and Gynecologists.

Data from Workowski KA, Berman S. Sexually transmitted diseases treatment guidelines, 2010. Centers for Disease Control and Prevention [published erratum appears in MMWR Morb

(continued)

Table 3-12. Diseases Characterized by Cervicitis or Urethritis* *(continued)*

Mortal Wkly Rep 2011;60:18]. MMWR Recomm Rep 2010;59:1–110; Update to CDC's Sexually transmitted diseases treatment guidelines, 2010: oral cephalosporins no longer a recommended treatment for gonococcal infections. Centers for Disease Control and Prevention. MMWR Morb Mortal Wkly Rep 2012;61:590–4; *and* Papp JR, Schachter J, Gaydos CA, Van Der Pol B. Recommendations for the laboratory-based detection of Chlamydia trachomatis and Neisseria gonorrhoeae–2014. Division of STD Prevention, National Center for HIV/AIDS, Viral Hepatitis, STD, and TB Prevention, CDC. MMWR Recomm Rep 2014;63(RR02):1–19.

made. The CDC also notes that clinicians should consider availability, cost, patient acceptance, and antimicrobial susceptibility when selecting a treatment regimen.

Outpatient therapy can provide similar outcomes to inpatient therapy for women with mild or moderate PID. It is important to assess response to treatment when outpatient therapy is provided. The decision to hospitalize must be individualized. The CDC has listed suggested criteria for hospitalization (see Box 3-23). Adolescents with PID often are hospitalized, but data do not substantiate that they benefit from inpatient therapy

---

Box 3-23. Suggested Criteria for Hospitalization for Pelvic Inflammatory Disease*

- Surgical emergencies (eg, appendicitis) cannot be excluded.
- The patient is pregnant.
- The patient does not respond clinically to oral antimicrobial therapy.
- The patient is unable to follow or tolerate an outpatient oral regimen.
- The patient has severe illness, nausea and vomiting, or high fever.
- The patient has a tuboovarian abscess.

*These criteria are from the *2010 Sexually Transmitted Diseases Treatment Guidelines* from the Centers for Disease Control and Prevention. A revision of these guidelines was underway during the production of the fourth edition of *Guidelines for Women's Health Care*. For the most up-to-date guidance, please refer to the current Centers for Disease Control and Prevention guidelines, available at www.cdc.gov/std/.

Reprinted from Workowski KA, Berman S. Sexually transmitted diseases treatment guidelines, 2010. Centers for Disease Control and Prevention [published erratum appears in MMWR Morb Mortal Wkly Rep 2011;60:18]. MMWR Recomm Rep 2010;59:1–110.

more than other age groups. Young women with mild-to-moderate disease have similar outcomes with either inpatient therapy or outpatient therapy, and response to outpatient therapy is similar across age groups. The CDC recommends that the same criteria used to determine the need for hospitalization of older women be used for adolescents with acute PID.

HUMAN PAPILLOMAVIRUS INFECTION

Infection with one or more HPV subtypes is extremely common, occurring in up to 80% of sexually active women by age 50 years. It appears that most young, sexually active men and women are, or have been, infected with this organism. Most cervical HPV infections appear to be transient, but the proportion of women whose infections are resolved decreases with age. In one prospective study, the time required for 50% of prevalent cases to become HPV DNA–negative was 4.8 months for nononcogenic types and 8.1 months for oncogenic types. This finding may not reflect the true duration of infection because it is unknown how long the women had been infected at the time of enrollment in the study. Infections of the cervix often are diagnosed through assessment of cervical cytology (see also the "Well-Woman Annual Health Assessment" section earlier in Part 3).

Some subtypes (particularly the nononcogenic types, such as types 6 and 11) are associated with the development of genital warts. In most cases, external warts can be treated with the topical application of podofilox, imiquimod, trichloroacetic or bichloroacetic acid, or podophyllin resin or the use of cryotherapy, laser ablation, or electrocautery. Treatment should be guided by the preference of the patient and the experience of the clinician. Patients who fail to respond to treatment may be immunosuppressed and should be counseled about, and offered, testing for HIV. Patients known to be immunosuppressed (eg, transplant patients, chronic steroid users, and HIV-positive patients) should receive HPV and STI prevention counseling.

INFECTIOUS HEPATITIS

Infection with hepatitis B virus (HBV) is contracted more often by other routes of exposure, although some studies have suggested that up to 60% of all such infections result from sexual transmission. Women who have active HBV infections or women who are HBV carriers should be counseled to have their partners use condoms during intercourse. They should avoid oral–genital contact. Patients with STIs, all adolescents not previously immunized, and others who are considered to be at high risk (see ACOG Annual Women's Health Care www.acog.org/About_ACOG/ACOG_Departments/Annual_Womens_Health_Care/High-Risk_Factors) should be offered HBV vaccination. Hepatitis B vaccination also should be initiated in nonimmunized sexual assault victims.

HUMAN IMMUNODEFICIENCY VIRUS INFECTION

The CDC estimates that approximately 40,000–50,000 new HIV infections occurred annually in the United States from 2006 to 2009. Almost one in five (18.1%) of all individuals infected with HIV are unaware of their HIV status. Heterosexual contact is the leading mode of HIV transmission in women. Women with STIs have an increased risk of HIV infection. In 2010, women accounted for more than 22% of new HIV infections diagnosed.

Women should be counseled routinely regarding HIV infection. The obstetrician–gynecologist should be prepared to educate patients about the modes of transmission of the virus, means of protection from infection, and the significance of HIV infection in pregnancy. Prevention of HIV infection should be a priority. Voluntary and confidential HIV testing should be available to any woman who wishes to be tested.

Physicians should be aware of, and follow, their states' HIV testing requirements. Clinicians should consult their state medical associations for more information on state laws governing HIV testing and test results. The CDC recommends that patients be notified that testing will be performed, but separate written consent and prevention counseling should not be required.

The CDC recommends that HIV-negative test results may be conveyed without direct personal contact with the patient. Individuals known to be at high risk of HIV infection should be advised of the need for periodic retesting and should be offered, or be referred for, prevention counseling. Individuals with HIV-positive test results should receive confidential communication of test results through personal contact by a clinician, nurse, midlevel practitioner, counselor, or other skilled staff member. Individuals who test positive for HIV should receive, or be referred for, clinical care promptly.

Several U.S. Food and Drug Administration-approved rapid HIV tests are available. With rapid HIV testing, results are available in 10–30 minutes if given at the point of care. Currently, blood and oral fluid rapid tests are used. Positive screening test results should be confirmed. Point-of-care testing facilitates screening in settings with limited access to laboratories but also allows patients in all settings, including the routine visit, to learn their test results during that visit. Such immediate notice not only reduces the number of individuals who do not return to learn their test results but also allows for prompt entry into care. The CDC recommends rapid HIV testing in settings such as emergency departments, STI clinics, and annual visits. Clinicians should develop resources to allow them to provide appropriate counseling and support services if they use rapid testing.

It is unethical for an obstetrician–gynecologist to refuse to accept as patients or to refuse to continue to care for individuals solely because they are, or are thought to be, seropositive for HIV. Health care providers should observe standard precautions to minimize skin, mucous membrane, and percutaneous exposure to blood, secretions, and body fluids from all patients to protect against a variety of pathogens, including HIV. In making decisions about patient-care activities, a health care worker infected with HIV should adhere to the fundamental professional obligation to avoid harm to patients (see also the "Human Resources" section in Part 1).

Sexual Health Risks of Noncoital Sexual Activity

Noncoital sexual behaviors, including activities such as mutual masturbation, oral sex, and anal sex, are common. Although these behaviors carry little to no risk of pregnancy, patients should be counseled that noncoital sexual activity is not necessarily "safe sex." Anal sex poses a particularly high risk because tissues in the rectum break easily, and organisms can be transmitted through breaks in skin and mucosal surfaces. Oral–genital sex is known to be a method of transmission of several STIs. Because people define sexuality in a variety of ways and may not report noncoital sexual activity, it is important that clinicians ask direct questions regarding sexual activity, including whether the patient has sex with men, women, or both; the number of sexual partners and her partners' sexual behavior; and frequency of oral and anal sex and mutual masturbation.

Counseling about noncoital sexual activity should address the risk of STIs during noncoital sexual activity and encourage STI prevention efforts. Clinicians also should consider the patient's history of STIs and patterns of barrier method use with each partner, as well as the local prevalence of STIs (available from local health departments). Use of latex or synthetic condoms during anal–genital intercourse to reduce the risk of STIs should be encouraged. Use of barrier protection during oral sex also should be encouraged. Latex sheets have been approved by the U.S. Food and Drug Administration for use to reduce the risk of transmission of STIs during oral sex; however, no effectiveness data are available. Dental dams (or oral dams), household plastic wrap, and condoms adapted to form a barrier sheet are other options for barrier protection for oral sex; however, these products have not been evaluated or cleared by the U.S. Food and Drug Administration for this use and no effectiveness data are available. Counseling also should include the risk of STI transmission with the use of sex toys and encourage cleaning of and condom use on sex toys.

Bibliography

Adams DA, Gallagher KM, Jajosky RA, Kriseman J, Sharp P, Anderson WJ, et al. Summary of Notifiable Diseases – United States, 2011. Division of Notifiable Diseases and Healthcare Information, Office of Surveillance, Epidemiology, and Laboratory Services, CDC. MMWR Morb Mortal Wkly Rep 2013;60:1–117.

Addressing health risks of noncoital sexual activity. Committee Opinion No. 582. American College of Obstetricians and Gynecologists. Obstet Gynecol 2013; 122:1378–83.

American College of Obstetricians and Gynecologists. Sexually transmitted infections in adolescents. In: Guidelines for adolescent health care [CD-ROM]. 2nd ed. Washington, DC: American College of Obstetricians and Gynecologists; 2011. p. 64–72.

American College of Obstetricians and Gynecologists. Annual women's health care. Available at: http://www.acog.org/wellwoman. Retrieved October 1, 2013.

American College of Obstetricians and Gynecologists. Annual women's health care: high risk factors. Available at: http://www.acog.org/About_ACOG/ACOG_Depart ments/Annual_Womens_Health_Care/High-Risk_Factors. Retrieved October 1, 2013.

Calonge N. Screening for syphilis infection: recommendation statement. U.S. Preventive Services Task Force [published erratum appears in Ann Fam Med 2004;2:517]. Ann Fam Med 2004;2:362–5.

Centers for Disease Control and Prevention. Expedited partner therapy in the management of sexually transmitted diseases: review and guidance. Atlanta (GA): CDC; 2006. Available at: http://www.cdc.gov/std/treatment/eptfinalreport2006.pdf. Retrieved July 29, 2013.

Centers for Disease Control and Prevention. Guidance on the use of expedited partner therapy in the treatment of gonorrhea. Atlanta (GA): CDC; 2012. Available at: http://www.cdc.gov/std/ept/GC-EPT-GuidanceNov-2012.pdf. Retrieved July 29, 2013.

Centers for Disease Control and Prevention. Monitoring selected national HIV prevention and care objectives by using HIV surveillance data—United States and 6 U.S. dependent areas—2010. HIV Surveillance Supplemental Report 2012;17 (No. 3, part A). Atlanta (GA): CDC; 2012. Available at: http://www.cdc.gov/hiv/pdf/statistics_2010_HIV_Surveillance_Report_vol_17_no_3.pdf. Retrieved December 11, 2013.

Centers for Disease Control and Prevention. Sexually transmitted diseases. Available at: http://www.cdc.gov/std/. Retrieved July 29, 2013.

Expedited partner therapy in the management of gonorrhea and chlamydia by obstetrician-gynecologists. Committee Opinion No. 506. American College of Obstetricians and Gynecologists. Obstet Gynecol 2011;118:761–6.

Gynecologic herpes simplex virus infections. ACOG Practice Bulletin No. 57. American College of Obstetricians and Gynecologists. Obstet Gynecol 2004;104:1111–8.

Human immunodeficiency virus and acquired immunodeficiency syndrome and women of color. Committee Opinion No. 536. American College of Obstetricians and Gynecologists. Obstet Gynecol 2012;120:735–9.

Human papillomavirus vaccination. Committee Opinion No. 588. American College of Obstetricians and Gynecologists. Obstet Gynecol 2014;123:712–8.

Marrazzo JM, Cates W. Interventions to prevent sexually transmitted infections, including HIV infection. Clin Infect Dis 2011;53 Suppl 3:S64–78.

Papp JR, Schachter J, Gaydos CA, Van Der Pol B. Recommendations for the laboratory-based detection of Chlamydia trachomatis and Neisseria gonorrhoeae–2014. Division of STD Prevention, National Center for HIV/AIDS, Viral Hepatitis, STD, and TB Prevention, CDC. MMWR Recomm Rep 2014;63(RR02):1–19.

Prejean J, Song R, Hernandez A, Ziebell R, Green T, Walker F, et al. Estimated HIV incidence in the United States, 2006-2009. HIV Incidence Surveillance Group. PLoS One 2011;6:e17502.

Routine human immunodeficiency virus screening. Committee Opinion No. 596. American College of Obstetricians and Gynecologists. Obstet Gynecol 2014; 123:1137–9.

Screening for chlamydial infection: U.S. Preventive Services Task Force recommendation statement. U.S. Preventive Services Task Force. Ann Intern Med 2007;147:128–34.

Screening for gonorrhea: recommendation statement. U.S. Preventive Services Task Force. Ann Fam Med 2005;3:263–7.

Smith BD, Morgan RL, Beckett GA, Falck-Ytter Y, Holtzman D, Teo CG, et al. Recommendations for the identification of chronic hepatitis C virus infection among persons born during 1945–1965. Centers for Disease Control and Prevention [published erratum appears in MMWR Recomm Rep 2012;61:886]. MMWR Recomm Rep 2012;61:1–32.

Update to CDC's Sexually transmitted diseases treatment guidelines, 2010: oral cephalosporins no longer a recommended treatment for gonococcal infections. Centers for Disease Control and Prevention. MMWR Morb Mortal Wkly Rep 2012;61:590–4.

Workowski KA, Berman S. Sexually transmitted diseases treatment guidelines, 2010. Centers for Disease Control and Prevention [published erratum appears in MMWR Morb Mortal Wkly Rep 2011;60:18]. MMWR Recomm Rep 2010;59:1–110.

Resources

American College of Obstetricians and Gynecologists. Annual women's health care: high risk factors. Available at: http://www.acog.org/About_ACOG/ACOG_ Departments/Annual_Womens_Health_Care/High-Risk_Factors. Retrieved October 1, 2013.

American College of Obstetricians and Gynecologists. Barrier methods of contraception. Patient Education Pamphlet AP022. Washington, DC: American College of Obstetricians and Gynecologists; 2011.

American College of Obstetricians and Gynecologists. Genital herpes. ACOG Patient Education Pamphlet AP054. Washington, DC: ACOG; 2008.

American College of Obstetricians and Gynecologists. Gonorrhea, chlamydia, and syphilis. Patient Education Pamphlet AP071. Washington, DC: American College of Obstetricians and Gynecologists; 2013.

American College of Obstetricians and Gynecologists. HIV and women. ACOG Patient Education Pamphlet AP082. Washington, DC: ACOG; 2008.

American College of Obstetricians and Gynecologists. How to prevent sexually transmitted diseases. Patient Education Pamphlet AP009. Washington, DC: American College of Obstetricians and Gynecologists; 2013.

American College of Obstetricians and Gynecologists. Human papillomavirus infection. Patient Education Pamphlet AP073. Washington, DC: American College of Obstetricians and Gynecologists; 2013.

American College of Obstetricians and Gynecologists. Pelvic inflammatory disease. Patient Education Pamphlet AP077. Washington, DC: American College of Obstetricians and Gynecologists; 2010.

Branson BM, Handsfield HH, Lampe MA, Janssen RS, Taylor AW, Lyss SB, et al. Revised recommendations for HIV testing of adults, adolescents, and pregnant women in health-care settings. Centers for Disease Control and Prevention. MMWR Recomm Rep 2006;55(RR-14):1–17; quiz CE1–4.

Centers for Disease Control and Prevention. Expedited partner therapy. Available at: http://www.cdc.gov/std/ept/default.htm. Retrieved July 29, 2013.

Centers for Disease Control and Prevention. HIV/AIDS. Available at: http://www.cdc.gov/hiv. Retrieved July 29, 2013.

Centers for Disease Control and Prevention. National Center for HIV/AIDS, Viral Hepatitis, STD, and TB Prevention. Available at: http://www.cdc.gov/nchhstp/Default.htm. Retrieved July 30, 2013.

Centers for Disease Control and Prevention. Peer review plan for "US PHS preexposure prophylaxis for the prevention of HIV infection in the United States–2013: a clinical practice guideline and US PHS preexposure prophylaxis for the prevention of HIV infection in the United States–2013: clinical providers' supplement." Atlanta (GA): CDC; 2013. Available at: http://www.cdc.gov/hiv/pdf/policies_PRP_PrEP.2.pdf. Retrieved March 28, 2014.

Chou R, Selph S, Dana T, Bougatsos C, Zakher B, Blazina I, et al. Screening for HIV: systematic review to update the U.S. Preventive Services Task Force recommendation. Evidence Synthesis No. 95. AHRQ Publication No. 12-05173-EF-1. Rockville (MD): Agency for Healthcare Research and Quality; 2012. Available at: http://www.uspreventiveservicestaskforce.org/uspstf13/hiv/hivadultes.pdf. Retrieved July 30, 2013.

Interim guidance for clinicians considering the use of preexposure prophylaxis for the prevention of HIV infection in heterosexually active adults. Centers for Disease Control and Prevention. MMWR Morb Mortal Wkly Rep 2012;61:586–9.

Mast EE, Weinbaum CM, Fiore AE, Alter MJ, Bell BP, Finelli L, et al. A comprehensive immunization strategy to eliminate transmission of hepatitis B virus infection in the United States: recommendations of the Advisory Committee on Immunization Practices (ACIP) Part II: immunization of adults. Advisory Committee on Immunization Practices (ACIP).Centers for Disease Control and Prevention [published erratum appears in MMWR Morb Mortal Wkly Rep 2007; 56:1114]. MMWR Recomm Rep 2006;55(RR-16):1–33; quiz CE1–4.

Moyer VA. Screening for HIV: U.S. Preventive Services Task Force Recommendation Statement. U.S. Preventive Services Task Force. Ann Intern Med 2013;159:51–60.

Smith DK, Grohskopf LA, Black RJ, Auerbach JD, Veronese F, Struble KA, et al. Antiretroviral postexposure prophylaxis after sexual, injection-drug use, or other nonoccupational exposure to HIV in the United States: recommendations from the U.S. Department of Health and Human Services. U.S. Department of Health and Human Services. MMWR Recomm Rep 2005;54(RR-2):1–20.

University of California San Francisco. National HIV/AIDS Clinicians' Consultation Center. Available at: http://www.nccc.ucsf.edu/. Retrieved July 30, 2013.

PEDIATRIC GYNECOLOGY

Pediatric gynecology includes the care of prepubertal and peripubertal girls. A small percentage of this group will come to the attention of the obstetrician–gynecologist. The most common presenting problem is vulvovaginitis. Other problems include labial adhesions and labial agglutination, prepubertal bleeding (usually not caused by precocious puberty), and sexual abuse.

The Pediatric Gynecologic Examination

Pediatric gynecologic examinations should be conducted with patience and sensitivity by health care providers with interest and experience in this area. The examination in prepubertal girls is approached differently from that in reproductive-aged women, but it still may include examination of the vagina and internal genital organs. A speculum examination is generally not indicated during the office examination of a prepubertal girl. Forcible restraint never is indicated, and sedation rarely is necessary. The American Academy of Pediatrics recommends that, in general, the examination of a younger girl should be chaperoned by the girl's parent or caregiver. As girls become older, their caregivers and the children themselves should participate in the decision of whether to use a chaperone. As with adults, a full explanation of the examination and the reason for it is always warranted. The American Academy of Pediatricians states that it is wise for male health care providers to have a chaperone during female genital examinations.

The clinician should be familiar with state statutes regarding the need for consent by a parent or guardian for a pediatric gynecologic examination. All states require that findings of signs of physical or sexual abuse in minors be reported to state authorities.

A girl can be positioned in a froglike or lithotomy position, depending on her age. Gentle lateral and downward traction of the labia with the examiner's fingers will allow visualization of the external genitalia, including the hymeneal tissue. The vagina can be examined by placing the child in a knee–chest position (see Fig. 3-3). In this position, the vagina fills with air and generally can be visualized with an otoscope, which acts as a magnifying lens and light source but is not inserted into the vagina. Visualization is enhanced by lateral and superior traction of the labia majora.

A gentle digital rectal examination can be performed, if necessary given the patient's symptoms. It allows for assessment of the cervix, uterus, solid foreign bodies, or other masses. Cultures of the vagina can be accomplished by using small cotton-tipped swabs moistened with nonbacteriostatic saline or by using lavage systems.

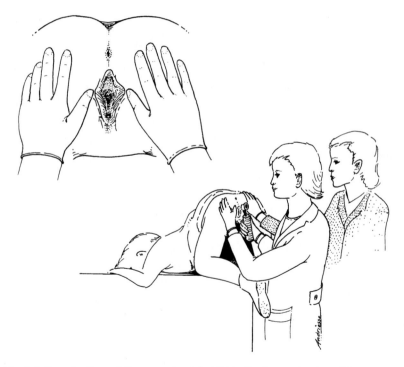

Fig. 3-3. Examination of the prepubertal child in the knee-chest position.
(Reprinted with permission from Emans SJ, Laufer MR, Goldstein DP, editors. Pediatric and adolescent gynecology. 5th ed. Philadelphia [PA]: Lippincott Williams & Wilkins; 2005. p. 13.)

Vulvovaginitis

The most common pediatric gynecologic problem an obstetrician–gynecologist is likely to encounter is vulvovaginitis, an inflammatory process that involves the vulva and vagina. Symptoms involve the vulva more than the vagina—the opposite of what is typically seen in reproductive-aged females. Girls may present with a variety of symptoms, including irritation, discomfort, pruritus, dysuria, and discharge.

Vulvovaginitis can be divided into two groups based on etiology: 1) nonspecific vulvovaginitis, and 2) specific infectious vulvovaginitis. Most cases are nonspecific. Yeast is not a common cause of vulvovaginitis in this age group because the prepubertal nonglycogenated vagina is alkaline and generally does not support fungal growth.

NONSPECIFIC VULVOVAGINITIS

Nonspecific vulvovaginitis is common in prepubertal girls and has been attributed to the proximity of the anus and vulva, poor hygiene, and the hypoestrogenic state. Chemical irritants, such as soaps, laundry detergents, and chemicals associated with the use of swimming pools or hot tubs, also may play a role. Nonspecific vulvovaginitis is a diagnosis of exclusion after pathogens have been ruled out. In a child with no history of vulvovaginitis, no purulent discharge, and no historical findings suggestive of abuse, the obstetrician–gynecologist may opt to treat the patient for nonspecific vulvovaginitis, avoiding the cost of cultures. However, many pediatric patients with symptoms of vulvovaginitis who visit gynecologists have had a previous evaluation and failed treatment, and they deserve a thorough evaluation with cultures and testing, as well as consideration of the presence of a foreign body.

Treatment is primarily aimed at improving perineal hygiene, such as careful wiping from front to back after bowel movements. Using sitz baths and avoiding chemical or traumatic irritation also are important. Regular bathing, as opposed to taking showers, is beneficial to perineal hygiene in prepubescent girls. Young girls also should be advised to wear cotton-only underwear and limit time spent in tights, leotards, and wet swimsuits.

INFECTIOUS VULVOVAGINITIS

Infectious vulvovaginitis, in which a specific pathogen is isolated as the cause of symptoms, may be caused by fecal or respiratory pathogens, such as *Escherichia coli, Streptococcus pyogenes, Staphylococcus aureus, Haemophilus influenzae,* and rarely *Candida species.* These organisms may be transmitted by the child using improper toilet hygiene and manually from the nasopharynx to the vagina. *Neisseria gonorrhoeae* or *Chlamydia trachomatis* also are causes of specific infectious vulvovaginitis, the presence of which strongly suggests sexual abuse (see "Sexual Abuse" later in this section). *Trichomonas vaginalis* is an uncommon cause of specific infectious vulvovaginitis in the unestrogenized prepubertal female. Other causes of infectious vulvovaginitis include *Shigella* species (which often presents with a blood-tinged purulent discharge) and *Yersinia* species of bacteria. Pinworms are the most common helminthic infestation in the United States, with the highest rates in school-aged and preschool children. Perianal itching may lead to excoriation and, rarely, bleeding. Vulvar and perianal erythema often is present.

Cultures with sensitivities to test for specific pathogens may be obtained with cotton swabs or urethral (calcium alginate tipped applicator) swabs moistened with nonbacteriostatic saline. Use of a swab can cause discomfort or, rarely, minimal bleeding. To distract the patient, the child can be asked to cough. A topical anesthetic can be applied before placing the swab into the vagina. Alternatively, a small feeding tube attached to a syringe with a small amount of saline for vaginal wash and aspiration can be used. This allows for examination of the fluid under the microscope as well as sending the fluid off for culture. A minimal amount of normal saline should be used to avoid dilution of the specimen. The CDC recommends performing a culture instead of a nucleic acid amplification test (NAAT) for the detection of *C trachomatis* and *N gonorrhoeae* in girls because data are limited on the use of NAATs in children. (For more information, see the CDC guidelines for the detection of *C trachomatis* and *N gonorrhoeae* at http://www.cdc.gov/std/.) Tests for *Shigella* may require special media and collection procedures. If pinworms are suspected, transparent adhesive tape or an anal swab should be applied to the anal region in the morning before defecation or bathing and then placed on a slide. Eggs seen on microscopic examination confirm the diagnosis.

The treatment of specific vulvovaginitis should be directed at the organism causing the symptoms. Treatment guidelines are available from the CDC, the North American Society for Pediatric and Adolescent Gynecology, and the American Academy of Pediatrics (see Resources).

Vulvar Disorders

Vulvar disorders in children may be infectious (eg, molluscum contagiosum, condyloma, or herpes) or noninfectious (eg, labial agglutination, lichen sclerosus, psoriasis, atopic dermatitis, contact dermatitis, or seborrheic dermatitis). The diagnosis and management of these disorders are discussed here.

INFECTIOUS VULVAR DISORDERS

Molluscum contagiosum is characterized by 1–5-mm discrete, skin-colored, dome-shaped, smooth papules with a central cheesy plug, sometimes referred to as "umbilicated lesions." The area surrounding the lesions may be erythematous or pruritic. It is common in school-aged children, especially among those who live in overcrowded areas or have poor hygiene. Secondary spread of lesions may occur by autoinoculation. Diagnosis usually is made by visual inspection. The disease generally is self-limited and the lesions may resolve spontaneously and, for this reason, treatment usually is not necessary in the young child. If treatment is indicated, however, it should not be excessive or overly aggressive. Treatment choices in children may include cryosurgery, application of topical anesthetic and curettage, and topical silver nitrate. Successful use of topical 5% imiquimod cream also has been reported and it is approved by the U.S. Food and Drug Administration for use in patients 12 years and older.

Condyloma acuminata, or warts, result from perinatal transmission of the human papillomavirus (HPV) or close sexual or nonsexual contact with an infected individual or object. Diagnosis usually is made by visual inspection. Biopsy has a limited place in management and should be reserved for those cases in which the diagnosis is in question or operative treatment is planned. Human papillomavirus DNA testing is not helpful. Nonintervention is a reasonable approach in asymptomatic children because lesions may resolve spontaneously or decrease in size over time.

A variety of treatment options are available for symptomatic children, although none are uniformly effective, and the recurrence risk is high with all modalities. Destructive and excisional options, which may require general or local anesthesia, include topical trichloroacetic acid, local cryotherapy, electrocautery, excision by scalpel or scissors, and laser ablation. Successful use of topical 5% imiquimod cream also has been widely reported. Referral to a specialist should be considered for children in need of extensive treatment. Because condylomata acuminata frequently are sexually transmitted, the possibility of sexual abuse should be addressed (see "Sexual Abuse" later in this section).

The herpes simplex virus (HSV) can spread by autoinoculation or close nonsexual or sexual contact. Beyond the neonatal period, the presence of genital HSV indicates the need for a sexual abuse evaluation. Herpes simplex virus type 1 and HSV type 2 may involve the genitalia. The condition begins as clusters of painful vesicles on an erythematous base that may be accompanied by malaise, fever, and myalgia. Rupture results in ulcerations covered with a hemorrhagic yellowish-gray crust. According to the CDC, cell culture and polymerase chain reaction are the preferred HSV tests for individuals who seek medical treatment for genital ulcers. Viral culture isolates and polymerase chain reaction samples should be typed to determine which type of HSV is causing the infection. Accurate type-specific HSV serologic assays are based on HSV-specific glycoprotein G2 (HSV-2) and glycoprotein G1 (HSV-1). Children older than 2 years may be treated with oral acyclovir. If HSV is not detected as the etiologic agent, other possible causes of genital ulcers include cytomegalovirus, Epstein-Barr virus, and Behcet disease.

NONINFECTIOUS VULVAR DISORDERS

Labial adhesions are not uncommon in prepubertal girls and have been noted in children as young as 3 months old. They typically resolve spontaneously by menarche. The combination of vulvar irritation and hypoestrogenic environment can lead to labial adhesions. On examination, the line of agglutination can be visualized between the two labia minora. Labial adhesions should be observed unless they are symptomatic. If the condition produces symptoms (eg, frequent urinary tract infections, dysuria, or inability to void), the usual treatment is topical estrogen cream applied twice daily for 6 weeks directly over the line of agglutination. The caregiver should be instructed how to apply the cream, taking care to apply only a small amount to the semitranslucent line of adhesions by rubbing the cream into the skin using a cotton swab while applying gentle labial traction. Girls should be monitored for adverse effects of estrogen therapy, including breast budding and vaginal bleeding. To decrease the risk of recurrence and to prevent reagglutination of raw opposing skin surfaces, an emollient can be applied nightly for at least 1 month after the initial separation. Labial adhesions should not be separated manually in the office without anesthesia, as it can be very painful and may preclude subsequent examinations because of fear of pain.

Lichen sclerosus produces a sclerotic, atrophic, parchment-like plaque with an hourglass or keyhole appearance that can affect the vulvar, perianal, or perineal skin. The affected area breaks down easily; thus, girls may present with vulvar bleeding. Accompanying subepithelial hemorrhages may be misinterpreted as sexual abuse or trauma. Alternatively, the patient may experience perineal itching, soreness, or dysuria. The etiology of lichen sclerosus is unknown, although a relationship to autoimmune disease is currently the most accepted theory. In the past, it was believed that childhood lichen sclerosus resolved at puberty; however, there are now many reports of childhood lichen sclerosus persisting into adulthood (see also "Vulvar Skin Disorders" in Part 4). Treatment includes avoidance of trauma by having the patient avoid irritation to the vulvar area. Ultrapotent topical corticosteroids are considered first-line therapy. Once symptoms are under control, the patient should be tapered off the drug unless therapy is required for a flare-up.

Precocious Puberty

Onset of puberty is affected by race, family history, birth weight, nutrition, international adoption, and exposure to estrogenic chemicals. Precocious puberty was defined previously as sexual development in girls younger than 8 years. However, the Lawson Wilkins Pediatric Endocrine Society guidelines for the evaluation of premature development state that pubic hair or breast development requires evaluation only when it occurs before age 7 years in non-African American girls and before age 6 years in African American girls.

Precocious puberty is classified based on the underlying pathologic mechanism. Central precocious puberty, also known as gonadotropin-releasing hormone (GnRH)–dependent precocious puberty, results from early reactivation of the hypothalamic–pituitary–gonadal axis. Peripheral (or GnRH-independent) precocious puberty is the result of excess estrogen or androgen from overproduction by the ovaries or adrenal glands or from external sources. Possible causes of each type are listed in Box 3-24.

Box 3-24. Causes and Classifications of Sexual Precocity in Females

Complete Isosexual Precocious Puberty (GnRH-dependent)
Familial
Idiopathic
Central nervous system tumors
- Harmartoma of the tuber cinereum
- Neurofibromatosis type I (cranioptic glioma)
- Hypothalamic astrocytoma
- Ependymoma

Other central nervous system disorders
Infections (eg, encephalitis or abscess)
Infiltrative disease (eg, sarcoid or tuberculousis)
Trauma
High intracranial pressures (eg, hydrocephalus or subarachnoid cyst)
Radiation
Androgen exposure (late onset congenital adrenal hyperplasia)
Children adopted from developing countries

Incomplete Isosexual Precocious Puberty (GnRH-independent)
Gonadotropin-secretory tumors
- Central nervous system (eg, germinoma)
- Not related to the central nervous system (eg, choriocarcinoma)

Excess androgen production
- Congenital adrenal hyperplasia
- Adrenal neoplasm
- Leydig cell adenoma

(continued)

Box 3-24. Causes and Classifications of Sexual Precocity in Females *(continued)*

Excess estrogen production
- Ovarian cysts and follicles
- Estrogen producing neoplasms of the ovary or adrenal gland
- McCune–Albright syndrome
- Peutz–Jeghers syndrome

Exogenous (eg, steroid hormones or foods)

Hypothyroidism

Variants
- Premature thelarche or adrenarche
- Premature isolated menarche

Abbreviation: GnRH, gonadotropin-releasing hormone.
Modified with permission from Styne DM, Cuttler L. Abnormal pubertal development. In: Rudolph CD, Rudolph AM, Lister GE, First LR, and Gershon AA, editors. Rudolph's pediatrics. 22nd ed. New York (NY): McGraw-Hill Medical; 2011. p. 2077–86.

The clinician should strive to determine the cause and mechanism by evaluation of clinical findings and laboratory testing or refer the patient to a pediatric gynecologist or pediatric endocrinologist for diagnosis and management. The child may require observation of progression from one stage of pubertal development to the next in less than 3–6 months. Diagnostic studies include measurement of accelerated growth velocity demonstrated by growth charts and advanced bone age. Pelvic ultrasonography may show presence of ovarian or adrenal pathology or uterine maturation. Serum estradiol levels should be measured. A level above 100 pg/mL may be associated with an ovarian cyst or tumor. It is appropriate to check basal and GnRH-stimulated luteinizing hormone levels. Pubertal girls should show no, or minimal, increase in luteinizing hormone and follicle-stimulating hormone in response to GnRH. An increase in luteinizing hormone into the adult range occurs in central precocious puberty. In all cases of central precocious puberty, magnetic resonance imaging of the brain is needed to determine if a central nervous system lesion is present. Treatment is dependent on cause and includes medical suppression of puberty with GnRH agonists or surgery for pelvic or pituitary tumors.

Benign variants of precocious puberty include isolated secondary sexual characteristics without increased growth velocity. Isolated precocious thelarche refers to unilateral or bilateral breast development. Isolated precocious pubarche is associated with pubic hair development, adult body odor, axillary hair, or mild acne with normal cortisol precursors in serum, including normal 17α-hydroxyprogesterone level after corticotrophin stimulation. Isolated precocious menarche—defined as vaginal bleeding without breast or pubic hair development, a vaginal lesion (tumor or foreign body), or trauma—is a rare event and usually is attributed to transient ovarian activity. Patients with benign variants of precocious puberty have normal prepubertal pelvic anatomy by ultrasonography and prepubertal hormonal responses to stimulation studies. Follow-up is recommended because progression can occur.

Sexual Abuse

Approximately one in five girls is a victim of some type of sexual abuse during childhood. Most perpetrators are males who are known and trusted by the family (eg, fathers, male relatives, friends of the family, and babysitters). Abductions and abuse by strangers are rare.

Urgent evaluation is required for collection of forensic evidence if the reported abuse has occurred within 72 hours. It is critical to vigorously pursue the collection of clothing and linens. In one study of children evaluated for sexual abuse in the emergency department, most of the forensic evidence collected 24 hours or more after the assault was obtained from clothing and linens. If the abuse occurred more than 72 hours earlier and the child is currently not in danger and free from injuries, she can be evaluated on a nonemergent basis.

The obstetrician–gynecologist should be aware of resources in the community for the evaluation of sexual abuse. Often, departments of children's services or local pediatric hospitals can help refer the child and her family to professionals with experience in interviewing and examining children suspected to be victims of sexual abuse.

Every state requires suspected and known sexual abuse to be reported. In situations in which the gynecologist is unsure if a report should be filed, local child protective service personnel can be helpful. A goal is to avoid filing vague and unnecessary reports that overburden the system but to file borderline reports when any child's safety is unclear. Many signs and symptoms consistent with abuse, such as nightmares or prepubertal bleeding, also have other causes. The state statutes do not imply that every observation of these signs and symptoms in a child requires a report of possible sexual abuse. The American Academy of Pediatrics has developed guidelines on appropriate filing (see Resources). Liability issues related to false reporting have not been problematic and should never impede filing.

Most children who have been sexually abused will have normal findings on examination. Findings that suggest abuse include lacerations of the vulva, posterior fourchette, or anus and transection of the hymen. However, hymen diameters are not a reliable marker of abuse. Prepubertal bleeding may be seen but usually is not present in abused children.

Approximately 5% of abused children will acquire a sexually transmitted infection; the clinician must decide if culturing for sexually transmitted infections is appropriate by evaluating the individual situation and taking into account community standards. Children with gonorrhea or chlamydial infection generally are symptomatic and have vaginal discharge. Gonorrhea and chlamydial infection cause vaginitis (not cervicitis) in children, so if a culture is performed, it should be taken from the vagina rather than the endocervix. If testing is done, the CDC recommends performing a culture instead of indirect or DNA testing (specifically, NAATs) because there are limited data on the use of these tests in children and these tests may not be admissible in courts because they are not labeled for use in children.

Psychologic support and therapy with a qualified mental health professional are often critical. For more information see the "Abuse" section later in Part 3.

Bibliography

American College of Obstetricians and Gynecologists. General management of pediatric gynecology patients. In: Guidelines for Adolescent Health Care. Washington, DC: ACOG; 2011. pp. 172–192.

Bayerl C, Feller G, Goerdt S. Experience in treating molluscum contagiosum in children with imiquimod 5% cream. Br J Dermatol 2003;149 Suppl 66:25–9.

Carel JC, Eugster EA, Rogol A, Ghizzoni L, Palmert MR, Antoniazzi F, et al. Consensus statement on the use of gonadotropin-releasing hormone analogs in children. ESPE-LWPES GnRH Analogs Consensus Conference Group. Pediatrics 2009;123:e752–62.

Davis AJ, Emans SJ. Human papilloma virus infection in the pediatric and adolescent patient. J Pediatr 1989;115:1–9.

Emans SJ, Laufer MR, Goldstein DP. Pediatric and adolescent gynecology. 5th ed. Philadelphia (PA): Lippincott Williams & Wilkins; 2005.

Kaplowitz PB. Treatment of central precocious puberty. Curr Opin Endocrinol Diabetes Obes 2009;16:31–6.

Kaplowitz PB, Oberfield SE. Reexamination of the age limit for defining when puberty is precocious in girls in the United States: implications for evaluation and treatment. Drug and Therapeutics and Executive Committees of the Lawson Wilkins Pediatric Endocrine Society. Pediatrics 1999;104:936–41.

Lewin LC. Sexually transmitted infections in preadolescent children. J Pediatr Health Care 2007;21:153–61.

Liota E, Smith KJ, Buckley R, Menon P, Skelton H. Imiquimod therapy for molluscum contagiosum. J Cutan Med Surg 2000;4:76–82.

Majewski S, Pniewski T, Malejczyk M, Jablonska S. Imiquimod is highly effective for extensive, hyperproliferative condyloma in children. Pediatr Dermatol 2003;20:440–42.

Nelson KC, Morrell DS. Spreading bumps: molluscum contagiosum in the pediatric population. Pediatr Ann 2007;36:814, 816–8.

Papp JR, Schachter J, Gaydos CA, Van Der Pol B. Recommendations for the laboratory-based detection of Chlamydia trachomatis and Neisseria gonorrhoeae–2014. Division of STD Prevention, National Center for HIV/AIDS, Viral Hepatitis, STD, and TB Prevention, CDC. MMWR Recomm Rep 2014;63(RR02):1–19.

Poindexter G, Morrell DS. Anogenital pruritus: lichen sclerosus in children. Pediatr Ann 2007;36:785–91.

Protecting children from sexual abuse by health care providers. American Academy of Pediatrics Committee on Child Abuse and Neglect. Pediatrics 2011;128:407–26.

Sanfilippo JS, Lara-Torre E, Edmonds DK, Templeman C, editors. Clinical pediatric and adolescent gynecology. New York (NY): Informa Healthcare; 2009.

Siegfried EC, Frasier LD. Anogenital warts in children. Adv Dermatol 1997;12:141–66; discussion 167.

Smolinski KN, Yan AC. How and when to treat molluscum contagiosum and warts in children. Pediatr Ann 2005;34:211–21.

Styne DM, Cuttler L. Abnormal pubertal development. In: Rudolph CD, Rudolph AM, Lister GE, First LR, Gershon AA, editors. Rudolph's pediatrics. 22nd ed. New York (NY): McGraw Hill Medical; 2011. p. 2077–86.

Tschudy MM, Arcara KM, editors. The Harriet Lane handbook: a manual for pediatric house officers. The Harriet Lane Service, Children's Medical and Surgical Center of the Johns Hopkins Hospital. 19th ed. Philadelphia (PA): Elsevier Mosby; 2012.

Vaginitis. ACOG Practice Bulletin No. 72. American College of Obstetricians and Gynecologists. Obstet Gynecol 2006;107:1195–206.

Resources

American Academy of Pediatrics. Bright Futures™. Available at: http://brightfutures.aap.org/index.html. Retrieved September 27, 2013.

American Academy of Pediatrics. Red book: report of the Committee on Infectious Diseases. 29th ed. Elk Grove Village (IL): American Academy of Pediatrics; 2012.

Kellogg N. The evaluation of sexual abuse in children. American Academy of Pediatrics Committee on Child Abuse and Neglect. Pediatrics 2005;116:506–12.

North American Society for Pediatric and Adolescent Gynecology. Available at: http://www.naspag.org. Retrieved September 27, 2013.

Sexual assault. Committee Opinion No. 592. American College of Obstetricians and Gynecologists. Obstet Gynecol 2014;123:905–9.

Workowski KA, Berman S. Sexually transmitted diseases treatment guidelines, 2010. Centers for Disease Control and Prevention [published erratum appears in MMWR Morb Mortal Wkly Rep 2011;60:18]. MMWR Recomm Rep 2010;59:1–110.

ADOLESCENTS

Assessment of an adolescent's developmental stage is necessary to guide the provision of appropriate preventive health care. Adolescents of the same age are often at different stages of pubertal, psychosocial, and cognitive development. Understanding these stages, providing anticipatory guidance about these stages to patients and their parents or guardians, and tailoring care to the patient's developmental stage is essential to obstetrician–gynecologists and all other health care providers who treat adolescents.

Adolescent Development

Adolescence is a time of psychosocial, cognitive, and physical development as young people make the transition from childhood to adulthood. Physical and cognitive development usually occur on different timetables and are rarely synchronous. Therefore, the obstetrician–gynecologist may encounter adolescents who have matured physically but not cognitively. Most young adolescents (12–14-year-olds) should be expected to be concrete thinkers with poor or inconsistent abstract reasoning or problem-solving skills. Middle-aged adolescents (15–17-year-olds) often assume they are invulnerable. They may assume, for example, that risks apply to their friends but not to themselves. Generally, older adolescents (18–21-year-olds) have acquired problem-solving abilities and have relatively consistent abstract reasoning. Thus, the clinical approach to counseling a cognitively younger adolescent will differ from the approach taken with a cognitively older adolescent or an adult.

An adolescent's initial visit for reproductive health guidance, screening, and provision of preventive services should take place between the ages of 13 years and 15 years. The exact timing and scope of the initial visit will depend on the individual girl and her physical and emotional development. Gynecologic problems may necessitate a visit at an earlier age (see also the "Pediatric Gynecology" section earlier in Part 3). The initial visit primarily establishes rapport between the obstetrician–gynecologist and the young woman; it generally does not include an internal pelvic examination. However, a full pelvic examination may be necessary when indicated by the medical history (eg, pubertal aberrancy, abnormal bleeding, or pelvic pain) (see Box 3-25 and Box 3-26). The timing of subsequent visits should be based on need but should include an annual visit for health guidance and assessment.

The primary health risks for adolescents are behavioral, such as a sedentary lifestyle, poor diet, smoking, alcohol and drug use, driving under the influence of drugs or alcohol, violence, early initiation of sexual activity, and poor use of contraception and sexually transmitted infection (STI) protection. Evidence indicates that knowledge-based education is not as successful in altering these behaviors as skill-based, communication-based, or activity-related strategies. For example, the gynecologist faced with a 15-year-old with an STI may have more success in preventing future infection by role-playing teen-to-teen communication strategies or discussing avoidance strategies (such as avoiding parties that serve alcohol), or discussing how to acquire and use condoms if the patient plans on continuing to be sexually active. The same amount of time spent discussing only the hazards of sexual activity (eg, potential for pregnancy and STIs) is likely to be less effective. Health care providers should provide the best possible

---

Box 3-25. Normal Menstrual Cycles in Young Females

Menarche (median age):	12.43 years
Mean cycle interval:	32.2 days in first gynecologic year
Menstrual cycle interval:	typically 21–45 days
Menstrual flow length:	7 days or less
Menstrual product use:	three to six pads or tampons per day

Reprinted from Menstruation in girls and adolescents: using the menstrual cycle as a vital sign. ACOG Committee Opinion No. 349. American College of Obstetricians and Gynecologists. Obstet Gynecol 2006;108:1323–8.

Box 3-26. Menstrual Conditions That May Require Evaluation

Menstrual periods that
- have not started within 3 years of thelarche
- have not started by 13 years of age with no signs of pubertal development
- have not started by 14 years of age with signs of hirsutism
- have not started by 14 years of age with a history or examination suggestive of excessive exercise or eating disorder
- have not started by 14 years of age with concerns about genital outflow tract obstruction or anomaly
- have not started by 15 years of age
- are regular, occurring monthly, and then become markedly irregular
- occur more frequently than every 21 days or less frequently than every 45 days
- occur 90 days apart even for one cycle
- last more than 7 days
- require frequent pad or tampon changes (soaking more than one every 1–2 hours)

Reprinted from Menstruation in girls and adolescents: using the menstrual cycle as a vital sign. ACOG Committee Opinion No. 349. American College of Obstetricians and Gynecologists. Obstet Gynecol 2006;108:1323–8.

care to respond to the needs of their adolescent patients. This care, at a minimum, should include comprehensive reproductive health services, such as sexuality education; counseling; mental health assessment; diagnosis and treatment regarding pubertal development; access to contraceptives and abortion; pregnancy-related care; and the prevention, diagnosis, and treatment of STIs. Efforts to include partners in services and counseling when appropriate may be helpful to the adolescent. If the patient is sexually active, appropriate screening should be performed (see also "The Physical Examination and Screening" later in this section).

Because the primary health risks to adolescents are behavioral, screening for behavioral risk factors is critical. In addition, it is important to screen for eating disorders and other weight issues, blood pressure problems, and mental health disturbances (such as anxiety; depression; and physical, sexual, and emotional abuse). Other components of the visit should include a review of immunization status and provision of appropriate vaccinations, including the human papillomavirus vaccine. Many practices use written screening questionnaires. It may be helpful to use a questionnaire developed specifically for adolescents. The American College of Obstetricians and Gynecologists (the College) provides an adolescent visit record and adolescent visit and parent questionnaire in Appendix A of *Guidelines for Adolescent Health Care* (see Bibliography).

Ideally, the adolescent preventive visit also involves a parent or guardian. Parents can be counseled on normal adolescent development issues and strategies to deal with adolescent behavioral health risks. The College recommends parental counseling sessions three times during the adolescent years as part of preventive care: at least once during their child's early adolescence, once during middle adolescence, and preferably once during late adolescence.

Confidentiality and Consent in Adolescent Health Care

Confidentiality refers to protection of the privileged and private nature of information shared during a health care encounter and other information and records about the encounter. Concerns about confidentiality are a major obstacle to the delivery of health care to adolescents. Although ensuring confidentiality is relatively simple when providing services to adults, providing the same degree of confidentiality protection to adolescents is usually less straightforward. The legal status of a minor and legal requirements for parental consent before the provision of medical services often encumber the patient–clinician relationship or place limits on the potential for protection of confidentiality. Confidentiality sometimes is interpreted to be a type of secrecy. This philosophy is counterproductive. Parents and physicians share a common goal—the health and well-being of the adolescent. The philosophy should be one of collaboration to maximize the likelihood of raising a healthy adolescent.

A confidential relationship can facilitate the open disclosure of health histories and risky behaviors that require medical intervention and might otherwise be hidden. However, concerns about confidentiality can be significant barriers to adolescents seeking reproductive care and providing accurate historical information. Common risk-taking behaviors and problems that adolescents may not share with their parents include eating disorders, tobacco use, substance use, sexual activity, and date rape. Many parents of sexually active adolescents are aware of the fact that, or strongly suspect that, their child is sexually active. In some cases and with the adolescent's permission, the clinician can facilitate the adolescent's discussing this activity with her parent(s) or guardian(s). However, some sexually active adolescents would avoid a reproductive health visit or not disclose sexual activity if the clinician did not clarify that this information was confidential.

Adolescent confidentiality also may be compromised by economic considerations because few adolescents have the ability to pay for health care services without the aid of a parent or other adult. Moreover, explanations of benefit forms issued by insurers are sent to the policyholders, usually the parent, which also could compromise the confidentiality of care received by adolescents.

Physicians should work with their office staff to establish office procedures and routines that safeguard the privacy of their adolescent patients whenever possible. Office personnel should recognize the issues of confidentiality relating to billing, reviewing claims, and reporting laboratory results. The handling of these issues should be communicated clearly to the adolescent and any involved parents or guardians during the visit. When these mechanisms and procedures compromise a patient's request for confidentiality, policies should be implemented that allow payment alternatives, such as reduced fees, sliding scales, and timed installment payments; patient referral to a practice or agency where subsidized care is offered; or both.

LEGAL CONSIDERATIONS

Clinicians should be familiar with federal and state laws that affect confidentiality and the current state statutes on the rights of minors to consent to health care services. State laws mandate the reporting of suspected physical or sexual abuse of minors to the appropriate authority. All states require consent for the treatment of a minor from a person legally entitled to authorize such care. Exceptions to this requirement for consent vary by state. Examples of exceptions include the following:

- Emergencies, when immediate treatment is needed to safeguard the life or health of the minor

- Treatment of "emancipated minors," including minors who are married, who are members of the armed forces, who live apart from their parents and are self-supporting, and who are themselves parents

- Specific health care services, such as contraceptive services, prenatal care and delivery, STI services, human immunodeficiency virus (HIV) testing and treatment, treatment for drug and alcohol abuse, and mental health treatment, when protected by state law

In these cases, minors generally have the right to privacy and the right to prevent clinicians from disclosing information about the care they receive. Each state has different regulations, and clinicians should become aware of those that apply to their practices. A listing of state laws that is updated monthly is available (www.guttmacher.org/statecenter/); state medical societies also may be able to provide useful resources (www.ama-assn.org/ama/pub/about-ama/our-people/the-federation-medicine/state-medical-society-websites.page).

Courts have increasingly recognized the growing independence of minors and the seriousness of their health care needs. Case law in some jurisdictions has established the right of a "mature minor" to consent to some forms of health care without prior parental consent. A mature minor generally is defined as an adolescent younger than the age of majority—set at 18 years in most states—who, although living at home as a dependent, demonstrates the cognitive maturity to give informed consent. When deciding whether to accept a court-determined mature minor as a patient, clinicians should evaluate their personal views. If their own views on autonomy and confidentiality would conflict with the provision of medical care to a minor declared independent by the courts, the patient would be better served by a referral to a physician experienced in such care. A minor's right to obtain an abortion without parental consent or notification is one area in which the rights of a minor frequently have been restricted statutorily. Many states have adopted mandatory parental consent or notification laws of some form, with an alternative allowing for judicial bypass in lieu of involving a parent or guardian.

ADDRESSING CONFIDENTIALITY

Adolescents are more likely to develop trusting relationships with their health care providers when the issue of confidentiality has been addressed satisfactorily. Clinicians should discuss confidentiality with each adolescent and, as appropriate, with her parent(s) or guardian(s) during the initial visit, which helps establish rapport and outline expectations. Table 3-13 describes the logistics of an adolescent office visit that supports confidentiality.

Parents and adolescents should be informed that they each have a private relationship with the clinician and should be made aware of any restrictions on confidentiality. For example, it should be explained that if the adolescent discloses any risk of significant bodily harm to herself or others, or if the clinician suspects physical or sexual abuse, the clinician will breach confidentiality. Practitioners should encourage and facilitate communication between a minor and her parent(s) or guardian(s) and should emphasize their shared goal of the health and well-being of the minor. During the course of the visit, clinicians are encouraged to speak individually with the adolescent and her parent(s) or guardian(s), allowing for maximal information to be shared and for each to feel included in decision making. Physicians should reassure parents that they will encourage the adolescent to include her parents in important health decisions. The goal is to encourage and facilitate family communication; maintaining confidentiality need not preclude working toward this goal.

The Physical Examination and Screening

Appropriate physical examination, laboratory testing, and immunizations are outlined in the periodic assessment for 13–18-year-olds (see also

Table 3-13. An Adolescent Office Visit That Supports Confidentiality

In Consultation With	The Physician Should
Patient and parent(s) or guardian(s)	Outline structure of visit
	Obtain general medical and family history
	Discuss confidentiality
	Address parental concerns*
Patient	Obtain health history, including risk-taking behaviors
	Address patient concerns
	Provide health guidance
	Address billing issues
Patient†	Perform physical examination, as indicated
Patient	Summarize findings and recommendations
	Determine parental involvement
	Determine method of notification of laboratory results
	Summarize findings and recommendations, as appropriate
Patient and parent(s) or guardian(s)	Provide guidance about adolescent development to parent
	Address confidentiality issues regarding billing issues

*If the parent wishes to speak with you about her concerns privately, this should be done before the confidential visit with the patient.

†Parent may be present, at patient's discretion.

Reprinted from American College of Obstetricians and Gynecologists. Confidentiality in adolescent health care. In: Guidelines for adolescent health care [CD-ROM]. 2nd ed. ed. Washington, DC: American College of Obstetricians and Gynecologists; 2011. p. 9–17.

"Well-Woman Care: Assessments & Recommendations" at www.acog.org/wellwoman). Pelvic examination is not a routine part of the annual assessment in females 13–18 years of age unless medically indicated. The College recommends beginning cervical cytology screening at age 21 years, irrespective of the sexual activity of the patient. This is based on the current understanding of human papillomavirus (HPV) infection in the adolescent patient and the pathophysiology of cervical cancer (see also the "Well-Woman Annual Health Assessment" and "Cancer Screening and Prevention" sections earlier in Part 3 and the "Abnormal Cervical Cytology" section in Part 4). Testing for STIs is recommended for all sexually active adolescents and can be performed without the need for cervical sampling (see also "Sexually Transmitted Infections" later in this section).

Tanner staging of breast and pubic hair development should be included in the recommended physical examination. The College publishes pamphlets to educate the adolescent about her changing body, menstruation, and the first gynecologic visit (see Resources). Evaluation of the menstrual cycle should be included. Clinicians should ask at every visit for the first date of the patient's last menstrual period.

PUBERTAL PROGRESS AND MENSTRUAL HISTORY

Pubertal progress and menstrual history should be obtained. A variety of menstrual conditions should prompt evaluation, including absence of menses with no signs of pubertal development by age 13 years; absence of menses within 3 years of thelarche; and absence of menses by age 15 years. Absence of menses by age 14 years with signs of hirsutism or concerns of excessive exercise, eating disorders, or genital outflow tract abnormalities also deserves evaluation (see Box 3-26).

Obstetrician–gynecologists should counsel adolescent patients about the proper use of tampons to decrease the risk of toxic shock syndrome. Patients should be advised to use tampons with the lowest absorbency needed to absorb their menstrual flow, change their tampon at least every 4–8 hours (or more often on the first days of their period), read all of the instructions that come with tampons, and avoid the use of tampons when they do not have their period.

HYPERTENSION

All adolescents should be screened annually for hypertension. Guidelines for blood pressure screening in adolescents have been developed by the National Heart, Lung, and Blood Institute National High Blood Pressure Education Program Working Group on High Blood Pressure in Children and Adolescents. Hypertension in adolescence is diagnosed after three consecutive blood pressure readings are above the 95th percentile on three separate occasions. Body size directly affects normal blood pressure, so a blood pressure interpreted as normal in a mature reproductive female may represent hypertension in a young adolescent.

LIPID DISORDERS

To determine their risk of developing hyperlipidemia and adult coronary heart disease, adolescents should be screened by history and selected adolescents should undergo lipid testing. For more information, see the guidelines developed by the National Heart, Lung, and Blood Institute Expert Panel on Blood Cholesterol in Children and Adolescents in the Bibliography.

OBESITY AND EATING DISORDERS

All adolescents should be screened annually for obesity and eating disorders by determining weight and stature, calculating a body mass index (BMI) for age, and asking about body image, eating patterns, activity levels, and sedentary behavior.

Obesity

The Centers for Disease Control and Prevention (CDC) defines an adolescent as obese if she has a BMI in or above the 95th percentile for her age. An adolescent whose BMI is equal to or greater than the 85th percentile-for-age, but less than the 95th percentile-for-age is considered to be overweight. A calculator that determines adolescent BMI for age percentile is available at http://apps.nccd.cdc.gov/dnpabmi/Calculator.aspx. Adolescents with a BMI in or above the 95th percentile for age should have an in-depth dietary and health assessment to determine psychosocial morbidity and the risk of obesity-related disease. Early referral to a nutrition program skilled in caring for adolescents and an exercise specialist may be warranted.

Overweight adolescents also should have a dietary and health assessment to determine psychosocial morbidity and risk of future cardiovascular disease if they have any of the following:

- Their BMI has increased by two or more units during the previous 12 months

- There is a family history of premature heart disease, obesity, hypertension, or diabetes mellitus
- They express concern about their weight
- They have elevated blood pressure or serum cholesterol levels

Obstetrician–gynecologists are strongly encouraged to provide these assessments. It is important to note that weight loss is recommended for adolescents only in certain circumstances. Older overweight and obese adolescents who have completed linear growth or those with comorbidities (such as polycystic ovary syndrome) who are obese, for example, may require weight loss. More often, among adolescents who are still growing in height, the goal is to slow the rate of weight gain while achieving normal growth and development.

Eating Disorders

All adolescents should be screened annually for eating disorders, using common symptoms and weight formulas as a guide. Substantial weight loss or patient preoccupation with dieting should alert the obstetrician–gynecologist to the possibility of an eating disorder. In addition, results of vital sign testing and a careful cardiac examination to listen for arrhythmias may help to confirm the presence of eating disorders and identify patients who need emergency hospitalization (see also the "Psychosocial Issues" section later in Part 3).

SEXUALLY TRANSMITTED INFECTIONS

All sexually active adolescents should be counseled regarding safe sex practices and contraception. In addition, routine screening for chlamydial infection, gonorrhea, and HIV is recommended for all sexually active adolescents. Urine screening for chlamydial infection and gonorrhea should be done if pelvic examination is otherwise not indicated or circumstances do not allow for the examination. Despite these recommendations, which are consistent with the CDC and other major medical professional groups, only 40% of eligible women who receive their medical care from commercial or Medicaid health plans are screened for chlamydial infection annually.

Expedited partner therapy is the clinical practice of treating the sex partners of patients, in whom STIs are diagnosed, by providing prescriptions or medications to the patient to take to his or her partner(s) without the health care provider first examining the partner(s). Expedited partner therapy is recommended in the management of gonorrhea and chlamydial infections when the partner is unlikely or unable to otherwise receive in-person evaluation and appropriate treatment. The changes to CDC treatment recommendations to require an intramuscular cephalosporin as first-line treatment for gonorrhea will be an impediment to expedited partner therapy (see Bibliography). In addition, the legality of expedited partner therapy is ambiguous in some states and overt legal impediments exist in others. Clinicians who practice in states where expedited partner therapy is legal should use it for eligible patients (see also the "Sexually Transmitted Infections" section earlier in Part 3).

HUMAN PAPILLOMAVIRUS VACCINATION

Vaccination against HPV is now part of the recommended immunization of young women (see also "Well-Woman Care: Assessments & Recommendations" at www.acog.org/wellwoman). The College recommends HPV vaccination for females aged 9–26 years. Cervical cytology screening recommendations are not affected by HPV vaccination status and should be followed regardless of vaccination status (see also the "Immunizations" section and the "Sexually Transmitted Infections" section earlier in Part 3).

CERVICAL CYTOLOGY SCREENING

Recommendations regarding cervical cytology screening in adolescents underwent marked changes in 2009. It is now recommended that cervical cancer screening should begin at age 21 years, regardless of the sexual activity of the patient. Human papillomavirus infections are very commonly acquired by young women shortly after first intercourse, and most are cleared by the immune system within several years without producing neoplastic changes. Most types of cervical dysplasia in adolescents regress as well. Adolescents are more successful in clearing HPV as compared with older women.

For those adolescents who have previously undergone screening with abnormal results, health care providers should consult the most current guidelines from the American Society for Colposcopy and Cervical Pathology (see Resources). The rationale for the guidelines is that most cervical intraepithelial neoplasia grades 1 and 2 regress in adolescents. Surgical excision or destruction of cervical tissue in a nulliparous adolescent may be detrimental to future fertility and cervical competency (see also the "Abnormal Cervical Cytology" section in Part 4).

Counseling

Screening provides an excellent opportunity to counsel adolescents about healthy lifestyles. Counseling and guidance should be directed at the risk behaviors and issues identified by the history, screening questionnaire, and physical examination.

CALCIUM AND VITAMIN D INTAKE

Most bone mass is achieved between ages 12 years and 20 years. The Institute of Medicine has determined that the recommended dietary allowance of calcium for adolescents aged 9–18 years is 1,300 mg/d. The average calcium intake in adolescent girls is less than 900 mg/d. The preferred approach to meeting these recommendations is through dietary sources. Other approaches include supplements and calcium-fortified foods. Vitamin D has a role in calcium absorption, muscle performance, and balance. The most common sources are fortified milk, cereals, egg yolks, saltwater fish, and liver. The recommended daily allowance of vitamin D for adolescents is 600 international units daily. There are two different types of supplemental vitamin D—vitamin D_3 (cholecalciferol) and vitamin D_2 (ergocalciferol)—which have recently been determined to be equally effective for bone health.

SMOKING

Approximately one quarter of high school seniors currently use tobacco. Females are as likely as males to be smokers. All adolescents should be asked annually about their use of tobacco products, and a cessation plan should be provided for adolescents who smoke or use any tobacco products. The Public Health Service recommends providing adolescent smokers with counseling interventions to aid them in quitting smoking. Because of an adolescent's preoccupation with body image, all adolescents should be counseled on the effects of smoking and other tobacco products on their hair, skin, fingernails, teeth, and breath, as well as on athletic performance. Parents who smoke should be encouraged to stop for their and their children's health benefit. For more information and resources, see also the "Substance Use and Abuse" section earlier in Part 3.

ALCOHOL AND SUBSTANCE ABUSE

Substance and alcohol use are major factors in injuries and deaths in adolescents. They contribute to accidents, homicide, and suicide, which represent the first, third, and fourth leading causes of death in this age group. In addition, adolescents using alcohol and substances are more likely to make poor decisions regarding sexuality or to be involved in date rape situations. All health care providers, including obstetrician–gynecologists, can reduce the harmful effects of substance use and abuse by routinely asking about such use, providing education about substances, assisting patients who wish to discontinue use, and referring when there is evidence of substance abuse or dependence.

Screening is critical. All adolescents should be asked annually about their use of alcohol, illicit drugs, prescription and nonprescription medications, and performance-enhancing drugs. This should be done in private after providing assurances of confidentiality and indications of the limits of confidentiality (eg, evidence of serious harm to self or others). Many state laws protect the confidentiality of minors with regard to substance abuse detection and treatment. Urine screening for drug use without the adolescent's knowledge and consent is not recommended and is illegal in many states. The American Academy of Pediatrics recommends that parental permission is not sufficient for involuntary drug testing of the adolescent with decisional capacity and that testing should be conducted noncovertly, confidentially, and with informed consent in the same context as for other medical conditions.

Adolescents whose substance use endangers their health should receive substance abuse counseling and treatment and be assessed for co-occurring depression, anxiety, and other mental disorders. The American Academy of Pediatrics recommends that parents receive information on how to monitor and prevent alcohol consumption in adolescents. If parents consume alcohol themselves, they should be encouraged to do so in moderation and to restrict their children from consuming their supplies (see also the "Substance Use and Abuse" section earlier in Part 3).

BODY PIERCING AND TATTOOS

Body piercing and tattoos are relatively common. Among adolescents and young adults, body piercings are more common than tattoos. Body piercing may involve the eyebrow, nipple, nasal septum, tongue, lips, navel, labia, and clitoral hood. The evolution of tattoos and body piercing into a more mainstream practice has been propelled by media stars and professional athletes. Studies among adolescents and young adults indicate that the driving forces behind body art include a desire for a form of decoration, enhancement of self-identity, peer acceptance, and group membership. However, in some adolescents, tattoos and piercings may serve as markers for other high-risk behaviors, including violence, substance abuse, and unprotected sexual activity. If an adolescent is planning on having piercings or tattoos, she should be strongly counseled about the potential risks to her health. Piercings and tattoos carry the risk of exposure to viral infections, including HPV, herpes virus, hepatitis B, hepatitis C, hepatitis D, and HIV, although transmission of HIV has not been documented. And, the presence of genital jewelry may increase condom breakage. Noninfectious complications include metal allergies, keloids, sarcoidal tissue reaction, epidermal cyst, torn earlobes, urethral obstruction, and airway obstruction. Based on limited evidence, there also is concern that the piercing of lower back tattoos for epidural anesthesia administration may transfer pigment dyes to the epidural space.

DEPRESSION AND SUICIDE

Depression is common in adolescents, and suicide is the third leading cause of death in this age group. Risk factors for suicide are listed in Box 3-27. Risk is highest when the adolescent can describe a plan for time, location, and means of suicide and has easy access to the means, especially medications or firearms. If an adolescent has any of these risk factors, the follow-up questions noted in Box 3-28 are appropriate. Adolescents who

Box 3-27. Risk Factors for Suicide or Suicide Attempts

- Previous suicide attempts
- Family history of suicide and mental health disorders
- History of self-injurious behavior, such as cutting
- History of alcohol or other substance abuse
- Exposure to other youth who have attempted or committed suicide
- Feelings of sadness, hopelessness, and helplessness
- Expression of thoughts of suicide, death, or dying or strong interest in the afterlife
- Being in a sexual minority (gay, lesbian, bisexual, transgender, and questioning youth) or culturally alienated (eg, recent immigrant)

Reprinted from American College of Obstetricians and Gynecologists. Mental health disorders in adolescents. In: Guidelines for adolescent health care [CD-ROM]. 2nd ed. ed. Washington, DC: American College of Obstetricians and Gynecologists; 2011. p. 85–96.

Box 3-28. Sample Follow-up Questions to Assess Suicide Risk of Adolescents With Risk Factors for Suicide

Questions should be asked in a nonjudgmental, direct, and nonthreatening manner. The clinician may begin with, "Sometimes adolescents dealing with similar issues or problems get very down and start to question life itself. Does this happen to you?"

A positive answer should be followed with questions such as the following:
- "Have you ever thought about suicide or harming yourself?"
- "Are you thinking about suicide now?"
- "Do you have a plan for suicide?" If yes, ask details of the plan.
- "Have you ever attempted suicide in the past?"

When any risk of suicide attempt is identified or admitted, the adolescent should be referred to a crisis mental health agency or emergency department for assessment by a mental health professional.

Reprinted from American College of Obstetricians and Gynecologists. Mental health disorders in adolescents. In: Guidelines for adolescent health care [CD-ROM]. 2nd ed. ed. Washington, DC: American College of Obstetricians and Gynecologists; 2011. p. 85–96.

are suicidal require emergency referral to a mental health professional. Parents should be counseled that children and adolescents should not have access to weapons or firearms or potentially lethal medications. One group of adolescents that deserves special concern and very careful screening are lesbian and bisexual teens who have a high relative risk of depression (see also the "Lesbians and Bisexual Women" section later in Part 3).

Adolescents with severe or recurrent depression should be referred to a mental health professional for therapy. Depression in adolescents is serious in terms of morbidity and mortality. It never should be assumed to be part of normal adolescent moodiness (see also the "Depression" section later in Part 3).

MOTOR VEHICLE ACCIDENTS

Parents and adolescents should be counseled on the prevention of motor vehicle accidents and related injuries, including the use of seat belts and avoiding riding with a driver who is under the influence of drugs or alcohol. A form developed by Students Against Destructive Decisions formalizes an agreement on how adolescents would deal with difficult situations and fosters a discussion with parents on this subject. This form is available through the organization's web site at www.sadd.org/contract.htm. Distracted driving is another growing cause of motor vehicle accidents among teenagers. Adolescents underestimate the dangers associated with distracted driving and overestimate their driving abilities. According to the 2011 Youth Risk Behavior Survey, 32.8% of high school students nationwide had sent text messages or e-mailed while driving a car or other vehicle on at least 1 day during the 30 days before the survey. For more information on education and prevention, see www.sadd.org/issues_distracted.htm.

VIOLENCE

Approximately one third of adolescent murder victims are female, and of them, one third are killed with a firearm. Nearly one half of all violent juvenile rapes, robberies, and assaults occur between noon and 6 PM. Violence perpetrated by girls is increasing. Excessive exposure to the media can cause increased violent behavior and callousness toward violence. Some advocates advise that parents and families reduce the risk by using violence rating systems for television and games and limiting access to media violence. Limiting firearm access and closely supervising adolescents are critical measures for prevention, and encouraging involvement in family activities, clubs, sports, and school also is recommended.

Sexuality

SEXUAL IDENTITY

Children as young as 10 years can recognize their sexual orientation as attraction to a particular sex. By high school, approximately 10% of Minnesota youth responding to a statewide health questionnaire said they were unsure about their orientation, with 4.5% reporting lesbian attraction and 1% reporting lesbian behavior. Lesbian adolescents must navigate the same developmental tasks as heterosexual peers. These tasks include accepting their sexual identity and deciding about sexual behaviors.

Clinicians should word questions regarding sexuality carefully to include same-sex relationships. Referring to a partner rather than a boyfriend is one strategy. The screening questionnaire may include queries on sexual orientation. Clinicians should be aware that the suicide risk is twofold to sixfold greater in gay and lesbian youth, and these adolescents account for almost one third of all completed adolescent suicides. Youth who self-identify as lesbian or gay during high school are also at higher risk of victimization and substance abuse at an earlier age. In addition, they are more likely to engage in sexual risk behaviors than their heterosexual peers. Therefore, screening for STIs is important.

Adolescents who are lesbians face additional challenges in development as they learn to accept their sexual identity. They may find it difficult to ask for, or they may not receive, understanding and acceptance from their parents, family, and friends. Appropriate referrals for counseling and support groups for the lesbian adolescent and her family should be considered (see also the "Lesbians and Bisexual Women" section later in Part 3).

SEXUALITY EDUCATION

The College strongly encourages parents to be involved actively in educating their children about sexuality and employing strategies that reduce the likelihood of adolescent pregnancy. Providing supervision and encouraging family and community activities are excellent strategies.

The College supports the inclusion of comprehensive, medically accurate, age-appropriate sexuality education from kindergarten through 12th grade as an integral part of health education in schools and communities. Sexuality education should encourage young people to delay becoming sexually active and, if sexually active, to use contraception and barrier protection to prevent unintended pregnancy and STIs. These twin goals are essential in all sexuality education programs. The College encourages its members to advocate for, and participate in, sexuality education.

Since the mid-1990s, sexuality education in the United States increasingly has emphasized sexual abstinence and restricted information about contraception and risk reduction. Federal support from 1996 to 2010 for abstinence-only education, along with other factors, had contributed to a growing emphasis on limiting sexuality education so as to exclude accurate instruction about contraception, abortion, and sexual orientation. Abstinence-only education has been criticized for withholding information on contraception and other aspects of human sexuality and for providing information that is not medically accurate. Comprehensive sexuality educational curricula, by contrast, not only promote abstinence but also incorporate reproductive health information, including both the risks and benefits of various methods of contraception, STI prevention, and forms of sexual expression that provide alternatives to intercourse.

Most research of abstinence-only education has shown no effect on delaying sexual initiation, return to abstinence, or number of sexual partners. However, one theory-based abstinence-only program that was not moralistic and did not emphasize abstinence until marriage reduced initiation of sex over the next 2 years. Two thirds of 48 selected comprehensive programs that supported abstinence and the use of condoms and contraceptives for sexually active teens have shown positive effects on behavior, including delayed initiation of sex, decreased number of sexual partners, and increased condom or contraceptive use. None increased sexual activity. However, positive effects across settings depend on carrying out all the original program components rather than implementing only some of them.

The College supports the efforts of communities to implement effective comprehensive sexuality education for adolescents that includes the following components:

- Parental involvement in children's sexuality education
- Scientifically accurate information about sexuality, STIs, contraception, and preventive health care
- Encouragement of abstinence from sexual intercourse as a healthy choice for adolescents, particularly young adolescents
- Efforts to increase effective use of contraceptives, including latex condoms and dual use of condoms with other effective contraceptive methods, by sexually active adolescents
- Efforts to increase availability and use of long-acting reversible contraceptive methods by sexually active adolescents
- Ongoing rigorous evaluation of the effectiveness of a variety of forms of sexuality education in terms of their effects on sexual behavior and contraceptive use, as well as unintended pregnancy and abortion rates

Obstetrician–gynecologists can be resources for support and assistance to sexuality education programs in their communities. Sexuality education is an important component of efforts to decrease unintended pregnancy and STIs. In addition, increased availability of confidential reproductive health services—including family planning; abortion; and services for the prevention, diagnosis, and treatment of STIs—is critical. For more information on sexuality education, see the College's resource *Guidelines for Adolescent Health Care*.

RISK OF PREGNANCY AND DISEASE

Each year in the United States, an estimated 757,000 adolescents become pregnant. More than one half of these pregnancies (56%) end in a live birth, 28% end by abortion, and 15% end by miscarriage or stillbirth. Few adolescents choose to place their children for adoption; most choose to parent their children, a decision that has lifelong consequences. Although

U.S. adolescent pregnancy rates have declined from a previous high of more than 1 million per year, rates still are the highest of any developed nation. The decline in adolescent pregnancy can be attributed to slight declines in sexual activity and increased use of contraception.

The percentage of high school students who reported ever having sexual intercourse declined during 1991–2001 (54.1–45.6%), although it did not change significantly from 2001 to 2011 (45.6–47.4%). The prevalence of high school students reporting current sexual activity decreased from 37.5% in 1991 to 33.7% in 2011. The percentage of high school students who had engaged in sexual intercourse with four or more partners during their lifetime decreased during 1991–2001 (18.7%–14.2%) and then did not change significantly from 2001 to 2011 (14.2–15.3%). Data show that the likelihood of having experienced sexual intercourse increases steadily with age.

Condom use at last coitus among sexually active adolescents increased from 46.2 % in 1991 to 60.2% in 2011. More contraceptive options are also available to adolescent women. Most notably, the use of intrauterine devices among adolescents has been found to be safe and effective. Intrauterine devices and contraceptive implants can be offered to adolescents as a reliable form of birth control. Emergency contraception may be used to prevent pregnancy after an unprotected or inadequately protected act of sexual intercourse (see also the "Family Planning" section earlier in Part 3).

Girls from higher-income households are more likely than those from lower-income households to use contraception at first coitus and to abort their pregnancy. The combination of these factors results in fewer pregnant adolescents in affluent schools compared with schools in lower socioeconomic areas, sometimes giving the erroneous impression that coital activity is significantly less common in adolescents from higher socioeconomic backgrounds.

It has been estimated that although young people aged 15–24 years represent only 25% of the sexually experienced population, they acquire nearly one half of all new STIs. The CDC estimates that more than 1 in 10 sexually active female adolescents have chlamydial infections. It also is estimated that at least one half of all new HIV infections in the United

States are among individuals younger than 25 years. Adolescent females are at greatest risk of STIs because they often fail to use condoms correctly and consistently, are biologically more susceptible to infection, frequently have multiple sequential sexual partners, and face many obstacles to the use of health care (see also the "Sexually Transmitted Infections" section earlier in Part 3).

Noncoital sexual activity most commonly co-occurs with coital activity. Oral and anal sex are more common among adolescents who have already had vaginal coitus. According to the 2006–2008 National Survey of Family Growth, 45% of females aged 15–19 years reported having had oral sex with an opposite-sex partner. Most adolescents do not use barrier protection for noncoital sexual activities. It is critical to screen adolescents for noncoital sexual activity and to educate them that these activities carry a risk of acquiring STIs and about ways to protect themselves. Adolescents may not consider themselves "sexually active" if they are engaging only in noncoital sexual activity (see also the "Sexually Transmitted Infections" section earlier in Part 3).

Unintended Pregnancy Options Counseling

Rates of unintended pregnancy are higher for adolescents than for any other age group. In the event of an unintended pregnancy, the adolescent who is ambivalent about her pregnancy, like any patient, should be counseled about her options: continuing the pregnancy to term and raising the infant, continuing the pregnancy to term and placing the infant for legal adoption, or terminating the pregnancy. In cases of conscientious objection, where a clinician declines to provide requested care to a patient for moral or religious reasons, transfer of primary clinical responsibility to another clinician is in the patient's best interest. The discussion with the patient also should determine her wishes as to what counseling resources should be offered to her partner, if any, or what information should be given to her parents (if she is a dependent adolescent). Some states require parental notification or consent before a minor can obtain an abortion. In some states, pregnancy in individuals younger than a certain age is considered child abuse and must be reported. All health care providers should be aware of their state laws in this regard.

SEXUAL AND REPRODUCTIVE COERCION, SEXUAL ASSAULT, AND SEXUAL ABUSE

Sexual and reproductive coercion, sexual assault, and sexual abuse are widespread in the adolescent population. Obstetrician–gynecologists are in a unique position to address these issues and provide screening and clinical interventions to improve health outcomes. Because evidence demonstrates that violence and poor reproductive health outcomes are strongly linked, health care providers should screen adolescent girls for intimate partner violence and reproductive and sexual coercion at periodic intervals, such as annual examinations and new patient visits. Health care providers also should screen routinely for a history of sexual assault.

Sexual and Reproductive Coercion

Sexual coercion includes a range of behaviors that a partner may use related to sexual decision making to pressure or coerce a person to have sex without using physical force. These behaviors include repeatedly pressuring a partner to have sex; threatening to end a relationship if the person does not have sex; forcing sex without a condom or not allowing other prophylaxis use; intentionally exposing a partner to an STI, including HIV; or threatening retaliation if notified of a positive STI test result. In the 2006–2010 National Survey of Family Growth, females aged 18–24 years whose first coitus was before age 20 years were asked about whether or not their first sexual intercourse experience was desired. Of women whose age at first coitus was 17 years or younger, 27.8% reported that their first sex was not voluntary. For those who had first sex at age 14 years or younger, 18% reported that they "really didn't want it to happen,"compared with 8.9% among those who delayed first sex to age 18 years or 19 years.

Reproductive coercion is related to behavior that interferes with contraception use and pregnancy. The most common forms of reproductive coercion include sabotage of contraceptive methods, pregnancy coercion, and pregnancy pressure. In a qualitative study of adolescent females, 25% reported that their abusive male partners were trying to get them pregnant through interference with planned contraception, forcing the female partners to hide their contraceptive methods.

Sexual Assault and Abuse

Sexual assault is a crime of violence and aggression and encompasses a continuum of sexual activity that ranges from sexual coercion to contact abuse (unwanted kissing, touching, or fondling) to rape. Because definitions vary among states, sexual assault is sometimes used interchangeably with rape. The Federal Bureau of Investigation uses the following recently revised, more comprehensive definition of rape to track statistics for the annual Uniform Crime Report: "Penetration, no matter how slight, of the vagina or anus with any body part or object, or oral penetration by a sex organ of another person, without the consent of the victim." The Federal Bureau of Investigation's change does not affect definitions under federal or state criminal laws; the new definition only applies for statistical purposes, so that crimes under existing state laws will now be counted by the federal government.

Methods of obtaining data influence estimates of the incidence and prevalence of rape and sexual assault. Data compiled from reports to law enforcement officials underestimate the incidence of sexual assault. The 2010 National Intimate Partner and Sexual Violence Survey reported that 42% of female rape victims experienced their first completed rape before the age of 18 years.

Victims of sexual assault who are of reproductive age are at risk of unintended pregnancy and STIs. Unintended pregnancy is especially high among adolescents who are assaulted because of their relatively low use of contraception. Therefore, emergency contraception and prophylaxis for STIs should be available and provided. Health care providers who have an objection to providing emergency contraception should arrange for provision of emergency contraception, as indicated. Sexual assault victims are also at risk of mental health conditions, such as posttraumatic stress disorder. The physician who examines victims of sexual assault has a responsibility to be aware of state and local statutory or policy requirements that may involve the use of evidence-gathering kits.

The age at which an adolescent may consent to sexual intercourse varies by state and is generally 16–18 years. Sexual assault that occurs in childhood, defined by most states as younger than 14 years, is considered child abuse. Laws requiring the reporting of child abuse, including sexual abuse, exist in every state. The College, along with the American Academy of Family Physicians, the American Academy of Pediatrics, and the Society for Adolescent Health and Medicine, support the following guidance:

- Sexual activity and sexual abuse are not synonymous. It should not be assumed that adolescents who are sexually active are, by definition, being abused. Many adolescents have consensual sexual relationships.

- It is critical that adolescents who are sexually active receive appropriate confidential health care and counseling.

- Open and confidential communication between the health care provider and the adolescent patient, together with careful clinical assessment, can identify most sexual abuse cases.

- Physicians and other health providers must know their state laws and report cases of sexual abuse to the proper authority, in accordance with those laws, after discussion with the adolescent and parent, as appropriate.

It is critical to empower adolescents with preventive strategies in an attempt to avoid future violence. This must be done with skill for patients who have already been abused, as they may conclude they should or could have prevented the previous abuse and put blame on themselves rather than the perpetrator. Many adolescents have not developed the skills to recognize and avoid potentially dangerous dating or social situations. It is important to counsel adolescents that alcohol and substance use increases vulnerability to sexual assault. Adolescents should be aware of the dangers of date rape drugs and know how to avoid being a victim (see Resources). Some adolescents have distorted perceptions of violence and fail to recognize a partner's behavior as violent. (For more information on sexual assault and abuse, see the "Abuse" section later in Part 3.)

Adolescents With Disabilities

Adolescence is a time of transition for all teenagers and their families. For an adolescent with physical or intellectual and developmental disabilities, the onset of menstrual cycles, the expression of sexuality, and the possibility of pregnancy can provide significant challenges for the patient and her caregivers. Adolescent girls, particularly those who have had a disability from early childhood, require a smooth transition from the care of the pediatrician or family physician, who often provided and coordinated all health care services, to a multitude of health care providers, who may not offer health care management services. It is incumbent upon the obstetrician–gynecologist to participate in service coordination for the adolescent with disabilities, as well as to provide direct gynecologic and reproductive care. A positive, respectful experience in early adolescence can affect the adolescent's self-esteem and willingness to seek out future reproductive health services.

Knowledge of the adolescent's preferred mode of communication and the health care provider's patience are critical to ensure optimal health care delivery. It is important to make every attempt to address and communicate with the adolescent directly as well as with her caregiver.

Ascertaining the capacity of the adolescent with intellectual and developmental disabilities to provide informed consent can be complex. Multiple interviews over the course of time and involving a person trained in communication with a person with intellectual and developmental disabilities may be required to ascertain the patient's comprehension of the nature of the procedure and its effect on her. Even when it is determined that the adolescent does not have the capacity to consent, it is important to gain her assent before commencing a procedure. The determination of the capacity to consent should be made based on the level of risk to the patient. Increased scrutiny is necessary with more invasive or risky procedures. As with all adolescents, it is important for the health care provider to be aware of state regulations regarding the nature of the activities to which an adolescent can legally consent and to note that these statutes can vary from state to state.

Guidelines for primary and preventive reproductive health care—such as cervical cytology screening, STI screening, pelvic examination, psychosocial risk screening, and review of immunization status—are the same as those for adolescents without disabilities (see also "The Physical Examination and Screening" earlier in this section). If an external genital examination, speculum examination, or bimanual examination is clinically indicated in an adolescent with disabilities, it may be necessary to alter the position and method of examination. (For more information, see the "Women With Disabilities" section later in Part 3). As for all adolescents, the patient's medical history should include screening for the following: eating disorders; tobacco, alcohol, and drug use; depression; abuse; sexual activity; and sexual abuse. Immunizations are important for all adolescents with disabilities and could be especially important for those who have immunosuppression issues. In general, the patient's pediatrician will have followed the recommended schedule of vaccinations by age. Because of the high risk of sexual assault for adolescents with disabilities, HPV vaccination is strongly recommended as early as possible, beginning at age 9 years.

Frequently, caregivers may look to the obstetrician–gynecologist for guidance about menstrual issues. Requests for amenorrhea for menstrual manipulation are frequent, and the health care provider should offer information and counseling in this area. Abnormal uterine bleeding assessment and therapy in adolescents with disabilities follows the same general approach as that of patients without disabilities except for special considerations, such as menstrual hygiene and the higher risk of abnormal bleeding that is due to medical conditions. A menstrual history should be discussed in detail to determine the effects on the patient's health and well-being. Possible causes of menstrual difficulties in adolescents with disabilities include obesity, thyroid disease, genetic disorders, antiepileptic and psychiatric medications, polycystic ovary syndrome, and cervicitis. The most important issue to determine is how the bleeding, whether it is normal or irregular, affects the adolescent's life. Clinicians also should always consider the possibility that any patients with irregular bleeding could be pregnant. If, after evaluation, the adolescent, her family, and the health care provider decide that limiting menstruation is warranted, the least invasive, least harmful, and most reversible intervention should be used. Hysterectomy is very rarely indicated for adolescents with disabilities (eg, for cancer treatment). Abnormal bleeding is almost always managed medically for a teenager without disabilities. The same should be true for adolescents with disabilities. For more information on evaluation and management, see the "Abnormal Genital Bleeding" section in Part 4.

The obstetrician–gynecologist can offer guidance regarding the expression of healthy, safe, and consensual sexual activity for adolescents with disabilities and address parental concerns about their vulnerability to abuse and pregnancy. If the adolescent indicates she is interested in sexual activity, the clinician should assess her ability to consent to voluntary sexual activity and her history of sexual activity. Abuse is often a concern of families when an adolescent with disabilities, with or without cognitive impairment, reaches puberty and menarche. Rates of sexual assault are high among individuals with disabilities. Clinicians must be vigilant in looking for signs, symptoms, or changes in behavior that may be indicators of sexual abuse in those patients who may not be able to communicate details of their abuse.

The degree of cognitive impairment and physical disability of the adolescent and access to appropriate education and supervision greatly affects the contraception methods that best meet the needs of adolescent with disabilities. It is critical to assess who is requesting the contraception and to assess the adolescent's safety as well as her ability to consent to sexual activity. Pregnancy and parenting for adolescents with physical or intellectual and developmental disabilities may have unique medical and social aspects, but rarely are precluded by the disability itself. Discussions regarding the implications of pregnancy and parenting should be initiated with all adolescents in the context of the educational sessions on sexuality and contraception.

The onset of menses and the awakening of sexuality can be unsettling to patients and their families. Obstetricians–gynecologists have the obligation to do no harm, involve the adolescent with disabilities as much as possible in any decisions, and ensure that she is comfortable, safe, and prepared for her life as a woman of reproductive age, whatever her abilities may be. Please see the College's resource *Reproductive Health Care for Adolescents With Disabilities* for more information.

Bibliography

Access to emergency contraception. Committee Opinion No. 542. American College of Obstetricians and Gynecologists. Obstet Gynecol 2012;120:1250–3.

Addressing health risks of noncoital sexual activity. Committee Opinion No. 582. American College of Obstetricians and Gynecologists. Obstet Gynecol 2013;122:1378–83.

Adolescents and long-acting reversible contraception: implants and intrauterine devices. Committee Opinion No. 539. American College of Obstetricians and Gynecologists. Obstet Gynecol 2012;120:983–8.

Adoption. Committee Opinion No. 528. American College of Obstetricians and Gynecologists. Obstet Gynecol 2012;119:1320–4.

American College of Obstetricians and Gynecologists. Guidelines for adolescent health care [CD-ROM]. 2nd ed. ed. Washington, DC: American College of Obstetricians and Gynecologists; 2011.

American College of Obstetricians and Gynecologists. Reproductive health care for adolescents with disabilities: supplement to Guidelines for adolescent health care. 2nd ed. ed. Washington, DC: American College of Obstetricians and Gynecologists; 2012. Available at: http://www.acog.org/Resources_And_Publications/Guidelines_for_Adolescent_Health_Care/Reproductive_Health_Care_for_Adolescents_With_Disabilities. Retrieved July 23, 2013.

American Medical Association. State medical society websites. Available at: http://www.ama-assn.org/ama/pub/about-ama/our-people/the-federation-medicine/state-medical-society-websites.page. Retrieved September 26, 2013.

Black MC, Basile KC, Breiding MJ, Smith SG, Walters ML, Merrick MT, et al. The National Intimate Partner and Sexual Violence Survey (NISVS): 2010 summary report. Atlanta (GA): National Center for Injury Prevention and Control; Centers for Disease Control and Prevention; 2011. Available at: http://www.cdc.gov/ViolencePrevention/pdf/NISVS_Report2010-a.pdf. Retrieved July 30, 2013.

Centers for Disease Control and Prevention. Guidance on the use of expedited partner therapy in the treatment of gonorrhea. Atlanta (GA): CDC; 2012. Available at: http://www.cdc.gov/std/ept/GC-EPT-GuidanceNov-2012.pdf. Retrieved July 29, 2013.

Chamberlain L, Levenson R. Addressing intimate partner violence, reproductive and sexual coercion: a guide for obstetric, gynecologic and reproductive health care settings. 2nd ed. Washington, DC: San Francisco (CA): American College of Obstetricians and Gynecologists; Futures Without Violence; 2012. Available at: http://www.futureswithoutviolence.org/userfiles/file/HealthCare/reproguidelines_low_res_FINAL.pdf. Retrieved September 10, 2013.

Chandra A, Mosher WD, Copen C, Sionean C. Sexual behavior, sexual attraction, and sexual identity in the United States: data from the 2006–2008 National Survey of Family Growth. Natl Health Stat Report 2011;36:1–36.

Copen CE, Chandra A, Martinez G. Prevalence and timing of oral sex with opposite-sex partners among females and males aged 15-24 years: United States, 2007–2010. Natl Health Stat Report 2012;56:1–16.

Department of Health and Human Services. Impacts of four Title V, Section 510 abstinence education programs: final report. Washington, DC: HHS; 2007. Available at: http://aspe.hhs.gov/hsp/abstinence07/report.pdf. Retrieved September 27, 2013.

Department of Health and Human Services, Office on Women's Health. Date rape drugs. Washington, DC: HHS; 2008. Available at: http://www.womenshealth.gov/ publications/our-publications/fact-sheet/date-rape-drugs.pdf. Retrieved September 27, 2013.

Eaton DK, Kann L, Kinchen S, Shanklin S, Flint KH, Hawkins J, et al. Youth risk behavior surveillance—United States, 2011. Centers for Disease Control and Prevention. MMWR Surveill Summ 2012;61(4):1–162.

English A, Ford CA. The HIPAA privacy rule and adolescents: legal questions and clinical challenges. Perspect Sex Reprod Health 2004;36:80-6.

Expedited partner therapy in the management of gonorrhea and chlamydia by obstetrician-gynecologists. Committee Opinion No. 506. American College of Obstetricians and Gynecologists. Obstet Gynecol 2011;118:761–6.

Federal Bureau of Investigation. Summary Reporting System (SRS) user manual version 1.0. Criminal Justice Information Services (CJIS) Division, Uniform Crime Reporting (UCR) Program. Washington, DC: FBI; 2013. Available at: http:// www.fbi.gov/about-us/cjis/ucr/nibrs/summary-reporting-system-srs-user-manual. Retrieved November 25, 2013.

Fiore MC, Jaen CR, Baker TB, Bailey WC, Benowitz NL, Curry SJ, et al. Treating tobacco use and dependence: 2008 update. Clinical Practice Guideline. Rockville (MD): U.S. Department of Health and Human Services, Public Health Service; 2008. Available at: http://www.ahrq.gov/professionals/clinicians-providers/guide lines-recommendations/tobacco/clinicians/treating_tobacco_use08.pdf. Retrieved July 26, 2013.

Ford C, English A, Sigman G. Confidential Health Care for Adolescents: position paper for the society for adolescent medicine. J Adolesc Health 2004;35:160-7.

Guttmacher Institute. State center. Available at: http://www.guttmacher.org/state-center/. Retrieved September 27, 2013.

Human papillomavirus vaccination. Committee Opinion No. 588. American College of Obstetricians and Gynecologists. Obstet Gynecol 2014;123:712–8.

Institute of Medicine. Dietary reference intakes tables and application. Available at: http://www.iom.edu/Activities/Nutrition/SummaryDRIs/DRI-Tables.aspx. Retrieved July 24, 2013.

Martinez G, Copen CE, Abma JC. Teenagers in the United States: sexual activity, contraceptive use, and childbearing, 2006–2010 national survey of family growth. Vital Health Stat 23 2011;(31):1-35.

Menstrual manipulation for adolescents with disabilities. ACOG Committee Opinion No. 448. American College of Obstetricians and Gynecologists. Obstet Gynecol 2009;114:1428–31.

Menstruation in girls and adolescents: using the menstrual cycle as a vital sign. ACOG Committee Opinion No. 349. American College of Obstetricians and Gynecologists. Obstet Gynecol 2006;108:1323–8.

Miller E, Decker MR, Reed E, Raj A, Hathaway JE, Silverman JG. Male partner pregnancy-promoting behaviors and adolescent partner violence: findings from a qualitative study with adolescent females. Ambul Pediatr 2007;7:360–6.

Nicoletti A. Perspectives on pediatric and adolescent gynecology from the allied health care professional. Teens, tattoos and body piercing. J Pediatr Adolesc Gynecol 2004;17:215–6.

Report of the Expert Panel on Blood Cholesterol Levels in Children and Adolescents. National Cholesterol Education Program. Pediatrics 1992;89(part 2):525–84.

Reproductive and sexual coercion. Committee Opinion No. 554. American College of Obstetricians and Gynecologists. Obstet Gynecol 2013;121:411–5.

Sexual assault. Committee Opinion No. 592. American College of Obstetricians and Gynecologists. Obstet Gynecol 2014;123:905–9.

Shain BN. Suicide and suicide attempts in adolescents. American Academy of Pediatrics Committee on Adolescence. Pediatrics 2007;120:669–76.

Sterilization of women, including those with mental disabilities. ACOG Committee Opinion No. 371. American College of Obstetricians and Gynecologists. Obstet Gynecol 2007;110:217–20.

Students Against Destructive Decisions. Distracted driving. Available at: http://sadd. org/issues_distracted.htm. Retrieved September 27, 2013.

The fourth report on the diagnosis, evaluation, and treatment of high blood pressure in children and adolescents. National High Blood Pressure Education Program Working Group on High Blood Pressure in Children and Adolescents. Pediatrics 2004;114:555–76.

The initial reproductive health visit. Committee Opinion No. 598. American College of Obstetricians and Gynecologists. Obstet Gynecol 2014;123:1143–7.

Weinstock H, Berman S, Cates W Jr. Sexually transmitted diseases among American youth: incidence and prevalence estimates, 2000. Perspect Sex Reprod Health 2004;36:6–10.

Welliver D, Welliver M, Carroll T, James P. Lumbar epidural catheter placement in the presence of low back tattoos: a review of the safety concerns. AANA J 2010;78:197–201.

Resources

Adolescent confidentiality and electronic health records. Committee Opinion No. 599. American College of Obstetricians and Gynecologists. Obstet Gynecol 2014;123:1148–50.

American Academy of Pediatrics. AAP policy. Available at: http://pediatrics.aappub lications.org/site/aappolicy/index.xhtml. Retrieved September 27, 2013.

American College of Obstetricians and Gynecologists. Adolescent health care. Washington, DC: American College of Obstetricians and Gynecologists; 2013. Available at: http://www.acog.org/About_ACOG/ACOG_Departments/Adolescent_ Health_Care. Retrieved September 30, 2013.

American College of Obstetricians and Gynecologists. Birth control–especially for teens. Patient Education Pamphlet AP112. American College of Obstetricians and Gynecologists; 2013.

American College of Obstetricians and Gynecologists. Having a baby–especially for teens. Patient Education Pamphlet AP103. Washington, DC: American College of Obstetricians and Gynecologists; 2013.

American College of Obstetricians and Gynecologists. Annual women's health care. Available at: http://www.acog.org/wellwoman. Retrieved October 1, 2013.

American College of Obstetricians and Gynecologists. You and your sexuality– especially for teens. Patient Education Pamphlet AP042. Washington, DC: American College of Obstetricians and Gynecologists; 2013.

American College of Obstetricians and Gynecologists. Your changing body– especially for teens. Patient Education Pamphlet AP041. Washington, DC: American College of Obstetricians and Gynecologists; 2012.

American College of Obstetricians and Gynecologists. Your first gynecologic visit– especially for teens. Patient Education Pamphlet AP150. Washington, DC: American College of Obstetricians and Gynecologists; 2011.

American Medical Association. Confidential care for minors. In: Code of medical ethics of the American Medical Association: current opinions and annotations. 2012-2013 ed. Chicago (IL): AMA; 2012. p. 185-7.

American Society for Colposcopy and Cervical Pathology. Updated consensus guidelines on the management of women with abnormal cervical cancer screening tests and cancer precursors. Frederick (MD): ASCCP; 2013. Available at: http://www. asccp.org/Guidelines. Retrieved September 27, 2013.

Bright Futures. American Academy of Pediatrics. Available at: http://brightfutures. aap.org. Retrieved July 20, 2013.

Center for Adolescent Health and the Law. Available at: http://www.cahl.org. Retrieved September 27, 2013.

English A, Bass L, Boyle AD, Eshragh F. State minor consent laws; a summary. 3rd ed. Chapel Hill (NC): Center for Adolescent Health & the Law; 2010.

Food and Drug Administration. Inked and regretful: removing tattoos. Available at: http://www.fda.gov/ForConsumers/ConsumerUpdates/ucm336842.htm. Retrieved July 30, 2013.

Future of Sex Education Initiative. National sexuality education standards core content and skills, K–12. Available at: http://www.futureofsexeducation.org/docu ments/josh-fose-standards-web.pdf. Retrieved July 30, 2013.

Guide to Community Preventive Services. Preventing HIV/AIDS, other STIs, and teen pregnancy: group-based abstinence education interventions for adolescents. Available at: http://www.thecommunityguide.org/hiv/abstinence_ed.html. Retrieved July 30, 2013.

Guttmacher Institute. Adolescents. Available at: http://www.guttmacher.org/sec tions/adolescents.php. Retrieved September 27, 2013.

Massad LS, Einstein MH, Huh WK, Katki HA, Kinney WK, Schiffman M, et al. 2012 updated consensus guidelines for the management of abnormal cervical cancer screening tests and cancer precursors. 2012 ASCCP Consensus Guidelines Conference; Obstet Gynecol 2013;121:829–46.

Morreale MC, Stinnett AJ, Dowling EC, editors. Policy compendium on confidential health services for adolescents. 2nd ed. Chapel Hill (NC): Center for Adolescent Health & the Law; 2005.

National Campaign to Prevent Teen and Unplanned Pregnancy. Available at: http://www.thenationalcampaign.org. Retrieved September 27, 2013.

North American Society for Pediatric and Adolescent Gynecology. Tools for the clinician. Available at: http://www.naspag.org/index.php/professionalspage/6-tools-fortheclinician. Retrieved September 27, 2013.

Reproductive health care for adolescents with human immunodeficiency virus. Committee Opinion No. 572. American College of Obstetricians and Gynecologists. Obstet Gynecol 2013;122:721–6.

Students Against Destructive Decisions. Contract for life. Available at: http://www.sadd.org/contract.htm. Retrieved July 30, 2013.

MENOPAUSE

Menopause is the permanent cessation of menstruation that occurs 1 year after the last menstrual period and marks the end of a women's reproductive ability. In North America, the median age of menopause is 51 years. Medical intervention in menopausal women should focus on primary and preventive health care and counseling and address diet, fitness, use of alcohol, smoking cessation, cancer screening, and the role of hormone therapy (HT) (see also the "Well-Woman Annual Health Assessment" section and specific health topics earlier in Part 3).

Most women go through a period of irregular menstrual activity before menopause. Common symptoms of menopause include vasomotor symptoms (hot flushes) and vaginal dryness. Atrophic changes of the external genitalia commonly occur with time. Certain medical conditions occur more often in this age group. These conditions include cancer, osteoporosis, coronary artery disease, cerebrovascular disease, diabetes mellitus, pulmonary disorders, Alzheimer disease, and adult macular degeneration. Many of these conditions are associated with aging and low estrogen levels after menopause.

The North American Menopause Society (NAMS) notes that women who experience premature menopause (at age 40 years or earlier) or primary ovarian insufficiency are medically a distinctly different group from women who reach menopause at the median age. According to NAMS, the data regarding HT in women who experience menopause at the median age should not be extrapolated to women who initiate HT at the time of premature menopause. Given the potential harmful effects of estrogen deficiency on bone mass and the severity of vasomotor symptoms in young women, NAMS recommends the use of HT or oral contraceptives—if not contraindicated—until the median age of natural menopause, with periodic reassessment.

Counseling

Counseling should be provided as described in the "Well-Woman Annual Health Assessment" section and in the sections on specific health topics earlier in Part 3. The following recommendations are of particular importance.

Patients in the perimenopausal period should be given information about the normal events of aging, including specific information regarding the reduction of ovarian hormonal function and the manifestations of these ovarian changes. In addition, women should be apprised that positive modifications in lifestyle, such as improvements in dietary and exercise habits, may benefit their overall health during menopause. Smoking cessation, lipid monitoring, blood pressure monitoring, weight management, and annual health care maintenance should be emphasized. Recommendations for cancer screening, such as cervical cancer testing and mammography, should be reviewed (see also the "Well-Woman Annual Health Assessment" section and the "Cancer Screening and Prevention" section earlier in Part 3). Discussions regarding elder abuse and intimate partner and domestic violence should be considered (see also the "Abuse" section later in Part 3).

Menopausal women should be counseled about the benefits of exercise, proper nutrition, and avoidance of certain lifestyle factors (cigarettes and alcohol) in preventing or slowing development of osteoporosis. They also should be informed about special dietary needs, including the importance of calcium intake. The 2011 Institute of Medicine recommended dietary allowance for calcium is 1,000 mg per day for individuals aged 19–50 years and 1,200 mg per day for those aged 51 years and older. The vitamin D recommended dietary allowance now ranges from 600 international units per day for most of life to 800 international units per day after age 70 years. Routine screening for vitamin D levels is not recommended. However, screening is recommended for individuals at high risk of vitamin D deficiency, such as those with certain medical conditions that may affect vitamin D absorption and those taking medications that affect vitamin D levels. Women who are at risk of fractures should be informed of the importance of accident prevention and safety issues (see also the "Osteoporosis" section earlier in Part 3).

Hormone Therapy

At least three treatment regimens are used for the administration of menopausal HT:

1. Cyclic. Estrogen is given for 25 days or more, with the addition of a cyclic progestin.
2. Combined. Estrogen and a low dose of progestin are given daily or through the levonorgestrel intrauterine system (levonorgestrel intrauterine device).
3. Estrogen only. Estrogen is given for 25 days per month or more.

Endometrial sampling is not necessary before instituting therapy in asymptomatic patients. In women who have an intact uterus, the use of an estrogen–progestin regimen is recommended to reduce the risk of endometrial hyperplasia and endometrial cancer. Consideration also may be given to the use of the levonorgestrel intrauterine system as an alternative delivery method for the progestin component of combined HT.

BENEFITS AND RISKS ASSOCIATED WITH HORMONE THERAPY

The benefits and risks of menopausal HT—either combined HT or estrogen therapy—should be discussed in detail with each patient before the initiation of therapy and when renewing her annual prescription so that she can make the best decision for her own health. After a thorough discussion regarding the risks and benefits of menopausal HT, the patient should undergo a medical evaluation before the initiation of treatment.

Benefits

Estrogens alone or estrogens plus progestins are highly effective for the alleviation of hot flushes and night sweats. For patients with severe symptoms that affect quality of life, estrogens are the most effective treatment. Estrogen is effective for the treatment of patients with vaginal dryness and atrophic changes that impede sexual function. Topical and systemic estrogens appear to be equally effective in relieving vaginal atrophy and associated dyspareunia. Because some women aged 65 years and older may continue to need systemic HT for the management of vasomotor symptoms, the American College of Obstetricians and Gynecologists recommends against routine discontinuation of systemic estrogen at age 65 years. As with younger women, the use of combined HT or estrogen therapy should be individualized based on each woman's risk–benefit ratio and clinical presentation.

Hormone therapy (either estrogen therapy or combined therapy) has a beneficial effect on bone health and is approved for the prevention of osteoporosis in women at an increased risk of osteoporosis and fracture (see also the "Osteoporosis" section earlier in Part 3). The benefit of HT for bone health is dose related, and today's lower doses may not be as effective for fracture prevention as the higher doses used in the past. If use of HT for bone health is being considered, the clinician must work closely with the patient to determine what is in her best interest.

Risks

The following are some concerns patients may have regarding HT:

- Endometrial neoplasia. Unopposed systematic estrogen use increases the risk of endometrial cancer. Treatment with a combination of progestin and estrogen eliminates this increased risk.

- Ovarian neoplasia. There are conflicting data pertaining to the association of HT and ovarian cancer. Current HT users who had been on the therapy for less than 5 years did not have an increased risk of ovarian cancer, whereas data did suggest a small increased risk of ovarian cancer with use for longer than 5 years.

- Breast neoplasia. Current data suggest that combined estrogen and progestin therapy can be used for 3–5 years before encountering an increased risk of breast cancer. Estrogen therapy can be used for a longer period of time, in the absence of other risk factors, because of the delayed risk of breast cancer seen with estrogen therapy.

- Cholelithiasis. Women should be cautioned about the increased risks of gallstones and biliary tract surgery with the use of menopausal HT.

- Thromboembolic disease. Combined HT or estrogen therapy for the management of menopausal symptoms and related disorders is associated with an increased risk of venous thromboembolism. In healthy women with a negative risk history, the probability of venous thromboembolism is generally low. This risk increases with age and the presence of additional risk factors, including cardiovascular disease, obesity, fracture, renal disease, and congenital and acquired thrombophilic disorders. It is prudent for the prescriber to carefully assess the personal and family history of patients before prescribing combined HT or estrogen therapy. Recent studies suggest that orally administered estrogen may exert a prothrombotic effect, whereas transdermally administered estrogen has little or no effect in elevating prothrombotic substances and may have beneficial effects on proinflammatory markers. When prescribing estrogen therapy, the gynecologist should take into consideration the possible thrombosis-sparing properties of transdermal forms of estrogen therapy.

- Hypertension. Hormone therapy modestly lowers blood pressure; however, in a few women it may induce or exacerbate hypertension. Routine blood pressure monitoring is appropriate.

- Cardiovascular. Hormone therapy should not be initiated or continued for primary or secondary prevention of coronary heart disease. Evidence is insufficient to conclude that long-term estrogen therapy or combined HT use improves cardiovascular outcomes. In addition, in the Women's Health Initiative trial, women taking combined estrogen and progestin therapy and those taking an estrogen-only regimen had an increased risk of stroke. Recent evidence suggests that women in early menopause who are in good cardiovascular health are at low risk of adverse cardiovascular outcomes and should be considered candidates for the use of estrogen therapy or conjugated equine estrogen plus a progestin for relief of menopausal symptoms.

CONTRAINDICATIONS TO HORMONE THERAPY

Contraindications to estrogen therapy include the following:

- Undiagnosed abnormal genital bleeding
- Known or suspected estrogen-dependent neoplasia except in appropriately selected patients

- Active deep vein thrombosis, pulmonary embolism, or a history of these conditions
- Active or recent arterial thromboembolic disease (stroke, myocardial infarction)
- Liver dysfunction or liver disease
- Known or suspected pregnancy
- Hypersensitivity to estrogen therapy preparations

The safety of estrogen therapy or combined HT for the treatment of vasomotor symptoms in breast cancer survivors is unknown. Randomized controlled trials in the 1990s were terminated early when findings indicated increases in breast cancer recurrences. This is still a controversial area because a large quantitative review of published data that evaluated the use of menopausal HT in women with a history of breast cancer showed that HT was not associated with an increased risk of recurrence, cancer-related mortality, or total mortality. Given the conflicting reports, the use of HT generally is contraindicated in patients with hormone-positive breast cancer.

A history of endometrial cancer generally also is considered to be a contraindication to HT. This opinion is based on the fact that adenocarcinoma is considered an estrogen-dependent neoplasm. Although this contraindication is widely accepted, there is a lack of scientific evidence to support the theory that estrogen therapy is potentially dangerous for endometrial cancer patients who have had a hysterectomy.

COMPOUNDED BIOIDENTICAL HORMONE THERAPY

Compounded bioidentical menopausal HT consists of plant-derived hormones that are prepared by a pharmacist and can be custom made for a patient according to a physician's specifications. Evidence is lacking to support superiority claims of compounded bioidentical hormones over conventional menopausal HT. Most compounded products have not undergone rigorous clinical testing for safety or efficacy. These preparations have variable purity and potency and lack efficacy and safety data. Although it is required that manufactured drugs be consistent from batch to batch, there are no similar quality control measures for compounded drugs to ensure that the bioavailability of active ingredients is consistent, such that underdosage and overdosage are possible. Therefore, although interest in and requests for compounded pharmaceutical products appear to be increasing, physicians and patients should exercise caution in prescribing and using them. Conventional HT is preferred over compounded HT given the available data. Advocates and compounders of bioidentical hormones also recommend the use of hormone level testing as a means of offering individualized therapy. Despite claims to the contrary, evidence is inadequate to support increased efficacy or safety for individualized HT regimens based on salivary, serum, or urinary testing.

Nonhormonal Therapy

Management of menopausal symptoms often can be accomplished through nonhormonal options. Treatments for vasomotor symptoms include pharmacologic agents, complementary and alternative therapies, and lifestyle and behavioral alterations. Safety and efficacy data on herbal treatments are unclear, and more data are needed on the efficacy of lifestyle changes and alternative therapies. Nonhormonal treatment options for vaginal symptoms include vaginal lubricants and moisturizers. For patients in whom nonhormonal treatments fail, the use of low-dose estrogen methods (vaginal, topical, ring, and tablets) may be considered. Hormone therapy generally is contraindicated in women with a history of hormone-sensitive cancer, and consideration of its use should be made in consultation with an expert in cancer treatment such as an oncologist.

PHARMACOLOGIC AGENTS

A variety of low-dose antidepressant medications or the anticonvulsant gabapentin can be used to manage vasomotor symptoms, although this use is generally off label. Selective serotonin reuptake inhibitors (eg, citalopram or fluoxetine) and serotonin-norepinephrine reuptake inhibitors (eg, venlafaxine) have been shown to be safe and effective in reducing the severity of hot flushes in menopausal women and patients with breast cancer, although caution must be used when these agents are used in conjunction with tamoxifen; serotonin-norepinephrine reuptake inhibitors are generally preferable to selective serotonin reuptake inhibitors in women using tamoxifen. A lower-dose form of paroxetine was recently approved by the

U.S. Food and Drug Administration (FDA) as the first nonhormonal treatment for moderate-to-severe vasomotor symptoms associated with menopause. As with other antidepressants, the lower-dose paroxetine carries a black box warning regarding suicidality. Other options for management of vasomotor symptoms in women who cannot use estrogens or progestins or choose not to use these methods include gabapentin and clonidine, although these agents are not FDA-approved for this indication.

COMPLEMENTARY AND ALTERNATIVE THERAPIES

Several natural products have been used for the management of vasomotor symptoms. In the United States, none of these complementary therapies are regulated by the FDA and have not been tested for safety, efficacy, or purity because they are considered nutritional supplements. Data do not show that phytoestrogens (eg, soy products) and herbal supplements (eg, Chinese herbal medicine, black cohosh, ginseng, St. John's wort, and ginkgo biloba) are efficacious for the treatment of vasomotor symptoms. There also are insufficient data to support the use of soy products or herbal remedies for the treatment of vaginal symptoms.

Acupuncture has shown no benefit over placebo for the management of vasomotor symptoms. Similarly, reflexology has not been shown to significantly reduce vasomotor symptoms compared with nonspecific foot massage. There are some preliminary data to suggest that local injection of anesthetic into the stellate ganglion may reduce vasomotor symptoms in women with contraindications to HT. However, additional studies are needed to assess the safety and effectiveness of this novel technique.

LIFESTYLE AND BEHAVIORAL ALTERATIONS

Despite limited supporting data, common-sense lifestyle solutions such as layering of clothing, maintaining a lower ambient temperature, and consuming cool drinks are reasonable measures for the management of vasomotor symptoms. Women also may be advised to avoid consumption of alcohol and caffeine, which have been associated with increased severity and frequency of vasomotor symptoms. Although there is some evidence that aerobic exercise may improve quality of life and mood in women with vasomotor symptoms, there are insufficient data to recommend exercise for the treatment of vasomotor symptoms.

VAGINAL LUBRICANTS AND MOISTURIZERS

Nonestrogen water-based or silicone-based vaginal lubricants and moisturizers may alleviate vaginal symptoms related to menopause. These products may be particularly helpful in women who do not wish to use hormonal therapies. Vaginal lubricants are intended to be used to relieve friction and dyspareunia related to vaginal dryness during intercourse and are applied to the vaginal introitus before intercourse. Vaginal moisturizers are intended to trap moisture and provide long-term relief of vaginal dryness. Although there are limited data regarding the effectiveness of these products, prospective studies have demonstrated that vaginal moisturizers improve vaginal dryness, pH balance, and elasticity and reduce vaginal itching, irritation, and dyspareunia, and many women have found nonhormonal vaginal lubricants and moisturizers to be effective in managing vaginal dryness.

Bibliography

Compounded bioidentical menopausal hormone therapy. Committee Opinion No. 532. American College of Obstetricians and Gynecologists and the American Society for Reproductive Medicine. Obstet Gynecol 2012;120:411–5.

Elective and risk-reducing salpingo-oophorectomy. ACOG Practice Bulletin No. 89. American College of Obstetricians and Gynecologists. Obstet Gynecol 2008; 111:231–41.

Estrogen and progestogen therapy in postmenopausal women. Practice Committee of the American Society for Reproductive Medicine. Fertil Steril 2008;90:S88–102.

Food and Drug Administration. FDA approves the first non-hormonal treatment for hot flashes associated with menopause. Silver Spring (MD): FDA; 2013. Available at: http://www.fda.gov/NewsEvents/Newsroom/PressAnnouncements/ucm359030.htm. Retrieved September 27, 2013.

Hormone therapy and heart disease. Committee Opinion No. 565. American College of Obstetricians and Gynecologists. Obstet Gynecol 2013;121:1407–10.

Institute of Medicine. Dietary reference intakes tables and application. Available at: http://www.iom.edu/Activities/Nutrition/SummaryDRIs/DRI-Tables.aspx. Retrieved July 24, 2013.

Lethaby A, Marjoribanks J, Kronenberg F, Roberts H, Eden J, Brown J. Phytoestrogens for vasomotor menopausal symptoms. Cochrane Database of Systematic Reviews 2007, Issue 4. Art. No.: CD001395. DOI: 10.1002/14651858.CD001395.pub3.

Management of menopausal symptoms. Practice Bulletin No. 141. American College of Obstetricians and Gynecologists. Obstet Gynecol 2014;123:202–16.

Management of gynecologic issues in women with breast cancer. Practice Bulletin No. 126. American College of Obstetricians and Gynecologists. Obstet Gynecol 2012; 119:666–82.

Nelson HD, Vesco KK, Haney E, Fu R, Nedrow A, Miller J, et al. Nonhormonal therapies for menopausal hot flashes: systematic review and meta-analysis. JAMA 2006;295:2057–71.

Osteoporosis. Practice Bulletin No. 129. American College of Obstetricians and Gynecologists. Obstet Gynecol 2012;120:718–34.

Postmenopausal estrogen therapy: route of administration and risk of venous thromboembolism. Committee Opinion No. 556. American College of Obstetricians and Gynecologists. Obstet Gynecol 2013;121:887–90.

The 2012 hormone therapy position statement of the North American Menopause Society. North American Menopause Society. Menopause 2012;19:257–71.

The menopausal transition. Practice Committee of the American Society for Reproductive Medicine. Fertil Steril 2008;90:S61–5.

Resources

American College of Obstetricians and Gynecologists. Osteoporosis. Patient Education Pamphlet AP048. Washington, DC: American College of Obstetricians and Gynecologists; 2013.

American College of Obstetricians and Gynecologists. Perimenopausal bleeding and bleeding after menopause. Patient Education Pamphlet AP162. Washington, DC: American College of Obstetricians and Gynecologists; 2010.

American College of Obstetricians and Gynecologists. The menopause years. Patient Education Pamphlet AP047. Washington, DC: American College of Obstetricians and Gynecologists; 2013.

Food and Drug Administration. Estrogen and estrogen with progestin therapies for postmenopausal women. Available at: http://www.fda.gov/Drugs/DrugSafety/InformationbyDrugClass/ucm135318.htm. Retrieved July 30, 2013.

Moyer VA. Menopausal hormone therapy for the primary prevention of chronic conditions: U.S. Preventive Services Task Force recommendation statement. U.S. Preventive Services Task Force. Ann Intern Med 2013;158:47–54.

North American Menopause Society. Menopause practice: a clinician's guide. 4th ed. Mayfield Heights (OH): NAMS; 2010.

WOMEN 65 YEARS AND OLDER

Currently, 13.3% of the U.S. population is 65 years of age or older. It is projected that this number will double to 88.5 million people by 2050, more than double original estimates. This increase in the older population is due in large part to the "baby boomers," who began to turn age 65 years in 2011. This aging process is frequently associated with the development of chronic medical conditions and disabilities, which can be exhibited as behavioral, emotional, and functional changes that may affect independence, self-sufficiency, and autonomy. Limited and fixed incomes compound these issues for individuals if their available funds are inadequate to purchase services and medication. Obstetrician–gynecologists and other health care providers should aim to ensure that this segment of the population remains as healthy as possible and to provide appropriate health care. Clinicians can begin to meet these goals during the routine annual visit by providing age-appropriate screening (see also "Well-Woman Care: Assessments & Recommendations" at www.acog.org/wellwoman) and addressing the special needs of this population of patients.

Communication Issues

Communication with elderly patients can present special challenges. Visual and hearing deficits are more common in these patients and can detract from effective communication. It is important to be alert to inattention, inappropriate questions, and lack of response. Ask early in the visit whether there is an issue with hearing or vision, and assess mental status. Appropriate adjustments can then be made that will make the visit more effective and reduce frustration and stress on all parties involved.

In the elderly, memory for short, logically associated material usually is good; however, this may not be true for more complex material.

Comprehension can be improved by the following:

- Reducing and screening out distractions
- Alerting the patient to changes of subject
- Stating clearly the important information to be learned
- Keeping new information brief and relevant
- Providing written instructions (in large print size)
- Reviewing and repeating salient points several times
- Utilizing a teach-back method of counseling

Functional Assessment

There is wide variation in the mental, social, and physical status of older women. In addition, medical problems may be made more complex by the physiologic changes that accompany aging; for example, changes in height, weight, and posture may cause pain and the need for pain-relief medications, which can then affect cognition. Other changes, such as altered regulation of homeostasis, can contribute to more serious medical problems, to altered metabolism of drugs with increased sensitivity to medications, and to increased susceptibility to infection, all of which can contribute to slower, more complicated recovery from illnesses and surgical procedures.

Loss of independence and inability to perform daily living activities are realistic fears of older people. For many, a time comes in which a decision must be made about independent living and the need for assistance with daily life activities. Although remaining in their homes is a preference for many older people at this life stage, personal safety must be considered when addressing these issues. It is important for the elderly to maintain their dignity, independence, and ability to make major life decisions as long as possible while remaining in a safe environment. An assessment of the woman's ability to function in the home setting is critical. Identification, prevention, and minimization of disorders associated with decreased mobility are good initial steps to ensure patient safety. Evaluation of functional assessment findings, coupled with appropriate management, referrals, or both can assist the elderly woman to live independently and maintain her health. A functional assessment also should be carried out before any medical intervention or surgery.

The following functions should be evaluated:

- Cognitive and affective mental function
- Vision
- Hearing
- Motor function
- Gait and balance
- Bowel and bladder function
- Environmental risks and support systems

Numerous screening and assessment tools for functional assessment have been developed and tested (see Resources).

COGNITIVE FUNCTION

Cognitive changes in aging women are subject to significant variation. Some changes may be age related, whereas others may be related to underlying (often unidentified) illnesses, medications, depression, or a combination of these factors. An important first step in caring for aging women and others who may have impaired cognitive function is to assess the patient's ability to make health care decisions. At times this is not clear. A woman's capacity to make a decision depends on her ability to understand information and appreciate the implications of that information, and assessing her capacity may require the assistance of professionals with expertise in making such determinations. Surrogate decision makers should be identified for patients who are incapable of making health care decisions or who have been found legally incompetent (see also the "End-of-Life Considerations" section later in Part 3).

Some deterioration of mental status commonly occurs with aging. Marked changes in mental status usually are associated with dementia. Depression may be preexisting in a patient, but it also can be initiated, exacerbated, or both in old age by social and family isolation, inactivity, inability to mobilize, elder abuse, and neglect. Delirium, although often confused with dementia, usually is transient and frequently is associated with a treatable medical condition or with drug toxicity, drug interaction, or both.

There are several etiologies of cortical dementias. The most common are as follows:

- Alzheimer disease
- Dementia associated with cerebrovascular disease
- Previous head trauma

Alzheimer disease is the most common form of dementia, with an estimated 11% of the U.S. population 65 years and older believed to have the disease. The lifetime risk of developing Alzheimer disease for women older than 65 years without signs of dementia is one in five. Alzheimer disease is associated with aging: 38% of affected individuals are 85 years or older, whereas only 4% are younger than 65 years. There also are a number of causes of noncortical dementias, related to the following:

- Drug toxicity
- Drug interaction
- Alcohol and other substance abuse
- Systemic infections
- Renal failure
- Heart failure
- Metabolic diseases
  — Malnutrition
  — Iron deficiency
  — Hypothyroidism
  — Vitamin B_{12} and folate deficiencies

Delirium is characterized by an acute and fluctuating course and is an impairment of cognition that is not attributable to prior or progressive dementia. Any disturbance in consciousness or environment can be a risk factor for development of delirium, including the following: recent anesthesia or surgery; use of sleep medications; an idiosyncratic response to medication; a change in living arrangements; or an underlying untreated, poorly treated, or inadequately treated medical condition.

HEARING AND VISION

Early identification and management of hearing and visual difficulties can improve emotional and physical morbidity. Hearing disorders afflict more than one third of women older than 65 years. Hearing difficulties may appear as tinnitus, high-frequency hearing loss (difficulty understanding women and children), difficulty locating the source of sounds, and vertigo. Visual problems occur in just under one fifth of women of this age, even when eyeglasses or contacts are used. The primary signs and symptoms are night blindness, reading difficulty, eye pain, blurred central vision, and diminished awareness of peripheral objects.

BLADDER AND BOWEL FUNCTION

Depending on the definition used and the population queried, urinary incontinence affects 10–70% of women living in a community setting and up to 50% of nursing home residents. The prevalence of incontinence appears to increase gradually during young adult life, has a broad peak around middle age, and then steadily increases in the elderly. In addition to causes intrinsic to the lower urinary tract, the following factors may be involved: delirium, infection, atrophic urethritis or vaginitis, medications, depression, excessive urine output (eg, that is due to hyperglycemia or medications to treat congestive heart failure), restricted mobility, and stool impaction. Asymptomatic bacteriuria is a common incidental finding and does not require treatment.

Approximately 20% of elderly people report problems with bowel function. Normal bowel habits include formed stools every 1–3 days. Constipation can be related to a low-fiber diet, medications, low fluid intake, colorectal dysmotility, irritable bowel syndrome, obstruction, hypothyroidism, sedentary lifestyle, or inadequate toilet facilities. Diarrhea may result from infection, medications, laxative abuse, irritable bowel syndrome, or interventions to alleviate bowel impaction.

Common Medical Conditions

There are a number of medical conditions that are seen more frequently in the elderly. These include cardiovascular disease, fractures, cancer, and infections. In addition, nutritional deficiencies may occur.

CARDIOVASCULAR DISEASE

Cardiovascular disease is the leading cause of death among women, with an overall increase in heart attacks occurring about 10 years after menopause, according to the American Heart Association. Changes in women's physiology after menopause—including increases in blood pressure, triglyceride, and low-density lipoprotein cholesterol levels; decreases in high-density lipoprotein cholesterol; and declining estrogen levels—contribute to an increased risk of cardiovascular disease. Gender differences in the presenting signs and symptoms of cardiovascular disease also exist. Often, the indicators of cardiovascular disease are more subtle in women than in men and require a high index of suspicion to diagnose. Delay in evaluation and diagnosis of symptoms is a major contributor to women's increased morbidity and mortality from the disease. Late onset of hypertension, especially isolated systolic hypertension, increases the incidence of stroke and myocardial infarction; therefore, early detection and treatment are important (see also the "Cardiovascular Disorders" section earlier in Part 3).

FRACTURES

Fracture is a major health hazard in women 65 years and older. Morbidity and loss of function can occur with all fractures and consequently present a significant burden to the patient, the family, and society. Vertebral and hip fractures are common and are associated with morbidity and mortality. These fractures lead to immobility, surgical procedures, prolonged rehabilitation, and, potentially, placement in a long-term care facility. Morbidity and mortality are especially high with hip fractures. Of women older than 80 years who have had a hip fracture, only 56% could walk independently after 1 year. Approximately 3–6% of women die of complications while hospitalized for hip fracture, an outcome often correlated with comorbidity and age. In addition, patient immobility following hip fracture surgery can lead to complications, such as phlebitis and pulmonary emboli, and can be exacerbated by other age-related visual or auditory impairments. Full mobility may not be realized and the individual may need to use a walker, acquire an unstable gait, and be at risk of another fall. Osteoporosis increases the risk of fractures; for more information, see also the "Osteoporosis" section earlier in Part 3.

CANCER

Cancer is the second leading cause of death in women 65 years or older. Appropriate screening and preventive counseling should take place (see also the "Cancer Screening and Prevention" section earlier in Part 3). Increasingly, however, screening is no longer recommended in older women for types of cancer that are slow to develop because limited life expectancy may minimize patients' ability to benefit from screening. For example, cervical cancer screening should be discontinued at age 65 years for women at average risk who have a history of adequate recent screening and no history of advanced cervical abnormalities. Screening for breast cancer has been particularly controversial. There is no consensus as to whether there is an age at which the risks of mammography outweigh the benefits. Medical comorbidity and life expectancy should be considered in a breast cancer screening program for women aged 75 years or older because the benefit of screening mammography decreases compared with the harms of overtreatment with advancing age. Women aged 75 years or older should, in consultation with their physicians, decide whether or not to continue mammographic screening.

INFECTIONS

Infections account for mortality in approximately one third of older women. The most common ones are urinary tract infections, pneumonia, influenza, herpes zoster infections, and tuberculosis, especially in institutionalized women. Appropriate immunizations should be recommended and administered (see also the "Immunizations" section earlier in Part 3). Women who are 65 years or older who are vaccinated against the flu can receive either the standard-dose or high-dose inactivated influenza vaccine.

A stronger immune response occurs with the high-dose vaccine than with the standard-dose vaccine, but it is not known whether the improved immune response leads to greater protection against influenza.

NUTRITIONAL DEFICIENCIES

Nutritional requirements and metabolism change with aging. Illness and chronic medical conditions can lead to nutritional deficiencies. A simple and easily implemented solution to this problem is to increase intake of foods that naturally contain large amounts of vitamins and minerals, such as complex carbohydrates (eg, grains, legumes, potatoes, and fruit). A diet rich in complex carbohydrates (55–60%) will increase nutrient intake.

Fewer calories are needed to maintain good health as women age. Women should be encouraged to maintain their weight in the normal range by adjusting their diet accordingly and to follow a regular exercise program for weight regulation, bone health, and for other health benefits (see also the "Fitness" section earlier in Part 3). Serial measures of weight, a dietary history, or both may reveal potential problems and warrant additional diagnostic testing. When all laboratory values have been received, medical conditions that have been uncovered should be treated. Management should include nutrition counseling and an evaluation of the individual's support system, including any financial issues, with social service referrals as necessary.

Common Psychosocial Concerns

In addition to variations in cognitive function, many older women are at increased risk of psychosocial problems. Depression is very common in elderly women and often is unrecognized and untreated. Women should be screened for suicide risk factors, symptoms of depression, abnormal bereavement, and changes in cognitive function and be offered treatment as indicated. Sleep disorders in aging women are associated with menopausal symptoms, dementia, depression, sleep apnea, daytime medication use, and pain syndromes.

Alcoholism, sexual dysfunction, and complications that arise from multiple medication use increase and often are undiagnosed in this age group.

Health care providers should be aware of signs and symptoms of physical or emotional abuse and of neglect. The woman's social support system is critical for her health, recovery, and functioning. Patients should be asked about family and other support systems, as well as whether they have formal or informal help at home.

Medication Use

Older women experience adverse events that relate to drug therapy more frequently and in more unexpected ways than younger women. Polypharmacy, or the administration of many drugs from many sources, is not uncommon. Over-the-counter medications, including complementary and alternative supplements, often are not included by women in their recall of medications. To verify what drugs and other agents are being used, have the patient or a family member bring all medications, including vitamins and over-the-counter medications, to the office visit. Health care providers should obtain information on the medications that each patient currently is taking, either at scheduled times or on an as-needed basis. This should include information about allergies or drug sensitivities. As part of its National Patient Safety Goals, The Joint Commission recommends that this information be compared with the new medications ordered for the patient in the hospital or outpatient setting to identify and resolve discrepancies. This process of comparing a patient's new medication orders with all of the medications the patient currently is taking is called medication reconciliation. The Joint Commission also recommends that patients be provided with written information on the medications they should be taking when they are discharged from the hospital or at the end of the outpatient visit.

Often, older women have poor medication adherence because of multiple medications, misunderstanding of instructions, diminished hearing, impaired vision, or poor short-term memory. Difficulties also may result from a lack of access to a pharmacy, inability to pay for medications, or difficulty opening medications (eg, childproof bottles). In addition, borrowed medication can make up a substantial percentage of medication taken by older women.

The physiologic changes that accompany aging result in alterations in the processes of drug absorption, distribution, metabolism, and elimination (pharmacokinetics), and can alter drug bioavailability. In addition, the biochemical and physiologic effects of the drugs themselves and their mechanisms of action (pharmacodynamics) appear to change in aging women. The elderly often are more sensitive or responsive to the effects of a drug and require smaller doses. This altered responsiveness ranges from increased therapeutic effects to serious adverse drug reactions. Adverse effects in the elderly may present atypically as subtle changes in mental status or an acute decline in functional status. Serious drug reactions in the elderly most commonly are caused by psychotropic drugs, diuretics, and cardiovascular agents.

A reduction in the number of drugs prescribed may minimize adverse drug reactions and interactions. Medical conditions should be managed without medications whenever appropriate. It is critical to monitor for multiple medications prescribed by different physicians and to develop a coordinated medication plan for elderly patients. The cornerstone of a medication plan is an accurate list of everything the patient is taking, including over-the-counter and borrowed medications. This list requires review, updating, and evaluation of adherence and drug-taking patterns at every visit. Many new drugs have not been evaluated thoroughly in elderly women and may need to be used with caution.

A variety of techniques may improve a patient's adherence to medication regimens. They include actively involving the patient in the decision to use a medication, simplifying the dosing regimen as much as possible, eliminating unnecessary medications, evaluating the woman's functional ability to take the medications, using assistance devices such as easy-to-open bottles and prefilled medication boxes, and encouraging the woman to report any adverse reactions immediately.

The American Geriatric Society publishes the Beers Criteria for Potentially Inappropriate Medication Use in Older Adults as a means to inform clinical decision making concerning the prescribing of medication for older adults in order to improve safety and quality of care. It recommends against the use of systemic estrogen, with or without progestins, in patients 65 years and older, because of evidence of carcinogenic potential (breast and endometrium) and lack of cardioprotective effect and cognitive protection in older women. Because some women aged 65 years and older may continue to need systemic hormone therapy for the management of vaso-motor symptoms, the American College of Obstetricians and Gynecologists recommends against routine discontinuation of systemic estrogen at age 65 years. As with younger women, use of combined hormone therapy or estrogen therapy should be individualized based on each woman's risk–benefit ratio and clinical presentation. Vaginal estrogen may be an option for women whose chief concern is vaginal atrophy (see also the "Menopause" section earlier in Part 3).

Bibliography

Alzheimer's Association. 2013 Alzheimer's disease facts and figures. Chicago (IL): Alzheimer's Association; 2013. Available at: http://www.alz.org/downloads/facts_figures_2013.pdf. Retrieved July 30, 2013.

American College of Obstetricians and Gynecologists. Immunization for women. Washington, DC: American College of Obstetricians and Gynecologists; 2012. Available at: http://www.immunizationforwomen.org/. Retrieved September 4, 2013.

American College of Obstetricians and Gynecologists. Annual women's health care. Available at: http://www.acog.org/wellwoman. Retrieved October 1, 2013.

American Geriatrics Society updated Beers Criteria for potentially inappropriate medication use in older adults. American Geriatrics Society 2012 Beers Criteria Update Expert Panel. J Am Geriatr Soc 2012;60:616–31.

American Heart Association. Menopause and heart disease. Available at: http://www.heart.org/HEARTORG/Conditions/More/MyHeartandStrokeNews/Menopause-and-Heart-Disease_UCM_448432_Article.jsp. Retrieved September 27, 2013.

Boonen S, Autier P, Barette M, Vanderschueren D, Lips P, Haentjens P. Functional outcome and quality of life following hip fracture in elderly women: a prospective controlled study. Osteoporos Int 2004;15:87–94.

Breast cancer screening. Practice Bulletin No. 122. American College of Obstetricians and Gynecologists. Obstet Gynecol 2011;118:372–82.

Burge R, Dawson-Hughes B, Solomon DH, Wong JB, King A, Tosteson A. Incidence and economic burden of osteoporosis-related fractures in the United States, 2005–2025. J Bone Miner Res 2007;22:465–75.

Centers for Disease Control and Prevention. Immunization schedules. Available at: http://www.cdc.gov/vaccines/schedules/index.html. Retrieved July 23, 2013.

Cooper C, Atkinson EJ, Jacobsen SJ, O'Fallon WM, Melton LJ,3rd. Population-based study of survival after osteoporotic fractures. Am J Epidemiol 1993;137:1001–5.

Corrada MM, Brookmeyer R, Paganini-Hill A, Berlau D, Kawas CH. Dementia incidence continues to increase with age in the oldest old: the 90+ study. Ann Neurol 2010;67:114–21.

Hormone therapy and heart disease. Committee Opinion No. 565. American College of Obstetricians and Gynecologists. Obstet Gynecol 2013;121:1407–10.

Informed consent. ACOG Committee Opinion No. 439. American College of Obstetricians and Gynecologists. Obstet Gynecol 2009;114:401–8.

Osteoporosis. Practice Bulletin No. 129. American College of Obstetricians and Gynecologists. Obstet Gynecol 2012;120:718–34.

Screening for cervical cancer. Practice Bulletin No. 131. American College of Obstetricians and Gynecologists. Obstet Gynecol 2012;120:1222–38.

The Joint Commission. Comprehensive accreditation manual for hospitals : CAMH. Oakbrook Terrace (IL): The Commission; 2014.

U.S. Census Bureau. Population estimates. Available at: http://www.census.gov/popest. Retrieved July 30, 2013.

Urinary incontinence in women. ACOG Practice Bulletin No. 63. American College of Obstetricians and Gynecologists. Obstet Gynecol 2005;105:1533–45.

Vincent GK, Velkoff VA. The next four decades: the older population in the United States: 2010 to 2050 population estimates and projections. Current Population Reports. Washington, DC: U.S. Census Bureau; 2010. Available at: http://www.census.gov/prod/2010pubs/p25-1138.pdf. Retrieved July 30, 2013.

Resources

Alzheimer's Association. Provider tools for identifying and managing cognitive impairment. Available at: http://www.alz.org/documents/mndak/toolkitsinglemarch13.pdf. Retrieved July 31, 2013.

American College of Obstetricians and Gynecologists. Healthy eating. Patient Education Pamphlet AP130. Washington, DC: American College of Obstetricians and Gynecologists; 2013.

American Geriatrics Society, British Geriatrics Society. Prevention of falls in older persons. AGS/BGS clinical practice guideline. New York (NY): AGS; London: BGS; 2010. Available at: http://www.medcats.com/FALLS/frameset.htm. Retrieved September 16, 2013.

American Geriatrics Society. A guide to dementia diagnosis and treatment. Available at: http://dementia.americangeriatrics.org/documents/AGS_PC_Dementia_Sheet_2010v2.pdf. Retrieved July 30, 2013.

California Workgroup on Guidelines for Alzheimer's Disease Management. Guideline for Alzheimer's disease management: final report. Sacramento (CA): State of California, Department of Public Health; 2008. Available at: http://www.cdph. ca.gov/programs/alzheimers/Documents/professional_GuidelineFullReport.pdf.

Elder abuse and women's health. Committee Opinion No. 568. American College of Obstetricians and Gynecologists. Obstet Gynecol 2013;122:187–91.

National Heart, Lung, and Blood Institute. Women's Health Initiative. Available at: http://www.nhlbi.nih.gov/whi. Retrieved July 31, 2013.

North American Menopause Society. Available at: http://www.menopause.org. Retrieved July 31, 2013.

Pharmacological management of persistent pain in older persons. American Geriatrics Society Panel on Pharmacological Management of Persistent Pain in Older Persons. J Am Geriatr Soc 2009;57:1331–46.

FEMALE GENITAL CUTTING

Female genital cutting, also known as female genital mutilation or female circumcision, is genital alteration performed on girls and young women for nontherapeutic reasons. Although opposition to it has increased, the practice is still widespread. According to the World Health Organization, approximately 140 million girls and women worldwide have undergone these procedures. Although practiced primarily in Africa, variations of female genital cutting have been found in the Middle East and Southeast Asia. In the United States, it is a federal crime to perform any medically unnecessary surgery on the genitalia of a girl younger than 18 years; however, women who have undergone the procedure may immigrate to this country. The African Women's Health Center at Brigham and Women's Hospital estimates that 228,000 women and girls in the United States have undergone, or are at risk of, female genital cutting.

Many different phrases have been used to describe female genital cutting. When talking with any woman who has undergone female genital cutting, it is important to determine how she refers to the procedure and adopt that terminology. The intent of this practice is circumcision, the cutting of genitals, based on cultural beliefs. The term mutilation emphasizes the degree of damage caused by this practice. It is important to recognize that most women who have undergone female genital cutting do not consider themselves to be mutilated and may be offended by such a suggestion.

There is no scientific basis for the practice of female genital cutting. Reasons given by families for the performance of female genital cutting include the following:

- Psychosexual reasons—attenuation of sexual desire in the female, insurance of chastity and virginity before marriage and fidelity within marriage, and increased male sexual pleasure

- Sociologic and cultural reasons—identification with the cultural heritage, initiation of girls into womanhood, social integration, and maintenance of social cohesion; removal of external genitals, which some cultures consider dirty and unsightly
- Myths—enhancement of fertility and promotion of child survival
- Religious reasons—mistaken belief by practitioners that female genital cutting has religious support and is required by the religious scripture

Many forms of female genital cutting are practiced. The most common type, which accounts for up to 90% of cases, involves the removal of the clitoris and partial or total excision of the labia minora. The most extreme form, infibulation, involves excision of part or all of the external genitalia and stitching or narrowing of the vaginal opening; this constitutes about 10% of all procedures.

Female genital cutting is performed predominantly on girls aged 0–15 years by medically untrained individuals under high-risk, unsterile conditions using crude instruments and no anesthetics. Immediate complications may include severe pain, infection (including human immunodeficiency virus [HIV]), tetanus, shock, hemorrhage, difficulty in passing urine, genital ulceration, injury to adjacent tissue, and death. Long-term complications may include the following:

- Chronic infection of the genital or urinary tracts
- HIV
- Chronic pain
- Keloids and other scarring abnormalities
- Vulvar abscesses
- Fistulae
- Menstrual abnormalities
- Infertility
- Urinary incontinence or voiding difficulty
- Depression, anxiety, and posttraumatic stress disorder

- Sexual dysfunction and dyspareunia
- Obstetric complications
  — Prolonged labor
  — Cesarean delivery
  — Extensive lacerations
  — Postpartum hemorrhage
  — Fetal asphyxia or death
  — Sepsis

The American College of Obstetricians and Gynecologists joins many other organizations (the World Health Organization, United Nations International Children's Emergency Fund, International Federation of Gynecology and Obstetrics, American Academy of Pediatrics, and the American Medical Association) in opposing all forms of medically unnecessary surgical modification of the female genitalia. The American College of Obstetricians and Gynecologists further recommends that the issue be addressed by the following:

- Treating patients who have undergone female genital cutting with sensitivity and compassion
- Tailoring obstetric and gynecologic care to the special physical and psychosocial needs of these patients
- Promoting awareness among the public
- Promoting awareness among health care providers
- Developing methods for educating physicians regarding the gynecologic and obstetric care of women who have undergone this procedure

Any general health care provider should do the following to address female genital cutting:

- Know the demographics of the local patient population to determine if female genital cutting is a medical issue that is likely to arise.
- Communicate effectively with this patient population with awareness and sensitivity.

- Work with interpreters and social workers, as necessary, to address the special needs of immigrants and refugees within this patient population.
- Review with patients the basics of female anatomy and reproductive function.
- Provide health education about female genital cutting and its physical and psychosexual consequences.
- Review with patients any special gynecologic issues, including menstrual, urinary, and sexual functions; family planning; and cancer screening.
- Offer alternatives to vaginal treatments or medications because the patient may not be comfortable with inserting, or may be unable to insert, anything in the vagina.
- Understand techniques for performing a pelvic examination on a woman who has had female genital cutting, including alternative procedures, as necessary:
  — Small or narrow speculum
  — Single-digit bimanual examination
  — Rectal examination to assess pelvic organs
  — Ultrasonographic evaluation

Specialized care of the patient who has undergone female genital cutting may include the following:

- Referral to a physician with special interest in pelvic or vaginal reconstructive surgery or a clinician practicing in an area of high prevalence of female genital cutting
- Familiarity with the types of female genital cutting and ensuing complications of each type
- Understanding of surgical therapies available, including the following:
  — Excision of cysts
  — Revision of introital or urethral scarring
  — Defibulation (opening the area that has been surgically closed)

— Repair of fistulae

— Procedures for correcting vaginal stenosis

- Counseling the patient before and after surgical correction about the new appearance of her anatomy and the expected changes in her urinary, menstrual, and sexual function

- Eliciting the help of social workers and psychiatric professionals

- Communication with policy makers, community groups, and women's groups about this issue

- Awareness of the current research on female genital cutting and on the safest timing and techniques for repair and reconstruction

Bibliography

American College of Obstetricians and Gynecologists. Female genital cutting: clinical management of circumcised women [CD-Rom]. 2nd ed. Washington, DC: ACOG; 2008.

Brigham and Women's Hospital. African Women's Health Center. Available at: http://www.brighamandwomens.org/Departments_and_Services/obgyn/services/africanwomenscenter/default.aspx. Retrieved July 31, 2013.

World Health Organization. Eliminating female genital mutilation: an interagency statement UNAIDS, UNDP, UNECA, UNESCO, UNFPA, UNHCHR, UNHCR, UNICEF, UNIFEM, WHO. Geneva: WHO; 2008. Available at: http://whqlibdoc. who.int/publications/2008/9789241596442_eng.pdf. Retrieved September 12, 2013.

World Health Organization. Female genital mutilation. Fact sheet No. 241. Geneva: WHO; 2013. Available at: http://www.who.int/mediacentre/factsheets/fs241/en. Retrieved July 31, 2013.

Resources

Biller-Andorno N, Wild V. The ethics of evidence. Hastings Cent Rep 2012;42:29-30.

Macklin R. Aesthetic enhancement? Or human rights violation? Hastings Cent Rep 2012;42:28–9.

Nour NM. Using facts to moderate the message. Hastings Cent Rep 2012;42:30–1.

Rosenberg LB, Gibson K, Shulman JF. When cultures collide: female genital cutting and U.S. obstetric practice. Obstet Gynecol 2009;113:931–4.

Seven things to know about female genital surgeries in Africa. Public Policy Advisory Network on Female Genital Surgeries in Africa. Hastings Cent Rep 2012;42:19–27.

World Health Organization. Female genital mutilation. Available at: http://www. who.int/topics/female_genital_mutilation/en. Retrieved July 31, 2013.

LESBIANS AND BISEXUAL WOMEN

Lesbians and bisexual women are as diverse as the general population of all women. They are represented among all ages, racial and ethnic groups, and socioeconomic strata. Given this diversity, obstetrician–gynecologists will encounter lesbian and bisexual patients, although not all will disclose their sexual orientation. Practitioners have the responsibility to provide quality care to all women regardless of sexual orientation.

Finding accepting, supportive, and culturally competent health and mental health practitioners may be difficult for lesbians and bisexual women. For this reason, lesbians may forgo needed health care or may not disclose their sexual identity to health care providers. To address more fully the health care needs of lesbians, clinicians should educate themselves and examine their own biases, developing responses to disclosure that are positive, respectful, and therapeutic.

Barriers to Health Care

Lesbians and bisexual women may experience barriers to health care, including the following:

- Confidentiality and disclosure concerns, especially in the adolescent population
- Lack of insurance coverage, because many are not able to participate in their partners' employment benefits package as would a married spouse
- Caregiver attitudes that cause them to hesitate in obtaining health care
- Limited understanding as to what their health risks may be

Routine Health Visits

Providers of reproductive health care and family planning services should not assume that patients, even if pregnant, are heterosexual. Likewise, they should not assume that women who say they are lesbians or bisexual are not in need of routine gynecologic care, including family planning and sexually transmitted infection (STI) and human immunodeficiency virus (HIV) screening and prevention counseling. Being a lesbian or bisexual woman does not inherently affect an individual's health status. There are no known physiologic differences between lesbians and heterosexual women. Standard comprehensive obstetric and gynecologic care is recommended for lesbians and bisexual women.

Many practitioners incorrectly presume that lesbian patients do not require screening for cervical cancer because they are at low risk. However, most lesbians have been sexually active with men at some point in their lives, and human papillomavirus transmission and cervical dysplasia may occur even with sexual contact exclusively among women. The usual recommendations from the American College of Obstetricians and Gynecologists should be followed to determine the onset and interval for cervical cancer screening (see also the "Well-Woman Annual Health Assessment" section earlier in Part 3).

Lesbians and bisexual women should be screened for STIs and HIV based on the same risk factors as other women (see also the "Sexually Transmitted Infections" section earlier in Part 3). Again, because most lesbians have been sexually active with men at some point in their lives and because some STIs can be transmitted by sexual activity exclusively among women, it should not be assumed that STI screening is unnecessary. All patients, regardless of their sexual orientation, should be encouraged to practice safer sex. Safer sex practices for lesbians include using gloves and dental dams, using condoms on sex toys, avoiding sharing of sex toys, and avoiding contact with a partner's menstrual blood and any visible genital lesions.

Psychosocial Concerns

Clinicians should be alert to the signs and symptoms of depression, substance abuse, and violence (including intimate partner violence) in all patients and conduct appropriate screening and intervention. Lesbians and bisexual women may be at greater risk of depressive disorders and drug or alcohol dependency. Violence and fear of violence because of sexual orientation can confer emotional sequelae, including depression, diminished self-esteem, and suicidal thoughts. Mental health concerns also apply to youth who self-identify as lesbian, gay, or bisexual. Counseling may be very helpful for adolescents who are uncertain about their sexual orientation or have difficulty expressing their sexuality and can assist a lesbian or bisexual adolescent in coping with difficulties faced at home, school, or in the community (see also the "Adolescents" section earlier in Part 3).

Legal Considerations

Most lesbians are in long-term relationships. Lesbians and their partners would be well advised to contact an attorney to keep abreast of legal decisions in their state regarding health care powers of attorney for each other. Sexual orientation should not be a barrier to receiving fertility services to achieve a pregnancy. Lesbians should have equal access to co-parenting and second parent adoption rights. This view also is supported by the American Academy of Pediatrics and the American Medical Association. Lesbians in same-sex parent families should be encouraged to confer with an attorney because the laws on adoption vary by state and continue to evolve. The American College of Obstetricians and Gynecologists supports equitable treatment for lesbians and their families, not only for direct health needs but also for indirect health issues, which include the same legal protections afforded married couples.

Creating a Welcoming Patient Care Environment

Obstetrician–gynecologists can make their practices more receptive to lesbian and bisexual patients by offering the following:

- Education and appropriate training of office staff to ensure a welcoming and respectful environment
- Registration forms and questionnaires that give patients the opportunity to identify sexual relationships and behaviors (see the "Well-Woman Annual Health Assessment" section earlier in Part 3 and the "Sexual Function and Dysfunction" section in Part 4)

- Posted nondiscrimination policies
- Use of inclusive language such as partner or spouse
- Use of nonjudgmental methods for inquiring about sexual orientation and behavior:
  - "Are you single, partnered, married, widowed, or divorced, or do you have a domestic partner?"
  - "Are you or have you been sexually active with anyone—male, female, or both—or are you not sexually active?"
  - "Who are you sexually attracted to—men, women, or both?"
- Reassurances regarding confidentiality, including the offer not to record information about sexual orientation in writing in the patient's records or to code the information
- Display of educational materials about sexual orientation and gender issues for patients and their families (see Resources)
- Referrals to counseling and support groups for patients and their families (see Resources)

Bibliography

Addressing health risks of noncoital sexual activity. Committee Opinion No. 582. American College of Obstetricians and Gynecologists. Obstet Gynecol 2013; 122:1378–83.

Health care for lesbians and bisexual women. Committee Opinion No. 525. American College of Obstetricians and Gynecologists. Obstet Gynecol 2012;119:1077–80.

Marriage equality for same-sex couples. Committee Opinion No. 574. American College Obstetricians and Gynecologists. Obstet Gynecol 2013;122:729–32.

Resources

Gates GJ. How many people are lesbian, gay, bisexual, and transgender? Los Angeles (CA): The Williams Institute, UCLA School of Law; 2011. Available at: http://williamsinstitute.law.ucla.edu/wp-content/uploads/Gates-How-Many-People-LGBT-Apr-2011.pdf. Retrieved July 31, 2013.

Gay and Lesbian Medical Association. Available at: http://www.glma.org. Retrieved July 31, 2013.

Parents, Family, and Friends of Lesbians and Gays. Available at: http://community.pflag.org. Retrieved July 31, 2013.

Whitman–Walker Health. Mautner Project of Whitman–Walker Health. Available at: http://www.whitman-walker.org/mautnerproject. Retrieved April 10, 2014.

▌TRANSGENDER INDIVIDUALS

"Transgender" is a broad term used for people whose gender identity or gender expression differs from their assigned sex at birth. However, there is no universally accepted definition of the word transgender because of the lack of agreement regarding what groups of people are considered transgender. The spectrum of transgender identity includes transsexual, crossdresser, bi-gendered, intersex, female-to-male, and male-to-female (Box 3-29). Transgender individuals may live full-time or part-time in their chosen gender. Regardless, all transgender individuals should be referred to by their chosen pronoun.

Estimates of the prevalence of transgender individuals are limited by the lack of centralized reporting and are not clearly established; however, studies suggest that transgender individuals constitute a small but substantial population. This low prevalence likely further contributes to their social marginalization and the scarcity of scientific data about their health care needs.

Barriers to Health Care

Transgender individuals are at increased risk of experiences with discrimination and violence and of poor health outcomes. A 2006 Internet survey of 446 female-to-male transgender individuals showed that they have diminished quality of life compared with other men and women in the United States. Fears about judgment or discrimination from health care providers may prevent transgender patients from revealing their chosen gender identity or from seeking health care at all. In 1999, the American Public Health Association passed a resolution that recognizes the unique health care needs of transgender individuals and urges researchers and health care providers to provide transgender individuals with sensitive and culturally competent health care. Insensitivity of health

Box 3-29. Transgender Definitions

Transsexual—an individual who strongly identifies with the other sex and seeks hormones, gender-affirmation surgery, or both to feminize or masculinize the body; may live full-time in the crossgender role.*

Crossdresser—an individual who dresses in the clothing of the opposite sex for reasons that include a need to express femininity or masculinity, artistic expression, performance, or erotic pleasure, but do not identify as that gender. The term transvestite was previously used to describe a crossdresser, but it is now considered pejorative and should not be used.[†]

Bigendered—individuals who identify as both or alternatively male and female, as no gender, or as a gender outside the male or female binary.[†]

Intersex—individuals with a set of congenital variations of the reproductive system that are not considered typical for either male or female. This includes newborns with ambiguous genitalia, a condition that affects 1 in 2,000 newborns in the United States each year.[‡]

Female-to-male—refers to someone who was identified as female at birth but who identifies and portrays his gender as male. This term often is used after the individual has taken some steps to express his gender as male, or after medically transitioning through hormones or surgery. Also known as FTM or transman.[†]

Male-to-female—refers to someone who was identified as male at birth but who identifies and portrays her gender as female. This term often is used after the individual has taken some steps to express her gender as female, or after medically transitioning through hormones or surgery. Also known as MTF or transwoman.[†]

---

*The health of lesbian, gay, bisexual, and transgender people: building a foundation for better understanding. Washington, DC: National Academies Press; 2011. Available at: http://www.nap.edu/openbook.php?record_id=13128&page=R1. Retrieved July 31, 2013.

[†]Fenway Health. Glossary of gender and transgender terms. Boston (MA): Fenway Health; 2010. Available at: http://www.fenwayhealth.org/site/DocServer/Handout_7-C_Glossary_of_Gender_and_Transgender_Terms__fi.pdf. Retrieved July 31, 2013.

[‡]Dreger AD. "Ambiguous sex"—or ambivalent medicine? Ethical issues in the treatment of intersexuality. Hastings Cent Rep 1998;28:24–35.

Reprinted from Health care for transgender individuals. Committee Opinion No. 512. American College of Obstetricians and Gynecologists. Obstet Gynecol 2011;118:1454–8.

care providers around transgender issues, such as not using appropriate pronouns or not acknowledging the chosen gender identity, has been reported and is frequently cited as a reason for avoiding health care services. Other factors that may inhibit individuals from seeking health care include low self-esteem from a negative body image and fear that their transgender status will be revealed. Maintaining privacy is critical when treating transgender patients, as concerns about breaches in confidentiality also are often reported as a barrier to care.

Caring for Transgender Individuals

The obstetrician–gynecologist should be prepared to provide or refer transgender patients for routine health maintenance and preventive care as well as hormonal and surgical therapies. Basic preventive services, such as sexually transmitted infection (STI) testing and cancer screening can be provided without any specific training in transgender care. Physical examination and screening tests should be based on the organ systems present rather than the perceived gender of the patient.

FEMALE-TO-MALE TRANSGENDER INDIVIDUALS

Discomfort with the female aspects of their physical body may make female-to-male transgender individuals less likely to seek gynecologic care. In one study of 122 female-to-male transgender individuals, 49% did not undergo annual pelvic examinations, with 40% citing "discomfort with the exam due to gender issues" as the reason. The presence of breasts is a source of significant gender identity conflict for female-to-male transgender patients, which may lead to avoidance of breast cancer screening. In addition, because of social marginalization, transgender individuals may be at increased risk of STIs and human immunodeficiency virus (HIV) and, therefore, require appropriate safe sex counseling and STI testing. Female-to-male transgender patients with male sexual partners may be at risk of pregnancy, and contraception should be discussed. Age-appropriate screening for breast and cervical cancer should be continued unless mastectomy has been performed or the cervix has been removed.

More than one half of female-to-male patients undergo testosterone therapy, which may put them at increased risk of hyperlipidemia, cardiovascular disease, liver disease, and breast cancer. Female-to-male transgender individuals who use androgens and have not had a hysterectomy may be at increased risk of endometrial cancer and ovarian cancer. The use of illicitly obtained testosterone is associated with an increase in needle sharing, which also puts these patients at increased risk of infection with HIV or hepatitis.

Supplemental calcium and vitamin D should be recommended according to current osteoporosis-prevention guidelines to help maintain bone density (see also the "Osteoporosis" section earlier in Part 3). This is especially true for female-to-male patients who are taking testosterone (because of its unknown effect on bone density) or who have had, or are considering, oophorectomy.

MALE-TO-FEMALE TRANSGENDER INDIVIDUALS

Age-appropriate screening for breast cancer (see also the "Cancer Screening and Prevention" section earlier in Part 3) and prostate cancer should be provided to male-to-female transgender patients. Opinions vary regarding the need for Pap testing in this population. In patients who have a neo-cervix created from the glans penis, routine cytologic examination of the neocervix may be indicated. It also is recommended that male-to-female transgender patients who receive estrogen therapy have an annual prolactin level assessment and visual field examination to screen for prolactinoma.

Creating a Welcoming Patient Care Environment

Most importantly, health care providers should treat transgender individuals with respect and dignity. Office and support staff should develop and maintain sensitive attitudes and practices for all patients, including transgender individuals, as well as for their families and significant others. Patient forms should be made inclusive and less discriminatory by including additional options for gender identification and relationship status. Questions should be framed in ways that do not make assumptions about gender identity, sexual orientation, or behavior. It is more appropriate for clinicians to ask their patients which terms they prefer. Language should be inclusive to allow the patient to decide when and what to disclose. Care of transgender individuals often requires special considerations that can be addressed best by physicians with expertise and experience in this area, although experts are mostly limited to large urban areas. Transgender individuals are entitled to compassionate and culturally appropriate care. Health care providers who are morally opposed to providing care to this population should refer them elsewhere.

Bibliography

American Public Health Association. The need for acknowledging transgendered individuals within research and clinical practice. APHA Policy Statement 9933. Washington, DC: APHA; 1999. Available at: http://www.apha.org/advocacy/policy/policysearch/default.htm?id=204. Retrieved September 12, 2013.

Dreger AD. "Ambiguous sex"–or ambivalent medicine? Ethical issues in the treatment of intersexuality. Hastings Cent Rep 1998;28:24–35.

Dutton L, Koenig K, Fennie K. Gynecologic care of the female-to-male transgender man. J Midwifery Womens Health 2008;53:331–7.

Fenway Health. Glossary of gender and transgender terms. Boston (MA): Fenway Health; 2010. Available at: http://www.fenwayhealth.org/site/DocServer/Handout_7-C_Glossary_of_Gender_and_Transgender_Terms__fi.pdf. Retrieved July 31, 2013.

Health care for transgender individuals. Committee Opinion No. 512. American College of Obstetricians and Gynecologists. Obstet Gynecol 2011;118:1454–8.

Institute of Medicine. The health of lesbian, gay, bisexual, and transgender people: building a foundation for better understanding. Washington, DC: National Academies Press; 2011.

McKay B. Lesbian, gay, bisexual, and transgender health issues, disparities, and information resources. Med Ref Serv Q 2011;30:393–401.

Moore E, Wisniewski A, Dobs A. Endocrine treatment of transsexual people: a review of treatment regimens, outcomes, and adverse effects. J Clin Endocrinol Metab 2003;88:3467–73.

Rachlin K, Green J, Lombardi E. Utilization of health care among female-to-male transgender individuals in the United States. J Homosex 2008;54:243–58.

Resources

Centers for Disease Control and Prevention. Lesbian, gay, bisexual and transgender health. Available at: http://www.cdc.gov/lgbthealth/index.htm. Retrieved September 17, 2013.

Gay and Lesbian Medical Association. Available at: www.glma.org. Retrieved September 17, 2013.

Gay, Lesbian, Bisexual, and Transgender (GLBT) Health Access Project. Available at: http://www.glbthealth.org. Retrieved September 17, 2013.

Lesbian Health and Research Center. Available at: http://lesbianhealthinfo.org. Retrieved September 17, 2013.

National Coalition for LGBT Health. Available at: http://lgbthealth.webolutionary. com. Retrieved September 17, 2013.

National Library of Medicine. MedlinePlus: gay, lesbian, bisexual and transgender health. Available at: http://www.nlm.nih.gov/medlineplus/gaylesbianbisexualand transgenderhealth.html. Retrieved September 17, 2013.

University of California, San Francisco. Center of Excellence for Transgender Health. Available at: http://www.transhealth.ucsf.edu. Retrieved September 17, 2013.

World Professional Association for Transgender Health. Available at: www.wpath. org. Retrieved September 17, 2013.

WOMEN WITH DISABILITIES

Disability, as defined by the Americans With Disabilities Act of 1990, is a "physical or mental impairment that substantially limits one or more of the major life activities of an individual, a record of such impairment, or being regarded as having such an impairment." Physical, developmental, sensory, cognitive, and psychiatric impairments may affect the quality and availability of health care services for women. Women with disabilities have unique gynecologic needs that require practitioner awareness, sensitivity, and skill. As for all women, the optimal health care of women with disabilities is comprehensive, affirms the patient's dignity, maximizes the patient's interests, and avoids harm.

Health care providers have a societal and professional ethical responsibility to accommodate and individualize the care of women with special needs. In addition, Title III of the Americans With Disabilities Act requires that a public accommodation operated by a private entity, including professional offices of health care providers, take steps to ensure that no individual with a disability is discriminated against on the basis of the disabling limitation (see also Appendix G). Physical limitations and communication difficulties that might hinder the health care of women with disabilities can be overcome by alternative positioning, modification of examinations, knowledge of the issues, technology, sensitivity, and patience (see Box 3-30).

In addition to physical barriers, a woman with disabilities may experience knowledge and attitudinal barriers in her physician's office. In the health care setting, not infrequently, women with disabilities report feeling that they are viewed as asexual and unlikely to be lovers, wives, or mothers. Sexuality issues that women with disabilities face need to be addressed; these issues include the desire and ability for consensual sexual relationships and childbearing. Pregnancy and parenting for women with physical disabilities may have unique medical and social aspects but rarely are precluded by the disability itself.

511

Box 3-30. Suggestions for Office Practices That Serve Women With Disabilities

Before scheduling an appointment for the patient, the following steps are recommended:

- Become familiar with health care provider responsibilities stipulated in the Americans With Disabilities Act. Assess the medical practice environment and make appropriate modifications in layout, equipment, and staff training. If possible, include women with disabilities in the assessment and development of service delivery plans.
- Identify a point person within the practice to research local disability resources and be responsible for assuring the development and documentation of a plan of care for each woman with disabilities.

The following steps are recommended when scheduling an appointment for the patient:

- Ask about the special needs of the patient, including extra time, access considerations, and communication requirements.
- Determine at the time the appointment is made whether or not the patient usually gives consent for examination or treatment. If the patient is not able, the legal guardian or authorized (documented) caregiver should be asked to accompany the patient to the appointment.
- Contact, with consent, the primary care physician to ascertain medical history and gain advice or direction concerning the following:
  — Psychosocial factors, such as living arrangements, and the reliability of patient and caretakers to follow through with advice and medical treatment; the most effective methods of health education; and the availability of community resources for the patient
  — Physical factors, such as the patient's ability to use a standard examination table; best method of transfer (for patients with physical disabilities); best position for examination; most appropriate person to accompany the patient during examination; the extent of examination possible without sedation; the patient's history of examination under sedation or anesthesia
- Determine the patient's mode of transportation to the office and, if she is dependent on a public disability transport system, allow for some time flexibility.
- Scan the office or clinic to determine the accessibility of the reception areas, restroom, examination room, consultation room, X-ray and laboratory area, and other equipment for the patient.

(continued)

Box 3-30. Suggestions for Office Practices That Serve Women With Disabilities *(continued)*

- Determine the need for assistants to aid in transferring, positioning, and supporting the patient.
- Determine the need to arrange for an interpreter (sign language or other).
- Determine the patient's desire to have a chaperone present during the examination, and schedule the examination to accommodate this need.
- Schedule, if possible, the patient's appointment at a time of light patient volume and maximum staffing.

The following steps are recommended before or at the time of the appointment:

- Discuss the patient's appointment with office staff before the appointment, and designate a point person for facilitation.
- Allow the patient to determine who, if anyone, is to accompany her during the examination.
- Allow time before the examination for the patient to become familiar with the examination room and the health care provider.
- Be alert to cold or hard instruments and loud noises because the patient may be extremely sensitive to tactile and auditory stimulation.
- Be alert to signs of physical and sexual abuse, such as statements by the patient or physical signs of abuse, including the presence of sexually transmitted infections and bruising or swelling of the genitals. Reporting requirements on abuse differ in each state.

The following steps are recommended for providing health education:

- Stock the office with health education resources and materials available for women with physical and developmental disabilities.
- Patients who live in a group situation may have multiple caregivers. For these women, all printed health education, instruction, and treatment information is best delivered in lower literacy English (other language as indicated) as well as orally to the accompanying attendant. Consider using visiting nurses to ensure instructions or treatment regimens are understood and followed.

Modified from American College of Obstetricians and Gynecologists. Access to reproductive health care for women with disabilities. In: Special issues in women's health. Washington, DC: ACOG; 2005. p. 39–59.

Before examination and treatment of a woman with developmental disabilities, it should be determined who will give consent (see also the "Ethical Issues" section in Part 1). It is important to ascertain if the patient is capable of understanding findings and recommendations or whether this information needs to be concurrently transmitted to an identified guardian or caregiver.

Women with developmental disabilities may present with a broad range of health concerns, including difficulty maintaining preventive care, poor hygiene, unanticipated pubertal development, the need for contraception, pregnancy, abnormal uterine bleeding, or menopausal issues. They may have unidentified sexual activity and need to be screened routinely for sexually transmitted infections. Psychosocial factors must be considered to determine an appropriate treatment plan that offers individualized reproductive health care and education to this group of women and their caregivers.

Health care providers should familiarize themselves with the nature of the woman's disability because the conditions may affect directly the decisions made in her reproductive health care. For example, women with physical or developmental disabilities may take medication for spasms and seizures. An understanding of such medications, possible interactions, and their effects on gynecologic issues also is important.

Women with disabilities often undergo screening for cervical and breast cancer less frequently than recommended. If possible, screening for cancer should be performed according to standard recommendations from the American College of Obstetricians and Gynecologists (see also the "Cancer Screening and Prevention" section earlier in Part 3). In women with developmental disabilities, it may be necessary to perform the pelvic examination under general anesthesia. Before examination, it is important to ascertain from the patient if she has previously experienced autonomic dysreflexia, the reaction of the autonomic nervous system to noxious stimuli, including manipulation of visceral organs, constipation, distended bladder, and skin lesions. Symptoms include extreme hypertension, flushing, diaphoresis, and piloerection. Autonomic dysreflexia has a rapid onset and can result in seizures, intracranial hemorrhage, coma, and death. It often can be avoided by emptying the bladder before the examination, using an anesthetic gel, and performing slow and gentle internal examinations with a warmed speculum. Autonomic dysreflexia usually can be managed by stopping the stimuli, raising the patient's head, and monitoring blood pressure.

Women with disabilities are at risk of abuse by family members, institutional workers, and those who provide personal care and services. This abuse may include withholding of assistance or assistive devices. Women who rely on others for their personal and household needs may be reluctant to disclose concerns about abuse or violence for fear of retaliation or loss of these essential services performed by an abusive health care provider.

Contraceptive options should be discussed with all reproductive-aged women with disabilities. Considerations include the following: pharmacologic interactions of the contraception with other medications; actual or potential conditions of the woman; the amount of assistance available to, and required for, the woman; her lifestyle and self-care needs; and her desires for future pregnancy. Of particular value are contraceptive methods that are not administered frequently or that have a relatively long duration. Menstrual suppression through use of hormonal contraception may be useful for women with developmental or physical disabilities that make menstrual hygiene problematic. Adverse effects, such as unscheduled bleeding, must be considered. In most cases, the chosen method of contraception should be the least restrictive in preserving future reproductive options. It is imperative that physicians comply with the highest ethical standards—as well as to federal, state, and local laws and regulations—when considering sterilization for women with developmental disabilities.

Bibliography

American College of Obstetricians and Gynecologists. Access to reproductive health care for women with disabilities. In: Special issues in women's health. Washington, DC: ACOG; 2005. p. 39–59.

Informed consent. ACOG Committee Opinion No. 439. American College of Obstetricians and Gynecologists. Obstet Gynecol 2009;114:401–8.

Sterilization of women, including those with mental disabilities. ACOG Committee Opinion No. 371. American College of Obstetricians and Gynecologists. Obstet Gynecol 2007;110:217–20.

Resources

Heaton C, Roberts BS, Murphy L, Meagher M, Randall D. Let's talk about health: what every woman should know. North Brunswick (NJ): The ARC of New Jersey; 1994.

American College of Obstetricians and Gynecologists. Reproductive health care for women with disabilities. Interactive site for clinicians serving women with disabilities. Available at: http://www.acog.org/About_ACOG/ACOG_Departments/Women_with_Disabilities/Interactive_site_for_clinicians_serving_women_with_disabilities. Retrieved September 17, 2013.

Center for Research on Women with Disabilities. Baylor College of Medicine. Available at http://www.bcm.edu/crowd/. Retrieved September 17, 2013.

Centers for Disease Control and Prevention. Mammography use and women with disabilities: a tip sheet for public health professionals. Available at: http://www.cdc.gov/ncbddd/documents/mammography-tip-sheet-_-php_1a_1.pdf. Retrieved July 31, 2013.

END-OF-LIFE CONSIDERATIONS

Obstetricians and gynecologists, including those in training, care for women throughout their life span and not infrequently need to participate in end-of-life decision making. Tragic accidents occasionally threaten the life of a pregnant woman and her fetus, and terminal outcomes occur for some patients with gynecologic cancer. As a result, physicians are expected to present options and guide patients as they make decisions in advance of, as well as in the face of, such events. Life-threatening situations are never easy to deal with, even for the well trained.

Regardless of a patient's age, the opportunity to formulate advance directives allows her to express her choices about the treatment she would like to receive in the event she becomes unable to participate in decisions concerning her care and to identify the person she wishes to have act as her surrogate decision-maker. Physician orders for life-sustaining treatment (also known as medical orders for life-sustaining treatment) are available once a patient develops serious, progressive, chronic illnesses that may require standing medical orders. Familiarity with the ethical, legal, and psychosocial aspects of providing end-of-life care and with the facilitation of end-of-life decision making will assist clinicians in providing the most appropriate care to their patients and their families.

The first step in advance care planning and caring for a critically ill or terminally ill patient is to identify her values and beliefs through shared and ongoing communication between the clinician, patient, and her family, when applicable. Comprehensive and ongoing communication not only advances patient self-determination but also may help prevent ethical conflict and crisis. Clinicians should be especially careful not to impose their beliefs about benefits and risks on a patient or coerce her to achieve goals that are not in accordance with her values and beliefs. For instance, the harms associated with ongoing therapeutic interventions may not be acceptable to some patients. Respect for a woman's autonomy should guide the manner of care that she wishes to receive at the end of life. Her wishes should be respected, as relayed by her surrogate decision maker if she has not previously voiced or documented any wishes and does not have the capacity to make her own health care decisions. If physicians have moral reservations about providing certain forms of care or about stopping treatment, they should (if appropriate to the circumstances) make that known, in accordance with existing guidance about conscientious objection. If decisions made by a woman or made on her behalf by her surrogate decision maker cause the physician to experience significant moral distress or ethical conflict, the physician has the right to transfer care to a physician who has more expertise and is more comfortable with these choices (see also the "Ethical Issues" section in Part 1).

Many clinicians are uncomfortable with the prospect of providing care for a patient at the end of her life. The ethos that has shaped U.S. medical research and practice for the past half century regards the use of interventions to promote cure and prolong life as the clinician's primary obligation. But palliative strategies, such as pain relief, attentive and responsive communication with the patient about her health status, and the facilitation of communication with the patient's family, also are essential components of care. There is a growing role for multidisciplinary health care teams when a care plan transitions towards palliation, including specialists from palliative medicine, spiritual care, and social work. As part of an ongoing effort to provide care even when therapeutic interventions are no longer warranted, it is important to note that neither the presence of a "do not attempt resuscitation" or "allow natural death" order nor specific directives regarding limitation of other treatments remove the responsibility for providing palliative and comfort care. For the generalist whose patient is, or has been, under the care of a specialist, palliative care often is the most valuable service that can be offered. The idea that "nothing more can be done" improperly equates care with cure and should be avoided. It undervalues the considerable importance of the clinician in providing comfort to the critically ill or terminally ill patient.

Legal Rights

The federal Patient Self-Determination Act of 1990 requires that all hospitals and other medical programs that receive federal Medicare and Medicaid money create a formal procedure to inform patients, on admission to the facility or at the time of enrollment in a health maintenance organization, about their rights under state law regarding health care decision making. This information includes the rights to refuse treatment and to formulate advance directives. An advance directive is the formal mechanism by which a patient may express her values regarding her future health status or appoint a surrogate decision maker for medical decisions. Facilities also are required to document in the patient's record whether or not an advance directive was executed. Noncompliance with these requirements can mean the loss of eligibility to receive Medicaid and Medicare funds. Every state and the District of Columbia also have laws allowing for advance directives. State law will determine what an advance directive may contain and how and when it is followed.

A living will and a health care power of attorney are the two most common types of advance directives. Although both address issues of end-of-life decision-making, these documents serve different purposes and clinicians should be aware of their distinct functions. Depending on the laws in a particular state, a patient may decide that either a living will or a health care power of attorney is better suited to her needs. She also may have both types of directives or a single document that combines the aspects of both. Although legal advice to prepare an advance directive is not necessary, patients may want to consult with an attorney for guidance.

A living will is a written statement that tells the health care team and family in advance what types of health care the patient would accept or refuse if she were to lack decision-making capacity and be unable to express her wishes. A living will goes into effect only if the patient is unable to make decisions for herself. Until this time, the patient can change her mind at any time about what she has written. The laws about living wills vary from state to state, but in general, living wills address the following issues:

- Life-sustaining treatments, including cardiopulmonary resuscitation and respirator use

- Artificial nutrition and hydration if required as the main treatment to keep patients alive
- The degree and type of pain relief
- Major surgery and other major interventions, such as renal dialysis

Laws in some states are more restrictive than in others regarding when a living will can be used. Most states limit the rights of pregnant patients to refuse certain treatments through a living will because of the need to protect the developing fetus. Knowledge of local regulations is important. In addition, although physicians are legally obligated to honor a patient's living will, they may not be required to do so if they believe in good faith that under particular concrete circumstances the request is not sound.

Standard, easy-to-complete patient forms for living wills usually are available from hospitals, insurance companies, physician offices, and health departments. Many forms also allow the patient to express her wishes regarding organ donation if she is a suitable candidate. When using a standard form, it is important to confirm that the form is valid under state law and to follow the instructions, including those that require witnesses or notarization.

In a health care power of attorney, the patient authorizes a health care agent to act as a surrogate decision maker and make medical decisions for her when she no longer is able to do so. A patient may indicate in her health care power of attorney her wishes about her medical care, and she should discuss them with her surrogate decision maker, who will be expected to make decisions consistent with the patient's wishes. In a health care power of attorney, the patient might specify what powers she is giving her surrogate decision maker. These powers may include the power to choose physicians, the right to decide whether to hospitalize the patient, and the right to accept or refuse treatment. The patient also may give the surrogate decision maker instructions as to whether she wishes to be an organ donor, if eligible. Because the health care power of attorney designates a surrogate decision-maker to elect or decline a number of different interventions, it generally is applicable in more situations than a living will. As with living wills, many states have restrictions on a surrogate decision maker who is appointed to make decisions on behalf of a pregnant woman.

After a living will, health care power of attorney, or both are completed, several copies should be made to provide to physicians, an attorney, and relevant family or friends. If the patient has designated a surrogate decision maker, this individual should have copies of all advance directives. Patients should keep the originals in a secure place and provide a copy to the hospital when admitted. Patients also might want to keep in their wallet or purse a small card indicating that they have an advance directive, where the advance directive can be found, and the name and address of their surrogate decision maker, if any.

Unfortunately, only a small number of adults have prepared advance directives. Most patients do not want to think about becoming ill and being unable to care for themselves. It is best to prepare an advance directive when healthy. No one knows when a serious accident will happen. For these reasons, it is important that the medical team make the options of advance directives known and available to all patients regardless of age or medical status. A good opportunity to initiate the discussion of end-of-life caregiving goals is during well-woman care at the time of the periodic examination or early in prenatal care. To facilitate these discussions, the patient history form could contain questions about a patient's execution of an advance directive.

Because a patient's wishes regarding care might change over time or under different conditions of illness, these discussions should include occasional reevaluation of values and goals and, if necessary, updating of the advance directive. Decision making should be treated as a process rather than as an event.

Terminal Care

PROVISIONS FOR CARE: HOSPITAL, HOSPICE, HOME

Several options for the provision of terminal care commonly exist for dying patients and their families. Among the levels of care available are care in the hospital, care in a residential hospice, and care in the home with or without hospice support.

Seriously ill people generally seek out hospital care in the hope of avoiding death, pain, and suffering. However, when death is imminent, the anticipation of death in a hospital may be accompanied by the fear that medical care is less focused on human suffering and dignity than on medical logic and vital functions. In 1989, the Study to Understand Prognosis and Preferences for Outcomes and Risks of Treatment was undertaken in an effort to understand the characteristics of dying in U.S. hospitals. The baseline study showed that much terminal care in the United States is inappropriate. Many patients died after prolonged hospitalization or intensive care; many suffered from unrelieved pain. Several reasons exist for these problems. Clinicians may be uncertain about patient prognosis, may not agree with other members of the health care team about the course of care, may not know the patient's preferences regarding life-sustaining interventions, or may have failed to discuss care options with patients and families.

Hospitalized patients and their families should be granted real decision-making powers concerning terminal care. Recommendations to grant patients more powers in these decisions include the following suggestions:

- Patients and families should be provided with explicit prognostic information.
- Discussions about life-sustaining care need to occur frequently. Typically, patients look to their physicians to take the lead in these discussions.
- The quality of discussions about life-sustaining interventions should be improved. These discussions should include information about providing or withholding therapy, with special attention to the patient's values and concerns.

Hospice refers to a concept of care rather than a specific place for care. Hospice care provides support for people in the last phases of incurable diseases in the hope that they will live as fully or comfortably as possible. Care is provided in home-based and facility-based settings. No specific supportive therapy is excluded from consideration, and treatments generally are based on agreements among the patient, physician, and hospice team. The expected outcome is relief from symptoms and enhancement of quality of life. The patient's and family's needs should be considered when deciding between home-based and residential hospice care.

The core team providing hospice care typically consists of the patient's attending and hospice physicians, registered nurses, social workers, spiritual counselors, family members, and trained volunteers. Hospice care also uses specialized team members to meet specific patient care needs. These team members may include allied therapists, art and music therapists, dietitians, pharmacists, nurses, and nursing assistants.

The hospice interdisciplinary team collaborates with the patient's attending physician to develop a patient-directed, individualized plan of care. The plan of care is based on team assessments that recognize the patient's and family's psychologic and social values. At a minimum, the plan generally includes the following parameters:

- Problems and needs of the patient and her family
- Realistic and achievable goals and objectives
- Agreed-on outcomes
- Required medical equipment
- The use of advance directives in care plan development

Medicare coverage includes hospice benefits. Today, many private insurers and Medicaid also offer hospice benefits, a recognition of the compassion associated with hospice care and its cost-effective delivery.

PAIN MANAGEMENT

Pain often is undertreated, particularly at the end of life. Current protocols often specify principles such as the idea that no terminally ill patient should be in pain. Studies indicate that concerned family members generally are satisfied with life-sustaining treatment decisions, but their primary concerns are with failures in communication and pain control. Pain relief is one of the primary goals (for the patient and her family) of terminal care (see also the "Acute and Chronic Pain Management" section in Part 4).

Posthumous Reproduction

A last consideration for the obstetrician–gynecologist who provides end-of-life care is use of gametes and embryos for posthumous reproduction.

In the course of fertility treatment and assisted reproduction, reproductive tissue (including oocytes, sperm, and embryos) may be cryopreserved. Patients should be strongly encouraged to state in writing their decisions regarding the disposition of their stored gametes and embryos in the case that one, or if partnered, both individuals die before the gametes or embryos are used. Options include transferring dispositional control of the gametes or embryos to a surviving partner or to a third party, donating to research, or discarding them. Such decisions should be honored. Occasionally, family members or surrogate decision makers may ask physicians to invasively procure posthumous gametes for reproductive purposes. The American Society for Reproductive Medicine states that a request to obtain oocytes after a woman's death without the woman's prior consent or known wishes need not be honored.

Bibliography

Dying well in the hospital: lessons from SUPPORT. Hastings Cent Rep 1995;25(6): S1–S36.

End-of-life decision making. ACOG Committee Opinion No. 403. American College of Obstetricians and Gynecologists. Obstet Gynecol 2008;111:1021–7.

Finnerty JF, Fuerst CW, Karns LB, Pinkerton JV. End-of-life discussions for the primary care obstetrician/gynecologist. Am J Obstet Gynecol 2002;187:296–301.

Hofmann JC, Wenger NS, Davis RB, Teno J, Connors AF, Jr, Desbiens N, et al. Patient preferences for communication with physicians about end-of-life decisions. SUPPORT Investigators. Study to Understand Prognoses and Preference for Outcomes and Risks of Treatment. Ann Intern Med 1997;127:1–12.

Jennings B. Preface: Improving end of life care: why has it been so difficult? Hastings Cent Rep 2005;Spec No:S2–4.

Medical futility. ACOG Committee Opinion No. 362. American College of Obstetricians and Gynecologists. Obstet Gynecol 2007;109:791–4.

Posthumous reproduction. Ethics Committee of the American Society for Reproductive Medicine. Fertil Steril 2004;82(suppl):S260-2.

Roberts JA, Brown D, Elkins T, Larson DB. Factors influencing views of patients with gynecologic cancer about end-of-life decisions. Am J Obstet Gynecol 1997; 176:166–72.

Resources

American Cancer Society. Available at: www.cancer.org. Retrieved September 17, 2013.

American Hospice Foundation. www.americanhospice.org. Retrieved on September 17, 2013.

American Medical Association. Advance care planning. In: Code of medical ethics of the American Medical Association: current opinions and annotations. 2012–2013 ed. Chicago (IL): AMA; 2012. p. 92–3.

American Medical Association. Sedation to unconsciousness in end-of-life-care. In: Code of medical ethics of the American Medical Association: current opinions and annotations. 2012–2013 ed. Chicago (IL): AMA; 2012. p. 113–4.

American Society of Clinical Oncology. Advanced cancer care planning: what patients and families need to know about their choices when facing serious illness. Alexandria (VA): ASCO; 2011. Available at: http://www.cancer.net/sites/cancer.net/files/vignette/Advanced_Cancer_Care_Planning.pdf. Retrieved July 31, 2013.

Center to Advance Palliative Care. Available at: www.capc.org. Retrieved July 31, 2013.

Children's Hospice International. Available at: www.chionline.org. Retrieved July 31, 2013.

Dunn GP, Martensen R, Weissman D, editors. Surgical palliative care: A resident's guide. Chicago (IL); Essex (CT): American College of Surgeons; Cunniff-Dixon Foundation; 2009. Available at: http://www.facs.org/palliativecare/surgicalpalliativecareresidents.pdf. Retrieved September 30, 2013.

EPEC Project Robert Wood Johnson Foundation. EPEC: education for physicians on end-of-life care: participant's handbook: plenary 3: elements and models of end-of-life care. Princeton (NJ): EPEC Project RWJF; 1999. Available at: http://www.ama-assn.org/ethic/epec/download/plenary_3.pdf. Retrieved September 13, 2013.

Family Caregiver Alliance. Available at: www.caregiver.org. Retrieved July 31, 2013.

Find Law. State living wills laws. Available at: http://statelaws.findlaw.com/estate-planning-laws/living-wills.html. Retrieved September 27, 2013.

Get Palliative Care. Center to Advance Palliative Care. Available at: www.getpalliativecare.org. Retrieved July 31, 2013.

Hospice and Palliative Nurses Association. Available at: www.hpna.org. Retrieved July 31, 2013.

Hospice Foundation of America. Available at: http://www.hospicefoundation.org. Retrieved July 31, 2013.

Kearney MK, Weininger RB, Vachon ML, Harrison RL, Mount BM. Self-care of physicians caring for patients at the end of life: "Being connected... a key to my survival." JAMA 2009;301:1155–64, E1.

National Association for Home Care and Hospice. Available at: www.nahc.org. Retrieved on July 31, 2013.

National Healthcare Decisions Day. Available at: http://www.nhdd.org/. Retrieved July 31, 2013.

National Hospice and Palliative Care Organization. Available at: http://www. nhpco.org. Retrieved July 31, 2013.

National Hospice and Palliative Care Organization. Download your state's advance directives. Available at: http://www.caringinfo.org/i4a/pages/index.cfm?pageid= 3289. Retrieved July 31, 2013.

National Hospice and Palliative Care Organization. Standards of practice for hospice programs. Alexandria (VA): NHPCO; 2010. Available at: http://www.nhpco. org/sites/default/files/public/quality/Standards/NHPCO_STANDARDS_2010CD. pdf. Retrieved September 13, 2013.

National Institute on Aging. Available at: www.nia.nih.gov. Retrieved July 31, 2013.

National POLST Paradigm Task Force. Oregon Health & Science University. Center for Ethics in Health Care. Available at: http://www.polst.org. Retrieved September 27, 2013.

Searight HR, Gafford J. Cultural diversity at the end of life: issues and guidelines for family physicians. Am Fam Physician 2005;71:515–22.

PSYCHOSOCIAL ISSUES

Communication and counseling skills are an important aspect of women's health care; psychosocial well-being is an important element of overall health. Some of the psychosocial issues most commonly encountered by obstetrician–gynecologists are discussed here.

Stress

Stress can be a reaction to a short-lived situation or it can be long lasting and due to relationship problems or other serious situations. Distress occurs when an individual does not adapt well to stress. Stress may interfere with a patient's ability to live a normal life. It may manifest itself in an inability to concentrate, irritability, fatigue, and other physical symptoms.

Stress secondary to partner and relationship problems may manifest as sexual dysfunction. Although stress may be associated with sexual dysfunction and some estimates indicate that up to 43% of women have a form of sexual dysfunction at some point in their life, only 12 % of women report having sexual dysfunction and feeling distressed about it. Similarly, it is unclear whether the stress related to sexual dysfunction is a contributing factor in some of the behaviors and psychosocial disorders described later in this section, or if it is an associated symptom. For example, women who present with various forms of eating disorders were reported to have a higher incidence of sexual dysfunction than women without an eating disorder. In a study of women with various types of eating disorders, those with the restricting type or the binge-eating and purging type of anorexia nervosa had the highest percentage of loss of libido—75% and 74%, respectively. Stress-reduction techniques, such as mindfulness, meditation, yoga, prayer, and progressive muscle relaxation, may reduce fatigue and low-libido symptoms (see also the "Sexual Function and Dysfunction" section in Part 4).

Feeding and Eating Disorders

A woman's health is enhanced by maintaining a healthy weight and good eating habits. Various psychosocial factors can affect the maintenance of proper nutrition and a healthy body weight. More than 5 million people in the United States are affected by feeding and eating disorders each year. Extremes in eating behavior are a manifestation of eating disorders. Extreme reduction of food intake or extreme overeating is associated with feelings of distress or concern about weight or body appearance. Early detection of unhealthy situations and therapeutic intervention can improve quality of life and prevent medical complications.

TYPES

Feeding and eating disorders in the fifth edition of the *Diagnostic and Statistical Manual of Mental Disorders* include anorexia nervosa, bulimia nervosa, binge-eating disorder, pica, rumination disorder, and avoidant/ restrictive food intake disorder. The first three types are the disorders most frequently encountered in the age group cared for by obstetrician– gynecologists and are discussed as follows. It is important to note that the patient may move from one category to another during the course of the eating disorder.

Anorexia Nervosa

Anorexia nervosa is defined by three essential features: 1) persistent energy intake restriction, which leads to a significantly low body weight in the context of age, sex, developmental trajectory, and physical health; 2) an intense fear of gaining weight or of becoming fat, or persistent behavior that interferes with weight gain; and 3) a disturbance in self-perceived body weight or shape. Notably, "amenorrhea for more than three menstrual cycles" has been eliminated as a diagnostic criterion for anorexia in the fifth edition of the *Diagnostic and Statistical Manual of Mental Disorders*. Although amenorrhea or other menstrual irregularity may be a present- ing symptom, it is not an applicable diagnostic criterion in all situations (eg, premenarchal females, oral contraceptive users, and postmenopausal women). In addition, some individuals may meet all other diagnostic requirements for anorexia but still report some menstrual activity. Subtypes of anorexia nervosa are shown in Box 3-31.

Individuals with anorexia nervosa commonly control body weight through voluntary starvation, excessive exercise, or other weight control measures, such as diet pills or diuretic drugs. The overwhelming majority of patients (95%) with diagnosed anorexia nervosa are female. Individuals 12–18 years of age are most frequently affected, but anorexia nervosa does occur in older women and has been reported in young children.

Bulimia Nervosa

Bulimia nervosa is defined as recurrent episodes of binge eating accompanied by the following: eating, in a discrete period of time (eg, within any 2-hour period), an amount of food that is definitely larger than what most individuals would eat in a similar period of time under similar circumstances; and the sense of lack of control over the amount being eaten or the ability to stop. Patients with bulimia nervosa are unduly influenced in their self-evaluation by body shape and weight. These individuals do not deny themselves food but rather engage in excess food consumption and then purge it out of their systems using laxatives, self-induced vomiting,

---

Box 3-31. Subtypes of Anorexia Nervosa

Binge-eating/purging—During the past 3 months, the patient has engaged in recurrent episodes of binge eating or purging behavior, with purging accomplished through self-induced vomiting or the misuse of laxatives, diuretics, or enemas.

Restricting—During the past 3 months, the patient has not engaged in recurrent episodes of binge-eating or purging behavior; weight loss is accomplished through dieting, fasting, excessive exercise, or two or more of these three.

Some patients engage in cycles of binge eating and purging in addition to frequent fasting.

Adapted from American Psychiatric Association. Diagnostic and statistical manual of mental disorders: DSM-5. 5th ed. Washington, DC: APA; 2013.

and other behaviors. Individuals with bulimia nervosa may be of average weight, underweight, or overweight.

Binge-Eating Disorder

Binge-eating disorder is defined as eating large amounts of food in a discrete period of time and is characterized by marked distress regarding binge eating and a sense of lack of control. The binge eating occurs, on average, at least once a week for 3 months. In this way, it is a variant of bulimia nervosa. However, binge eaters do not routinely engage in purging behaviors or compensatory behaviors, such as excessive exercise or prolonged fasting. Research has shown that dieting (fasting), chronic restrained eating, and excessive exercise may be important triggers for binge-eating disorder.

HEALTH CONSEQUENCES

Eating disorders can have life-threatening consequences. Anorexia nervosa ranks third among common chronic disorders in adolescents, surpassed only by asthma and obesity. It can cause psychologic, physiologic, endocrine, and gynecologic problems (see Box 3-32). Medical complications of anorexia nervosa include cardiac abnormalities, dangerously low blood pressure and body temperature, low white blood cell count, chronic constipation, osteoporosis, slowed adolescent growth or development, short stature, loss of menstrual periods, infertility, hair loss, and fingernail destruction. Morbidity may reach 10–15%. Deaths are from causes such as starvation, cardiac arrhythmias, cardiac failure, and suicide.

The medical complications of bulimia nervosa can be life threatening and include electrolyte abnormalities that can lead to heart rhythm disturbances, dehydration, dangerously low blood pressure, menstrual cycle abnormalities, enlarged parotid glands, destruction of dental enamel, dental cavities, and bowel abnormalities. Pulmonary complications of aspiration pneumonia and pneumomediastinum can result from vomiting. Irreversible cardiomyopathy may occur in patients with bulimia who use ipecac to induce vomiting.

Binge-eating disorder has a persistent course and often is associated with comorbid psychopathology (eg, depression), which contributes to medical complications. Because patients with binge-eating disorder are not purging, they do not have the risks associated with vomiting and the use of laxatives and diuretics. Massive caloric intake often results in obesity with its associated complications.

Box 3-32. Common Presentations of Eating Disorders

Gynecologic presentations
- Amenorrhea
- Menstrual irregularity
- Constipation or abdominal pain
- Sexually transmitted infections
- Contraceptive needs
- Pelvic pain
- Atrophic vaginitis
- Breast atrophy

Other presentations
- Depression
- Weakness
- Sports injuries and fractures
- Mouth sores
- Pharyngeal trauma
- Dental caries
- Heartburn
- Chest pain
- Muscle cramps
- Bloody diarrhea
- Bleeding or easy bruising
- Fainting
- Routine medical care

Reprinted from American College of Obstetricians and Gynecologists. Eating disorders in adolescents. In: Guidelines for adolescent health care [CD-ROM]. 2nd ed. Washington, DC: American College of Obstetricians and Gynecologists; 2011. p. 134–47.

SCREENING AND ASSESSMENT

The American College of Obstetricians and Gynecologists recommends that all women be counseled on dietary and nutrition issues on a yearly basis or as appropriate. All adolescents should be screened annually for eating disorders and obesity by determining actual weight and stature, calculating body mass index, and asking about body image and eating patterns. A screening tool, such as the SCOFF questionnaire or the EAT-26 questionnaire, also may be used (see Resources). Vital sign abnormalities, including abnormal blood pressure or pulse rate, may be the initial finding that alerts a clinician to a potential eating disorder.

Women and adolescents should be assessed for organic disease, anorexia nervosa, or bulimia nervosa if any of the following conditions or behaviors is found:

- Restriction of energy intake relative to requirements, leading to a significantly low body weight in the context of age, sex, developmental trajectory, and physical health
- Recurrent dieting when not overweight
- Amenorrhea or abnormal menses
- Use of self-induced emesis, laxatives, starvation, or diuretics to lose weight
- Undue influence of body weight or shape on self-evaluation
- Body mass index below the 5th percentile
- Hypotension, bradycardia, cardiac arrhythmia, or hypothermia
- Excessive exercising
- Recurrent constipation or unexplained pelvic abdominal pain
- Marked perianal erythema (may be secondary to laxative abuse)

The clinician who finds indications of an eating disorder in a patient should discuss their concerns with the patient and consider the following diagnostic studies:

- Complete blood count (usually normal; white blood cell count possibly low)

- Thyroid function tests (levels of thyroxine and triiodothyronine usually are low in patients with anorexia)
- Electrocardiography (cardiac abnormalities: eg, slow heart rate or disturbances of heart rhythm)
- Electrolyte evaluation (abnormal findings related to purging)
- Follicle-stimulating hormone and luteinizing hormone tests

MANAGEMENT

Once an eating disorder has been suspected or diagnosed, the clinician should assess his or her ability to identify and manage continuing problems and join with a multidisciplinary team of specialists or refer the patient to another practitioner when needed. The presence of suicidal ideation should indicate the need for immediate referral to a mental health practitioner experienced in treating this psychiatric condition. At the least, the treatment team should consist of a medical practitioner, a mental health therapist, and a nutritionist or dietitian. Supporting services may include psychiatric or eating disorder programs or facilities, if available. In the case of the diagnosis in a child or adolescent, clinicians should be familiar with any state regulations regarding confidentiality and parental consent for treatment. If an adolescent patient is living at home and if appropriate, the clinician should include the parents in the discussion of the diagnosis and management recommendations. (For more information on informed consent and confidentiality in the treatment of adolescent patients, see the "Adolescents" section earlier in Part 3.)

Management of eating disorders may include hospitalization, nutritional rehabilitation, psychosocial therapy, medications, the use of the addiction model, or a combination of psychosocial and medication strategies. Patients with anorexia nervosa often have concurrent hypoestrogenism. Merely providing the patient who has anorexia nervosa with hormones does not treat this complex disease adequately and may exacerbate patient concerns about weight gain and body image. Other interventions, as already indicated, are much more critical to prevent mortality and morbidity.

Nonsuicidal Self-Injury Behavior and Related Disorders

Nonsuicidal self-injury behavior disorder is characterized by repetitive infliction of shallow yet painful injuries to the surface of one's body with a sharp object with the intent to relieve negative emotions. Patients who repeatedly cut or burn themselves or do other damage to their bodies but lack suicidal intent may be displaying signs of nonsuicidal self-injury behavior. Although tattooing and body piercing has become more popular in today's society, a compulsive approach to these activities may indicate the need to screen for nonsuicidal self-injury behavior.

Although self-injury behavior can occur in any population, it is more often found in adolescent females with a history of physical, emotional, or sexual abuse. These individuals have a higher incidence of substance abuse and eating disorders. Patients who practice self-injury have often been raised in families that discouraged expression of anger and so they subsequently have a lack of skills to express their emotions, and they may also lack a good social support network.

Other disorders characterized by self-injury behavior include trichotillomania, stereotypic self-injury disorder, excoriation, and borderline personality disorder. Trichotillomania involves self-injurious behavior focused on pulling out one's hair (commonly from the scalp, eyebrows, or eyelashes) during periods of relaxation. Stereotypic self-injury behavior disorder includes head banging, self-biting, or self-hitting during periods of intense concentration and often is associated with developmental delay. Excoriation disorder is characterized by skin-picking (without an implement) of self-deemed unsightly or blemished sites, typically on the face, arms, and hands. Borderline personality disorder is a serious mental illness characterized by instability in interpersonal relationships and impulsivity. Although self-injury behavior is a common symptom of borderline personality disorder, individuals with nonsuicidal self-injury behavior typically do not display the intense bouts of aggressive and hostile behavior that is characteristic of borderline personality disorder.

Recognition of self-injury behavior requires referral to a mental health professional experienced in its diagnosis and treatment. Management includes psychotherapy, group therapy, and pharmacologic agents.

Bibliography

American College of Obstetricians and Gynecologists. Eating disorders in adolescents. In: Guidelines for adolescent health care [CD-ROM]. 2nd ed. Washington, DC: American College of Obstetricians and Gynecologists; 2011. p. 134–47.

American Psychiatric Association. Diagnostic and statistical manual of mental disorders: DSM-5. 5th ed. Washington, DC: APA; 2013.

Andersen AE, Ryan GL. Eating disorders in the obstetric and gynecologic patient population. Obstet Gynecol 2009;114:1353–67.

Laumann EO, Paik A, Rosen RC. Sexual dysfunction in the United States: prevalence and predictors. JAMA 1999;281:537–44.

Pinheiro AP, Raney TJ, Thornton LM, Fichter MM, Berrettini WH, Goldman D, et al. Sexual functioning in women with eating disorders. Int J Eat Disord 2010;43:123–9.

Rome ES, Ammerman S, Rosen DS, Keller RJ, Lock J, Mammel KA, et al. Children and adolescents with eating disorders: the state of the art. Pediatrics 2003;111: e98–108.

Rosen DS. Identification and management of eating disorders in children and adolescents. American Academy of Pediatrics Committee on Adolescence. Pediatrics 2010;126:1240–53.

Resources

American College of Obstetricians and Gynecologists, District II. Finding solutions for female sexual dysfunction. Albany (NY): American College of Obstetricians and Gynecologists, District II; 2010. Available at: http://mail.ny.acog.org/website/FSDResourceGuide.pdf. Retrieved September 14, 2013.

American College of Obstetricians and Gynecologists. Adolescent visit record and adolescent visit and parent questionnaires. Washington, DC: American College of Obstetricians and Gynecologists; 2010.

American College of Obstetricians and Gynecologists. Annual women's health care. Available at: http://www.acog.org/wellwoman. Retrieved October 1, 2013.

American College of Obstetricians and Gynecologists. Weight control: eating right and keeping fit. Patient Education Pamphlet AP064. Washington, DC: American College of Obstetricians and Gynecologists; 2013.

American Psychological Association. Psychology topics: sexuality. Available at: http://www.apa.org/topics/sexuality/index.aspx. Retrieved July 31, 2013.

Dell D. Mood and anxiety disorders. In: Clin Update Womens Health Care. 2008. p.1–98.

Eating Attitudes Test (EAT-26). Available at: http://www.eat-26.com/index.php. Retrieved July 31, 2013.

ECRI Institute. Bulimia nervosa resource guide. Available at: http://www.bulimiagu ide.org. Retrieved July 31, 2013.

Herzog DB, Franks DL, Cable P. Unlocking the mysteries of eating disorders: a life-saving guide to your child's treatment and recovery. New York (NY): McGraw-Hill; 2008.

Morgan JF, Reid F, Lacey JH. The SCOFF questionnaire: a new screening tool for eating disorders. West J Med 2000;172:164–5.

National Eating Disorders Association. Available at: https://www.nationaleatingdis orders.org/. Retrieved September 14, 2013.

National Institute of Mental Health. Eating disorders. Bethesda (MD): NIMH; 2011. Available at: http://www.nimh.nih.gov/health/publications/eating-disorders/ eating-disorders.pdf. Retrieved September 14, 2013.

National Institutes of Mental Health. Borderline personality disorder. Available at: http://www.nimh.nih.gov/health/publications/borderline-personality-disorder/ index.shtml. Retrieved July 31, 2013.

Sadock BJ, Sadock VA, Ruiz P. Kaplan & Sadock's synopsis of psychiatry: behavioral sciences/clinical psychiatry. 11th ed. Philadelphia (PA): Lippincott Williams & Wilkins; 2014.

Sidran Institute. Available at: www.sidran.org. Retrieved September 14, 2013.

Zerbe KJ, Rosenberg J. Eating disorders. In: Clin. Update Womens Health Care. 2008. p.1–86.

ABUSE

Violence and abuse are important problems that affect women and adolescents, and they often have serious short-term and long-term health consequences. Abuse may be verbal, physical, or sexual and can manifest as intimate partner violence, child abuse, rape, sexual assault, elder abuse, or neglect. Clinicians should be alert to signs of patients' exposure to violence or abuse. However, because patients may be asymptomatic, it is important that physicians conduct screening for past and present abuse with all patients. Universal screening is best conducted while obtaining a patient's health history. Practitioners should ask patients directly about current or past intimate partner or domestic violence, rape or sexual assault, and childhood physical and sexual abuse. Screening should be done in a comfortable and private environment. Arrangements should be made for referral to appropriate community services as needed. Clinicians should be familiar with any local and state requirements to report intimate partner violence, domestic violence, child abuse or assault (physical or sexual), and elder neglect or abuse.

Intimate Partner Violence and Domestic Violence

Although there is no single definition of intimate partner violence that satisfies all medical, social, and criminal justice purposes, the term typically refers to violence perpetrated against adolescent and adult women within the context of past or current intimate relationships. Intimate partner violence encompass subjection of a partner to physical abuse, psychologic abuse, sexual violence, and reproductive and sexual coercion (see also "Sexual Assault or Rape" and "Reproductive and Sexual Coercion" later in this section). The term domestic violence also is used by many people to describe intimate partner violence. The term domestic violence, however, encompasses other forms of violence, including abuse of older individuals and children (see also "Elder Abuse" and "Child Abuse, Child Sexual Abuse, and the Adult Manifestations of Childhood Sexual Abuse" later in this section).

Domestic violence is a widespread social and public health problem that disproportionately affects women of all age, racial, educational, and socioeconomic groups and covers a broad spectrum of behaviors. It encompasses a pattern of actual or threatened physical, sexual, or psychologic abuse between family members or intimate partners and can range from intimidating behaviors to life-threatening actions. Although the true extent of intimate partner violence and domestic violence is difficult to ascertain, prevalence studies estimate that each year in the United States, 2 million women are abused by someone they know, and the prevalence of intimate partner violence goes up during pregnancy. According to the U.S. Department of Justice, violence by an intimate partner accounts for approximately 22% of all the violent crime experienced by women.

PATTERNS OF ABUSE

No one is immune from intimate partner or domestic violence, regardless of age, socioeconomic status, profession, religion, ethnicity, education, or sexual orientation. There is no typical victim, nor is there a typical abuser. Most frequently, the abuse is directed at a woman by a man. Often, perpetrators are violent only with family members and have different public and private images. They minimize the seriousness of the violence and refuse to take responsibility for their behavior, accusing the victim of provoking them. The hallmark of their behavior is coercive control, including isolation of the victim.

Women with disabilities are vulnerable to physical, sexual, or emotional abuse, as well as neglect and exploitation. The abuse can include withholding necessary assistive devices, care, or treatment. Immigrant and refugee women are at risk of violence and abuse because of isolation and manipulation by their partners, language and cultural differences, and lack of awareness of their rights and legal and social resources.

CONSEQUENCES

Research confirms that ongoing or past violence can lead to long-term physical and psychologic consequences. As a result, patients may acquire additional health care problems, which may subsequently lead to overuse of health care resources. The estimated costs of intimate partner violence against women exceed $5.8 billion each year.

Violence between intimate partners may be the most important risk factor for child abuse. Child abuse occurs at a rate 15 times higher in families with intimate partner violence than in families without violence. Witnessing or experiencing abuse in the home is associated with higher levels of behavioral and emotional problems, as well as poor social interaction and school performance. Adolescents are at risk of physical and sexual abuse by parents, family members, peers, and dating partners. Adolescent exposure to violence is associated with anger, depression, anxiety, and posttraumatic stress. Growing up in an abusive household increases a woman's risk of abuse in adulthood.

ROLE OF HEALTH CARE PROVIDERS

The clinician's role is to know the signs and symptoms of intimate partner and domestic violence, ask all patients about past or present exposure to violence, assess the patient's risk of danger, and intervene and refer as appropriate (Box 3-33).

Nonacute presentations of abuse include reports of chronic headaches, sleep and appetite disturbances, palpitations, chronic pelvic pain, urinary frequency or urgency, irritable bowel syndrome, sexual dysfunction, abdominal symptoms, and recurrent vaginal infections. These nonacute symptoms often represent clinical manifestations of internalized stress (ie, somatization). Diagnostic clues to intimate partner and domestic violence include nonspecific stress-related symptoms (eg, depression and chronic pain) or injuries in various stages of healing for which the explanation is inconsistent with the findings. There may be other evidence of abuse identified from a reproductive history, including recurrent abortions. Although the results of most physical examinations of individuals affected by domestic violence or intimate partner violence are normal, the physical examination may reveal bruises, burns, bite marks, and other injuries, particularly on the head, neck, breasts, abdomen, and groin.

There may be no pathognomonic signs or symptoms of intimate partner violence or domestic violence; hence, universal screening is warranted.

Box 3-33. The RADAR Model of the Physician's Approach to Domestic Violence

R: Remember to ask routinely about partner violence in your own practice.

A: Ask directly about violence with such questions as "At any time, has a partner hit, kicked, or otherwise hurt or frightened you?" Interview your patient in private at all times.

D: Document information about "suspected domestic violence" or "partner violence" in the patient's chart, and file reports when required by law.

A: Assess your patient's safety. Is it safe to return home? Find out if any weapons are kept in the house, if the children are in danger, and if the violence is escalating.

R: Review options with your patients. Know about the types of referral options (eg, shelters, support groups, legal advocates).

Reprinted with permission from Intimate Partner violence: how to recognize and treat victims of abuse. 4th ed, pg 25. Massachusetts Medical Society. Copyright 2004 Massachusetts Medical Society. All rights reserved.

Because of the prevalence of violence, all women should be screened for domestic violence at periodic intervals, such as annual examinations and new patient visits. Although patients may be reluctant to bring up their abuse, they often are responsive to direct inquiry. Questions must be asked in privacy and in a nonjudgmental manner. At the beginning of the assessment, offer a framing statement to show that screening is done universally and not because intimate partner violence is suspected. Also, inform patients of the confidentiality of the discussion and exactly what state law mandates that a physician must disclose. The following four questions are easily incorporated into a routine review of systems:

1. "Has anyone close to you ever threatened to hurt you?"
2. "Has anyone ever hit, slapped, kicked, or hurt you physically?"
3. "Has anyone, including your partner or a family member, pressured or forced you to do something sexually that you did not want to do?"
4. "Are you ever afraid of your partner or anyone at home?"

When there are injuries, it is appropriate to ask the direct question: "Did someone cause these injuries?" The patient's answer will provide direction to pursue a series of questions relating to issues of safety for the woman and her children, the role of friends and family, and the range of available options.

When a patient confides that she has been abused, it is important to acknowledge the trauma and reinforce the fact that the patient is not to blame. The clinician should reinforce that the patient has done nothing to deserve the abuse and that intimate partner violence and domestic violence are crimes. The physician must be prepared to discuss the abuse with the woman and establish a plan to deal with medical needs, psychosocial needs, and emergent issues. It is useful to have a protocol for physicians to follow that incorporates available resources.

Once intimate partner or domestic violence has been identified and acknowledged, the next step is to assess immediate safety. If the patient will be returning to an unsafe home, safety planning should be conducted. If she is afraid for her safety, she should be offered shelter immediately. With the patient's consent, social-work services, women's shelters, or community services for victims of violence should be immediately contacted. (See Box 3-34 for suggested steps for patients to take when they are ready to leave an abusive situation.) If the patient is not in need of immediate shelter or concerned that a sudden departure from her home environment may cause more threat of harm to herself or other family members, she should be advised that shelter is available if needed in the future. She should be provided with information on community resources and referred for continued assistance and support. Community resources include emergency housing (usually in shelters), peer group and individual counseling, and legal and social services advocacy. Most communities have agencies and programs to help abused women and families seek viable alternatives. Clinicians should remember that a woman is always the best judge of her safety. Respect must be given for a decision to stay or leave the abuser. Clinicians should remind the patient that they remain resources. Of the women who ultimately leave their abuser, the majority do not leave the first time a physician asks them about the violence.

Box 3-34. Making an Exit Plan to Leave an Abusive Relationship

Making a decision to leave an abusive relationship can be difficult. Clinicians can assist by providing concrete, practical guidance. Women can be encouraged to call a woman's shelter for more help with a safety plan and be assured that such calls would be anonymous. If the woman is ready to leave, the following tips may be helpful:

- Pack a bag in advance, and leave it at a neighbor's or friend's house. Include cash or credit cards and extra clothes for yourself and your children. Take each child's favorite toy or plaything.

- Hide an extra set of car and house keys outside of the house in case you have to leave quickly.

- Take important papers, such as the following:

  — Birth certificate (including children's)

  — Health insurance cards and medicine

  — Deed or lease to the house or apartment

  — Checkbook and extra checks

  — Social Security number or green card or work permit

  — Court papers or orders

  — Driver's license or photograph identification

  — Pay stubs

Modified from American College of Obstetricians and Gynecologists. Leaving the violence. Available at: http://www.acog.org/About_ACOG/ACOG_Departments/Violence_Against_Women/Leaving_the_Violence. Retrieved September 27, 2013.

In particularly distressed women, an assessment of suicide risk may be indicated. Obviously, in acute crisis situations that involve serious risks to the life of the victim, her children, or others, crisis intervention resources should be used.

Psychologic and social assistance are best provided by services that are "trauma specific," meaning that the practitioners are experienced in treating victims of domestic violence or intimate partner abuse. Most agencies for battered women and rape crisis centers are expert in dealing with all forms of violence against women.

Perpetrators often retaliate when they suspect disclosure of abuse. Thus, every effort should be made to maintain confidentiality, especially regarding telephone calls, and to minimize paper materials, such as bills or brochures, given to the patient. The clinician and patient should discuss acceptable methods of communication and exchange of information. Office staff must be informed about the importance of confidentiality in any contact with the patient's home.

Laws regarding reporting obligations vary widely among states; therefore, familiarity with local laws and policies is critical. In all states, physicians are required by law to report suspected child abuse. Mandatory reporting of intimate partner or domestic violence is required by some states, but it remains a controversial issue, especially with regard to issues of patient safety and confidentiality. Information regarding state reporting requirements is available through state medical associations, local violence prevention or service programs, or the state attorney general's office. A summary of state laws can be found at www.futureswithoutviolence.org/userfiles/file/HealthCare/MandReport2007FINALMMS.pdf.

Elder Abuse

Elder abuse, or elder mistreatment, refers to intentional acts that result in harm or create a risk of harm or distress, and failure by a caregiver to satisfy the elder's basic needs or protect the elder from harm. An estimated 1–2 million U.S. citizens aged 65 years or older have been injured, exploited, or mistreated by someone caring for them; and most elders who experience abuse are women. However, it is acknowledged that these findings represent the most overt cases and that elder abuse is underreported.

The American College of Obstetricians and Gynecologists supports screening of patients older than 60 years to help identify victims of abuse and provide them with appropriate medical and psychosocial care and referrals. Evaluation should include a thorough social history to assess family structure, the stability of social supports, financial stressors, and substance abuse or mental health history. Health care providers should directly question their patients about present and past abuse (see Box 3-35). Multiple falls or fractures, multiple emergency department visits or hospitalizations,

---

Box 3-35. Performing an Elder Mistreatment Assessment

- Interview the patient separately and be aware that family members and caregivers may be abusers
- Start with general, open-ended questions and progress to more specific questions
- Note inconsistent or frequently changing stories
- Observe patient's reactions to accompanying family members or caregivers
- Remain empathic

Sample Screening Questions for Patients
- Do you feel safe in your home?
- Are you afraid of anyone in your home?
- Has anyone threatened you or verbally assaulted you?
- Has anyone touched you without your permission?
- Does anyone ever ask you to sign documents that you do not understand?
- Has anyone ever taken your things without your permission?
- Are you alone a lot?
- Has anyone ever failed to help you when you were unable to help yourself?
- Do you have anyone to share your worries with?

Data from Stanford School of Medicine. Elder abuse: how to screen. Available at http://elderabuse.stanford.edu/screening/how_screen.html. Retrieved July 11, 2013.

---

or chronic poorly controlled medical problems should prompt clinicians to consider an unstable social situation and abuse. Signs of neglect also can be subtle, including poor hygiene and nail care, weight loss, unkempt appearance, missing assistive devices (eg, hearing aids, glasses, or dentures), and inappropriate attire. Poor medication adherence or laboratory values reflecting dehydration, malnutrition, or abnormal medication levels also may suggest neglect.

When cases of abuse are confirmed, most states mandate that health care providers report the case to Adult Protective Services. Health care providers should become familiar with their individual state mandates regarding the reporting of abuse because it varies from state to state. A list of the most up-to-date reporting requirements can be found at www. ncea.aoa.gov/stop_abuse/get_help/state/index.aspx. Partnering or having a referral relationship with social workers, nurses, and psychiatrists for outpatient referrals is an important step for health care providers. A team approach to the problem is the best way to ensure that the multiple psychosocial, medical, and legal aspects of a case are addressed.

Child Abuse, Child Sexual Abuse, and the Adult Manifestations of Childhood Sexual Abuse

Child abuse generally is categorized in four ways: 1) physical abuse, 2) emotional or psychologic abuse, 3) sexual abuse, and 4) neglect. In 2010, The U.S. Department of Health and Human Services estimated that about 1.25 million children were victims of abuse or neglect, a decrease from 1.55 million in 1996, which is nevertheless considered statistically marginal. Every state and the District of Columbia require physicians to report suspected child abuse.

Most nonsexual physical abuse of children involves boys, whereas girls are sexually abused three times more often than boys. Young single mothers who were themselves abused are at risk of physically abusing and neglecting their children. Most perpetrators of child sexual assault are males, and it is estimated that the risk of a child being abused is 15 times greater in families that experience intimate partner violence.

Sexual assault that occurs in childhood, defined by most states as younger than 14 years, is considered child abuse. Childhood sexual abuse may be further defined as any exposure to sexual acts imposed on children, who inherently lack the emotional, maturational, and cognitive development to understand or to consent to such acts. These acts do not always involve sexual intercourse or physical force. Instead, they may involve manipulation and trickery.

The actual incidence of childhood sexual abuse in the United States is unknown, but the Department of Health and Human Services estimates that approximately 135,300 children are sexually abused each year. However, for some abusive actions, the National Incidence Study of Child

Abuse and Neglect definitions count children as sexually abused only if they experienced moderate injury or harm (physical, emotional, or behavioral) from that maltreatment. Therefore, it can be assumed that the actual rate of childhood sexual abuse is higher.

Adult manifestations of childhood abuse may include depression; anxiety; posttraumatic stress symptoms; eating disorders; alcohol, drug, and tobacco use and abuse; suicide attempts or ideation; poor self-care; and somatic disorders (eg, chronic pelvic pain, migraine, and gastrointestinal disorders). Adolescents and adult women with such histories are at increased risk of sexually transmitted infections (STIs) (including human immunodeficiency virus [HIV] infection). These patients are less likely to have regular cervical cytology screening. Adult survivors of childhood sexual abuse also may have histories that include early, unplanned pregnancy; recurrent abortions; and little or no prenatal care (see Box 3-36).

With recognition of the extent of family violence, it is strongly recommended that all women be screened for a history of sexual abuse. Patients overwhelmingly favor universal inquiry about sexual assault because they report a reluctance to initiate a discussion of this subject. If the physician suspects abuse, but the patient does not disclose it, the obstetrician–gynecologist should remain open and reassuring. Patients may bring up the subject at a later visit if they have developed trust in the obstetrician–gynecologist. Not asking about sexual abuse may give tacit support to the survivor's belief that abuse does not matter or does not have medical relevance and the opportunity for intervention is lost.

Once identified, there are a number of ways that the obstetrician–gynecologist can offer support to survivors of abuse. These include techniques to increase patient comfort during the gynecologic or obstetric visit and examination, the use of empowering messages, and the provision of counseling referrals.

- Visits and examinations. All procedures should be explained in advance, and whenever possible, the patient should be allowed to suggest ways to lessen her fear. It is important to ask permission to touch the patient. Techniques to increase the patient's comfort include talking her through the steps, maintaining eye contact, allowing her to control the pace, allowing her to see more (eg, use of a mirror in

Box 3-36. Common Symptoms in Adult Survivors of Childhood Sexual Abuse

Physical Presentations
- Chronic and diffuse pain (especially abdominal or pelvic)
- Gynecologic problems (dyspareunia, vaginismus, and nonspecific vaginitis)
- Obesity, eating disorders
- Insomnia, sleep disorders
- Sexual dysfunction
- Addiction
- Low pain threshold
- Self-neglect

Psychologic and Behavioral Presentations
- Depression and anxiety
- Posttraumatic stress disorder symptoms
- Distorted self-perception
- Abuse of alcohol and illicit drugs
- Smoking
- Physically inactive
- Poor contraceptive practices
- Compulsive sexual behaviors
- Early adolescent or unintended pregnancy
- Prostitution
- Sexual dysfunction
- Somatizing disorders
- Eating disorders
- Poor adherence to medical recommendations
- Tendency to be victimized

Data from Adult manifestations of childhood sexual abuse. Committee Opinion No. 498. American College of Obstetricians and Gynecologists. Obstet Gynecol 2011;118:392–5.

pelvic examinations), or having her assist during her examination (eg, putting her hand over the physician's to guide the examination).

- Positive messages. Some positive and healing responses to the disclosure of abuse include discussing with the patient that she is a survivor of abuse and is not to blame. She should be reassured that it took courage for her to disclose the abuse, and she has been heard and believed.

- Counseling referrals. Traumatized patients generally benefit from mental health care. The obstetrician–gynecologist can be a powerful ally in the patient's healing by offering support and referral. Efforts should be made to refer survivors to professionals with significant experience in abuse-related issues. Physicians should compile a list of experts with experience in abuse and have a list of appropriate crisis hotlines that operate in their communities.

Reproductive and Sexual Coercion

Reproductive and sexual coercion involve behavior intended to maintain power and control in a relationship related to reproductive health by someone who is, was, or wishes to be involved in an intimate or dating relationship with an adult or adolescent. Many women who experience reproductive and sexual coercion also experience physical or sexual violence.

Reproductive coercion is related to behavior that interferes with contraception use and pregnancy. The most common forms of reproductive coercion include sabotage of contraceptive methods, pregnancy coercion, and pregnancy pressure. Birth control sabotage is active interference with a partner's contraceptive methods in an attempt to promote pregnancy. Pregnancy pressure involves behavior intended to pressure a female partner to become pregnant when she does not wish to become pregnant. Pregnancy coercion involves coercive behavior, such as threats or acts of violence, if a partner does not comply with the perpetrator's wishes regarding the decision to terminate or continue a pregnancy. Homicide is a leading cause of pregnancy-associated mortality in the United States.

Sexual coercion includes a range of behavior that a partner may use related to sexual decision making to pressure or coerce a person to have sex without using physical force. This behavior includes repeatedly pressuring a partner to have sex, threatening to end a relationship if the person does not have sex, forcing sex without a condom or not allowing other prophylaxis use, intentionally exposing a partner to an STI, including HIV, or threatening retaliation if notified of a positive STI infection test result.

Because evidence demonstrates that violence and poor reproductive health are strongly linked, health care providers should screen women and adolescent girls for reproductive and sexual coercion and intimate partner violence at periodic intervals, such as annual examinations and new patient visits. In contrast to most intimate partner violence interventions, which significantly depend on programs or resources outside the clinical setting, women's health care providers can directly provide interventions that address reproductive and sexual coercion. Interventions include education on the effect of reproductive and sexual coercion and intimate partner violence on patients' health and choices, counseling on harm-reduction strategies, and prevention of unintended pregnancies by offering long-acting methods of contraception that are less detectable to partners. (For more information on screening and interventions, see the "Family Planning" section earlier in Part 3.)

Sexual Assault or Rape

Sexual assault is a crime of violence and aggression and encompasses a continuum of sexual activity that ranges from sexual coercion to contact abuse (unwanted kissing, touching, or fondling) to rape. Because definitions vary among states, the term sexual assault is sometimes used interchangeably with rape. The Federal Bureau of Investigation uses the following recently revised, more comprehensive definition of rape to track statistics for the annual Uniform Crime Report: "Penetration, no matter how slight, of the vagina or anus with any body part or object, or oral penetration by a sex organ of another person, without the consent of the victim." The Federal Bureau of Investigation's change does not affect definitions under federal or state criminal laws; the new definition only applies for statistical purposes, so that crimes under existing state laws will now be counted by the federal government.

Data compiled from reports to law enforcement officials underestimate the incidence of sexual assault because of varying definitions of sexual assault and underreporting by victims. Although the true prevalence of rape or sexual assault is unknown, estimates based on the 2010 National Intimate Partner and Sexual Violence Survey reveal that approximately 1.3 million rape-related physical assaults occur against women annually. Approximately 18% of women surveyed reported that they had been victims of a completed or attempted rape during their lifetime. Nearly 80% reported that they were first raped before age 25 years, and 42% before age 18 years. Among female victims, 51% reported that at least one perpetrator was a current or former intimate partner, 41% reported an acquaintance, 13% reported a family member, and 14% reported a stranger.

Health care providers should routinely screen all women for a history of sexual assault, paying particular attention to those who report pelvic pain, dysmenorrhea, or sexual dysfunction. Early identification of victims of sexual assault can lead to prevention of long-term and persistent physical and mental health consequences of abuse. Reproductive-aged victims of sexual assault are at risk of unintended pregnancy, sexually transmitted infections, and mental health conditions, including posttraumatic stress disorder.

Clinicians who evaluate a victim of sexual assault in the acute phase have a number of medical and legal responsibilities (see Box 3-37). Health care providers should offer victims emergency contraception and sexually transmitted infection prophylaxis. The health care provider who examines victims of sexual assault has a responsibility to comply with state and local statutory or policy requirements for the use of evidence-gathering kits. Clinicians also may want to consider including a toxicology screen in the workup of victims of sexual violence, particularly adolescents and young adults. Other health personnel, particularly those trained to respond to rape-trauma victims, should be consulted to provide immediate intervention if necessary and to facilitate counseling and follow-up. Generally, a visit for clinical and psychologic follow-up should take place within 1–2 weeks, with additional encounters scheduled thereafter as indicated by results and assessments.

Box 3-37. Physician's Role in Evaluation of Sexual Assault Victims

Medical Issues
- Obtain informed consent.
- Assess and treat physical injuries.
- Obtain past gynecologic history.
- Perform physical examination, including pelvic examination, with appropriate chaperone.
- Obtain appropriate specimens and serologic tests for sexually transmitted infection testing.
- Provide appropriate infectious disease prophylaxis as indicated.
- If the assailant's human immunodeficiency virus status is unknown, evaluate the risks and benefits of nonoccupational postexposure prophylaxis.
- Provide or arrange for provision of emergency contraception as indicated.
- Provide counseling regarding findings, recommendations, and prognosis.
- Arrange follow-up medical care and referrals for psychosocial needs.

Legal Issues*
- Provide accurate recording of events.
- Document injuries.
- Collect samples as indicated by local protocol or regulation.
- Identify the presence or absence of sperm in the vaginal fluids, and make appropriate slides.
- Report to authorities as required.
- Ensure security of chain of evidence.

---

*Many jurisdictions have prepackaged kits for the initial forensic examination of a rape that provide specific containers and instructions for the collection of physical evidence and for written and pictorial documentation of the victim's subjective and objective findings. See www.rainn.org/get-information/sexual-assault-recovery/rape-kit for more information on rape kits.

Data from Sexual assault. Committee Opinion No. 592. American College of Obstetricians and Gynecologists. Obstet Gynecol 2014;123:905–9.

Bibliography

Adult manifestations of childhood sexual abuse. Committee Opinion No. 498. American College of Obstetricians and Gynecologists. Obstet Gynecol 2011;118: 392–5.

Alpert EJ, editor. Intimate partner violence: the clinician's guide to identification, assessment, intervention, and prevention. Massachusetts Medical Society Committee on Violence, Intervention and Prevention. 5th ed. Waltham (MA): Massachusetts Medical Society; 2010.

American College of Obstetricians and Gynecologists. Leaving the violence. Available at: http://www.acog.org/About_ACOG/ACOG_Departments/Violence_Against_Women/Leaving_the_Violence. Retrieved September 27, 2013.

Black MC, Basile KC, Breiding MJ, Smith SG, Walters ML, Merrick MT, et al. The National Intimate Partner and Sexual Violence Survey (NISVS): 2010 summary report. Atlanta (GA): National Center for Injury Prevention and Control; Centers for Disease Control and Prevention; 2011. Available at: http://www.cdc.gov/ViolencePrevention/pdf/NISVS_Report2010-a.pdf. Retrieved July 30, 2013.

Elder abuse and women's health. Committee Opinion No. 568. American College of Obstetricians and Gynecologists. Obstet Gynecol 2013;122:187–91.

Federal Bureau of Investigation. Summary Reporting System (SRS) user manual version 1.0. Criminal Justice Information Services (CJIS) Division, Uniform Crime Reporting (UCR) Program. Washington, DC: FBI; 2013. Available at: http://www.fbi.gov/about-us/cjis/ucr/nibrs/summary-reporting-system-srs-user-manual. Retrieved November 25, 2013.

Intimate partner violence. Committee Opinion No. 518. American College of Obstetricians and Gynecologists. Obstet Gynecol 2012;119:412–7.

Kellogg N. The evaluation of sexual abuse in children. American Academy of Pediatrics Committee on Child Abuse and Neglect. Pediatrics 2005;116:506–12.

National Center on Elder Abuse. State resources. Available at: http://www.ncea.aoa.gov/stop_abuse/get_help/state/index.aspx. Retrieved September 27, 2013.

Nelson HD, Bougatsos C, Blazina I. Screening women for intimate partner violence: a systematic review to update the U.S. Preventive Services Task Force recommendation. Ann Intern Med 2012;156:796,808, W-279, W-280, W-281, W-282.

Reproductive and sexual coercion. Committee Opinion No. 554. American College of Obstetricians and Gynecologists. Obstet Gynecol 2013;121:411–5.

Sedlak AJ, Mettenburg J, Basena M, Petta I, McPherson K, Greene A, et al. Fourth national incidence study of child abuse and neglect (NIS-4): report to Congress. Washington, DC: U.S. Department of Health and Humans Services; 2010. Available at: http://www.acf.hhs.gov/sites/default/files/opre/nis4_report_congress_full_pdf_jan2010.pdf. Retrieved September 16, 2013.

Sexual assault. Committee Opinion No. 592. American College of Obstetricians and Gynecologists. Obstet Gynecol 2014;123:905–9.

Stanford School of Medicine. Elder abuse: how to screen. Available at: http://eldera-buse.stanford.edu/screening/how_screen.html. Retrieved September 27, 2013.

The Commonwealth Fund. Addressing domestic violence and its consequences: policy report of The Commonwealth Fund Commission on Women's Health with appendices. New York (NY): The Commonwealth Fund; 1998.

Tjaden P, Thoennes N. Full report of the prevalence, incidence, and consequences of violence against women. Washington, DC: U.S. Department of Justice, Office of Justice Programs; 2000. Available at: https://www.ncjrs.gov/pdffiles1/nij/183781.pdf. Retrieved September 16, 2013.

Resources

American College of Obstetricians and Gynecologists. Domestic violence. ACOG Patient Education Pamphlet AP083. Washington, DC: American College of Obstetricians and Gynecologists; 2008.

American College of Obstetricians and Gynecologists. Elder abuse: an introduction for the clinician. Available at: http://www.acog.org/About_ACOG/ACOG_Departments/Violence_Against_Women/Elder_Abuse__An_Introduction_for_the_Clinician. Retrieved September 17, 2013.

American College of Obstetricians and Gynecologists. Violence against women. Available at: http://www.acog.org/About_ACOG/ACOG_Departments/Violence_Against_Women. Retrieved September 17, 2013.

Centers for Disease Control and Prevention. Sexually transmitted diseases (STDs). Available at: http://www.cdc.gov/std. Retrieved January 30, 2014.

Chamberlain L, Levenson R. Addressing intimate partner violence, reproductive and sexual coercion: a guide for obstetric, gynecologic and reproductive health care settings. 2nd ed. Washington, DC: San Francisco (CA): American College of Obstetricians and Gynecologists; Futures Without Violence; 2012. Available at: http://www.futureswithoutviolence.org/userfiles/file/HealthCare/reproguidelines_low_res_FINAL.pdf. Retrieved September 10, 2013.

Futures Without Violence. Available at: http://www.futureswithoutviolence.org/. Retrieved September 10, 2013.

Futures Without Violence. State codes on intimate partner violence victimization reporting requirements for health care providers. San Francisco (CA): FWV; 2007. Available at: http://www.futureswithoutviolence.org/userfiles/file/HealthCare/MandReport2007FINALMMS.pdf. Retrieved September 27, 2013.

National Domestic Violence Hotline. 800-799-SAFE (7233) and 800-787-3224 (TTY). http://www.thehotline.org. Retrieved September 10, 2013.

DEPRESSION

Major depressive disorders may begin at any age, with the average age of onset in the mid-20s. In one half of women, the onset of depression occurs between age 20 years and 50 years. Depression can be overdiagnosed in women who have experienced grief reactions or who are undergoing situational stress. However, it can be underdiagnosed if clinicians do not maintain a high level of suspicion.

Mood disorders, especially depression, are among the most common psychiatric illnesses in women. Many patients treated by obstetrician–gynecologists will have a depressive illness. The lifetime prevalence of major depressive disorders in adults in the United States is 16.6%, and women are approximately 70% more likely than men to experience depression during their lifetime. The reasons for this disparity are multidimensional and may include biologic, social, and economic issues that are specific to women.

According to the World Health Organization, depression is the leading cause of disability in women, which accounts for $30 billion to $50 billion in lost productivity and direct medical costs in the United States each year. The lives of 19 million adults and millions more family members and friends are affected.

Health care providers who work with women have a unique advantage in identifying and diagnosing depression. Routine screening for depression is recommended in clinical practices that have systems in place to ensure accurate diagnosis, effective treatment, and follow-up. If depression is identified, it can be effectively treated in up to 85% of cases. It is estimated that nearly two thirds of individuals affected do not get the help they need. Treatment may include medication, psychotherapy, or both. Clinicians will need to provide follow-up care for any patients that have not been referred elsewhere. The likelihood of a recurrence is 50% after a major episode of depression, and it continues to increase with each occurrence.

Symptoms

The presenting symptoms of depressive disorders may be somatic or behavioral and sometimes can be attributed to an organic condition. In some cases, depression may be related to a condition for which a woman is receiving care, such as infertility, perinatal loss, postpartum depression, or other medical condition. Several tools utilizing a series of questions have been used to screen for depression and other mood disorders. Box 3-38 includes an example of an abbreviated tool and its sample questions that are appropriate for initial screening for depression in women. These questions may be included on a written screening questionnaire or asked as part of the interview process, particularly if other risk factors are present.

When the initial screening suggests a depressive disorder, a more comprehensive assessment is in order. Psychologic symptoms, such as depressed mood, crying spells, loss of interest or pleasure in usual activities, or suicidal thoughts, are obvious, but a high index of suspicion is needed in the differential diagnosis, regardless of symptoms. Diagnostic criteria, such as those provided in the American Psychiatric Association's *Diagnostic and Statistical Manual of Mental Disorders*, can be useful (see Box 3-39). Patients should be screened for psychosocial stressors.

Box 3-38. Sample Questions Appropriate for Depression Screening

Over the past 2 weeks, have you felt down, depressed, or hopeless?

Over the past 2 weeks, have you felt little interest or pleasure in doing things?

Not at all	Several days	More than half the days	Nearly every day
(0)	(1)	(2)	(3)

The recommended cutoff when used for screening is a score of 3 or greater.

Data from Whooley MA, Avins AL, Miranda J, Browner WS. Case-finding instruments for depression. Two questions are as good as many. J Gen Intern Med 1997;12:439-45., and Spitzer RL, Williams JB, Kroenke K, Linzer M, deGruy FV,3rd, Hahn SR, et al. Utility of a new procedure for diagnosing mental disorders in primary care. The PRIME-MD 1000 study. JAMA 1994;272:1749–56.

Box 3-39. Diagnostic Criteria for Major Depressive Disorder

A. Five (or more) of the following symptoms have been present during the same 2-week period and represent a change from previous functioning; at least one of the symptoms is either 1) depressed mood or 2) loss of interest or pleasure. Note: Do not include symptoms that are clearly attributable to another medical condition.

1. Depressed mood most of the day, nearly every day, as indicated by either subjective report (eg, feels sad, empty, or hopeless) or observation made by others (eg, appears tearful). (Note: In children and adolescents, can be irritable mood.)

2. Markedly diminished interest or pleasure in all, or almost all, activities most of the day, nearly every day (as indicated by either subjective account or observation).

3. Significant weight loss when not dieting or weight gain (eg, a change of more than 5% of body weight in a month) or decrease or increase in appetite nearly every day. (Note: In children, consider failure to make expected weight gains.)

4. Insomnia or hypersomnia nearly every day.

5. Psychomotor agitation or retardation nearly every day (observable by others, not merely subjective feelings of restlessness or being slowed down).

6. Fatigue or loss of energy nearly every day.

7. Feelings of worthlessness or excessive or inappropriate guilt (which may be delusional) nearly every day (not merely self-reproach or guilt about being sick).

8. Diminished ability to think or concentrate, or indecisiveness, nearly every day (either by subjective account or as observed by others).

9. Recurrent thoughts of death (not just fear of dying), recurrent suicidal ideation without a specific plan, or suicide attempt or a specific plan for committing suicide.

B. The symptoms cause clinically significant distress or impairment in social, occupational, or other important areas of functioning.

C. The episode is not attributable to the physiologic effects of a substance or to another medical condition.

(continued)

Box 3-39. Diagnostic Criteria for Major Depressive Disorder
(continued)

Note: Criteria A–C represent a major depressive episode.

Note: Responses to a significant loss (eg, bereavement, financial ruin, losses from a natural disaster, a serious medical illness or disability) may include the feelings of intense sadness rumination about the loss, insomnia, poor appetite, and weight loss noted in Criterion A, which may resemble a depressive episode. Although such symptoms may be understandable or considered appropriate to the loss, the presence of a major depressive episode in addition to the normal response to the significant loss should also be carefully considered. This decision inevitably requires the exercise of clinical judgment based on the individual's history and the cultural norms for the expression of distress in the context of loss.*

D. The occurrence of the major depressive episode is not better explained by schizoaffective disorder, schizophrenia, schizophreniform disorder, delusional disorder, or other specified and unspecified schizophrenia spectrum and other psychotic disorders.

E. There has never been a manic episode or a hypomanic episode. Note: This exclusion does not apply if all of the manic-like or hypomanic-like episodes are substance-induced or are attributable to the physiologic effects of another medical condition.

---

*In distinguishing grief from a major depressive episode, it is useful to consider that in grief the predominant effect is feelings of emptiness and loss, whereas in a major depressive episode it is a persistent depressed mood and the inability to anticipate happiness or pleasure. For more information on how to make the important distinction between the symptoms characteristic of bereavement and those of a major depressive episode, please see the *Diagnostic and Statistical Manual of Mental Disorders*, Fifth Edition.

Reprinted with permission from the Diagnostic and statistical manual of mental disorders: DSM-5. 5th ed. Washington, DC: APA. Copyright 2013 American Psychiatric Association. All rights reserved.

The history should include previous psychologic problems, including consultations with a mental health professional, previous psychiatric illness, or contemplation of suicide. The family history should include a question concerning depression in relatives, especially first-degree relatives.

The clinician should be alert for additional symptoms of depression, which may include, but are not limited to, the following:

- Persistent physical symptoms that do not respond to treatment or do not have an identifiable physical cause, such as headaches, digestive disorders, or chronic pain

- Exaggerated or prolonged depressive symptoms following common reproductive events, conditions, or procedures, such as miscarriage, stillbirth, premature delivery, infertility, hysterectomy, mastectomy, childbirth, or menopause

- Multiple somatic problems that may include dysmenorrhea, dyspareunia, sexual dysfunction, and fatigue

  — Chronic, clinically unconfirmed vulvovaginitis, idiopathic vulvodynia, or chronic vaginal pain and burning

  — Chronic pelvic or genitourinary tract pain

  — Severe, incapacitating premenstrual syndrome

All depressed patients should be evaluated for suicidal thinking and previous suicide attempts. This evaluation is best done by direct questioning. If a woman has specific plans or significant risk of suicide, such as prior attempts or hopelessness, a mental health specialist should be consulted immediately. Of all people hospitalized for depression, 15% will eventually take their own lives.

Differential Diagnosis

The clinician must keep in mind other conditions and distinguish them from depression; these conditions include bipolar disorder, grief, substance abuse, schizophrenia, dementia, medical illness, and medication effects. Patients who report symptoms of mania may have a bipolar disorder, and medical treatment will be different from the treatment for depression. Antidepressant medications can induce mania and should be used with caution in a patient previously treated for mania. In such cases, referral to a psychiatrist is recommended. Screening for medical conditions, such as thyroid dysfunction, should be considered because it has been found in up to 10% of patients with depression.

Management

The obstetrician–gynecologist may elect to treat depression in some individuals. Although some patients might be unable to participate in their treatment (eg, individuals who are severely depressed, who display psychotic features, or who have made suicide attempts), the selection of treatment should be a collaborative decision between practitioner and patient whenever possible. Such shared decision making is likely to increase adherence and, therefore, treatment effectiveness. Medications should be considered for patients with moderate or severe depression, prior positive response to medication, or recurrent depression, as well as for patients who prefer medication to psychotherapy. Obstetrician–gynecologists should be familiar with several drugs in different categories that they would feel comfortable prescribing. Psychotherapy alone often is effective in treating patients with mild or moderate depression, and a psychotherapy referral should be considered for patients with relatively mild depression when it is the patient's preference. Combined treatment with psychotherapy and medication should be considered when the depression is more severe, there is an important psychosocial issue that would respond to therapy, or the patient has a history of treatment nonadherence or recurrent depression. Referral generally is recommended for the following situations:

- Depression with suicide risk
- Bipolar disorder
- Depression with psychotic symptoms (hallucinations, delusions)
- Depression in a pediatric or adolescent patient (some medications may increase suicide risk in this age group) (see Bibliography)
- Failure to respond to previous interventions
- The need for combination or multiple medications
- Substance abuse (such patients are at higher risk of suicide and require additional therapeutic interventions)
- Practitioner's lack of comfort with treating the patient

The major categories of antidepressant medication are tricyclic agents, selective serotonin-reuptake inhibitors (SSRIs), heterocyclic agents, and monoamine oxidase inhibitors. No one antidepressant is clearly more effective than another. The choice of an appropriate antidepressant generally is made on the basis of safety, adverse effect profiles, and cost. Safety of the medication and lack of significant adverse effects make SSRIs a first choice in antidepressants. Tricyclic agents often are used because of lower initial cost and greater experience with their use. However, several studies indicate that SSRIs are as cost-effective as tricyclic agents because they have fewer adverse effects, require less frequent medication changes, and have a higher rate of adherence. An example in which an adverse effect profile may be important in selecting an antidepressant is avoidance of drugs that may cause sexual dysfunction.

Fluoxetine is a widely used medication for the treatment of depression. It also is used to treat premenstrual dysphoric disorder (see also the "Premenstrual Syndrome" section in Part 4). Like the SSRIs, bupropion, trazodone, and heterocyclic agents appear to be safer than tricyclic agents in cases of potential overdose. Clinicians should be aware that bupropion is marketed under the name Zyban for smoking cessation. Note that monoamine oxidase inhibitors can have adverse effects and fatal interactions with other medications; only practitioners with substantial experience with monoamine oxidase inhibitors should prescribe them.

The American Psychiatric Association advises that the recommended length of treatment with medication is until the patient is symptom free. This is generally up to 6 months for the first episode of depression; in the case of recurrent episodes, the duration of treatment generally will be at least as long as the previous episodes of treatment, but frequently will be longer. Frequent recurrences may require prolonged treatment of up to several years.

Bibliography

American Psychiatric Association. Diagnostic and statistical manual of mental disorders: DSM-5. 5th ed. Washington, DC: APA; 2013.

Gjerdingen DK, Yawn BP. Postpartum depression screening: importance, methods, barriers, and recommendations for practice. J Am Board Fam Med 2007;20:280–8.

Kessler RC, Berglund P, Demler O, Jin R, Merikangas KR, Walters EE. Lifetime prevalence and age-of-onset distributions of DSM-IV disorders in the National Comorbidity Survey Replication [published erratum appears in Arch Gen Psychiatry 2005;62:768]. Arch Gen Psychiatry 2005;62:593–602.

Lock J, Walker LR, Rickert VI, Katzman DK. Suicidality in adolescents being treated with antidepressant medications and the black box label: position paper of the Society for Adolescent Medicine. Society for Adolescent Medicine. J Adolesc Health 2005;36:92–3.

Screening for depression in adults: U.S. preventive services task force recommendation statement. U.S. Preventive Services Task Force. Ann Intern Med 2009;151: 784–92.

Spitzer RL, Williams JB, Kroenke K, Linzer M, deGruy FV,3rd, Hahn SR, et al. Utility of a new procedure for diagnosing mental disorders in primary care. The PRIME-MD 1000 study. JAMA 1994;272:1749–56.

Whooley MA, Avins AL, Miranda J, Browner WS. Case-finding instruments for depression. Two questions are as good as many. J Gen Intern Med 1997;12:439–45.

Resources

American College of Obstetricians and Gynecologists. Depression. Patient Education Pamphlet AP106. Washington, DC: American College of Obstetricians and Gynecologists; 2012.

American College of Obstetricians and Gynecologists. Mental health disorders in adolescents. Guidelines for adolescent health care [CD-ROM]. 2nd ed. ed. Washington, DC: American College of Obstetricians and Gynecologists; 2011. p. 85–96.

American College of Obstetricians and Gynecologists. Postpartum depression. ACOG Patient Education Pamphlet AP091. Washington, DC: American College of Obstetricians and Gynecologists; 2013.

American College of Obstetricians and Gynecologists. Primary and preventive health care for female adolescents. Guidelines for adolescent health care [CD-ROM]. 2nd ed. ed. Washington, DC: American College of Obstetricians and Gynecologists; 2011. p. 25–42.

American Psychiatric Association. Key topics: depression. Available at: http://www. psychiatry.org/mental-health/key-topics/depression. Retrieved July 31, 2013.

American Psychological Association. Psychology topics: depression. Available at: http://www.apa.org/topics/depress/index.aspx. Retrieved July 31, 2013.

Dell D. Mood and anxiety disorders. Clin Update Womens Health Care. 2008; VII(5):1–98.

Medicines for treating depression: a review of the research for adults. Effective Health Care Program. AHRQ Pub. No. 12-EHC012-A. Rockville (MD): Agency for Healthcare Research and Quality; 2012. Available at: http://effectivehealthcare.ahrq. gov/ehc/products/210/1142/sec_gen_anti_dep_cons_fin_to_post.pdf. Retrieved September 16, 2013.

Mental Health America. Available at: http://www.mentalhealthamerica.net. Retrieved July 31, 2013.

Second-generation antidepressants for treating adult depression: an update. Effective Health Care Program. AHRQ Pub. No. 12-EHC012-3. Rockville (MD): Agency for Healthcare Research and Quality; 2012. Available at: http://effectivehealthcare. ahrq.gov/ehc/products/210/1143/sec_gen_anti_dep_clin_fin_to_post.pdf. Retrieved September 16, 2013.

GYNECOLOGIC CARE

This part addresses management issues for women who have conditions that have a major effect on their health, such as endometriosis and urinary incontinence. Some of these conditions may be identified at the time of the well-woman examination but may exceed the expertise of the generalist. Sections include focused information on the diagnosis of these conditions and recommendations for management from the American College of Obstetricians and Gynecologists as well as other relevant medical and governmental organizations. The last section focuses on ambulatory gynecologic surgery and offers guidelines for the performance of invasive procedures in the office and other ambulatory settings.

AMENORRHEA

Amenorrhea, the absence or abnormal cessation of menstruation, affects 2–5% of all women of childbearing age in the United States. Primary amenorrhea is defined as no menarche by 16 years of age. Secondary amenorrhea occurs when menstruating women fail to menstruate for 3–6 months. Amenorrhea has variable etiologies and implications in patients depending on age, severity, and associated symptoms.

Normal Menstrual Cycles

The menstrual cycle is an important component in the assessment of overall health status, and the American College of Obstetricians and Gynecologists recommends including the menstrual cycle as an additional vital sign. The median age of menarche in the United States and other developed countries is between 12 years and 13 years of age, but because age at menarche may vary internationally, health care providers should be aware of potential differences within their populations. Menstrual cycles are often irregular through adolescence, but by the third year after menarche approximately 60–80% of cycles are 21–34 days long. After the onset of menarche, cycles should occur at least every 90 days; longer intervals may represent an underlying etiology.

Etiology

There are numerous etiologies for amenorrhea, but among the most common are polycystic ovary syndrome (PCOS), hypothalamic causes, primary ovarian insufficiency, and hyperprolactinemia (see also the "Polycystic Ovary Syndrome" section later in Part 4). Table 4-1 and Table 4-2 list the common causes of primary and secondary amenorrhea, respectively, by the frequency they are encountered in clinical practice.

Table 4-1. Common Causes of Primary Amenorrhea

Category	Approximate Frequency (%)
Breast development	30
Müllerian agenesis	10
Androgen insensitivity	9
Vaginal septum	2
Imperforate hymen	1
Constitutional delay	8
No breast development: high FSH	40
46,XX	15
46,XY	5
Abnormal karyotype	20
No breast development: low FSH	30
Constitutional delay	10
Prolactinomas	5
Kallmann syndrome	2
Other CNS	3
Stress, weight loss, anorexia	3
PCOS	3
Congenital adrenal hyperplasia	3
Other	1

Abbreviations: CNS, central nervous system; FSH, follicle-stimulating hormone; PCOS, polycystic ovary syndrome.

Modified from Current evaluation of amenorrhea. Practice Committee of American Society for Reproductive Medicine. Fertil Steril 2008;90:S222. Copyright 2008, with permission from Elsevier.

Evaluation

Because the evaluation and treatment of amenorrhea may vary depending on the underlying etiology, a thorough history, physical examination, and often laboratory evaluation are critical for appropriate care of these patients. Although primary amenorrhea has been defined as no menarche by 16 years of age, many diagnosable and treatable disorders can and should

Table 4-2. Common Causes of Secondary Amenorrhea

Category	Approximate Frequency (%)
Low or normal FSH	66
Weight loss, anorexia, or both	
Nonspecific hypothalamic	
Chronic anovulation including PCOS	
Hypothyroidism	
Cushing syndrome	
Pituitary tumor, empty sella, Sheehan syndrome	
Gonadal failure: high FSH	12
46,XX	
Abnormal karyotype	
High prolactin	13
Anatomic	7
Asherman syndrome	
Hyperandrogenic states	2
Ovarian tumor	
Nonclassic congenital adrenal hyperplasia	
Undiagnosed	

Abbreviations: FSH, follicle-stimulating hormone; PCOS, polycystic ovary syndrome.
Modified from Current evaluation of amenorrhea. Practice Committee of American Society for Reproductive Medicine. Fertil Steril 2008;90:S222. Copyright 2008, with permission from Elsevier.

be detected earlier. Thus, an evaluation for primary amenorrhea should be considered for any girl who has not reached menarche by 15 years of age or has not done so within 3 years of thelarche. Lack of breast development by 13 years of age also should be evaluated. The American Society for Reproductive Medicine recommends an evaluation for secondary amenorrhea after 3 months of amenorrhea in a regularly menstruating woman.

A thorough patient history should be taken and include inquiries about the following: past medical illnesses; date of last menstrual period; history of amenorrhea; exercise (amount per day and per week); dietary history (restrictions, special diets); eating disorders; medications; illicit drug use; psychiatric history; and a history of conditions such as hirsutism, acne, and galactorrhea.

Physical examination should include assessment of pubertal development (Tanner staging); evaluation of genital tract anatomy; presence of hirsutism, acne, or both; and measurement of body mass index. The need for imaging studies, such as ultrasonography, magnetic resonance imaging (MRI), and computed tomography, will depend on the patient's medical history and whether the evaluation is for primary or secondary amenorrhea.

Laboratory studies used in the assessment of amenorrhea include pregnancy testing and measurement of levels of thyroid-stimulating hormone, prolactin, and follicle-stimulating hormone (FSH). Thyroid-stimulating hormone level is evaluated to rule out subclinical hypothyroidism. A persistently elevated prolactin level may indicate a prolactinoma, and the American Society for Reproductive Medicine recommends follow-up evaluation with MRI. The most common diagnoses when FSH levels are normal or low are hypothalamic amenorrhea and PCOS (see also the "Polycystic Ovary Syndrome" section later in Part 4). An elevated FSH level in women younger than 40 years may signify primary ovarian insufficiency. Once confirmed by repeat testing, elevated FSH levels should prompt evaluation of autoimmune antibodies; the most commonly associated condition is autoimmune thyroiditis. The American Society for Reproductive Medicine recommends completion of a chromosomal analysis, including premutation analysis for Fragile X syndrome, in women in whom primary ovarian insufficiency is diagnosed.

Management

Management of amenorrhea depends on the etiology. Patients requiring therapy that is beyond the scope and expertise of the general obstetrician–gynecologist should be referred to appropriate health care providers for treatment.

Patients with primary amenorrhea that is due to constitutional delay require no treatment. Management of amenorrhea that is due to genetic (inherited) abnormalities includes supplemental hormone therapy (HT) to enable the development of normal secondary sex characteristics (breast development, pubic hair growth) and prevent osteoporosis. Patients with structural abnormalities (eg, vaginal agenesis) should be referred for treatment. Individuals who are found to have 46, XY karyotype are at increased risk of gonadal malignancy and will need to have gonads removed following breast development and attainment of adult stature.

The management of amenorrhea caused by primary ovarian insufficiency may involve HT and adequate consumption of calcium and vitamin D (see also the "Menopause" section in Part 3). Management of amenorrhea that is due to PCOS includes lifestyle modification, HT (such as combined oral contraceptive pills), and ovulation induction with clomiphene citrate when pregnancy is desired (see also the "Polycystic Ovary Syndrome" section later in Part 4). Patients with pituitary gland dysfunction, especially hyperprolactinemia, should be evaluated with MRI of the pituitary gland and referred for treatment, as needed.

Emotional or physical stress, eating disorders, restricted caloric intake, and increased or excessive exercise all may result in hypothalamic amenorrhea, though the treatment may vary greatly depending on the specific issue. All of these etiologies, however, may result in osteoporosis because of the effect of hypoestrogenism on bone remodeling. Current research indicates that the most effective means of improving bone mass is to treat the underlying condition; increasing caloric intake to improve energy availability has been shown to be critical for bone health (see also the "Osteoporosis" section in Part 3). If the underlying cause cannot be easily treated, the American Society for Reproductive Medicine recommends initiation of therapy with cyclic estrogen–progestin or oral contraceptives to prevent excessive bone loss. These treatments, however, do not normalize the metabolic factors that negatively affect bone health and have not been demonstrated to reduce the risk of fractures. Furthermore, there are no established guidelines addressing when, or if, HT should be used for the treatment of hypothalamic amenorrhea in females younger than 16 years. Hypothalamic amenorrhea that is due to other etiologies, such as disorders of the central nervous system, pituitary gland, or hypothalamus, requires referral to an appropriate specialist for management.

Bibliography

American College of Obstetricians and Gynecologists. Guidelines for adolescent health care [CD-ROM]. 2nd ed. ed. Washington, DC: American College of Obstetricians and Gynecologists; 2011.

Current evaluation of amenorrhea. Practice Committee of American Society for Reproductive Medicine. Fertil Steril 2008;90:S219–25.

Menstruation in girls and adolescents: using the menstrual cycle as a vital sign. ACOG Committee Opinion No. 349. American College of Obstetricians and Gynecologists. Obstet Gynecol 2006;108:1323–8.

Mullerian agenesis: diagnosis, management, and treatment. Committee Opinion No. 562. American College of Obstetricians and Gynecologists. Obstet Gynecol 2013;121:1134–7.

Rebar RW. Premature ovarian failure. Obstet Gynecol 2009;113:1355–63.

Resources

American College of Obstetricians and Gynecologists. Your first period—especially for teens. Patient Education Pamphlet AP049. Washington, DC: American College of Obstetricians and Gynecologists; 2012.

American Society for Reproductive Medicine. Abnormalities of the female reproductive tract (Müllerian defects). Birmingham (AL): ASRM; 2012. Available at: http://www.asrm.org/FACTSHEET_Abnormalities_of_the_Female_Reproductive_Tract. Retrieved April 10, 2014.

Eunice Kennedy Shriver National Institute of Child Health and Human Development. Amenorrhea: overview. Available at: https://www.nichd.nih.gov/health/topics/amenorrhea/Pages/default.aspx. Retrieved July 31, 2013.

Eunice Kennedy Shriver National Institute of Child Health and Human Development. Primary ovarian insufficiency. Available at: http://poi.nichd.nih.gov. Retrieved July 31, 2013.

Nattiv A, Loucks AB, Manore MM, Sanborn CF, Sundgot-Borgen J, Warren MP. American College of Sports Medicine position stand. The female athlete triad. American College of Sports Medicine. Med Sci Sports Exerc 2007;39:1867–82.

ABNORMAL GENITAL BLEEDING

Any bleeding other than what is expected in a normal ovulatory cycle is considered abnormal genital bleeding. Abnormal genital bleeding is one of the most common reasons for a woman to seek gynecologic care. The source of abnormal genital bleeding may be difficult to assess; it may be the rectum, the urinary tract, or the vulva, vagina, cervix, or uterus. The uterus is the source of most abnormal genital bleeding in adult women. Abnormal uterine bleeding (AUB) is a generic term that is a subclassification of genital bleeding. Physical examination readily distinguishes between the two, and each have a separate set of etiologies and treatments (see also "Abnormal Uterine Bleeding" later in this section).

A wide variety of conditions can cause the bleeding, including trauma, infection, endocrine or medical abnormalities, lesions, tumors, or neoplasm. It is also possible for contraception or pregnancy to be an etiologic factor. If genital bleeding is secondary to trauma, the differential diagnosis should include rape and abuse. Research into abnormal genital bleeding has been limited by a lack of widely accepted, high-quality and validated outcome measures that are objective and take into account patient quality of life measures. Nevertheless, there are a number of useful diagnostic tools and effective therapeutic options for the woman with abnormal genital bleeding.

Evaluation, Diagnosis, and Management

The following is an ordering of the differential diagnosis for abnormal genital bleeding, based on the age of the patient when symptoms occur:

- In children, the source of abnormal genital bleeding can include foreign bodies, vaginitis, urethral prolapse, neoplasm, trauma, and precocious puberty (see also the "Pediatric Gynecology" section in Part 3).

- In adolescents, abnormal genital bleeding most often occurs as a result of persistent anovulation, including anovulation caused by polycystic ovary syndrome (PCOS) and contraception. Pregnancy, pelvic infections, and coagulopathies (in as many as 19% of adolescents who require hospitalization) also are common in adolescents. Tumors also should be considered.

- Women in the second through fourth decades of life most often develop abnormal genital bleeding from pregnancy, structural lesions (eg, leiomyomas and polyps), anovulation (eg, PCOS), and hormonal contraception. Endometrial hyperplasia (or atrophy) and endometrial cancer also should be considered.

- Menopausal women most often develop bleeding from hormone therapy, endometrial atrophy, leiomyomas, endometrial hyperplasia, and malignancy.

Less common causes of abnormal genital bleeding include the following:

- Vascular anomalies of the uterus
- Infection
- Cirrhosis
- Drug therapy (ie, other than hormonal treatment)
- Thyroid dysfunction

An accurate diagnosis for the cause of bleeding should be established. Medical history should include a structured menstrual history that includes questions about heaviness of bleeding, duration, interval, regularity, and pain; family history of bleeding problems; and the use of medications or herbal supplements. A general physical examination, speculum examination, and bimanual examination should be completed. Proper evaluation of abnormal genital bleeding also may include the following:

- Evaluation for pregnancy
- Complete blood count and measurement of thyroid-stimulating hormone level
- Examination for lower genital tract lesions
- Cervical cytology

- Evaluation for infection or sexually transmitted infections
- Evaluation for endocrine dysfunction, such as PCOS
- Evaluation for bleeding disorder
- Evaluation for trauma or sexual assault (Clinicians should be familiar with any state reporting requirements regarding evidence of abuse or intimate partner violence and sexually transmitted infections; see also the "Sexually Transmitted Infections" section and the "Abuse" section in Part 3.)
- Endometrial biopsy
- Ultrasonography (transvaginal or transabdominal, depending on the patient's age and the indication)
- Sonohysterography
- Hysteroscopy

The management of abnormal genital bleeding varies greatly, depending on the underlying disorder. Medication, an office procedure, or surgery may be required, depending on the etiology, the patient's age, and the patient's reproductive status. A discussion of the evaluation and management of AUB follows.

Abnormal Uterine Bleeding

Abnormal uterine bleeding is any bleeding from the uterus that is abnormal in volume, duration, frequency, or regularity. It is a symptom with many different etiologies.

CLASSIFICATION AND ETIOLOGY OF ABNORMAL UTERINE BLEEDING

Descriptive terms that traditionally have been used to characterize abnormal menstrual bleeding patterns include menorrhagia, metrorrhagia, polymenorrhea, and oligomenorrhea. Menorrhagia, or heavy menstrual bleeding, is defined as menstrual blood loss greater than 80 mL. (However, this definition is used for research purposes and, in practice, excessive blood loss should be based on the patient's perception.) Metrorrhagia is defined as bleeding between periods. Polymenorrhea is defined as bleeding that occurs more often than every 21 days, and oligomenorrhea is defined as bleeding that occurs less frequently than every 35 days.

In 2011, to remedy the confusion surrounding nomenclature for AUB, the International Federation of Gynecology and Obstetrics (FIGO) introduced a new classification system, the adoption of which is supported by the American College of Obstetricians and Gynecologists. With this system, AUB is classified by pattern and etiology (Fig. 4-1). The term dysfunctional uterine bleeding, formerly used to describe AUB without a systematic or structural cause, should no longer be used.

A major cause of AUB (after pregnancy is ruled out) is uterine leiomyomas (commonly known as fibroids). These are the most common solid tumors in women and are the leading indication for hysterectomy, most often for AUB and pelvic pressure. An example of the PALM-COEIN

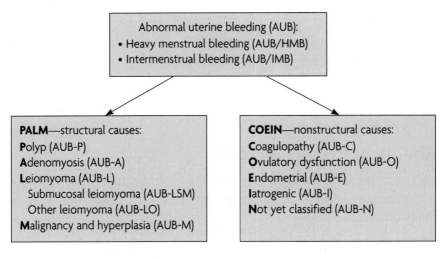

Fig. 4-1. Basic PALM–COEIN classification system for the causes of abnormal uterine bleeding in nonpregnant reproductive-aged women. This system, approved by the International Federation of Gynecology and Obstetrics, uses the term "abnormal uterine bleeding" paired with terms that describe associated bleeding patterns ("heavy menstrual bleeding" or "intermenstrual bleeding"), a qualifying letter (or letters) to indicate its etiology (or etiologies), or both. (Modified from Munro MG, Critchley HO, Broder MS, Fraser IS. FIGO classification system [PALM-COEIN] for causes of abnormal uterine bleeding in nongravid women of reproductive age. FIGO Working Group on Menstrual Disorders. Int J Gynaecol Obstet 2011;113:3–13.)

terminology used for symptomatic uterine leiomyomas is AUB-L (abnormal uterine bleeding-leiomyoma). Another very common, nonstructural cause of AUB is ovulatory dysfunction, which often is the result of an endocrinopathy, such as PCOS. The new terminology for this etiology is AUB-O (abnormal uterine bleeding-ovulatory dysfunction).

Women with undiagnosed coagulopathies may present initially with AUB. These disorders include defects in primary hemostasis, platelet deficiency (leukemia or idiopathic thrombocytopenia), platelet dysfunction (von Willebrand disease), and abnormalities of secondary hemostasis (congenital factor deficiencies). Von Willebrand disease is the most common inherited bleeding disorder among American women, with a prevalence of 0.6–1.3%. The overall prevalence is even greater among women with chronic heavy menstrual bleeding, and ranges from 5% to 24%. A diagnosis of von Willebrand disease will have significant implications for the woman's future gynecologic and obstetric care. Given the prevalence and the consequences of such a diagnosis, hematologic disorders should be considered in all patients presenting with AUB or heavy menstrual bleeding, especially adolescents with a sudden onset of AUB or heavy menstrual bleeding at menarche.

EVALUATION AND DIAGNOSIS OF ABNORMAL UTERINE BLEEDING

The initial evaluation of patients with AUB is similar to that for patients with abnormal genital bleeding and includes a thorough medical history and physical examination, appropriate laboratory and imaging tests, and consideration of age-related factors (see also "Evaluation, Diagnosis, and Management" of abnormal genital bleeding earlier in this section).

An initial screening for an underlying disorder of hemostasis should be performed. In all adolescents with heavy menstrual bleeding and adult patients with a positive screening history for a bleeding disorder, laboratory testing is indicated. Initial tests should include a complete blood count with platelets, prothrombin time, and partial thromboplastin time (fibrinogen or thrombin time are optional); bleeding time is neither sensitive nor specific, and is not indicated. Depending on the results of the initial tests, or if a patient's medical history is suggestive of an underlying bleeding condition, specific tests for von Willebrand disease or other coagulopathies may be indicated.

Any patient with an abnormal physical examination, such as an enlarged or globular uterus on bimanual examination, should undergo transvaginal ultrasonography to evaluate for myomas and adenomyosis. When symptoms persist despite treatment in the setting of a normal pelvic examination, further evaluation is indicated with transvaginal ultrasonography, biopsy, or both if not already performed. When there is clinical suspicion for endometrial polyps or submucosal leiomyomas, sonohysterography or hysteroscopy will enable better detection of lesions.

Endometrial tissue sampling should be performed in patients with AUB who are older than 45 years as a first-line test. Endometrial sampling also should be performed in patients younger than 45 years with a history of unopposed estrogen exposure (such as seen in obesity or PCOS), failed medical management, and persistent AUB. An office endometrial biopsy is the first-line procedure for tissue sampling in the evaluation of patients with AUB. Other evaluation methods, such as transvaginal ultrasonography, sonohysterography, or office hysteroscopy also may be necessary when the endometrial biopsy is insufficient, nondiagnostic, or cannot be performed.

Transvaginal ultrasonography in postmenopausal women with bleeding has an extremely high negative predictive value for endometrial cancer when 4 mm is used as a cut-off. An endometrial thickness of greater than 4 mm or inability to visualize thickness, however, should be evaluated with another method, such as endometrial biopsy, sonohysterography, or office hysteroscopy. Ultrasonographic measurement of endometrial thickness is of limited value in detecting benign abnormalities in the premenopausal woman as compared with its ability to exclude malignancy in the postmenopausal woman. Thus, measurement of endometrial thickness in premenopausal women is not helpful in the evaluation of AUB.

Sonohysterography is a procedure that can be performed in an office setting by a qualified individual. It has the ability to delineate abnormalities in the uterine cavity that may be missed with routine transvaginal ultrasonography and does so without radiation exposure or significant discomfort to the patient. It is important to ensure that the patient is not pregnant, so scheduling during the follicular phase or after a course of progestin should be considered.

Hysteroscopy may be performed in an office setting or in the operating room. Hysteroscopy allows direct visualization of endometrial cavity abnormalities and the ability to take directed biopsies. Hysteroscopy is highly accurate in diagnosing endometrial cancer but less useful for detecting hyperplasia.

Routine use of magnetic resonance imaging in the evaluation of AUB is not recommended. However, magnetic resonance imaging may be useful to guide the treatment of leiomyomas, particularly when the uterus is enlarged, contains multiple leiomyomas, or precise leiomyoma mapping is of clinical importance.

MANAGEMENT OF ABNORMAL UTERINE BLEEDING

The primary goal of management is to treat the underlying disorder. A universal single approach in the management of all patients with AUB is not feasible or appropriate. In general, treatment options depend on the following:

- Suspected etiology—an underlying coagulopathy should be considered in all patients (particularly adolescents) when AUB is not otherwise explained, does not respond to medical therapy, or both
- Frequency and quantity of bleeding
- Patient age
- Health status
- Reproductive plans

Many causes of AUB are amenable to medical management. Decisions should be based on the patient's medical history and contraindications to therapies. The treatment of choice for AUB-O if carcinoma is not a concern or has been ruled out is medical therapy. Medical treatment options for AUB-O include progestin therapy and combined hormonal contraception. Medical management should be the initial treatment for most patients with acute AUB, if clinically appropriate. Options include intravenous conjugated equine estrogen, multidose regimens of oral contraceptives or oral progestins, and tranexamic acid. Antifibrinolytic drugs, such as tranexamic acid, work by preventing fibrin degradation and are effective treatments for patients with chronic AUB.

The need for surgical treatment is based on the clinical stability of the patient, the severity of bleeding, contraindications to medical management, the patient's lack of response to medical management, and the underlying medical condition of the patient. Surgical options include dilation and curettage (D&C), endometrial ablation, uterine artery embolization, and hysterectomy. The choice of surgical modality (eg, D&C versus hysterectomy) is based on the aforementioned factors plus the patient's desire for future fertility. Specific treatments, such as hysteroscopy with D&C, polypectomy, or myomectomy, may be required if structural abnormalities are suspected as the cause of acute AUB (see also the "Leiomyomas" section later in Part 4). Dilation and curettage alone (without hysteroscopy) is an inadequate tool for evaluation of uterine disorders and may provide only a temporary reduction in bleeding (cycles after the D&C will not be improved). Dilation and curettage with concomitant hysteroscopy may be of value for those patients in whom intrauterine pathology is suspected or a tissue sample is desired. Case reports of uterine artery embolization and endometrial ablation show that these procedures successfully control acute AUB. Endometrial ablation, although readily available in most centers, should be considered only if other treatments have been ineffective or are contraindicated, and it should be performed only when a woman does not have plans for future childbearing and when the possibility of endometrial or uterine cancer has been reliably ruled out as the cause of the acute AUB. Hysterectomy, the definitive treatment for controlling heavy bleeding, may be necessary for patients who do not respond to medical therapy.

Bibliography

American College of Obstetricians and Gynecologists. General management of pediatric gynecology patients. Guidelines for adolescent health care [CD-ROM]. 2nd ed. ed. Washington, DC: American College of Obstetricians and Gynecologists; 2011. p. 172–92.

Diagnosis of abnormal uterine bleeding in reproductive-aged women. Practice Bulletin No. 128. American College of Obstetricians and Gynecologists. Obstet Gynecol 2012;120:197–206.

Endometrial ablation. ACOG Practice Bulletin No. 81. American College of Obstetricians and Gynecologists. Obstet Gynecol 2007;109:1233–48.

Fraser IS, Critchley HO, Munro MG, Broder M. A process designed to lead to international agreement on terminologies and definitions used to describe abnormalities of menstrual bleeding. Writing Group for this Menstrual Agreement Process. Fertil Steril 2007;87:466–76.

James AH. Obstetric management of adolescents with bleeding disorders. J Pediatr Adolesc Gynecol 2010;23:S31–7.

James AH. Von Willebrand disease. Obstet Gynecol Surv 2006;61:136–45.

Kadir RA, Economides DL, Sabin CA, Owens D, Lee CA. Frequency of inherited bleeding disorders in women with menorrhagia. Lancet 1998;351:485–9.

Long-acting reversible contraception: implants and intrauterine devices. Practice bulletin No. 121. American College of Obstetricians and Gynecologists. Obstet Gynecol 2011;118:184–96.

Management of abnormal uterine bleeding associated with ovulatory dysfunction. Practice Bulletin No. 136. American College of Obstetricians and Gynecologists. Obstet Gynecol 2013;122:176–85.

Management of acute abnormal uterine bleeding in nonpregnant reproductive-aged women. Committee Opinion No. 557. American College of Obstetricians and Gynecologists; Obstet Gynecol 2013;121:891–6.

Matteson KA, Boardman LA, Munro MG, Clark MA. Abnormal uterine bleeding: a review of patient-based outcome measures. Fertil Steril 2009;92:205–16.

Menstruation in girls and adolescents: using the menstrual cycle as a vital sign. ACOG Committee Opinion No. 349. American College of Obstetricians and Gynecologists. Obstet Gynecol 2006;108:1323–8.

Munro MG, Critchley HO, Broder MS, Fraser IS. FIGO classification system (PALM-COEIN) for causes of abnormal uterine bleeding in nongravid women of reproductive age. FIGO Working Group on Menstrual Disorders. Int J Gynaecol Obstet 2011;113:3–13.

Noncontraceptive uses of hormonal contraceptives. Practice Bulletin No. 110. American College of Obstetricians and Gynecologists. Obstet Gynecol 2010; 115:206–18.

Shankar M, Lee CA, Sabin CA, Economides DL, Kadir RA. von Willebrand disease in women with menorrhagia: a systematic review. BJOG 2004;111:734–40.

Sharp HT. Assessment of new technology in the treatment of idiopathic menorrhagia and uterine leiomyomata. Obstet Gynecol 2006;108:990–1003.

Sonohysterography. Technology Assessment in Obstetrics and Gynecology No. 8. American College of Obstetricians and Gynecologists. Obstet Gynecol 2012;119: 1325–8.

The role of transvaginal ultrasonography in the evaluation of postmenopausal bleeding. ACOG Committee Opinion No. 440. American College of Obstetricians and Gynecologists. Obstet Gynecol 2009;114:409–11.

Von Willebrand disease in women. Committee Opinion No. 580. American College of Obstetricians and Gynecologists. Obstet Gynecol 2013;122:1368–73.

Resources

American College of Obstetricians and Gynecologists. Abnormal uterine bleeding. Patient Education Pamphlet AP095. Washington, DC: American College of Obstetricians and Gynecologists; 2012.

American College of Obstetricians and Gynecologists. Endometrial ablation. Patient Education Pamphlet AP134. Washington, DC: American College of Obstetricians and Gynecologists; 2009.

American College of Obstetricians and Gynecologists. Perimenopausal bleeding and bleeding after menopause. Patient Education Pamphlet AP162. Washington, DC: American College of Obstetricians and Gynecologists; 2010.

Learman LA, Nakagawa S, Gregorich SE, Jackson RA, Jacoby A, Kuppermann M. Success of uterus-preserving treatments for abnormal uterine bleeding, chronic pelvic pain, and symptomatic fibroids: age and bridges to menopause. Am J Obstet Gynecol 2011;204:272.e1–7.

ENDOMETRIOSIS

Endometriosis, defined as the presence of endometrial tissue outside the uterine cavity, is a gynecologic condition that affects 6–10% of women of reproductive age, 50–60% of women and adolescent girls with pelvic pain, and up to 50% of women with infertility. A familial predisposition toward endometriosis via a proposed polygenic and multifactorial mechanism has been documented. A female patient who has an affected first-degree relative has a 7–10-fold increased risk of also developing the condition. The retrograde menstruation theory has gained widespread acceptance as an explanation for the dissemination of endometrial cells outside of the uterus. The exact factor or factors that lead to the survival and subsequent implantation of the displaced endometrium remain unknown but may include immune dysfunction, gene mutations, or both. Defects with obstructed outflow, such as cervical or vaginal atresia and incomplete müllerian fusion, commonly are associated with pelvic endometriosis, although regression usually occurs after surgical correction of the anomaly.

Endometriosis differs in presentation, findings on physical examination, and visibility at the time of laparoscopy between adolescents and adults (see also "Endometriosis in Adolescents" later in this section). Many experts have attempted to develop a classification system for endometriosis. The classification system developed by the American Society for Reproductive Medicine is commonly used (see Fig. 4-2). This system classifies endometriosis by the extent and location of disease.

AMERICAN SOCIETY FOR REPRODUCTIVE MEDICINE
REVISED CLASSIFICATION OF ENDOMETRIOSIS

Patient's Name _____   Date_____

Stage I   (Minimal) - 1-5
Stage II (Mild) - 6-15
Stage III (Moderate) - 16-40
Stage IV (Severe) - >40
Total_____

Laparoscopy_____ Laparotomy_____ Photography_____
Recommended Treatment_____

Prognosis_____

PERITONEUM	ENDOMETRIOSIS		<1cm	1-3cm	>3cm
		Superficial	1	2	4
		Deep	2	4	6
OVARY	R	Superficial	1	2	4
		Deep	4	16	20
	L	Superficial	1	2	4
		Deep	4	16	20

	POSTERIOR CULDESAC OBLITERATION	Partial	Complete
		4	40

	ADHESIONS		<1/3 Enclosure	1/3-2/3 Enclosure	>2/3 Enclosure
OVARY	R	Filmy	1	2	4
		Dense	4	8	16
	L	Filmy	1	2	4
		Dense	4	8	16
TUBE	R	Filmy	1	2	4
		Dense	4*	8*	16
	L	Filmy	1	2	4
		Dense	4*	8*	16

*If the fimbriated end of the fallopian tube is completely enclosed, change the point assignment to 16.

Denote appearance of superficial implant types as red [(R), red, red-pink, flamelike, vesicular blobs, clear vesicles], white [(W), opacifications, peritoneal defects, yellow-brown], or black [(B) black, hemosiderin deposits, blue]. Denote percent of total described as R___%, W___% and B___%. Total should equal 100%.

Additional Endometriosis: _____   Associated Pathology: _____
_____   _____
_____   _____

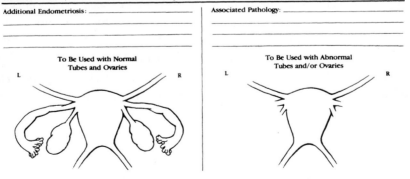

To Be Used with Normal
Tubes and Ovaries

To Be Used with Abnormal
Tubes and/or Ovaries

(continued)

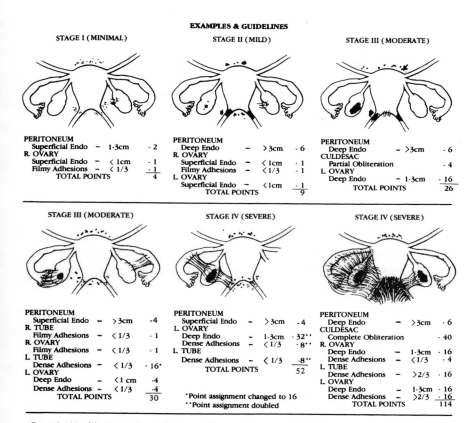

EXAMPLES & GUIDELINES

Determination of the stage or degree of endometrial involvement is based on a weighted point system. Distribution of points has been arbitrarily determined and may require further revision or refinement as knowledge of the disease increases.

To ensure complete evaluation, inspection of the pelvis in a clockwise or counterclockwise fashion is encouraged. Number, size and location of endometrial implants, plaques, endometriomas and/or adhesions are noted. For example, five separate 0.5cm superficial implants on the peritoneum (2.5 cm total) would be assigned 2 points. (The surface of the uterus should be considered peritoneum.) The severity of the endometriosis or adhesions should be assigned the highest score only for peritoneum, ovary, tube or culdesac. For example, a 4cm superficial and a 2cm deep implant of the peritoneum should be given a score of 6 (not 8). A 4cm deep endometrioma of the ovary associated with more than 3cm of superficial disease should be scored 20 (not 24).

In those patients with only one adnexa, points applied to disease of the remaining tube and ovary should be multiplied by two. **Points assigned may be circled and totaled. Aggregation of points indicates stage of disease (minimal, mild, moderate, or severe).

The presence of endometriosis of the bowel, urinary tract, fallopian tube, vagina, cervix, skin etc., should be documented under "additional endometriosis." Other pathology such as tubal occlusion, leiomyomata, uterine anomaly, etc., should be documented under "associated pathology." All pathology should be depicted as specifically as possible on the sketch of pelvic organs, and means of observation (laparoscopy or laparotomy) should be noted.

Fig. 4-2. Classification of endometriosis. (Reprinted from Fertility and Sterility Vol 67, American Society for Reproductive Medicine. Revised classification of endometriosis, p. 817–21. Copyright 1997, with permission from American Society for Reproductive Medicine.)

Symptoms

Symptoms and sequelae of endometriosis vary widely but include the following:

- Dysmenorrhea
- Adnexal mass (symptomatic or asymptomatic)
- Abnormal uterine bleeding
- Chronic pelvic pain
- Dyspareunia
- Infertility
- Uterosacral ligament nodularity

The most common symptom noted in published reviews is acquired or progressive dysmenorrhea. Pain often starts before the onset of menses. Other symptoms may include gastrointestinal symptoms, and a black–brown discharge before menses.

Evaluation and Diagnosis

The differential diagnosis for endometriosis includes primary dysmenorrhea, adenomyosis, irritable bowel syndrome, obstructive müllerian anomalies, pelvic inflammatory disease, interstitial cystitis, musculoskeletal disorders, and other problems associated with pelvic pain, such as sexual abuse. Clinicians should carefully evaluate women for these other causes of pelvic pain before initiating aggressive treatment for endometriosis and reconsider these etiologies in women who do not respond to standard endometriosis therapies.

A significant number of women with endometriosis remain asymptomatic. For example, endometriosis is found in women undergoing tubal ligation and hysterectomy who have no history of endometriosis or pelvic pain. Thus, clinicians should consider the possibility that patients with proven endometriosis also may have other conditions that cause pelvic pain (see also the "Acute and Chronic Pain Management" section later in Part 4).

Direct visualization of endometriosis lesions remains the preferred method for diagnosing endometriosis. Nonetheless, the need for a surgical procedure to determine a diagnosis of endometriosis as the cause of pelvic pain continues to be debated. Arguments against the requirement to perform surgery to definitively diagnose endometriosis include the imprecision of surgical diagnosis as well as the inherent risks of surgery.

Management

Medical and surgical modalities have been used for management. For pain management, evidence exists to support short-term benefits with either modality. No definitive data indicate the superiority of either modality for long-term management of pain, and a substantial proportion of women managed with either method experience a recurrence of symptoms. Medical suppressive therapies, such as oral contraceptives or gonadotropin-releasing hormone (GnRH) agonists for endometriosis-associated infertility, are ineffective according to a 2007 Cochrane review (see Bibliography).

Clinicians should recognize that endometriosis is a chronic disorder. In discussing treatment options with the patient, clinicians should plan long-term therapy based on the patient's age, presenting symptoms, severity of disease, and reproductive plans.

Nonsurgical Interventions

First-line therapy for women with presumed endometriosis who wish to preserve fertility includes combined oral contraceptives and nonsteroidal antiinflammatory drugs (NSAIDs). After failure of initial treatment, second-line therapies include empiric therapy with a 3-month course of a GnRH agonist, depot medroxyprogesterone acetate, the levonorgestrel intrauterine system (levonorgestrel intrauterine device [IUD]), and danazol. The role of aromatase inhibitors in the treatment of endometriosis is under investigation. Gonadotropin-releasing hormone agonists are highly effective in reducing the pain syndromes associated with endometriosis but are not superior to other methods, such as combined oral contraceptives as first-line therapy, and may have significant adverse effects, including hot flushes, vaginal dryness, and osteopenia. When a GnRH agonist is used for therapy, the administration of add-back therapy (using either sex-steroid hormones or other specific bone-sparing agents) may reduce or eliminate bothersome adverse effects and drug-induced bone mineral loss without reducing the efficacy of pain relief. Add-back regimens have been advocated for use in women undergoing long-term GnRH therapy (more than 6 months), but can be started immediately. In patients with laparoscopy-confirmed endometriosis and dysmenorrhea, combined oral contraceptives and oral norethindrone, depot medroxyprogesterone acetate or the levonorgestrel IUD are effective compared with placebo and are equivalent to more costly regimens, such as GnRH agonists. Nonpharmacologic therapeutic options to manage pain associated with endometriosis include pelvic biofeedback, physical therapy, hypnotherapy, cognitive and relaxation techniques, massage, and acupuncture (see also the "Complementary and Alternative Medicine" section in Part 3).

SURGICAL INTERVENTIONS

The efficacy of surgical therapy depends heavily on the experience and expertise of the surgeon. Excision of an endometrioma is superior to simple drainage and ablation of the cyst wall. Long-term (at least 24 months) oral contraceptive use is effective in reducing endometrioma recurrence as well as in reducing the frequency and severity of dysmenorrhea. As discussed previously, medical suppressive therapies appear ineffective in the treatment of endometriosis-related infertility. Although surgical management of endometriosis-related infertility does improve pregnancy rates, the magnitude of improvement is unclear.

When surgery is elected, operative laparoscopy has numerous advantages compared with laparotomy. However, no conservative surgical method has been shown to be superior in the treatment of endometriosis. A substantial number of women (44%) will experience recurrence of symptoms within 1 year postoperatively.

Surgical methods in use include the following:

- Ablation of lesions
- Excision
- Endocoagulation
- Electrocautery
- Laser vaporization

Hysterectomy, with or without bilateral oophorectomy, often is regarded as definitive therapy for pain control; however, symptoms may recur even after hysterectomy and oophorectomy. Ovarian conservation is associated with increased likelihood of recurrence of symptoms and additional surgery. Menopausal estrogen therapy is not contraindicated after bilateral salpingo-oophorectomy, but data on the recurrence of lesions and symptoms are limited.

CONSULTATION OR REFERRAL

Generalists should consider consultation or referral to a specialist if their level of expertise has been exceeded. The following referrals or support services may be needed:

- Reproductive endocrinologist
- Gynecologic surgeon
- Pain management unit
- Radiographic imaging
- Physical therapist
- Alternative therapies
    — Hypnotherapy
    — Relaxation techniques
    — Massage
    — Acupuncture

Endometriosis in Adolescents

Endometriosis can be a debilitating disease in adolescent females, and prompt evaluation and consideration of the adverse effects of endometriosis is essential in this age group. Gynecologists, pediatricians, and other adolescent health care providers should recognize that thelarche and the presence of endogenous estrogen can be considered a developmental milestone and benchmark for inclusion of endometriosis in the differential diagnosis of adolescent females with chronic pelvic pain or dysmenorrhea. A multidisciplinary team approach to the adolescent who has endometriosis may be the most rewarding for the adolescent, her family, and the clinician.

EVALUATION AND DIAGNOSIS

Adolescent patients typically present with progressive and severe dysmenorrhea, but also may present with noncyclic pelvic pain. A thorough review of a patient's history and physical examination are necessary to assess for the differential diagnoses of pelvic pain, such as appendicitis, pelvic inflammatory disease, müllerian anomalies or outflow obstruction, bowel disease, hernias, musculoskeletal disorders, and psychosocial complaints. It is important to evaluate the vagina and uterus for a possible obstructive anomaly and the ovaries for a possible ovarian mass. Findings of the physical examination of adolescents may vary from the adult population because uterosacral nodularity and endometriomas are found in more advanced disease and, thus, are uncommon in adolescents.

MANAGEMENT

Treatment should focus on conservative, fertility-sparing measures with medical and surgical interventions. The first line of therapy for an adolescent with presumed endometriosis should include combined oral contraceptive and NSAIDs. After a comprehensive evaluation and adequate trial of combined oral contraceptives and NSAIDs without improvement in pain, laparoscopy can be offered for diagnosing and treating presumed endometriosis in an adolescent. Laparoscopy can be safely performed in adolescents, but the benefits always should be considered relative to the risks of surgery. Gynecologic surgeons who perform laparoscopy in adolescents with pelvic pain should be familiar with the typical lesions of endometriosis in adolescents, which tend to be red, clear, or white, as opposed to the "powder-burn" lesions seen commonly in adults who have endometriosis.

All adolescents should be offered medical therapy after surgery until they have completed child-bearing to suppress pain and progression of disease. Treatment after surgery should involve the use of NSAIDs and menstrual suppression with continuous combined oral contraceptives, depot medroxyprogesterone acetate, or the levonorgestrel IUD. Gonadotropin-releasing hormone agonists are effective in the treatment of endometriosis-related pain in adolescents, but their use alone (without add-back therapy) is limited to 6 months because of adverse effects on bone mineral density. Because there are limited data on the long-term effects of GnRH agonists with add-back therapy, their use may be reserved for adolescents refractory to continuous combination hormonal therapy menstrual suppression. Long-term treatment should continue until desired family size is reached or fertility no longer needs to be preserved. For more information, please see the American College of Obstetricians and Gynecologists' resource *Guidelines for Adolescent Health Care.*

Bibliography

American College of Obstetricians and Gynecologists. Endometriosis in adolescents. Guidelines for adolescent health care [CD-ROM]. 2nd ed. Washington, DC: American College of Obstetricians and Gynecologists; 2011. p. 164–71.

Burney RO, Giudice LC. Pathogenesis and pathophysiology of endometriosis. Fertil Steril 2012;98:511–9.

Davis L, Kennedy SS, Moore J, Prentice A. Oral contraceptives for pain associated with endometriosis. Cochrane Database of Systematic Reviews 2007, Issue 3. Art. No.: CD001019. DOI: 10.1002/14651858.CD001019.pub2.

Elective and risk-reducing salpingo-oophorectomy. ACOG Practice Bulletin No. 89. American College of Obstetricians and Gynecologists. Obstet Gynecol 2008;111: 231–41.

Endometriosis and infertility: a committee opinion. Practice Committee of the American Society for Reproductive Medicine. Fertil Steril 2012;98:591–8.

Eskenazi B, Warner ML. Epidemiology of endometriosis. Obstet Gynecol Clin North Am 1997;24:235–58.

Goldstein DP, deCholnoky C, Emans SJ, Leventhal JM. Laparoscopy in the diagnosis and management of pelvic pain in adolescents. J Reprod Med 1980;24:251–6.

Hughes E, Brown J, Collins JJ, Farquhar C, Fedorkow DM, Vanderkerchove P. Ovulation suppression for endometriosis for women with subfertility. Cochrane Database of Systematic Reviews 2007, Issue 3. Art. No.: CD000155. DOI: 10.1002/14651858.CD000155.pub2.

Malinak LR, Buttram VC, Jr, Elias S, Simpson JL. Heritage aspects of endometriosis. II. Clinical characteristics of familial endometriosis. Am J Obstet Gynecol 1980;137:332–7.

Management of endometriosis. Practice bulletin No. 114. American College of Obstetricians and Gynecologists. Obstet Gynecol 2010;116:223–36.

Matalliotakis IM, Arici A, Cakmak H, Goumenou AG, Koumantakis G, Mahutte NG. Familial aggregation of endometriosis in the Yale Series. Arch Gynecol Obstet 2008;278:507–11.

Noncontraceptive uses of hormonal contraceptives. Practice Bulletin No. 110. American College of Obstetricians and Gynecologists. Obstet Gynecol 2010;115: 206–18.

Revised American Society for Reproductive Medicine classification of endometriosis: 1996. Fertil Steril 1997;67:817–21.

Treatment of pelvic pain associated with endometriosis. Practice Committee of American Society for Reproductive Medicine. Fertil Steril 2008;90:S260–9.

Resources

American College of Obstetricians and Gynecologists. Abnormal uterine bleeding. Patient Education Pamphlet AP095. Washington, DC: American College of Obstetricians and Gynecologists; 2012.

American College of Obstetricians and Gynecologists. Chronic pelvic pain. Patient Education Pamphlet AP099. Washington, DC: American College of Obstetricians and Gynecologists; 2010.

American College of Obstetricians and Gynecologists. Dysmenorrhea. Patient Education Pamphlet AP046. Washington, DC: American College of Obstetricians and Gynecologists; 2012.

American College of Obstetricians and Gynecologists. Endometriosis. Patient Education Pamphlet AP013. Washington, DC: American College of Obstetricians and Gynecologists; 2012.

American College of Obstetricians and Gynecologists. Evaluating infertility. Patient Education Pamphlet AP136. Washington, DC: American College of Obstetricians and Gynecologists; 2012.

American College of Obstetricians and Gynecologists. Treating infertility. Patient Education Pamphlet AP137. Washington, DC: American College of Obstetricians and Gynecologists; 2012.

American College of Obstetricians and Gynecologists. When sex is painful. Patient Education Pamphlet AP020. Washington, DC: American College of Obstetricians and Gynecologists; 2010.

American Society for Reproductive Medicine. Endometriosis. Available at: http://www.asrm.org/topics/detail.aspx?id=440. Retrieved July 31, 2013.

American Society for Reproductive Medicine. Endometriosis: a guide for patients. Birmingham (AL): ASRM; 2012. Available at: http://www.asrm.org/uploadedFiles/ASRM_Content/Resources/Patient_Resources/Fact_Sheets_and_Info_Booklets/endometriosis.pdf. Retrieved July 31, 2013.

Cochrane Collaboration. Cochrane reviews. Available at: http://www.cochrane.org/cochrane-reviews. Retrieved July 31, 2013.

LEIOMYOMAS

Uterine leiomyomas (commonly known as fibroids) are the most common solid pelvic tumors in women and the leading indication for hysterectomy. When including direct costs, lost work-hour costs, and costs related to obstetric complications, uterine leiomyomas are estimated to cost the United States $5.9–34.4 billion annually. Uterine leiomyomas are clinically apparent in 25–50% of women, although studies in which careful pathologic examination of the uterus is carried out suggest that the prevalence may be as high as 80%. These tumors originate from proliferation of a single myometrial cell and may be estrogen dependent. Factors responsible for the genesis of leiomyomas are unknown; family history, ethnicity, and diet may play a role.

Diagnosis

Leiomyomas are asymptomatic in most women and are an incidental finding on pelvic examination. Among women who seek treatment for their symptoms, abnormal genital bleeding and pelvic pressure are the most common. In affected women, not all abnormal bleeding is caused by the leiomyomas; therefore, other causes of abnormal bleeding in the presence of leiomyomas should be ruled out (see also the "Abnormal Genital Bleeding" section earlier in Part 4). A number of tests may be used to confirm the diagnosis, including ultrasonography, hysteroscopy, hysterosalpingography, sonohysterography, and laparoscopy. Imaging tests, such as magnetic resonance imaging and computed tomography, may be used but rarely are needed.

Management

Treatment options for leiomyomas should be based on the type and severity of symptoms, the size and location of the leiomyomas, and the patient's age and future reproductive plans. Uterine leiomyomas are usually benign and do not appear to have a malignant potential. As benign neoplasms, uterine leiomyomas usually require treatment only when they cause symptoms, lead to urinary obstruction, or appear to contribute to infertility. The clinical diagnosis of rapidly growing leiomyomas has not been shown to predict uterine sarcoma. Thus, it should not be used as the sole indication for myomectomy or hysterectomy.

Uterine size and symptoms may regress after menopause. Postmenopausal women with leiomyomas may have more bleeding problems, and some leiomyomas increase in size while hormone therapy is taken. However, there appears to be no reason to withhold this treatment from women who desire or need such therapy.

Medical Interventions

Medical therapies for leiomyomas include contraceptive steroids, gonadotropin-releasing hormone (GnRH) agonists, GnRH antagonists, aromatase inhibitors, and progesterone modulators.

Contraceptive Steroids

The use of hormonal contraceptive agents or hormone therapy (progestins alone or in combination with estrogen) may be useful for symptoms related to abnormal menstruation. However, treatment with contraceptive steroids tends to give only short-term relief, and the crossover rate to surgical therapies is high.

Gonadotropin-Releasing Hormone Agonists

Gonadotropin-releasing hormone agonists have been used to treat uterine leiomyomas. Their use preoperatively is beneficial, especially when improvement of hematologic status and reduction in size of the uterus are important goals. These agents usually are given 2–3 months preoperatively. Benefits of the use of GnRH agonists should be weighed against the cost and adverse effects for individual patients. Long-term use of these agents usually is not recommended. The use of steroid hormones as add-back therapy to attenuate bone loss has produced reasonable results and allowed longer treatment regimens. However, much of the reduction in uterine volume is regained by 24 months when add-back therapy is used (see also the "Endometriosis" section earlier in Part 4).

Gonadotropin-Releasing Hormone Antagonists

Although not approved by the U.S. Food and Drug Administration (FDA) for preoperative treatment of leiomyomas, GnRH antagonists have the advantage of not inducing an initial steroidal flare as seen with GnRH agonists. The rapid effect of the antagonist allows a shorter duration of adverse effects and quicker reduction in leiomyoma volume with presurgical treatment.

Aromatase Inhibitors and Progesterone Modulators

Aromatase inhibitors and progesterone modulators have been found to be beneficial in small studies and case reports, although they are not FDA approved for the treatment of leiomyomas. Overall, few data exist about the use of these medications to treat uterine leiomyomas, and further research is necessary to elucidate their clinical use.

SURGICAL INTERVENTIONS

Surgical options for treatment of leiomyomas include myomectomy, uterine artery embolization, endometrial ablation, magnetic resonance imaging-guided focused ultrasound surgery, and hysterectomy. Many women seek an alternative to hysterectomy for a variety of reasons, including a desire to preserve childbearing potential. As alternatives to hysterectomy become increasingly available, the efficacies of these treatments and their risks and potential problems become important considerations.

Myomectomy

Abdominal myomectomy is a safe and effective option for women who wish to retain their uterus. A woman who selects this option should be counseled preoperatively about the relatively high risk of reoperation. Laparoscopic myomectomy appears to be a safe and effective option for women with a small number of moderately-sized uterine leiomyomas. Hysteroscopic myomectomy is effective for controlling heavy menstrual bleeding in women with submucosal leiomyomas. The use of vasopressin at the time of myomectomy appears to limit blood loss.

Leiomyomas may be a factor in infertility for some patients and are present in as many as 5–10% of infertile couples. The issues are complex, and myomectomy should not be performed solely for an infertility indication without completion of a comprehensive fertility evaluation.

Uterine Artery Embolization

Uterine artery embolization for the treatment of patients with symptomatic uterine leiomyomas has become increasingly popular. Based on current evidence, it appears that uterine artery embolization, when performed by experienced physicians, provides good short-term relief of bulk-related symptoms and a reduction in menstrual flow. Compared with hysterectomy or myomectomy, uterine artery embolization offers a shorter hospital stay and a quicker return to routine activities. However, uterine artery embolization is associated with a higher rate of minor complications and an increased likelihood of required surgical intervention within 2–5 years of the initial procedure. Overall complication rates associated with the procedure are low, but in rare cases, complications can include hysterectomy and death. For women wishing to retain fertility, uterine artery embolization should be used with caution. Although successful pregnancies can occur after uterine artery embolization, there is concern regarding impairment of ovarian function and increased risk of pregnancy complications after uterine artery embolization. Women who wish to undergo uterine artery embolization should have a thorough evaluation with an obstetrician–gynecologist to help facilitate optimal collaboration with interventional radiologists and to ensure the appropriateness of this therapy.

Endometrial Ablation

Endometrial ablation appears to be effective in controlling heavy menstrual bleeding in women with submucosal leiomyomas measuring up to 3 cm in diameter. For women with larger submucosal leiomyomas and heavy menstrual bleeding, hysteroscopic resection can be combined with endometrial ablation.

Magnetic Resonance Imaging-Guided Focused Ultrasound Surgery

Magnetic resonance imaging-guided focused ultrasound surgery was approved by the FDA in 2004. It has been shown to be safe and moderately effective in short term-studies, but data on outcomes beyond 24 months are limited.

Hysterectomy

In women with symptomatic leiomyomas, hysterectomy provides a definitive cure. Approximately 600,000 hysterectomies are performed each year in the United States. The proportion of hysterectomies with an indication of uterine leiomyomas has decreased significantly from 44% in 2000 to 31% in 2008. Traditionally, most hysterectomies have been performed abdominally. However, vaginal hysterectomy is the preferred choice of approach when feasible given the lower costs and complication rate. The morbidity associated with abdominal hysterectomy includes infectious complications (10%); major injuries to the bowel, bladder, ovaries, or ureter (1%); and a postoperative recuperative time of 4–6 weeks. The supracervical abdominal technique of hysterectomy offers no clinical advantage with regard to surgical complications, urinary symptoms, or sexual function in women undergoing hysterectomy for symptomatic uterine leiomyomas or abnormal uterine bleeding. Laparoscopic or robot-assisted hysterectomy may be an alternative to abdominal hysterectomy for those patients in whom a vaginal hysterectomy is not indicated or feasible.

Bibliography

Alternatives to hysterectomy in the management of leiomyomas. ACOG Practice Bulletin No. 96. American College of Obstetricians and Gynecologists. Obstet Gynecol 2008;112:387–400.

Cardozo ER, Clark AD, Banks NK, Henne MB, Stegmann BJ, Segars JH. The estimated annual cost of uterine leiomyomata in the United States. Am J Obstet Gynecol 2012;206:211.e1–9.

Endometrial ablation. ACOG Practice Bulletin No. 81. American College of Obstetricians and Gynecologists. Obstet Gynecol 2007;109:1233–48.

Gupta JK, Sinha A, Lumsden MA, Hickey M. Uterine artery embolization for symptomatic uterine fibroids. Cochrane Database of Systematic Reviews 2012, Issue 5. Art. No.: CD005073. DOI: 10.1002/14651858.CD005073.pub3.

Myomas and reproductive function. Practice Committee of American Society for Reproductive Medicine in collaboration with Society of Reproductive Surgeons. Fertil Steril 2008;90:S125–30.

Sharp HT. Assessment of new technology in the treatment of idiopathic menorrhagia and uterine leiomyomata. Obstet Gynecol 2006;108:990–1003.

Supracervical hysterectomy. ACOG Committee Opinion No. 388. American College of Obstetricians and Gynecologists. Obstet Gynecol 2007;110:1215–7.

Resource

American College of Obstetricians and Gynecologists. Uterine fibroids. ACOG Patient Education Pamphlet AP074. Washington, DC: ACOG; 2009.

ACUTE AND CHRONIC PAIN MANAGEMENT

The heterogeneous patient population cared for by obstetricians and gynecologists results in a broad range of pain management challenges. The pain experienced by gynecologic patients ranges from acute pain, such as postoperative incisional pain, to chronic pain, such as chronic pelvic pain and pain experienced by many patients with cancer. Although the treatment of patients with acute postoperative pain is typically less challenging than the long-term management of chronic pain syndromes, studies have shown that even this acute pain often is not controlled optimally. Many patients respond adequately to the as-needed administration of an opioid, such as morphine or meperidine, whereas other patients require alternative medications, modification of the dosage, or different routes of administration to achieve optimal results. Studies have documented that 25–70% of general surgical patients have unrelieved postoperative pain. Surveys of patients with chronic cancer pain have documented that approximately two thirds of these patients also have acute pain transiently. It is clear that even though the treatments required to provide adequate relief of pain are widely available, they often are not used adequately. The fear of regulatory scrutiny is the most common reason physicians give for failing to provide adequate medication for chronic pain.

Pain Management Guidelines and Quality Indicators

One of the first quality improvement programs for pain management was developed by the American Pain Society in 1995. These quality improvement guidelines for the treatment of acute pain and cancer pain were refined and expanded in 2005 based on a systematic review of pain management quality improvement studies (Box 4-1). The emphasis has shifted from processes to outcomes.

Box 4-1. American Pain Society's Pain Management Guidelines and Quality Indicators

Guidelines

- Recognize and treat pain promptly
- Involve patients and families in pain management plan
- Improve treatment patterns
- Reassess and adjust pain management plan as needed
- Monitor processes and outcomes of pain management

Quality Indicators

Quality indicators focus on appropriate use of analgesics and outcomes:

- Intensity of pain is documented using a numeric (0–10) or descriptive (mild, moderate, severe) rating scale
- Pain intensity is documented at frequent intervals
- Pain is treated by route other than intramuscular
- Pain is treated with regularly administered analgesics, and when possible, multimodal approach. (Includes a combination of pain control strategies, such as opioids, nonsteroidal antiinflammatory drugs, and nonpharmacologic interventions.)
- Pain is prevented and controlled to a degree that facilitates function and quality of life
- Patients are adequately informed and knowledgeable about pain management

Data from Gordon DB, Dahl JL, Miaskowski C, McCarberg B, Todd KH, Paice JA, et al. American pain society recommendations for improving the quality of acute and cancer pain management: American Pain Society Quality of Care Task Force. Arch Intern Med 2005;165:1574–80 *and* Gordon DB, Pellino TA, Miaskowski C, McNeill JA, Paice JA, Laferriere D, et al. A 10-year review of quality improvement monitoring in pain management: recommendations for standardized outcome measures. Pain Manag Nurs 2002;3:116–30.

Many hospitals have established comprehensive pain services, which often are directed by anesthesiologists and provide expert assessment and multimodality therapy for patients with acute and chronic pain. They should be used especially for patients who have a history of difficult-to-manage pain in the perioperative setting or for patients who may have a neurologic component to their pain.

The Joint Commission provides standards on pain assessment and treatment for accredited ambulatory care facilities, behavioral health care organizations, critical access hospitals, home care providers, hospitals, office-based surgery practices, and long-term health care providers. These standards address the assessment and management of pain and require organizations to do the following:

- Recognize the rights of patients to appropriate assessment and management of pain.

- Screen patients for pain during their initial assessment and, when clinically required, during ongoing, periodic reassessments.

- Educate patients suffering from pain and their families about pain management.

Approaches to Pain Management

The ability to manage pain optimally requires comprehensive assessment of pain and information regarding temporal characteristics (stable versus constant course, severity, location, quality, provocative factors, and palliative factors). The clinician should be well versed in the various options for the management of pain. Whenever possible, therapy should be directed toward resolving the underlying condition.

Ideally, clinicians also should be familiar with the following approaches to pain management:

- Oral, intramuscular, and transdermal medications
  - Nonsteroidal antiinflammatory medications
  - Opioid medications

- Anesthesia administered
  — Nerve blocks
  — Continuous conduction anesthesia
- Neuromodulation
  — Transcutaneous electrical nerve stimulation
  — Acupuncture
  — Massage
- Mood modification
  — Aromatherapy
  — Imagery
- Neurosurgery

The use of pain scales (eg, rating pain from 0 to 10) may be helpful. Clinicians also should be aware of the option for patient-controlled analgesia.

In general, nonsteroidal antiinflammatory drugs are overused and provide minimal benefit to patients in severe acute and chronic pain, particularly patients experiencing pain secondary to metastatic cancer. Often these drugs are used instead of opioids with the concern that patients may become dependent. However, this class of medications generally does not control this pain, which can be severe, particularly at the end of life.

Guidelines for the treatment of patients with severe pain secondary to metastatic cancer suggest that long-acting opioids be administered around the clock and be supplemented with short-acting oral opioids for episodes of breakthrough pain. Opioid administration through oral, rectal, or transdermal routes can control 90% of cancer pain. Effective management requires recognition of drug pharmacokinetics and potential adverse effects that may be age-related.

Methods of neuromodulation, such as transcutaneous electrical nerve stimulation, acupuncture, and massage, are based on the gate theory of pain control. These treatments can be useful for pain control, particularly when the pain is severe. Imagery, aromatherapy, and other mood modifiers can provide an atmosphere of relaxation and comfort.

More invasive neurostimulation approaches to pain management may be used in patients with neuropathic pain that has been refractory to typical medical management. These approaches include peripheral nerve stimulation, nerve root stimulation, spinal cord stimulation, deep brain stimulation, and motor cortex stimulation. Use of these approaches has been validated for several conditions, including pelvic and perineal pain and chronic headache (peripheral nerve stimulation); pain secondary to brain lesions (deep brain stimulation); and chronic pain syndromes, such as failed back surgery syndrome (spinal cord stimulation). Consultation with pain management and neurosurgery specialists is imperative when considering these approaches.

Pain Management Legislation and Regulations

Clinicians should be familiar with any relevant pain treatment legislation adopted in their state. They also should be aware of requirements regarding the use of controlled substances. For example, under the Food and Drug Administration Amendments Act of 2007, the U.S. Food and Drug Administration (FDA) has the authority to require a manufacturer to develop a risk evaluation and mitigation strategy when further measures are needed to ensure that a drug's benefits outweigh its risks. The 2012 risk evaluation and mitigation strategy for extended-release and long-acting opioid analgesics requires extended-release and long-acting opioid analgesic companies to make available training on proper prescribing practices for health care providers who prescribe these analgesics and also to distribute educational materials to prescribers and patients on the safe use of these powerful pain medications. Health care providers should be aware of, and in compliance with, risk evaluation and mitigation strategy requirements. Current risk evaluation and mitigation strategy information is available from the FDA web site (see www.fda.gov/Drugs/DrugSafety/PostmarketDrugSafetyInformationforPatientsandProviders/ucm111350.htm?utm_campaign=Google2&utm_source=fdaSearch&utm_medium=website&utm_term=rems&utm_content=1). For more information on preventing prescription drug abuse, see the "Substance Use and Abuse" section in Part 3).

Bibliography

American Pain Society. Pain: current understanding of assessment, management, and treatments. Chicago (IL): APS; 2012. Available at: http://www.americanpain society.org/education/content/enduringmaterials.html. Retrieved July 31, 2013.

Current world literature. Curr Opin Anaesthesiol 2012;25:629–38.

Food and Drug Administration. Risk Evaluation and Mitigation Strategy (REMS) for extended-release and long-acting opioids. Available at: http://www.fda.gov/Drugs/ DrugSafety/InformationbyDrugClass/ucm163647.htm. Retrieved July 26, 2013.

Gordon DB, Dahl JL, Miaskowski C, McCarberg B, Todd KH, Paice JA, et al. American pain society recommendations for improving the quality of acute and cancer pain management: American Pain Society Quality of Care Task Force. Arch Intern Med 2005;165:1574–80.

Gordon DB, Pellino TA, Miaskowski C, McNeill JA, Paice JA, Laferriere D, et al. A 10-year review of quality improvement monitoring in pain management: recommendations for standardized outcome measures. Pain Manag Nurs 2002;3:116–30.

Optimizing the treatment of pain in patients with acute presentations. Policy statement. American Society for Pain Management Nursing (ASPMN), Emergency Nurses Association (ENA), American College of Emergency Physicians (ACEP), American Pain Society (APS). Ann Emerg Med 2010;56:77–9.

Quality improvement guidelines for the treatment of acute pain and cancer pain. American Pain Society Quality of Care Committee. JAMA 1995;274:1874–80.

The Joint Commission. Facts about pain management. Oakbrook Terrace (IL): Joint Commission; 2012. Available at: http://www.jointcommission.org/assets/1/18/ pain_management.pdf. Retrieved July 31, 2013.

Resources

Federation of State Medical Boards of the United States. Model policy for the use of controlled substances for the treatment of pain. Euless (TX): FSMB; 2004. Available at: http://www.fsmb.org/pdf/2004_grpol_Controlled_Substances.pdf. Retrieved July 31, 2013.

Food and Drug Administration. FDA blueprint for prescriber education for extended-release and long-acting opioid analgesics . Silver Spring (MD): FDA; 2013. Available at: http://www.fda.gov/downloads/Drugs/DrugSafety/InformationbyDrugClass/ UCM277916.pdf. Retrieved August 9, 2013.

Management of endometriosis. Practice Bulletin No. 114. American College of Obstetricians and Gynecologists. Obstet Gynecol 2010;116:223–36.

Martino AM. In search of a new ethic for treating patients with chronic pain: what can medical boards do? J Law Med Ethics 1998;26:332–49, 263.

National Cancer Institute. Pain (PDQ®). Bethesda (MD): NCI; 2013. Available at: http://www.cancer.gov/cancertopics/pdq/supportivecare/pain/HealthProfessional. Retrieved July 31, 2013.

National Vulvodynia Association. Vulvodynia treatment registry. Available at: http://www.nva.org/treatmentregistry.html. Retrieved August 9, 2013.

World Health Organization. WHO's pain ladder for adults. Available at: http://www.who.int/cancer/palliative/painladder/en. Retrieved August 9, 2013.

PREMENSTRUAL SYNDROME

Premenstrual syndrome (PMS) is the cyclic recurrence of symptoms that occur in the luteal phase of the menstrual cycle, are variable in intensity and effect on daily life, and cease shortly after the onset of menstruation. Emotional and physical changes occur premenstrually in up to 85% of women of reproductive age, although the vast majority of patients with these symptoms do not have PMS. It is estimated that 20–40% of these women regard their emotional and physical changes as difficult, and a smaller proportion report a significant effect on work, lifestyle, or relationships. Severe PMS that interferes with daily life affects approximately 3–5% of reproductive-aged women and is classified by the American Psychiatric Association's *Diagnostic and Statistical Manual of Mental Disorders* as premenstrual dysphoric disorder (PMDD) (see also "Premenstrual Dysphoric Disorder" later in this section).

The etiology of PMS remains ill defined. Levels of estrogen and progesterone are normal in women with PMS, although there may be an underlying neurobiologic vulnerability to normal fluctuations of one or more of these hormones. Stress does not appear to be a major risk factor for PMS.

Evaluation and Diagnosis

Diagnosis of PMS depends on the exclusion of other medical and psychiatric disorders and the demonstration, with a patient-completed prospective calendar, of true cyclicity of symptoms severe enough to impair the woman's life. The diagnostic criteria for PMS are outlined in Box 4-2. These symptoms should be documented prospectively in two or three calendar months.

Clinicians should be able to rule out disease processes and psychiatric problems through a careful history, physical examination, and laboratory testing as indicated. Laboratory testing is only rarely needed; for example, a thyroid function test might be ordered if hypothyroidism is suspected. Menstrual magnification or exacerbation of other medical or psychologic disorders (including migraines, asthma, depression, or an anxiety disorder) should be considered in the differential diagnosis and ruled out before PMS or PMDD is diagnosed.

Box 4-2. Diagnostic Criteria for Premenstrual Syndrome

Premenstrual syndrome can be diagnosed if the patient reports at least one of the following affective and somatic symptoms during the 5 days before menses in each of the three prior menstrual cycles:*

Affective

- Depression
- Angry outbursts
- Irritability
- Anxiety
- Confusion
- Social withdrawal

Somatic

- Breast tenderness or swelling
- Abdominal bloating
- Headache
- Joint or muscle pain
- Weight gain
- Swelling of extremities

---

*These symptoms are relieved within 4 days of the onset of menses, without recurrence until at least cycle day 13. The symptoms are present in the absence of any pharmacologic therapy, hormone ingestion, or drug or alcohol use. The symptoms occur reproducibly during two cycles of prospective recording. The patient exhibits identifiable dysfunction in social, academic, or work performance.

Modified with permission from Mortola JF, Girton L, Yen SS. Depressive episodes in premenstrual syndrome. Am J Obstet Gynecol 1989;161:1682–7.

Management

As an overall clinical approach, treatments should be used in increasing order of complexity. In most cases, therapy options should be considered in the following order:

Step 1. Supportive therapy, including a complex carbohydrate diet, aerobic exercise, nutrition supplements (eg, calcium), and spironolactone

Step 2. Administration of selective serotonin reuptake inhibitors; for women who do not respond, an anxiolytic agent can be considered to alleviate specific symptoms

Step 3. Hormonal ovulation suppression with oral contraceptives or gonadotropin-releasing hormone agonists

Lifestyle changes, including diet and aerobic exercise, should be recommended first. For additional supportive therapy, calcium supplements have been shown to be effective in the treatment of women with PMS. Magnesium, vitamin B_6, and vitamin E may have minimal effectiveness. The bulk of scientific evidence does not support the usefulness of natural progesterone or primrose oil in the treatment of patients with PMS. Spironolactone is the only diuretic that has been shown to be of benefit in PMS. Oral contraceptive pills that contain drospirenone, an analog of spironolactone, may help treat premenstrual symptoms, although studies have not conclusively demonstrated benefit over other oral contraceptive pills.

Drug therapy should be considered for women with severe symptoms or symptoms resistant to supportive interventions. Several available drugs have been found to be effective for PMS and can be prescribed. Selective serotonin reuptake inhibitors are the initial drugs of choice, and any of the following may be used:

- Fluoxetine (It usually is administered in the morning to reduce insomnia. This drug is the most studied of the selective serotonin reuptake inhibitors.)
- Sertraline
- Paroxetine

- Citalopram
- Other antidepressants
  — Clomipramine
  — Venlafaxine

Clinicians should follow adult dosage guidance and should be aware that because some of these medications are available as extended-release formulations, dose and frequency may vary. Although continuous administration and luteal-phase administration are effective, one meta-analysis found continuous administration to be slightly more effective. Likelihood of patient adherence, however, can help guide the regimen. Treatment with the anxiolytic alprazolam is effective in some patients who are not relieved by other interventions, but its adverse effects limit its use as first-line therapy.

Oral contraceptives may improve physical symptoms of PMS, but their effectiveness in relieving mood symptoms has not been as promising. Gonadotropin-releasing hormone agonists and surgical oophorectomy have been shown to be effective in treating women with PMS. However, the adverse effects of hypoestrogenism limit their usefulness in most patients.

Premenstrual Dysphoric Disorder

Premenstrual dysphoric disorder is defined by the American Psychiatric Association as the cyclic recurrence of severe, sometimes disabling changes in affect—such as mood lability, irritability, dysphoria, and anxiety—that occur in the luteal phase of a woman's menstrual cycle and subside around, or shortly after, the onset of menses. These symptoms may be accompanied by the common physical and behavioral symptoms of PMS (Box 4-2). The *Diagnostic and Statistical Manual of Mental Disorders*' diagnostic criteria for PMDD are shown in Box 4-3. Although many of the symptoms of PMS and PMDD may be similar, the primary distinction is that although the symptoms of PMS may be uncomfortable, the symptoms of PMDD are severe enough to interfere with a woman's ability to function, comparable with other mental disorders, such as a major depressive episode or generalized anxiety disorder. Treatments for PMDD may be similar to treatments for depression (see also the "Depression" section in Part 3).

Box 4-3. Diagnostic Criteria for Premenstrual Dysphoric Disorder

A. In the majority of menstrual cycles, at least five symptoms must be present in the final week before the onset of menses, start to improve within a few days after the onset of menses, and become minimal or absent in the week postmenses.

B. One (or more) of the following symptoms must be present:

 1. Marked affective lability (eg, mood swings; feeling suddenly sad or tearful or increased sensitivity to rejection).

 2. Marked irritability or anger or increased interpersonal conflicts.

 3. Marked depressed mood, feelings of hopelessness, or self-deprecating thoughts.

 4. Marked anxiety, tension, feelings of being keyed up, on edge, or both.

C. One (or more) of the following symptoms must additionally be present, to reach a totally of five symptoms when combined with symptoms from Criterion B above.

 1. Decreased interest in usual activities (eg, work, school, friends, hobbies).

 2. Subjective difficulty in concentration.

 3. Lethargy, easy fatigability, or marked lack of energy.

 4. Marked change in appetite, overeating, or specific food cravings.

 5. Hypersomnia or insomnia.

 6. A sense of being overwhelmed or out of control.

 7. Physical symptoms such as breast tenderness or swelling, joint or muscle pain, a sensation of "bloating," or weight gain.

Note: The symptoms in Criteria A–C must have been met for most menstrual cycles that occurred in the preceding year.

D. The symptoms are associated with clinically significant distress or interferences with work, school, usual social activities, or relationships with others (eg, avoidance of social activities; decreased productivity and efficiency at work, school, or home).

E. The disturbance is not merely an exacerbation of the symptoms of another disorder, such as major depressive disorder, panic disorder, persistent depressive disorder (dysthymia), or a personality disorder (although it may co-occur with any of these disorders).

(continued)

Box 4-3. Diagnostic Criteria for Premenstrual Dysphoric Disorder *(continued)*

F. Criteria A should be confirmed by prospective daily ratings during at least two symptomatic cycles. (Note: The diagnosis may be made provisionally prior to this confirmation.)

G. The symptoms are not attributable to the physiologic effects of a substance (eg, a drug of abuse, a medication, or other treatment) or another medical condition (eg, hyperthyroidism).

Bibliography

American Psychiatric Association. Diagnostic and statistical manual of mental disorders: DSM-5. 5th ed. Washington, DC: APA; 2013.

Jarvis CI, Lynch AM, Morin AK. Management strategies for premenstrual syndrome/premenstrual dysphoric disorder. Ann Pharmacother 2008;42:967–78.

Lopez LM, Kaptein AA, Helmerhorst FM. Oral contraceptives containing drospirenone for premenstrual syndrome. Cochrane Database of Systematic Reviews 2012, Issue 2. Art. No.: CD006586. DOI: 10.1002/14651858.CD006586.pub4.

Marjoribanks J, Brown J, O'Brien PMS, Wyatt K. Selective serotonin reuptake inhibitors for premenstrual syndrome. Cochrane Database of Systematic Reviews 2013, Issue 6. Art. No.: CD001396. DOI: 10.1002/14651858.CD001396.pub3.

Mortola JF, Girton L, Yen SS. Depressive episodes in premenstrual syndrome. Am J Obstet Gynecol 1989;161:1682–7.

Shah NR, Jones JB, Aperi J, Shemtov R, Karne A, Borenstein J. Selective serotonin reuptake inhibitors for premenstrual syndrome and premenstrual dysphoric disorder: a meta-analysis. Obstet Gynecol 2008;111:1175–82.

Yonkers KA, O'Brien PM, Eriksson E. Premenstrual syndrome. Lancet 2008;371: 1200–10.

Resources

American College of Obstetricians and Gynecologists. Premenstrual syndrome. Patient Education Pamphlet AP057. Washington, DC: American College of Obstetricians and Gynecologists; 2010.

Department of Health and Human Services, Office on Women's Health. Menstruation, menopause, and mental health. Available at: http://www.womenshealth.gov/mental-health/menstruation-menopause. Retrieved April 10, 2014.

Department of Health and Human Services, Office on Women's Health. Premenstrual syndrome (PMS) fact sheet. Available at: http://www.womenshealth.gov/publications/our-publications/fact-sheet/premenstrual-syndrome.html. Retrieved April 10, 2014.

VAGINITIS

Vaginitis is defined as the spectrum of conditions that cause vulvovaginal symptoms, such as itching, burning, irritation, and abnormal discharge. Vaginal symptoms are common in the general population and are one of the most frequent reasons for patient visits to obstetrician–gynecologists. The most common causes of vaginitis are bacterial vaginosis (22–50% of symptomatic women), vulvovaginal candidiasis (17–39%), and trichomoniasis (4–35%).* Vaginitis has a broad differential diagnosis, and successful treatment frequently rests on accurate diagnosis.

Evaluation of women with vaginitis should include a focused history about the entire spectrum of vaginal symptoms, including change in discharge, vaginal malodor, itching, irritation, burning, swelling, dyspareunia, and dysuria. Questions about the location of symptoms (the vulva, vagina, and anus), duration, relation to the menstrual cycle, response to prior treatment (including self-treatment and douching), and sexual history can yield important insights into the likely cause. Evaluation may be compromised by patient self-treatment with nonprescription medications. Because self-diagnosis of vaginitis is unreliable, clinical evaluation of women with vaginal symptoms should be encouraged, particularly for women who fail to respond to self-treatment with a nonprescription antifungal agent.

Because many patients with vaginitis have vulvar manifestations of disease, the physical examination should begin with a thorough evaluation of the vulva. During speculum examination, samples should be obtained for vaginal pH determination, an amine ("whiff") test, and saline (wet mount)

---

*The recommendations for the diagnosis and management of these vaginal infections that are provided in this section are based on the *2010 Sexually Transmitted Diseases Treatment Guidelines* from the Centers for Disease Control and Prevention. A revision of these guidelines was underway during the production of the fourth edition of *Guidelines for Women's Health Care*. For the most up-to-date guidance, please refer to www.cdc.gov/std/.

and 10% potassium hydroxide microscopy evaluation. The pH and amine testing can be performed either through direct measurement or by colorimetric testing. It is important that the swab for pH evaluation be obtained from the midportion of the vaginal side wall to avoid false elevations in pH results caused by cervical mucus, blood, semen, or other substances.

In selected patients, vaginal cultures or polymerase chain reaction tests for *Trichomonas* species or yeast are helpful. Vaginal Gram staining for Nugent scoring of the bacterial flora may help to identify patients with bacterial vaginosis. Other currently available ancillary tests for diagnosing vaginal infections include rapid tests for enzyme activity from bacterial vaginosis-associated organisms and for *Trichomonas vaginalis* antigen, along with point-of-care testing for DNA of *Gardnerella vaginalis*, *T vaginalis*, and *Candida* species. Depending on risk factors, DNA amplification tests can be obtained for *Neisseria gonorrhoeae* and *Chlamydia trachomatis*.

Bacterial Vaginosis

Bacterial vaginosis is a polymicrobial infection marked by a lack of hydrogen peroxide-producing lactobacilli and an overgrowth of facultative anaerobic organisms. Organisms that are found with greater frequency and numbers in women with bacterial vaginosis include *G vaginalis*, *Mycoplasma hominis*, *Bacteroides* species, *Peptostreptococcus* species, *Fusobacterium* species, *Prevotella* species, *Atopobium vaginae*, and other anaerobes. Because these organisms are part of the normal flora, the mere presence of them, especially of *G vaginalis*, on a culture does not mean that the patient has bacterial vaginosis.

Patients with bacterial vaginosis, when symptomatic, may report an abnormal vaginal discharge and a fishy odor, especially after sexual intercourse or completion of menses. A clinical diagnosis of bacterial vaginosis requires the presence of three of the four Amsel criteria:

1. Abnormal gray discharge

2. Vaginal pH higher than 4.5

3. A positive amine test result

4. Clue cells that compromise more than 20% of the epithelial cells

Because bacterial vaginosis is an overgrowth of facultative and obligate anaerobic bacteria derived from the patient's own endogenous vaginal flora, the intent of treatment is not to eradicate these bacteria but to reduce their numbers and allow for the lactobacilli to become dominant. Treatment for bacterial vaginosis before abortion or hysterectomy significantly decreases the risk of postoperative infectious complications. Preferred treatment includes oral or intravaginal metronidazole or intravaginal clindamycin. The recurrence rate is approximately 20–40% at 1 month.

Vulvovaginal Candidiasis

Physical manifestations of vulvovaginal candidiasis range from asymptomatic colonization to severe symptoms. Symptomatic women may report itching; burning; irritation; dyspareunia; burning with urination; and a whitish, thick discharge.

Multiple studies conclude that a reliable diagnosis cannot be made on the basis of history and physical examination alone. Diagnosis requires the presence of either of the following two criteria: 1) visualization of blastospores or pseudohyphae on saline or 10% potassium hydroxide microscopy or 2) a positive culture result in a symptomatic woman. The diagnosis can be classified further as uncomplicated or complicated vulvovaginal candidiasis (see Box 4-4). This classification system has treatment implications, because complicated vulvovaginal candidiasis is more likely to fail standard antifungal therapy.

UNCOMPLICATED VULVOVAGINAL CANDIDIASIS

Women with uncomplicated vulvovaginal candidiasis can be treated successfully with any of the prescription or over-the-counter options recommended by the Centers for Disease Control and Prevention (CDC). Preferred over-the-counter intravaginal preparations include butoconazole, clotrimazole, miconazole, and tioconazole. Recommended prescription treatments include the intravaginal agents butoconazole (single-dose preparation), nystatin, and terconazole and the oral agent fluconazole. Because all listed antifungal treatments seem to have comparable safety and efficacy, the choice of therapy should be individualized to the specific

---

Box 4-4. Classification of Vulvovaginal Candidiasis*

Uncomplicated (presence of any of the following):
    Sporadic or infrequent episodes
    Mild-to-moderate symptoms or findings
    Suspected *Candida albicans* infection
    Infection in nonimmunocompromised women
Complicated (presence of any of the following):
    Recurrent episodes (four or more per year)
    Severe symptoms or findings
    Non-*C albicans* infection
    Infection in women with uncontrolled diabetes, debilitation, or immunosuppression

---

*The following information is from the *2010 Sexually Transmitted Diseases Treatment Guidelines* from the Centers for Disease Control and Prevention. A revision of these guidelines was underway during the production of the fourth edition of *Guidelines for Women's Health Care*. For the most up-to-date guidance, please refer to www.cdc.gov/std/.

Modified from Workowski KA, Berman S. Sexually transmitted diseases treatment guidelines, 2010. Centers for Disease Control and Prevention [published erratum appears in MMWR Morb Mortal Wkly Rep 2011;60:18]. MMWR Recomm Rep 2010;59:1–110.

---

patient; factors such as cost, convenience, adherence, ease of use, history of response or adverse reactions to prior treatments, and patient preference all can be taken into consideration.

COMPLICATED VULVOVAGINAL CANDIDASIS

Patients with complicated vulvovaginal candidiasis require more aggressive therapy with extended use of fluconazole or a topical azole agent to achieve relief of symptoms. Women with recurrent vulvovaginitis may benefit from maintenance therapy with fluconazole. For patients who are unable or unwilling to take fluconazole, topical azole treatments used intermittently as a maintenance regimen can be considered.

Trichomoniasis

Vaginal trichomoniasis is a common sexually transmitted infection with an estimated annual incidence of 3.7 million cases in the United States. Symptomatic women with trichomoniasis may have an abnormal frothy gray or yellow–green discharge, itching, burning, or postcoital bleeding; some women are asymptomatic. The classic presentation of cervical petechiae ("strawberry cervix") occurs only in a minority of cases. Although many women with trichomoniasis have an elevated vaginal pH, diagnosis in clinical settings usually relies on visualization of motile trichomonads on saline microscopy. A wet mount has a sensitivity of 60–70% in diagnosing trichomoniasis and must be evaluated immediately for optimal results. Point-of-care diagnostics also are available to test for trichomoniasis, with results available in as little as 10 minutes. The CDC notes that these tests can be more sensitive than wet preparations but that false-positive results might occur, especially in populations of low prevalence. Polymerase chain reaction assays, similar to those used to detect gonorrhea and chlamydial infections, are available for use. Trichomonad culture is another sensitive and highly specific test that is available. The CDC recommends culturing vaginal secretions for T vaginalis when trichomoniasis is suspected but not confirmed by microscopy.

Although metronidazole has been the mainstay of treatment for uncomplicated trichomoniasis in the United States, tinidazole also has been approved for single-dose therapy. Both treatments seem to be equally effective. Trichomoniasis is almost always sexually transmitted. Male partners of women with trichomoniasis also should be treated. To prevent reinfection, women with trichomoniasis should avoid intercourse until they and their partners have received treatment.

Other Causes of Vaginal Symptoms

Although bacterial vaginosis, vulvovaginal candidiasis, and trichomoniasis are the predominant causes of vulvovaginal symptoms, other causes may include a broad range of conditions, such as vulvar diseases, atrophic vaginitis, foreign bodies, and rarer forms of vaginitis.

CONTACT OR IRRITANT VULVOVAGINITIS

If a patient reports pruritus and has a normal pH and negative potassium hydroxide microscopy test result and yeast vaginal culture findings, the diagnosis of contact or irritant vulvovaginitis should be considered. A wide variety of substances, from sweat to perfumes, may cause symptoms often mistaken for yeast infection before a thorough evaluation. Contact and irritant vulvovaginitis can be treated by eliminating the irritating substance (if it has been defined) and applying local topical steroid creams or ointments.

ATROPHIC VAGINITIS

Patients with atrophic vaginitis may have an abnormal vaginal discharge, dryness, itching, burning, or dyspareunia. Although more common in postmenopausal and perimenopausal women, atrophic vaginitis can occur in the setting of other hypoestrogenic states, such as lactation, treatment with gonadotropin-releasing hormone agonists, use of injectable depot medroxyprogesterone acetate, and, rarely, with oral contraceptives. Diagnosis can be made on the basis of an elevated vaginal pH and the presence of parabasal or intermediate cells on microscopy. An amine test result will be negative. Atrophic vaginitis is best treated with topical estrogen, but local water-based moisturizing preparations or systemic estrogen also can be used.

DESQUAMATIVE INFLAMMATORY VAGINITIS

Of the rarer forms of vaginitis, the best defined seems to be desquamative inflammatory vaginitis. Symptoms include burning, dyspareunia, and copious yellow or green discharge. Examination reveals a purulent discharge with varying amounts of vestibular and vaginal erythema. The vaginal pH is elevated, and the amine test result is negative. Microscopy reveals large amounts of polymorphonuclear cells and parabasal cells. This condition easily is mistaken for trichomoniasis; however, in cases of desquamative inflammatory vaginitis, no motile trichomonads are present, and cultures for T vaginalis are negative. Although no randomized, controlled studies have been performed, a 14-day course with a 2% clindamycin cream often achieves a cure. However, relapse after therapy is fairly common.

Bibliography

Centers for Disease Control and Prevention. Sexually transmitted disease surveillance 2011. Atlanta (GA): U.S. Department of Health and Human Services; 2012. Available at: http://www.cdc.gov/std/stats11/Surv2011.pdf. Retrieved September 18, 2013.

Vaginitis. ACOG Practice Bulletin No. 72. American College of Obstetricians and Gynecologists. Obstet Gynecol 2006;107:1195–206.

Workowski KA, Berman S. Sexually transmitted diseases treatment guidelines, 2010. Centers for Disease Control and Prevention [published erratum appears in MMWR Morb Mortal Wkly Rep 2011;60:18]. MMWR Recomm Rep 2010;59:1–110.

Resources

American College of Obstetricians and Gynecologists. Disorders of the vulva. Patient Education Pamphlet AP088. Washington, DC: American College of Obstetricians and Gynecologists; 2013.

American College of Obstetricians and Gynecologists. Vaginitis. Patient Education Pamphlet AP028. Washington, DC: American College of Obstetricians and Gynecologists; 2010.

Centers for Disease Control and Prevention. Bacterial vaginosis. CDC Fact Sheet. Available at: http://www.cdc.gov/std/bv/STDFact-Bacterial-Vaginosis.htm. Retrieved August 9, 2013.

Centers for Disease Control and Prevention. Genital/vulvovaginal candidiasis (VVC). Available at: http://www.cdc.gov/fungal/diseases/Candidiasis/genital/index.html. Retrieved August 9, 2013.

Centers for Disease Control and Prevention. Trichomoniasis. CDC Fact Sheet. Available at: http://www.cdc.gov/std/trichomonas/STDFact-Trichomoniasis.htm. Retrieved August 9, 2013.

CHRONIC GYNECOLOGIC PAIN

Many women experience vulvar or pelvic pain and discomfort that affect the quality of their lives. Vulvodynia, vaginismus, and chronic pelvic pain are common gynecologic pain disorders routinely encountered by obstetrician–gynecologists in their clinical practices.

Vulvodynia and Vaginismus

Vulvodynia is described by most patients as burning, stinging, irritation, or rawness of the vulva. It is a condition in which pain is present with a normal appearance of the vulva (other than erythema). Vaginismus is an involuntary spasm of the muscles surrounding the vagina; it sometimes coexists with vulvodynia, which compounds the problem. Symptoms of vulvovaginal disorders are common, often chronic, and can significantly interfere with women's sexual function and sense of well-being (see also the "Vulvar Skin Disorders" section later in Part 4).

CLASSIFICATION AND ETIOLOGY

The most recent terminology and classification of vulvar pain by the International Society for the Study of Vulvovaginal Disease defines vulvodynia as "vulvar discomfort, most often described as burning pain, occurring in the absence of relevant visible findings or a specific, clinically identifiable, neurologic disorder." Vulvodynia is not caused by infection (eg, candidiasis, human papillomavirus infection, or herpes), inflammation (caused by, for example, lichen planus or immunobullous disorder), neoplasia (eg, Paget disease or squamous cell carcinoma), or a neurologic disorder (eg, herpes neuralgia or spinal nerve compression). The classification of vulvodynia is based on the site of the pain, whether it is generalized or localized, and whether it is provoked, unprovoked, or mixed.

Several causes have been proposed for vulvodynia, including embryologic abnormalities, increased urinary oxalate levels, genetic or autoimmune factors, hormonal factors, inflammation, infection, and neuropathic changes. Most likely, there is no single cause. Because the etiology of vulvodynia is unknown, it is difficult to say whether localized vulvodynia (previously referred to as vestibulitis) and generalized vulvodynia are different manifestations of the same disease process. Distinguishing localized disease from generalized disease is fairly straightforward and is done by examination with a cotton swab, as described in "Evaluation and Diagnosis" in this section. Early classification to localized or generalized vulvodynia can facilitate more timely and appropriate treatment.

In vaginismus, the involuntary muscle spasm of the muscles surrounding the vagina may function to tighten the vaginal opening, making vaginal intercourse more difficult. Causes include past sexual trauma or abuse, psychologic factors, or a history of discomfort with sexual intercourse. Sometimes no cause can be found. The *Diagnostic and Statistical Manual of Mental Disorders*, Fifth Edition, defines genito-pelvic pain/penetration disorder as the persistent or recurrent presence of one or more of the following four symptoms for a minimum of 6 months, which causes significant distress in the individual: 1) difficulty having intercourse, 2) marked vulvovaginal or pelvic pain during intercourse or penetration attempts, 3) marked fear or anxiety about vulvovaginal or pelvic pain anticipating, during, or resulting from vaginal penetration, and 4) marked tensing or tightening of the pelvic floor muscles during attempted vaginal penetration (see also the "Sexual Function and Dysfunction" section later in Part 4).

Evaluation and Diagnosis

Vulvodynia is a diagnosis of exclusion—a pain syndrome with no other identified cause. A thorough history identifies the patient's duration of pain, prior treatments, allergies, medical and surgical history, and sexual history. Cotton swab testing (see Fig.4-3) is used to identify areas of localized pain and to classify the severity of the pain. A diagram of pain locations and rankings of pain severity may be helpful in assessing the pain over time and response to treatment. The vagina should be examined, and tests, including wet preparation, vaginal pH testing, and fungal culture, should be performed as indicated. Fungal culture may identify resistant

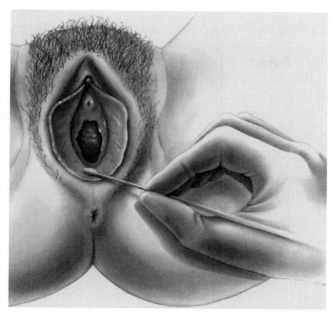

Fig. 4-3. Cotton swab testing. A cotton swab is used to test the vestibule for pain in diagnosing vestibulodynia. The vestibule is tested at the 2-, 4-, 6-, 8-, and 10-o'clock positions. When pain is present, the patient is asked to quantify it as mild, moderate, or severe. (Reprinted with permission from Haefner HK. Critique of new gynecologic surgical procedures: surgery for vulvar vestibulitis. Clin Obstet Gynecol 2000;43: 689–700.)

strains, but sensitivity testing generally is not required. Testing for human papillomavirus is unnecessary.

There are no definitive medical tests to diagnose vaginismus. As with vulvodynia, the diagnosis of vaginismus is made by exclusion of other causes. A thorough medical, social, and sexual history with complete physical examination, including a pelvic examination, are important to look for other causes of pain with sexual intercourse, such as dyspareunia.

Management

Many treatments have been used for patients with vulvodynia, including vulvar care measures (Box 4-5); topical, oral, and injectable medications;

Box 4-5. Vulvar Care Measures to Minimize Vulvar Irritation

- Wearing 100% cotton underwear (no underwear at night)
- Avoiding vulvar irritants (perfumes, dyes, shampoos, and detergents) and douching
- Using mild soaps for bathing, with none applied to the vulva
- Cleaning the vulva with water only
- Avoiding the use of hair dryers on the vulvar areas
- Patting the area dry after bathing and applying a preservative-free emollient (such as vegetable oil or plain petrolatum) topically to hold moisture in the skin and improve the barrier function
- Switching to 100% cotton menstrual pads (if regular pads are irritating)
- Using adequate lubrication for intercourse
- Applying cool gel packs to the vulvar area
- Rinsing and patting dry the vulva after urination

Data from Vulvodynia. ACOG Committee Opinion No. 345. American College of Obstetricians and Gynecologists. Obstet Gynecol 2006;108:1049–52.

biofeedback training; physical therapy; dietary modifications; cognitive behavioral therapy; sexual counseling; and surgery. Newer treatments include acupuncture, hypnotherapy, immunomodulation, neuromodulation, and botulinum toxin. Treatments for vaginismus include education, sex therapy, and specialized physical therapy (with or without vaginal dilators), in addition to the treatment of vulvodynia, if that also is present.

Vulvodynia and vaginismus can be difficult to treat, and rapid resolution is unusual, even with appropriate therapy. Decreases in pain may take weeks to months and may not be complete. No single treatment is successful in all women, and combinations of vulvar skin care and medical and behavioral therapies often are needed. Expectations for improvement need to be realistically addressed with the patient. Emotional and psychologic support is important for many patients, and sex therapy and counseling may be beneficial (see also the "Sexual Function and Dysfunction" section later in Part 4).

Chronic Pelvic Pain

Chronic pelvic pain is a common disorder of women that often presents a diagnostic dilemma for obstetrician–gynecologists, and requires a multidisciplinary approach to its evaluation, diagnosis, and treatment. There is no generally accepted definition of chronic pelvic pain. One proposed definition is noncyclic pain of 6 or more months' duration that localizes to the anatomic pelvis, the anterior abdominal wall at or below the umbilicus, the lumbosacral back, or the buttocks and is of sufficient severity to cause functional disability or lead to medical care.

A systematic, multisystem evaluation of potential sources is required, including the bladder, neurologic causes, psychologic causes, pain from birth trauma and pelvic surgery, as well as musculoskeletal and colorectal sources. Abuse is another important potential source to consider in women who present with chronic pelvic pain. Pelvic pain is highly associated with childhood or adult sexual abuse and intimate partner or domestic violence. Clinicians should screen for abuse and be familiar with any state requirements for reporting occurrences (see also the "Abuse" section in Part 3).

Chronic pelvic pain is frequently difficult to cure or manage adequately. A lack of physical examination findings does not negate the significance of a patient's pain, and normal examination results do not preclude the possibility of an abnormal pelvic condition. If a cause is found, management should be directed at treatment of the underlying condition causing the pain. Referral to an appropriate specialist should be provided if the source of the pain is found to be nongynecologic in nature. If no cause is identified, management should focus on pain relief (see also the "Acute and Chronic Pain Management" section earlier in Part 4).

Bibliography

American Psychiatric Association. Diagnostic and statistical manual of mental disorders: DSM-5. 5th ed. Washington, DC: APA; 2013.

Crowley T, Richardson D, Goldmeier D. Recommendations for the management of vaginismus: BASHH Special Interest Group for Sexual Dysfunction. Int J STD AIDS 2006;17:14–8.

Haefner HK, Collins ME, Davis GD, Edwards L, Foster DC, Hartmann ED, et al. The vulvodynia guideline. J Low Genit Tract Dis 2005;9:40–51.

Haefner HK. Critique of new gynecologic surgical procedures: surgery for vulvar vestibulitis. Clin Obstet Gynecol 2000;43:689–700.

Howard FM. Chronic pelvic pain. Obstet Gynecol 2003;101:594–611.

Lamont JA. Vaginismus. Am J Obstet Gynecol 1978;131:633–6.

National Library of Medicine. PubMed Health. Vaginismus. Available at: http://www.ncbi.nlm.nih.gov/pubmedhealth/PMH0002457. Retrieved August 9, 2013.

Nizard J, Raoul S, Nguyen JP, Lefaucheur JP. Invasive stimulation therapies for the treatment of refractory pain. Discov Med 2012;14:237–46.

Vulvodynia. ACOG Committee Opinion No. 345. American College of Obstetricians and Gynecologists. Obstet Gynecol 2006;108:1049–52.

Resources

American College of Obstetricians and Gynecologists. Chronic pelvic pain. Patient Education Pamphlet AP099. Washington, DC: American College of Obstetricians and Gynecologists; 2010.

American College of Obstetricians and Gynecologists. Vulvodynia. Patient Education Pamphlet AP127. Washington, DC: ACOG; 2014.

American College of Obstetricians and Gynecologists. When sex is painful. Patient Education Pamphlet AP020. Washington, DC: American College of Obstetricians and Gynecologists; 2010.

American Society for Colposcopy and Cervical Pathology. Vulvodynia: the basics. Frederick (MD): ASCCP; 2010. Available at: http://www.asccp.org/Portals/9/docs/pdfs/Practice%20Management/Vulvodynia%20Basics.pdf. Retrieved August 9, 2013.

Female sexual dysfunction. Practice Bulletin No. 119. American College of Obstetricians and Gynecologists. Obstet Gynecol 2011;117:996–1007.

National Vulvodynia Association. Available at: http://www.nva.org. Retrieved August 9, 2013.

VULVAR SKIN DISORDERS

In women who report symptoms of vulvar disorders, the most common diagnoses are dermatologic conditions and vulvodynia. Vulvar pruritus and vulvar pain may occur in the presence of obvious dermatologic disease or in conditions with few visible skin changes. Conditions commonly associated with vulvar pruritus are shown in Box 4-6. Vulvodynia, defined as burning, stinging, rawness, or soreness, with or without pruritus, can be further characterized by the site of the pain, whether it is generalized or localized, and whether it is provoked, spontaneous, or both. For a discussion of vulvodynia, see also the "Chronic Gynecologic Pain" section earlier in Part 4.

Evaluation

In evaluating vulvar pruritus, it can be helpful to group women into those conditions with acute symptoms and those with chronic symptoms (see Box 4-6). In cases of acute vulvar pruritus, common etiologies include vulvovaginal candidiasis and contact dermatitis. Chronic vulvar pruritus should prompt a search for underlying dermatoses, such as lichen sclerosus, lichen simplex chronicus, or psoriasis; neoplasia; or vulvar manifestations of systemic disease. Patients presenting with pain should first be evaluated to rule out underlying organic causes, including inflammatory conditions, neoplasia, infections, or neurologic disorders. When organic causes are ruled out, the diagnosis of vulvodynia can be made (see also "Chronic Gynecologic Pain" earlier in Part 4).

During evaluation, the medical history should include questions about the onset, duration, location, and nature of vulvar symptoms, as well as possible precipitating or known risk factors. The vulva and vagina should be carefully inspected as part of the pelvic examination. Microscopy of vaginal secretions, using saline and potassium hydroxide preparations in conjunction with vaginal pH determination, will help evaluate for infectious causes. Vaginal yeast cultures, culture for herpes simplex virus, and specific serologic tests may be necessary.

For autoimmune disorders, or in suspected cases of vulvar dermatoses (eg, lichen sclerosus and lichen planus) or neoplasia, a biopsy may be

---

Box 4-6. Conditions Commonly Associated With Vulvar Pruritus

Acute
- Infections
  - Fungal, including candidiasis and tinea cruris
  - Vulvovaginal candidiasis
  - Trichomoniasis
  - Molluscum contagiosum
  - Infestations, including scabies and pediculosis
- Contact dermatitis (allergic or irritant)

Chronic
- Dermatoses
  - Atopic and contact dermatitis
  - Lichen sclerosus, lichen planus, lichen simplex chronicus
  - Psoriasis
  - Genital atrophy
- Neoplasia
  - Vulvar intraepithelial neoplasia, vulvar cancer
  - Paget disease
- Infection
  - Vulvovaginal candidiasis, recurrent
  - Human papillomavirus infection
- Vulvar manifestations of systemic disease
  - Crohn disease

Modified from Diagnosis and management of vulvar skin disorders. ACOG Practice Bulletin No. 93. American College of Obstetricians and Gynecologists. Obstet Gynecol 2008;111:1243–53.

necessary for diagnosis. Findings, such as thickening, pebbling, hypopigmentation, or thinning of the epithelium, indicate a possible dermatologic process, and biopsy will aid in diagnosis and management. Biopsy of hyperpigmented or exophytic lesions, lesions with changes in vascular patterns, or unresolving lesions is particularly important and should be performed in order to rule out carcinoma. Diagnostic delays in identifying vulvar cancer are exceedingly common and have been linked to failures or procrastination in the performance of biopsies of abnormal-appearing vulvar skin.

Diagnosis and Management

Treatments of acute and chronic vulvar skin disorders are targeted toward the specific cause of the symptoms, based on history and physical examination, evaluation of vaginal secretions, cultures, and biopsy. Chronic or recurrent forms of vulvovaginal disease can be difficult to diagnose and treat.

VULVAR DERMATOSES

Lichen Sclerosus

A chronic disorder of the skin, lichen sclerosus is most commonly seen on the vulva, with extragenital lesions reported in up to 13% of women with vulvar disease. Patients presenting with lichen sclerosus most commonly report pruritus, followed by irritation, burning, dyspareunia, and tearing. On examination, typical lesions of lichen sclerosus are porcelain-white papules and plaques, often with areas of ecchymosis or purpura. The skin commonly appears thinned, whitened, and crinkling (leading to the description "cigarette paper"). Because other vulvar diseases can mimic lichen sclerosus, a biopsy is necessary to confirm the diagnosis, except in a prepubertal child.

Treatment for lichen sclerosus involves chronic treatment with a topical high-potency steroid, such as clobetasol propionate. A reasonable approach is to begin with once-daily application of ultrapotent topical steroids for 4 weeks, tapering to alternate days for 4 weeks, followed by 4 weeks of twice weekly application. Monitoring at 3 months and 6 months following initial therapy is recommended to assess the patient's response to therapy and to ensure proper application of the medication. Annual examinations are suggested for patients whose lichen sclerosus is well controlled, with more frequent visits for those with poorly controlled disease (for whom intralesional steroid injections also may be beneficial).

Lichen Planus

Lichen planus, an inflammatory disorder of the genital mucosa most likely related to cell-mediated immunity, exhibits a wide range of morphologies. The most common form and the most difficult to treat is the erosive form, which can lead to significant scarring and pain. The classic presentation of lichen planus on mucous membranes, including the buccal mucosa, is that of white, reticulate, lacy, or fernlike striae (Wickham striae). In erosive lichen planus, deep, painful, erythematous erosions appear in the posterior vestibule and often extend to the labia minora, which results in agglutination and resorption of the labial architecture. Symptoms commonly reported by patients with erosive vulvar lichen planus include dyspareunia, burning, and increased vaginal discharge.

Vulvovaginal lichen planus is a chronic, recurring disease that requires long-term maintenance. Although symptomatic improvement is possible, patients should be advised that complete control is not the norm. Treatment options include topical and systemic corticosteroids, topical and oral cyclosporine, topical tacrolimus, hydroxychloroquine, oral retinoids, methotrexate, azathioprine, and cyclophosphamide. In some cases, consultation with a dermatology colleague for long-term management may be appropriate.

SYMPTOMATIC VULVAR AND VAGINAL ATROPHY

It is estimated that up to 50% of all postmenopausal women experience vulvovaginal irritation, soreness, and dryness; lower urinary tract symptoms; recurrent cystitis; and dyspareunia. As women approach menopause, vulvar tissue becomes increasingly sensitive to irritants, and, in the absence of estrogen, the vaginal mucosa becomes pale, thin, and often dry. Vaginal pH becomes more alkaline and the vaginal flora is altered. Depending on symptomatology and after any indicated pathologic evaluation has been obtained, management options for urogenital atrophy in adult women include lifestyle modification strategies (eg, maintaining regular vaginal intercourse or masturbation), the use of vaginal moisturizers, and low-dose topical estradiol preparations. In 2013, a new oral medication, ospemifene, was approved by the U.S. Food and Drug Administration for the treatment of dyspareunia in postmenopausal women. Ospemifene is an estrogen agonist/antagonist that acts similarly to estrogen by increasing vaginal wall thickness, which results in a reduction in the amount of pain women experience with sexual intercourse.

VULVAR INTRAEPITHELIAL NEOPLASIA

Vulvar intraepithelial neoplasia (VIN) is an increasingly common problem, particularly among women in their 40s. The term VIN is used to denote high-grade squamous lesions and is subdivided into usual-type VIN (including warty, basaloid, and mixed VIN) and differentiated VIN. Usual-type VIN is commonly associated with carcinogenic genotypes of human papillomavirus (HPV) and other HPV persistence risk factors, such as cigarette smoking and immunocompromised status. Immunization with the quadrivalent HPV vaccine—which is effective against HPV genotypes 6, 11, 16, and 18—has been shown to decrease the risk of VIN and should be recommended for women in target populations (see also the "Immunizations" section in Part 3). Differentiated VIN usually is not associated with HPV and is more often associated with vulvar dermatologic conditions, such as lichen sclerosus.

Treatment is indicated for all cases of VIN. Wide local excision is recommended when cancer is suspected, despite a biopsy diagnosis of only VIN, to identify occult invasion. When occult invasion is not a concern, VIN can be treated with excision, laser ablation, or topical imiquimod (off-label use). Women with VIN should be considered at risk of recurrent VIN and vulvar cancer throughout their lifetimes. After resolution, women should be monitored at 6 months and 12 months and annually thereafter.

Bibliography

Diagnosis and management of vulvar skin disorders. ACOG Practice Bulletin No. 93. American College of Obstetricians and Gynecologists. Obstet Gynecol 2008;111:1243–53.

Food and Drug Administration. FDA approves Osphena for postmenopausal women experiencing pain during sex. Silver Spring (MD): FDA; 2013. Available at: http://www.fda.gov/newsevents/newsroom/pressannouncements/ucm341128.htm. Retrieved September 30, 2013.

Management of vulvar intraepithelial neoplasia. Committee Opinion No. 509. American College Obstetricians and Gynecologists. Obstet Gynecol 2011;118: 1192–4.

Resources

American College of Obstetricians and Gynecologists. Disorders of the vulva. Patient Education Pamphlet AP088. Washington, DC: American College of Obstetricians and Gynecologists; 2013.

British Association for Sexual Health and HIV. 2007 UK national guideline on the management of vulval conditions. Cheshire (UK): BASHH; 2007. Available at: http://www.bashh.org/documents/113/113.pdf. Retrieved August 9, 2013.

Rutanen EM, Heikkinen J, Halonen K, Komi J, Lammintausta R, Ylikorkala O. Effects of ospemifene, a novel SERM, on hormones, genital tract, climacteric symptoms, and quality of life in postmenopausal women: a double-blind, randomized trial. Menopause 2003;10:433–9.

ABNORMAL CERVICAL CYTOLOGY

Approximately 50 million cervical cytologic tests are performed in the United States each year. Of these tests, the findings of 3–10% will be reported as atypical squamous cells of undetermined significance, and another 2–5% will show evidence of more severe abnormalities (see also the "Cancer Screening and Prevention" section in Part 3).

Test Result Reporting

Effective cervical cancer prevention requires recognition and treatment of the precursors of invasive cancer and includes standardized terminology to report cervical cytologic and histologic test results. The 2001 Bethesda System of cervical cytologic test result reporting generally is accepted in the United States and describes the categories of epithelial cell abnormalities, including atypical squamous cells, atypical glandular cells, and low-grade squamous intraepithelial lesions or high-grade squamous intraepithelial lesions (HSIL) (see Box 4-7). Histologic diagnoses of cervical abnormalities are reported as cervical intraepithelial neoplasia (CIN) grades 1–3. However, in 2012, concerns about the diagnostic and management limitations of the CIN 2 categorization for lower anogenital human papillomavirus (HPV)-associated lesions led the College of American Pathologists and the American Society for Colposcopy and Cervical Pathology to adopt a unified histopathologic nomenclature with a single set of diagnostic terms for these lesions. The recommended terminology for HPV-associated squamous lesions of the lower anogenital tract is low-grade squamous intraepithelial lesions or HSIL, which may be further classified by the applicable –IN subcategorization. For example, cervical HSIL may be further qualified as (CIN 2) or (CIN 3). In addition, recommendations were made to describe the indications for the use of biomarkers to better define HPV-associated lesions of the lower anogenital tract and reduce interobserver variability in diagnosis.

Box 4-7. The 2001 Bethesda System for Reporting Cervical Cytology

Specimen Type
Indicate: conventional test (Pap test), liquid-based preparation, or other.

Specimen Adequacy
- Satisfactory for evaluation (describe presence/absence of endocervical/ transformation zone component and any other quality indicators, eg, partially obscuring blood, inflammation, etc.)
- Unsatisfactory for evaluation (specify reason)
  — Specimen rejected/not processed (specify reason)
  — Specimen processed and examined, but unsatisfactory for evaluation of epithelial abnormality because of (specify reason)

General Categorization (Optional)
- Negative for intraepithelial lesion or malignancy
- Other: see "Interpretation/Result" (eg, endometrial cells in a woman aged 40 years or older)
- Epithelial cell abnormality: See "Interpretation/Result" (specify "squamous" or "glandular" as appropriate)

Interpretation/Result
- Negative for intraepithelial lesion or malignancy (when there is no cellular evidence of neoplasia, state this in the "General Categorization" above, in the "Interpretation/Result" section of the report, or both, whether or not there are organisms or other nonneoplastic findings)
  — Organisms
    Trichomonas vaginalis
    Fungal organisms morphologically consistent with *Candida* species
    Shift in flora suggestive of bacterial vaginosis
    Bacteria morphologically consistent with *Actinomyces* species
    Cellular changes consistent with herpes simplex virus

(continued)

Box 4-7. The 2001 Bethesda System for Reporting Cervical Cytology *(continued)*

Interpretation/Result *(continued)*
— Other nonneoplastic findings (optional to report; list not inclusive)
  Reactive cellular changes associated with
    Inflammation (includes typical repair)
    Radiation
    Intrauterine device
  Glandular cells status posthysterectomy
  Atrophy
• Other (list not comprehensive)
  — Endometrial cells (in a woman aged 40 years or older) (specify if negative for squamous intraepithelial lesion)
• Epithelial cell abnormalities
  — Squamous cell
    Atypical squamous cells (ASC)
      Of undetermined significance (ASC-US)
      Cannot exclude HSIL (ASC-H)
    Low-grade squamous intraepithelial lesion (LSIL) (encompassing: human papillomavirus/mild dysplasia/cervical intraepithelial neoplasia (CIN) 1
    High-grade squamous intraepithelial lesion (HSIL) (encompassing: moderate and severe dysplasia, carcinoma in situ; CIN 2 and CIN 3)
    With features suspicious for invasion (if invasion is suspected)
    Squamous cell carcinoma
  — Glandular cell
    Atypical
      Endocervical cells (not otherwise specified or specify in comments)
      Endometrial cells (not otherwise specified or specify in comments)
      Glandular cells (not otherwise specified or specify in comments)

(continued)

Box 4-7. The 2001 Bethesda System for Reporting Cervical Cytology *(continued)*

Interpretation/Result *(continued)*
- Epithelial cell abnormalities *(continued)*
    - Atypical
        - Endocervical cells, favor neoplastic
        - Glandular cells, favor neoplastic
    - Endocervical adenocarcinoma in situ (AIS)
    - Adenocarcinoma
        - Endocervical
        - Endometrial
        - Extrauterine
        - Not otherwise specified
- Other malignant neoplasms (specify)

Ancillary Testing
Provide a brief description of the test method(s) and report the result so that it is easily understood by the clinician.

Automated Review
If case examined by automated device, specify device and result.

Educational Notes and Suggestions (Optional)
Suggestions should be concise and consistent with clinical follow-up guidelines published by professional organizations (references to relevant publications may be included).

Reprinted from Solomon D, Nayar R, editors. The Bethesda system for reporting cervical cytology : Definitions, criteria, and explanatory notes. 2nd ed. New York (NY): Springer; 2004, with kind permission of Springer Science+Media.

Evaluation and Management of Screening Results

Visual inspection of the vagina and cervix and a bimanual examination should follow a cytology report of abnormal findings. The first objective is to exclude the presence of invasive carcinoma. Once this has been accomplished, the objectives are to determine the grade and distribution of the intraepithelial lesion. Options for evaluation include repeat cytology, HPV DNA testing, colposcopy with directed biopsies, and endocervical assessment (see Table 4-3).

The expertise required to evaluate and manage patients with abnormal cytologic findings includes a thorough knowledge of the significance and natural history of cervical preinvasive disease. Additionally, the person responsible for evaluating the abnormal test result should be appropriately trained and experienced in colposcopy and aware of the various treatment options available for managing cervicovaginal abnormalities. Access to an appropriate cytologic and histopathologic laboratory is required. The following equipment may be needed for evaluation of the patient with an abnormal test result:

- Colposcope
- Acetic acid solution, 3–5%
- Hemostatic solution, such as Monsel's solution
- Instruments for the following:
  — Cervical biopsy
  — Endocervical sampling
- Appropriate fixative solution

The Clinical Laboratory Improvement Amendments have established requirements for the review of abnormal cervical cytology and follow-up of tests of identified high-risk patients (see also the "Compliance With Government Regulations" in Part 1, and Appendix E). In addition, clinicians should be familiar with any state requirements in this area.

In 2012, the American Society for Colposcopy and Cervical Pathology convened a consensus conference to update its recommendations on the appropriate management of women with cervical cytologic or histologic abnormalities (see Bibliography). These guidelines define when to return

Table 4-3. Management of Cervical Cancer Screening Results

Screening Method	Result	Management
Cytology screening alone	Cytology negative or ASC-US cytology and HPV negative	Screen again in 3 years
	All others	Refer to ASCCP guidelines*
Co-testing	Cytology negative, HPV negative	Screen again in 5 years
	ASC-US cytology and HPV negative	Refer to ASCCP guidelines*
	Cytology negative and HPV positive	Option 1: 12-month follow-up with co-testing
		Option 2: Test for HPV-16 or HPV-16/18 genotypes
		• If positive results from test for HPV-16 or HPV-16/18, referral for colposcopy
		• If negative results from test for HPV-16 or HPV-16/18, 12-month follow-up with co-testing
	All others	Refer to ASCCP guidelines*

Abbreviations: ASC-US, atypical squamous cells of undetermined significance; ASCCP, American Society for Colposcopy and Cervical Pathology; HPV, human papillomavirus.

* Massad LS, Einstein MH, Huh WK, Katki HA, Kinney WK, Schiffman M, et al. 2012 updated consensus guidelines for the management of abnormal cervical cancer screening tests and cancer precursors. 2012 ASCCP Consensus Guidelines Conference; Obstet Gynecol 2013;121:829–46.

Modified with permission from Saslow D, Solomon D, Lawson HW, Killackey M, Kulasingam SL, Cain J, et al. American Cancer Society, American Society for Colposcopy and Cervical Pathology, and American Society for Clinical Pathology screening guidelines for the prevention and early detection of cervical cancer. ACS-ASCCP-ASCP Cervical Cancer Guideline Committee. CA Cancer J Clin 2012;62:147–72.

to routine screening after treatment or resolution of abnormalities, given longer screening intervals than in the past; explain how to incorporate HPV testing; apply guidelines previously developed for adolescents to women aged 21–24 years; and integrate new data on risk of high-grade precursor lesions and cancer. A summary of these guidelines, including practice algorithms, is provided in the American College of Obstetricians and Gynecologists' Practice Bulletin No. 140 (see Bibliography).

Bibliography

Darragh TM, Colgan TJ, Cox JT, Heller DS, Henry MR, Luff RD, et al. The Lower Anogenital Squamous Terminology Standardization Project for HPV-Associated Lesions: background and consensus recommendations from the College of American Pathologists and the American Society for Colposcopy and Cervical Pathology. Members of LAST Project Work Groups [published erratum appears in J Low Genit Tract Dis 2013;17:368]. J Low Genit Tract Dis 2012;16:205–42.

Management of abnormal cervical cancer screening test results and cervical cancer precursors. Practice Bulletin No. 140. American College of Obstetricians and Gynecologists. Obstet Gynecol 2013;122: 1338–67.

Massad LS, Einstein MH, Huh WK, Katki HA, Kinney WK, Schiffman M, et al. 2012 updated consensus guidelines for the management of abnormal cervical cancer screening tests and cancer precursors. 2012 ASCCP Consensus Guidelines Conference; Obstet Gynecol 2013;121:829–46.

Saslow D, Solomon D, Lawson HW, Killackey M, Kulasingam SL, Cain J, et al. American Cancer Society, American Society for Colposcopy and Cervical Pathology, and American Society for Clinical Pathology screening guidelines for the prevention and early detection of cervical cancer. ACS-ASCCP-ASCP Cervical Cancer Guideline Committee. CA Cancer J Clin 2012;62:147–72.

Schiffman M, Wentzensen N. From human papillomavirus to cervical cancer. Obstet Gynecol 2010;116:177–85.

Screening for cervical cancer. Practice Bulletin No. 131. American College of Obstetricians and Gynecologists. Obstet Gynecol 2012;120:1222–38.

Solomon D, Nayar R, editors. The Bethesda system for reporting cervical cytology : Definitions, criteria, and explanatory notes. 2nd ed. New York (NY): Springer; 2004.

Resources

American College of Obstetricians and Gynecologists. Cervical cancer screening. Patient Education Pamphlet AP085. Washington, DC: American College of Obstetricians and Gynecologists; 2013.

American College of Obstetricians and Gynecologists. Colposcopy. Patient Education Pamphlet AP135. Washington, DC: American College of Obstetricians and Gynecologists; 2013.

American College of Obstetricians and Gynecologists. Understanding abnormal pap test results. ACOG Patient Education Pamphlet AP161. Washington, DC: American College of Obstetricians and Gynecologists; 2009.

American Society for Colposcopy and Cervical Pathology. Available at: http://www.asccp.org. Retrieved September 18, 2013.

CANCER DIAGNOSIS AND MANAGEMENT

Obstetrician–gynecologists play an important role in the identification and management of many forms of cancer that affect women, including cancer of the breast, cervix, vagina, endometrium, ovary, and vulva, in addition to gestational trophoblastic disease. Management typically includes the administration and interpretation of screening and diagnostic tests (see also the "Cancer Screening and Prevention" section in Part 3); initiation of prevention strategies; surveillance of at-risk patients; consultation with, and referral to, specialists as needed; and patient monitoring after treatment. In addition, it is important for women's health care providers to have an understanding of the effect of cancer treatments on common women's health issues, such as fertility, contraceptive management, sexual function, menopause, and osteoporosis, so that they can offer patients appropriate counseling and treatment.

Breast Cancer

In the United States, breast cancer is the most common cancer in women, with more than 232,000 new cases and approximately 40,000 deaths estimated in 2014. Breast cancer is the leading cause of death from cancer in women aged 20–59 years and is the second leading cause of cancer deaths overall, after lung cancer. The lifetime risk of developing breast cancer is approximately one in eight. The most common risk factors for developing breast cancer include advancing age and being female. Other risk factors include a personal or family history of breast cancer, nulliparity, early menarche, and late menopause. Mammography is the most effective method currently available for screening patients and reducing mortality (see also the "Cancer Screening and Prevention" section in Part 3).

EVALUATION AND DIAGNOSIS

Timely follow-up for an abnormal screening mammogram can optimize the diagnosis in, and treatment of, women with abnormal test results. Moreover, it is encouraged on an ethical basis and is consistent with the role of physicians as patient advocates.

The clinician should be able to elicit an accurate history and document risk factors that might increase the patient's risk of developing breast cancer, as well as perform a thorough and accurate clinical breast examination (see also the "Well-Woman Annual Health Assessment" section in Part 3). Based on personal as well as family history, women may be eligible for testing for *BRCA* gene mutations or for referral to a genetic counselor for further evaluation and consideration of testing.

Clinicians with the knowledge and experience to perform cyst aspiration and biopsy, when necessary, can facilitate their patients' prompt treatment. If a clinician is unable to provide this service, referral to a breast specialist or another clinician with this expertise is appropriate whenever an abnormality is noted on a mammogram or a mass is palpated on physical examination.

MANAGEMENT

The clinician should be familiar with the options for treating women with early and advanced breast cancer and should facilitate referrals for this treatment. The clinician also should be knowledgeable regarding the effect of breast cancer treatments and their potential gynecologic adverse effects.

Treatment options for breast cancer include chemotherapy, surgery, radiation therapy, and hormonal therapies. Typically, chemotherapy for breast cancer involves a combination of cytotoxic and biologic agents, which likely accounts for most of the ovarian toxicity and the adverse effects on ovarian function. Breast surgery involves either lumpectomy or mastectomy, with or without immediate or delayed reconstructive procedures. Some high-risk women undergoing breast cancer surgery may need, or choose, to have associated gynecologic surgery, including bilateral salpingo-oophorectomy, hysterectomy, or both to decrease their risk of other types of cancer. Radiation to the breast often is given after breast-conserving surgery to decrease the chance of recurrence or of metastasis to nearby lymph nodes. Radiation therapy also may be recommended after mastectomy or when cancer has metastasized to the lymph nodes, bones, or brain. Ovarian suppression with the use of gonadotropin-releasing hormone agonist or gonadotropin-releasing hormone antagonist therapy also can be used as part of breast cancer treatment in premenopausal women with hormone-receptor–positive (estrogen-receptor or progesterone-receptor) breast cancer and decreases the risk of recurrence.

Hormonal therapy for the treatment of hormone-responsive breast cancer includes aromatase inhibitors and estrogen agonists/antagonists (also known as selective estrogen receptor modulators), such as tamoxifen. Recent evidence supports a benefit for tamoxifen with use up to 10 years. In standard dosages, tamoxifen may be associated with endometrial proliferation, hyperplasia, polyp formation, invasive carcinoma, and uterine sarcoma. Postmenopausal women who take tamoxifen should be monitored closely for symptoms of endometrial hyperplasia or cancer and should have a gynecologic examination at least once every year. Premenopausal women treated with tamoxifen have no known increased risk of uterine cancer and as such require no additional monitoring beyond routine gynecologic care. Patients should be encouraged to report promptly any abnormal vaginal symptoms, including bloody discharge, spotting, or staining, and these symptoms should be investigated. Screening tests have not been effective in increasing the early detection of endometrial cancer in women who use tamoxifen and may lead to more invasive and costly diagnostic procedures; these tests are therefore not recommended. If atypical endometrial hyperplasia develops, appropriate gynecologic management should be instituted, and the use of tamoxifen should be reassessed. If tamoxifen therapy must be continued, hysterectomy should be considered in women with atypical endometrial hyperplasia. Tamoxifen use may be reinstituted after hysterectomy for endometrial carcinoma in consultation with the physician responsible for the woman's breast care.

Osteoporosis

Bone health may be adversely affected by many of the cancer treatment modalities, including chemotherapy, ovarian suppression, and aromatase inhibitors, which all result in lower estrogen levels, more bone loss, and increased risk of fracture. Bone loss is most rapid in premenopausal women undergoing ovarian suppression and taking aromatase inhibitors. Osteoporosis risk assessment in patients with breast cancer should include an assessment of clinical risk factors and bone mineral density testing and monitoring. The American Society of Clinical Oncology recommends bone mineral density monitoring by dual energy X-ray absorptiometry to assess and manage bone loss in patients with breast cancer at high risk of osteoporosis. First-line pharmacologic options approved by the U.S. Food and Drug Administration for the prevention and treatment of osteoporosis include bisphosphonates and raloxifene. Women also should be counseled about lifestyle changes to reduce the risk of bone loss and osteoporotic fractures, such as weight-bearing and muscle-strengthening exercises to reduce the risk of fractures and falls, other fall-prevention strategies, increasing vitamin D and calcium intake, cessation of smoking, and reducing alcohol intake (see also "Osteoporosis" in Part 3).

Menopause

Menopausal symptoms are common among patients with breast cancer, either as a result of temporary or permanent anovulation, ovarian suppression from chemotherapy, or as an adverse effect from hormonal therapies, such as tamoxifen. One of the most bothersome adverse effects is hot flushes. Systemic hormone therapy, based on studies to date, is not generally recommended in breast cancer survivors. Management of menopausal symptoms can be accomplished through nonhormonal options, including pharmacologic agents and lifestyle alterations. Selective serotonin reuptake inhibitors (SSRIs) (eg, citalopram or fluoxetine) and serotonin-norepinephrine reuptake inhibitors (eg, venlafaxine) have been shown to be safe and to reduce the severity of hot flushes in patients with breast cancer. In patients using tamoxifen, serotonin-norepinephrine reuptake inhibitors generally are preferable to SSRIs because of concerns that SSRIs may interfere with tamoxifen metabolism and thus block the drug's therapeutic benefit. Other options for management of vasomotor symptoms in breast cancer survivors who cannot use estrogens or progestins include gabapentin and clonidine. Common sense lifestyle solutions, such as layering of clothing, maintaining a lower ambient temperature, and consuming cool drinks, also are reasonable measures for the management of vasomotor symptoms. Lifestyle and behavioral changes to reduce vasomotor symptoms include paced-breathing, relaxation techniques, environmental modifications, and dietary changes. Although many patients with breast cancer also look to complementary and alternative modalities, such as acupuncture, phytoestrogens, and herbal supplements, data do not support their efficacy for the treatment of vasomotor symptoms (see also the "Complementary and Alternative Medicine" section and the "Menopause" section in Part 3).

Vaginal Dryness and Atrophy

Vaginal dryness and atrophy are common gynecologic issues in patients with breast cancer. For atrophic vaginitis in women with a history of hormone-sensitive breast cancer, nonhormonal methods should be considered first-line treatment. Nonhormonal options found to be effective and safe in breast cancer survivors include vaginal moisturizers and vaginal lubricants. Short-term use of hormonal methods may be considered for women with severe or refractory symptoms in whom other options have failed, following appropriate counseling with their oncologists about the potential risks. Although data regarding the safety of topical estrogen in breast cancer survivors are limited, small retrospective trials support the safety of topical estrogen products in this population. Low-dose, 10-microgram estradiol-17β vaginal tablets or the low-dose vaginal estradiol ring, compared with oral estradiol or estradiol vaginal cream, results in the lowest systemic absorption.

Contraception

Contraceptive options for patients with breast cancer include barrier methods, such as condoms and diaphragms, the copper intrauterine device, and sterilization. The U.S. Medical Eligibility Criteria for Contraceptive Use (U.S. MEC) published by the Centers for Disease Control and Prevention provides guidance on the safety of contraceptive method use for women with specific characteristics and medical conditions. For women who currently have breast cancer, all hormonal methods of contraception have a

U.S. MEC 4 rating and are contraindicated. For women with a history of breast cancer who have not had disease recurrence for 5 or more years, hormonal contraceptive methods have a U.S. MEC 3 rating, indicating that "the theoretical or proven risks usually outweigh the advantages" (see also the "Family Planning" section in Part 3).

SEXUAL FUNCTION

Breast surgery can have complex effects on sexual function that relate to perception of body image changes, attitudes before diagnosis of cancer, loss of sensation in breasts, sexual desire and ability to achieve orgasm, and feelings of loss of femininity and stability of a partnered relationship. Research also has consistently shown that patients with breast cancer who undergo chemotherapy are at higher risk of sexual dysfunction. For women who experience chemotherapy-induced menopause, vaginal dryness and sexual pain frequently are associated with sexual dissatisfaction. Despite the adverse effects of breast surgery and chemotherapy on sexual function, the most consistent predictor of satisfying sexual experiences in women with breast cancer is the quality of their relationship (see also the "Sexual Function and Dysfunction" section later in Part 4).

Fertility

Breast cancer treatments affect fertility primarily by the negative effect of chemotherapy on ovarian function. Most women who resume ovarian function experience a return of menses within 1 year of completing chemotherapy, although menstrual irregularities are common, and women are still at risk of premature menopause. Depending on a woman's age at diagnosis, a 5-year or more delay in fertility attempts may diminish ovarian reserve.

When breast cancer is diagnosed in a premenopausal woman, it is important to discuss her fertility concerns. Pregnancy after breast cancer is not thought to increase breast cancer recurrence. If future pregnancy is desired, appropriate consultation with fertility specialists should be offered (see also "Fertility Preservation" later in this section and the "Infertility" section later in Part 4).

Cervical and Vaginal Cancer

Despite the fact that use of the Pap test has been associated with a 70% decrease in deaths from cervical cancer during the past 50 years, many women still die from the disease, with an estimated 12,360 new cases of invasive cervical cancer and 4,020 deaths in the United States in 2014. Although the median age for the occurrence of invasive carcinoma has remained constant at 44–50 years, this malignancy is diagnosed in women of all ages. It has now been established that human papillomavirus is a major contributor to cervical malignancy. Although most women with human papillomavirus never will develop this cancer, 95% of cervical malignancies have been associated with it.

Most cases of serious disease are seen in women who have not had regular cervical cytology screening. Elderly women who have never been screened and older women who do not receive regular cervical cytology screening as recommended continue to be at high risk of developing this malignancy. Recommendations for cervical cytology screening and the management of abnormal cytology are outlined in Part 3 in the "Cancer Screening and Prevention" section and in Part 4 in the "Abnormal Cervical Cytology" section.

Primary vaginal cancer, which is the rarest of gynecologic malignancies, generally behaves and is diagnosed similarly to cervical cancer. Most of these lesions occur in postmenopausal women. Although preinvasive lesions of the vagina (vaginal intraepithelial neoplasia) sometimes can be detected by cytology tests in a manner identical to that for detecting cervical cancer, the Pap test is not a reliable means of routine screening for vaginal cancer. The American Cancer Society, the American Society for Colposcopy and Cervical Pathology, and the American Society for Clinical Pathology advise that women who have had a hysterectomy and have no history of cervical intraepithelial neoplasia grade 2 or higher are at very low risk of developing vaginal cancer and should not have vaginal cytology examinations. Continued vaginal cytology examinations in this population of women are not effective, particularly because of the very low risk of developing vaginal cancer, and will cause inconvenience, anxiety, and overtreatment. Women who had high-grade cervical intraepithelial lesions before hysterectomy can develop recurrent intraepithelial neoplasia or carcinoma at the vaginal cuff years after the procedure and should continue to follow age-appropriate cytology screening recommendations (see also the "Cancer Screening and Prevention" section in Part 3).

EVALUATION AND DIAGNOSIS

It is recommended that the staging system of the International Federation of Gynecology and Obstetrics (FIGO) be used. Staging of invasive cervical cancer with the FIGO system is achieved by clinical evaluation. Careful clinical examination should be performed by experienced examiners on all patients and may be performed with the patient under anesthesia. Although not required as part of FIGO staging procedures, various radiologic tests frequently are undertaken to help define the extent of tumor growth and guide therapy decisions, especially in patients with locally advanced disease.

MANAGEMENT

Very early invasive cancer usually is managed by surgery alone. Early carcinomas of the cervix usually can be managed by surgical techniques or radiation therapy. More advanced carcinomas require primary treatment with radiation therapy plus chemotherapy administered in small doses as a radiation sensitizer. After treatment for cervical carcinoma, patients should be monitored regularly (for example, with thrice-yearly follow-up examinations for the first 2 years and twice-yearly visits subsequently to year 5, with cervical cytology annually).

The clinician should be familiar with the options for treating women with early and advanced cervical cancer and should facilitate referrals for this treatment. Surgery or radiation therapy may be options for treatment, depending on the stage and size of the lesion. In most cases, women with diagnosed invasive cervical cancer should be referred to an obstetrician–gynecologist with advanced surgical training, experience, and demonstrated competence, such as a gynecologic oncologist, often in conjunction with a radiation oncologist.

Vaginal cancer is treated in a manner similar to cervical cancer. Most types of vaginal cancer require pelvic radiation therapy. Pelvic radiation therapy with surgery is typically reserved only for the few women with small stage I tumors.

Endometrial Cancer

Carcinoma of the endometrium is the most common genital tract malignancy in the United States, with an estimated 52,630 diagnosed cases and 8,590 deaths in 2014. It is found more frequently in women who have been exposed to unopposed estrogen, either endogenous or exogenous. A family history of endometrial or colorectal cancer confers increased risk. The use of combination oral contraceptives is associated with a decreased risk. Management and treatment of chronic anovulation decreases the risk of types of estrogen-dependent endometrial cancer.

RISK FACTORS

In the United States, the lifetime risk of developing endometrial cancer is 2.49%. White women have a 2.9% lifetime risk of developing endometrial cancer and a 0.49% risk of dying from the disease; African-American women have a 1.93% risk of developing the disease and a 0.75% risk of dying from it. Adenocarcinoma of the endometrium is predominantly a disease of postmenopausal women. Uterine sarcomas are rare. These tumors usually arise in the muscle of the uterine wall; rarely, they have arisen in uterine leiomyomas. Risk factors for the development of endometrial cancer include the following:

- Excess endogenous estrogen exposure
  - Obesity
  - Chronic anovulation (especially polycystic ovary syndrome)
  - Estrogen-secreting tumors
- Unopposed exogenous estrogen exposure
- Use of tamoxifen
- Early menarche, late menopause
- Personal history of breast, ovarian, or colon cancer
- Lynch syndrome (also known as hereditary nonpolyposis colorectal cancer)

EVALUATION AND DIAGNOSIS

Routine cervical cytology screening is not a reliable means of detecting endometrial cancer. There are no effective screening methods to detect endometrial cancer. Endometrial cancer should be suspected under the following circumstances:

- Bleeding in a postmenopausal woman
- Chronic anovulation and associated irregular bleeding in premenopausal women
- Perimenopausal women with the following:
  - Very heavy menstrual flow
  - Excessive intermenstrual bleeding

The clinician should be able to elicit an appropriate history and identify risk factors that would predispose patients to the development of endometrial cancer. Appropriate physical and pelvic examination should be done to determine the source of any abnormal bleeding and to rule out extrauterine causes. The clinician should have the appropriate expertise and equipment to perform outpatient endometrial biopsies and have the ability to obtain transvaginal ultrasonography to evaluate the endometrial thickness.

Women with postmenopausal bleeding may be assessed initially with either endometrial biopsy or transvaginal ultrasonography; this initial evaluation does not require performance of both tests. Transvaginal ultrasonography can be useful in the triage of patients in whom endometrial sampling was performed but tissue was insufficient for diagnosis. When transvaginal ultrasonography is performed for patients with postmenopausal bleeding and an endometrial thickness of less than or equal to 4 mm is found, endometrial sampling is not required. Meaningful assessment of the endometrium by ultrasonography is not possible in all patients. In such cases, alternative assessment should be completed. When bleeding persists despite negative initial evaluations, additional assessment usually is indicated.

Many patients with lesions that are well differentiated (grade 1) will have disease that has not spread beyond the uterus. The use of radiologic imaging, such as computed tomography or magnetic resonance imaging, is not recommended for routine preoperative evaluation. All other preoperative testing should be directed toward optimizing the surgical outcome.

MANAGEMENT

The clinician who plans to treat the patient with endometrial cancer must have the expertise to determine when full surgical staging is necessary and the ability to perform the required procedures, such as hysterectomy, bilateral salpingo-oophorectomy, and pelvic and paraaortic lymphadenectomy. A referral to, or consultation with, a gynecologic oncologist may be appropriate.

If a diagnosis of invasive endometrial cancer is made, surgical staging is still the gold standard. Most women with endometrial cancer should undergo systematic surgical staging, which includes biopsy of any suspicious lesions, obtaining intraperitoneal (abdominal cavity) samples for cytology (washings), bilateral pelvic and paraaortic lymphadenectomy, and complete resection of all disease. Exceptions include young or perimenopausal women with grade 1 endometrioid adenocarcinoma associated with atypical endometrial hyperplasia and women at increased risk of mortality secondary to comorbidities. Women who desire to maintain fertility may be candidates for treatment with progestins monitored by serial endometrial biopsy. Women who cannot undergo surgery because of comorbidities may be candidates for primary therapeutic radiation. However, radiation therapy may not eradicate the uterine cancer in 10–15% cases, thus careful preoperative evaluation and appropriate consultation should be undertaken before denying any woman the benefits of hysterectomy. More detailed treatment recommendations have been published by the American College of Obstetricians and Gynecologists, developed jointly with the Society of Gynecologic Oncology (see Bibliography).

When it is practical and feasible, consultation with a physician with advanced training and demonstrated competence, such as a gynecologic oncologist, may be recommended. Consultation may be particularly beneficial in the following situations:

- The ability to completely and adequately surgically stage the patient is not readily available at the time of her initial procedure.

- Preoperative histologic findings (eg, grade 3, papillary serous, clear cell, carcinosarcoma) suggest a high risk of extrauterine spread.
- The final pathology test result reveals an unexpected endometrial cancer after hysterectomy was performed for other indications.
- There is evidence of cervical or extrauterine disease.
- The pelvic washing results are positive for malignant cells.
- Recurrent disease is diagnosed or suspected.
- Nonoperative therapy is contemplated.

No definitive data support specific recommendations regarding the use of estrogen in women previously treated for endometrial cancer. At this time, the decision to use hormone therapy in these women should be individualized on the basis of potential benefit and risk to the patient.

Ovarian Cancer

Ovarian cancer is the leading cause of death from genital tract malignancy and the fifth leading cause of cancer-related death in U.S. women, with an estimated 21,980 new cases and 14,270 deaths in 2014. The main reason for these dismal statistics is the advanced stage of disease at diagnosis and an overall 5-year survival rate of only 20–30%. Most cases occur in women older than 50 years, but this disease also can affect younger women.

Much less common are malignancies that arise in the tissue that covers the ovary and lines the abdominal cavity (ie, the peritoneum). Primary peritoneal cancer behaves the same as ovarian cancer and is treated in a similar manner. The existence of primary peritoneal cancer explains why some tumors that look like ovarian cancer can develop even after bilateral oophorectomy.

The pathogenesis of ovarian carcinoma remains unclear. Pregnancy, breastfeeding, and oral contraceptive use are associated with a decreased risk of ovarian cancer. Only approximately 5–10% of patients with ovarian cancer have a significant family history for this malignancy. A woman with a germline mutation of *BRCA1* or *BRCA2* has a lifetime risk of 15–45% of developing ovarian cancer. There are no data demonstrating that screening improves early detection of ovarian cancer in this population. These women should be offered genetic counseling.

EVALUATION AND DIAGNOSIS

Currently, no available screening methods are appropriate for mass screening of the general population. The best way to detect ovarian cancer is for the patient and her clinician to have a high index of suspicion for the diagnosis in the symptomatic woman. This strategy requires education of physicians and patients as to the symptoms commonly associated with ovarian cancer. Factors that have been most significantly associated with ovarian cancer, if they occurred more than 12 days per month and for less than 1 year, were pelvic or abdominal pain, increase in abdominal size or bloating, and difficulty eating or feeling full.

In evaluating these symptoms, physicians should perform a physical examination, including a pelvic examination. Imaging studies (including transvaginal ultrasonography) may be helpful before making the diagnosis of irritable bowel syndrome, depression, stress, or other conditions. The use of an adjunctive qualitative serum test that measures the levels of five biomarkers associated with ovarian cancer (transthyretin, apolipoprotein A-1, β_2 microglobulin, transferrin, and CA 125 II) can help predict the malignancy potential of an already detected ovarian adnexal mass that requires surgery, and thus guide decisions regarding referral for surgical evaluation. In premenopausal women with symptoms, a CA 125 measurement alone has not been shown to be useful in most circumstances because elevated levels of CA 125 are associated with a variety of common benign conditions, including uterine leiomyomas, adenomyosis, pregnancy, and even menstruation. In postmenopausal women with a pelvic mass, a CA 125 measurement may be helpful in predicting a higher likelihood of a malignant tumor than a benign tumor, which may be useful in making consultation, referral decisions, or both; however, a normal CA 125 measurement alone does not rule out ovarian cancer.

Diagnostic criteria based on physical examination and imaging techniques that should be used to consider referral to, or consultation with, a physician trained to appropriately stage and debulk ovarian cancer (such as a gynecologic oncologist) are as follows:

- Postmenopausal women who have a pelvic mass that is suspicious for a malignant ovarian neoplasm, as suggested by at least one of the following indicators: an elevated CA 125 level, ascites, a nodular or fixed pelvic mass, or evidence of abdominal or distant metastasis

• Premenopausal women who have a pelvic mass that is suspicious for a malignant ovarian neoplasm, as suggested by at least one of the following indicators: a very elevated CA 125 level, ascites, evidence of abdominal or distant metastasis

MANAGEMENT

A woman with a suspicious or persistent adnexal mass requires surgical evaluation. In these circumstances, a physician trained to appropriately stage and debulk ovarian cancer, such as a gynecologic oncologist, should perform the operation. It should be done in a hospital facility that has the necessary support and consultative services (eg, pathology services) to optimize the patient's outcome. When a malignant ovarian tumor is discovered and the appropriate operation cannot be performed properly, a gynecologic oncologist should be consulted.

In addition to being able to perform comprehensive surgical staging and cytoreductive procedures when ovarian cancer is found, a treating physician also must understand the appropriate use of intraperitoneal chemotherapy. Evidence suggests that patients with optimally debulked stage III ovarian cancer may be candidates to receive part of their chemotherapy intraperitoneally. Combination intravenous and intraperitoneal chemotherapy may be an option for well-counseled, carefully selected patients with optimally debulked stage III ovarian cancer when provided by a physician with the requisite training and experience in administering this treatment. Combination intravenous and intraperitoneal treatment has been shown to be associated with higher rates of pain; fatigue; and hematologic, gastrointestinal, metabolic, and neurologic toxicities. Given the balance of efficacy, quality of life, and toxicity, the decision to use intraperitoneal chemotherapy must be individualized.

Vulvar Cancer

Vulvar cancer is fairly uncommon, accounting for approximately 5% of cases of all gynecologic malignancies, with an estimated 4,850 new cases and 1,030 deaths in the United States in 2014. The great majority of malignant vulvar lesions are types of squamous cell cancer. Less common malignancies of the vulva include melanoma, Bartholin gland carcinoma, and a variety of sarcomas. The prognostic factors for vulvar cancer recently have been defined more clearly. The development of more conservative surgical approaches, along with the combination of chemotherapy and radiation (chemoradiation), has contributed to improved quality of life in patients with this malignancy.

EVALUATION AND DIAGNOSIS

No screening strategies have been developed for the prevention of vulvar cancer through early detection of vulvar intraepithelial neoplasia (VIN). Diagnosis is limited to visual assessment. The appearance of VIN can vary. Biopsy is indicated for most pigmented vulvar lesions. Expert opinion is divided regarding the need for biopsy of all warty lesions, but biopsy should be performed in postmenopausal women with apparent genital warts and in women in whom topical therapies have failed (see also the "Vulvar Skin Disorders" section earlier in Part 4).

To avoid significant delay in diagnosis, the clinician should have a high index of suspicion of vulvar cancer when a woman, particularly one who is older, presents with vulvar symptoms or findings. The clinician also should be able to recognize the subtle findings associated with preinvasive and early invasive vulvar lesions and be able to perform appropriate diagnostic procedures, including colposcopy and vulvar biopsy, to confirm the diagnosis. If a diagnosis of extensive VIN or invasive cancer is made, referral of the patient to a gynecologic oncologist or a clinician with the requisite expertise to offer appropriate therapy (which is often multimodal) is required.

MANAGEMENT

Cases of vulvar cancer are managed individually based on the extent of the lesion and risk of inguinal lymph node metastasis. The type of surgical resection of the vulvar cancer is based on the size of the lesion as well as the site of the lesion. Assessment of the inguinal lymph nodes is determined by the stromal invasion of the vulvar cancer and its location. A locally advanced case of vulvar cancer may be initially treated with chemoradiation in order to limit the need for radical surgery.

Gestational Trophoblastic Disease

Gestational trophoblastic disease encompasses a spectrum of interrelated conditions originating from the placenta. These histologically distinct entities include complete and partial hydatidiform moles, invasive moles, placental site trophoblastic tumors, and gestational choriocarcinoma. With the currently available sensitive assays for human chorionic gonadotropin (hCG) to monitor the disease and with effective chemotherapy regimens (single agent and multiagent regimens), the previously observed morbidity and mortality from these disorders have been reduced greatly. With appropriate evaluation and treatment, most women with malignant gestational trophoblastic disease can be cured and their reproductive function preserved.

Estimates of the incidence of gestational trophoblastic disease vary widely. The following incidence rates apply to the United States:

- Hydatidiform mole is observed in 1 in 1,000 pregnancies. In approximately 5% of cases, a hydatidiform mole will develop into an invasive mole. Overall, invasive moles occur at an estimated rate of 1 in 15,000 pregnancies.

- Gestational choriocarcinoma occurs in approximately 2–7 of every 100,000 pregnancies: approximately 50% after molar pregnancies, 25% after term pregnancies, and the remainder after other gestational events.

- Overall, gestational trophoblastic tumors account for less than 1% of cases of female reproductive system cancers.

To allow optimal management, practicing obstetrician–gynecologists should be able to diagnose and manage primary molar pregnancies, diagnose and stage malignant gestational trophoblastic disease, and assess risk in women with malignant gestational trophoblastic disease to allow referral for appropriate initial treatment. Clinical experience, such as that acquired at regional gestational trophoblastic disease treatment centers, improves outcomes in the management of malignant gestational trophoblastic disease. Any woman for whom initial therapy for invasive mole has failed or who has a choriocarcinoma diagnosis should be referred to a physician or facility with training, expertise, and experience in managing the disease.

HYDATIDIFORM MOLE

Hydatidiform moles usually are diagnosed during the first trimester of pregnancy. The most common symptom is abnormal bleeding. Other signs and symptoms include uterine enlargement greater than expected for gestational age, absent fetal heart tones, cystic enlargement of the ovaries, hyperemesis gravidarum, and an abnormally high level of hCG for gestational age. The presence of these features in the first trimester should alert the clinician to the possibility of a molar gestation. Pregnancy-induced hypertension in the first half of pregnancy, although uncommon, is suggestive of hydatidiform mole. Ultrasonography has replaced all other noninvasive means of establishing the diagnosis. Molar tissue typically is identified as a diffuse mixed echogenic pattern replacing the placenta, produced by villi and intrauterine blood clots, but these findings may be subtle or lacking in cases of early complete or partial moles.

As long as hCG values are decreasing after molar evacuation, there is no role for chemotherapy. However, if hCG levels increase or plateau over several weeks, immediate evaluation and treatment for malignant postmolar gestational trophoblastic disease are indicated. Occasionally, the plateauing or increasing hCG levels represent a false-positive laboratory test result caused by heterophilic antibodies cross-reacting with the hCG test (phantom hCG).

MALIGNANT GESTATIONAL TROPHOBLASTIC DISEASE

Postmolar gestational trophoblastic disease most frequently is diagnosed on the basis of increasing or plateauing hCG values. Women with malignant gestational trophoblastic disease after nonmolar pregnancies may have subtle signs and symptoms of disease, which make the diagnosis difficult. Abnormal bleeding for more than 6 weeks after any pregnancy should be evaluated with hCG testing to exclude a new pregnancy or gestational trophoblastic disease. Gestational choriocarcinoma should be considered in any woman of reproductive age with metastatic disease from an unknown primary site. A serum hCG determination and exclusion of pregnancy are all that are required to diagnose metastatic gestational tro-phoblastic disease in these circumstances.

CONTRACEPTION AND FUTURE PREGNANCIES

Patients should be counseled to use a reliable form of hormonal contra-ception during the first year of remission. Oral contraceptives have been shown to be safe and effective during posttreatment monitoring based on randomized, controlled trials. According to U.S. MEC, intrauterine devices may pose too great a risk for use in women with decreasing or undetectable hCG levels (U.S. MEC 3) and are contraindicated in women with persis-tently elevated hCG levels or malignant disease (U.S. MEC 4; see also the "Family Planning" section in Part 3). Because of the 1–2% risk of a second mole in subsequent pregnancies, early ultrasonographic examination is recommended for all future pregnancies. There does not appear to be an increased risk of congenital malformations or other complications related to pregnancy.

Fertility Preservation

As more young women are cured of cancer with chemotherapy and radiotherapy, which can be gonadotoxic, interest is growing in treatments that may preserve fertility. In vitro fertilization with cryopreservation of embryos is currently the best option for fertility preservation when treat-ment for cancer is anticipated. The American Society for Reproductive Medicine considers oocyte cryopreservation a reasonable strategy for patients who are unable to cryopreserve embryos and recommends oocyte cryopreservation with appropriate counseling for women who are facing infertility that is due to chemotherapy or other gonadotoxic therapies.

When cancer is diagnosed in a premenopausal woman, it is important to discuss her fertility concerns. If future pregnancy is desired, appropriate consultation with fertility specialists should be offered to ascertain whether immediate assisted reproductive strategies are possible to preserve fertility. Certainly, the extent of the disease and prognosis may affect decision mak-ing (see also the "Infertility" section later in Part 4).

Bibliography

American Cancer Society. Radiation therapy for breast cancer. Available at: http://www.cancer.org/cancer/breastcancer/detailedguide/breast-cancer-treating-radiation. Retrieved August 9, 2013.

American Cancer Society. What are the key statistics about gestational trophoblastic disease? Available at: http://www.cancer.org/cancer/gestationaltrophoblasticdisease/detailedguide/gestational-trophoblastic-disease-key-statistics. Retrieved August 9, 2013.

Avoiding inappropriate clinical decisions based on false-positive human chorionic gonadotropin test results. ACOG. Committee Opinion No. 278. American College of Obstetricians and Gynecologists. Obstet Gynecol 2002;100:1057–9.

Breast cancer screening. Practice Bulletin No. 122. American College of Obstetricians and Gynecologists. Obstet Gynecol 2011;118:372–82.

Davies C, Pan H, Godwin J, Gray R, Arriagada R, Raina V, et al. Long-term effects of continuing adjuvant tamoxifen to 10 years versus stopping at 5 years after diagnosis of oestrogen receptor-positive breast cancer: ATLAS, a randomised trial. Adjuvant Tamoxifen: Longer Against Shorter (ATLAS) Collaborative Group [published erratum appears in Lancet 2013;381:804]. Lancet 2013;381:805-16.

Diagnosis and treatment of gestational trophoblastic disease. ACOG Practice Bulletin No. 53. American College of Obstetricians and Gynecologists. Obstet Gynecol 2004;103:1365–77.

Elective and risk-reducing salpingo-oophorectomy. ACOG Practice Bulletin No. 89. American College of Obstetricians and Gynecologists. Obstet Gynecol 2008;111:231–41.

Food and Drug Administration. FDA clears a test for ovarian cancer: test can help identify potential malignancies, guide surgical decisions. Silver Spring (MD): FDA; 2009. Available at: http://www.fda.gov/newsevents/newsroom/pressannouncements/ucm182057.htm. Retrieved September 30, 2013.

Hereditary breast and ovarian cancer syndrome. ACOG Practice Bulletin No. 103. American College of Obstetricians and Gynecologists and Society of Gynecologic Oncologists. Obstet Gynecol 2009;113:957–66.

Induced abortion and breast cancer risk. ACOG Committee Opinion No. 434. American College of Obstetricians and Gynecologists. Obstet Gynecol 2009;113:1417-8.

Management of abnormal cervical cancer screening test results and cervical cancer precursors. Practice Bulletin No. 140. American College of Obstetricians and Gynecologists. Obstet Gynecol 2013;122: 1338–67.

Management of adnexal masses. ACOG Practice Bulletin No. 83. American College of Obstetricians and Gynecologists. Obstet Gynecol 2007;110:201–14.

Management of endometrial cancer. ACOG Practice Bulletin No. 65. American College of Obstetricians and Gynecologists. Obstet Gynecol 2005;106:413–25.

Management of gynecologic issues in women with breast cancer. Practice Bulletin No. 126. American College of Obstetricians and Gynecologists. Obstet Gynecol 2012;119:666–82.

Mature oocyte cryopreservation: a guideline. Practice Committees of American Society for Reproductive Medicine. Society for Assisted Reproductive Technology. Fertil Steril 2013;99:37–43.

Oocyte cryopreservation. Committee Opinion No. 584. American College of Obstetricians and Gynecologists. Obstet Gynecol 2014;123:221–2.

Pecorelli S. Revised FIGO staging for carcinoma of the vulva, cervix, and endometrium [published erratum appears in Int J Gynaecol Obstet 2010;108:176]. Int J Gynaecol Obstet 2009;105:103–4.

Robson ME, Storm CD, Weitzel J, Wollins DS, Offit K. American Society of Clinical Oncology policy statement update: genetic and genomic testing for cancer susceptibility. American Society of Clinical Oncology. J Clin Oncol 2010;28:893–901.

Schiffman M, Wentzensen N. From human papillomavirus to cervical cancer. Obstet Gynecol 2010;116:177–85.

Siegel R, Ma J, Zou Z, Jemal A. Cancer Statistics, 2014. CA Cancer J Clin 2014;64: 9–29.

The role of the obstetrician-gynecologist in the early detection of epithelial ovarian cancer. Committee Opinion No. 477. American College of Obstetricians and Gynecologists. Obstet Gynecol 2011;117:742–6.

U.S. Medical Eligibility Criteria for Contraceptive Use, 2010. Centers for Disease Control and Prevention. MMWR Recomm Rep 2010;59 (RR-4):1–86.

Resources

American Cancer Society. Cancer treatment and survivorship facts & figures 2012-2013. Atlanta (GA): ACS; 2012. Available at: http://www.cancer.org/acs/groups/content/@epidemiologysurveilance/documents/document/acspc-033876.pdf. Retrieved September 18, 2013.

American College of Obstetricians and Gynecologists. Benign breast problems and conditions. Patient Education Pamphlet AP026. Washington, DC: American College of Obstetricians and Gynecologists; 2012.

American College of Obstetricians and Gynecologists. Cancer of the cervix. Patient Education Pamphlet AP163. Washington, DC: American College of Obstetricians and Gynecologists; 2013.

American College of Obstetricians and Gynecologists. Cancer of the ovary. Patient Education Pamphlet AP096. Washington, DC: American College of Obstetricians and Gynecologists; 2011.

American College of Obstetricians and Gynecologists. Cancer of the uterus. Patient Education Pamphlet AP097. Washington, DC: American College of Obstetricians and Gynecologists; 2008.

American College of Obstetricians and Gynecologists. Colposcopy. Patient Education Pamphlet AP135. Washington, DC: American College of Obstetricians and Gynecologists; 2013.

American College of Obstetricians and Gynecologists. Disorders of the vulva. Patient Education Pamphlet AP088. Washington, DC: American College of Obstetricians and Gynecologists; 2013.

CancerCare. Available at: http://www.cancercare.org. Retrieved on August 9, 2013.

Fertility preservation and reproduction in cancer patients. Ethics Committee of the American Society for Reproductive Medicine. Fertil Steril 2005;83:1622–8.

Foundation for Women's Cancer. Educational materials. Available at: http://www. foundationforwomenscancer.org/educational-materials. Retrieved August 12, 2013.

Kushi LH, Byers T, Doyle C, Bandera EV, McCullough M, McTiernan A, et al. American Cancer Society Guidelines on Nutrition and Physical Activity for cancer prevention: reducing the risk of cancer with healthy food choices and physical activity. American Cancer Society 2006 Nutrition and Physical Activity Guidelines Advisory Committee [published erratum appears in CA Cancer J Clin 2007;57:66]. CA Cancer J Clin 2006;56:254,81; quiz 313–4.

National Cancer Institute. Cancer survivorship research. Available at: http://cancer control.cancer.gov/ocs/index.html. Retrieved August 9, 2013.

National Coalition for Cancer Survivorship. Cancer survival toolbox. Available at: http://www.canceradvocacy.org/toolbox. Retrieved August 12, 2013.

National Colorectal Cancer Roundtable. Clinician's reference: fecal occult blood testing (FOBT) for colorectal cancer screening. Available at: http://nccrt.org/wp-content/uploads/FOBTCliniciansReferenceFinal.pdf. Retrieved August 12, 2013.

National Guideline Clearinghouse. Guideline syntheses. Available at: http://www. guideline.gov/syntheses/index.aspx. Retrieved August 12, 2013.

Rock CL, Doyle C, Demark-Wahnefried W, Meyerhardt J, Courneya KS, Schwartz AL, et al. Nutrition and physical activity guidelines for cancer survivors [published erratum appears in erratum in: CA Cancer J Clin 2013;63:215]. CA Cancer J Clin 2012;62:243–74.

Schorge JO, Modesitt SC, Coleman RL, Cohn DE, Kauff ND, Duska LR, et al. SGO White Paper on ovarian cancer: etiology, screening and surveillance. Gynecol Oncol 2010;119:7–17.

POLYCYSTIC OVARY SYNDROME

Polycystic ovary syndrome (PCOS) is a disorder characterized by hyperandrogenism, ovulatory dysfunction, and polycystic ovaries. Its etiology remains unknown, and treatment is largely symptom based and empirical. Polycystic ovary syndrome has the potential to cause substantial metabolic sequelae, including an increased risk of diabetes and cardiovascular disease, and these factors should be considered when determining long-term treatment.

Definition and Diagnostic Criteria

Polycystic ovary syndrome is a group of symptoms for which the definition has been somewhat controversial. In 1990, the National Institutes of Health (NIH) developed diagnostic criteria for PCOS, and subsequently revised criteria were proposed by the Rotterdam PCOS Consensus Workshop Group in 2003 and the Androgen Excess Society in 2006 (Table 4-4). The rationale behind the newer recommendations is that PCOS encompasses a broader clinical presentation than that defined by the NIH criteria. Critics of the Rotterdam criteria point out that polycystic ovaries demonstrated on ultrasonography are a nonspecific finding and may be found in women without endocrine or metabolic abnormalities. It should be noted that insulin resistance and elevated ratios of luteinizing hormone to follicle-stimulating hormone have been seen in many women with PCOS, but they are not part of any of the diagnostic criteria. In addition, medical conditions that can mimic and be confused with PCOS, such as nonclassical (late-onset) congenital adrenal hyperplasia, hyperprolactinemia, and androgen-secreting neoplasms, need to be ruled out (Box 4-8).

The suggested diagnostic evaluation for PCOS is included in Box 4-9. Although patients generally present to the obstetrician–gynecologist reporting symptoms, such as menstrual irregularity, infertility, or hirsutism,

Table 4-4. Recommended Diagnostic Schemes for Polycystic Ovary Syndrome by Varying Expert Groups

Signs and Symptoms*	National Institutes of Health Criteria[†] 1990 (both are required for diagnosis)	Rotterdam Consensus Criteria[‡] 2003 (two out of three are required for diagnosis)	Androgen Excess Society[§] 2006 (hyperandrogenism plus one out of remaining two are required for diagnosis)
Hyperandrogenism[‖]	R	NR	R
Oligomenorrhea or amenorrhea	R	NR	NR
Polycystic ovaries by ultrasound diagnosis		NR	NR

Abbreviations: R, required for diagnosis; NR, possible diagnostic criteria but not required to be present.

*All criteria recommend excluding other possible etiologies of these signs and symptoms and more than one of the factors present to make a diagnosis.

[†]Dunaif A, Givens JR, Haseletine FP, Merriam GR, editors. Polycystic ovary syndrome. Boston (MA): Blackwell Scientific Publications; 1992.

[‡]Revised 2003 consensus on diagnostic criteria and long-term health risks related to polycystic ovary syndrome. Rotterdam ESHRE/ASRM-Sponsored PCOS Consensus Workshop Group. Fertil Steril 2004;81:19–25.

[§]Azziz R, Carmina E, Dewailly D, Diamanti-Kandarakis E, Escobar-Morreale HF, Futterweit W, et al. Positions statement: criteria for defining polycystic ovary syndrome as a predominantly hyperandrogenic syndrome: an Androgen Excess Society guideline. Androgen Excess Society. J Clin Endocrinol Metab 2006;91:4237–45.

[‖]Hyperandrogenism may be either the presence of hirsutism or biochemical hyperandrogenemia.

Reprinted from Polycystic ovary syndrome. ACOG Practice Bulletin No. 108. American College of Obstetricians and Gynecologists. Obstet Gynecol 2009;114:936–49.

a critical element of caring for the patient with PCOS is addressing the substantial metabolic sequelae associated with the condition. Patients often develop diabetes or cardiovascular disease and have dyslipidemia; thus, all patients with PCOS should be screened for metabolic abnormalities. Patients also have an increased risk of endometrial carcinoma related to anovulation and unopposed estrogen.

Box 4-8. Factors to Consider in the Differential Diagnosis of Polycystic Ovary Syndrome

Androgen-secreting tumor

Exogenous androgens

Cushing syndrome

Nonclassical congenital adrenal hyperplasia

Acromegaly

Genetic defects in insulin action

Primary hypothalamic amenorrhea

Primary ovarian failure

Thyroid disease

Prolactin disorders

Reprinted from Polycystic ovary syndrome. ACOG Practice Bulletin No. 108. American College of Obstetricians and Gynecologists. Obstet Gynecol 2009;114:936–49.

Box 4-9. Suggested Evaluation for Patients With Polycystic Ovary Syndrome

Physical Examination

- Blood pressure
- Body mass index (calculated as weight in kilograms divided by height in meters squared): 25–29.9 = overweight; 30 or greater = obese
- Waist circumference: value greater than 35 in. = abnormal
- Presence of stigmata of hyperandrogenism and insulin resistance: acne, hirsutism, androgenic alopecia, acanthosis nigricans

Laboratory

- Documentation of biochemical hyperandrogenemia: total testosterone and sex hormone–binding globulin or bioavailable and free testosterone
- Exclusion of other causes of hyperandrogenism
    — Thyroid-stimulating hormone levels (thyroid dysfunction)
    — Prolactin (hyperprolactinemia)

(continued)

Box 4-9. Suggested Evaluation for Patients With Polycystic Ovary Syndrome *(continued)*

- Exclusion of other causes of hyperandrogenism *(continued)*
  - —17-hydroxyprogesterone (nonclassical congenital adrenal hyperplasia due to 21-hydroxylase deficiency)
    Random normal level less than 4 ng/mL or morning fasting level less than 2 ng/mL
  - —Consider screening for Cushing syndrome and other rare disorders, such as acromegaly
- Evaluation for metabolic abnormalities: 2-hour oral glucose tolerance test (fasting glucose less than 110 mg/dL = normal; 110–125 mg/dL = impaired; greater than 126 mg/dL = type 2 diabetes mellitus) followed by 75 g oral glucose ingestion and then 2-hour glucose level (less than 140 mg/dL = normal glucose tolerance; 140–199 mg/dL = impaired glucose tolerance; greater than 200 mg/dL = type 2 diabetes mellitus)
- Fasting lipid and lipoprotein level: total cholesterol greater than 200 mg/dL = abnormal, high-density lipoproteins less than 50 mg/dL = abnormal; triglycerides greater than 150 mg/dL = abnormal

Ultrasound Examination
- Determination of polycystic ovaries: in one or both ovaries, either 12 or more follicles measuring 2–9 mm in diameter, or increased ovarian volume (greater than 10 cm^3). If there is a follicle greater than 10 mm in diameter, the scan should be repeated at a time of ovarian quiescence in order to calculate volume and area. The presence of one polycystic ovary is sufficient to provide the diagnosis.
- Identification of endometrial abnormalities

Optional Tests to Consider
- Gonadotropin determinations to determine cause of amenorrhea
- Fasting insulin levels in younger women, those with diagnostic signs of insulin resistance and hyperandrogenism, or those undergoing ovulation induction
- 24-hour urinary free-cortisol excretion test or a low-dose dexamethasone suppression test in women with late onset of polycystic ovary syndrome symptoms or stigmata of Cushing syndrome

Modified from Polycystic ovary syndrome. ACOG Practice Bulletin No. 108. American College of Obstetricians and Gynecologists. Obstet Gynecol 2009;114:936–49.

Management

The treatment of patients with PCOS often depends on the presenting signs and symptoms.

OBESITY

In overweight and obese women, weight loss can result in spontaneous return of menses, improved pregnancy rates, decreased hirsutism, and improved glucose and lipid levels. Weight loss should be attempted first by exercise and nutrition interventions (see also the "Fitness" section in Part 3). Although weight loss of as little as 5% of initial weight has resulted in these benefits, the effects of weight loss in normal-weight women are not known. The use of pharmacologic weight-loss agents and gastric bypass surgery also has demonstrated benefit in women with reproductive and metabolic abnormalities.

RISK OF CARDIOVASCULAR DISEASE AND DIABETES

Overall, lifestyle modifications that include increased exercise and reduced caloric intake are the best first-line approach to decreasing the risk of cardiovascular disease and diabetes. Data are insufficient to recommend insulin-sensitizing agents to prevent diabetes in women with PCOS; women found to have impaired glucose tolerance or metabolic syndrome may, however, receive some benefit from active management with pharmacologic agents (see also the "Cardiovascular Disorders" section and the "Diabetes Mellitus" section in Part 3).

MENSTRUAL DISORDERS

In women not attempting to conceive, low-dose combined oral contraceptives remain the mainstay of long-term treatment for menstrual irregularities because they provide a progestin, suppress androgen secretion, increase sex hormone–binding globulin, and reduce the potential for endometrial cancer. There is insufficient evidence to determine the most effective combined hormonal contraceptive to treat menstrual disorders in women with PCOS. Progestin-only contraceptives or progestin-containing intrauterine devices are an alternative for endometrial protection, but they are associated with abnormal bleeding patterns in 50–89% of users. Small studies over 3–6 months using metformin have shown an improvement in ovulatory function in approximately one half the women studied. Serious but rare adverse effects of metformin may include lactic acidosis, but this is seen chiefly in patients with preexisting renal or hepatic disease, which are contraindications to this medication. Lactic acidosis also may occur with marked dehydration. Metformin administration should be discontinued before radiologic procedures that use iodinated contrast material, such as intravenous pyelography. Common adverse effects of metformin, such as bloating and diarrhea, may be decreased by initiating therapy at low doses and gradually increasing the amounts until therapeutic levels are attained.

There is currently no single accepted algorithm to guide ovulation induction in women with PCOS who are attempting to conceive. Patients should always first be counseled about lifestyle modification with weight loss and exercise. Clomiphene citrate is still the recommended first-line pharmacologic agent for ovulation induction. The third joint consensus conference on PCOS sponsored by the American Society for Reproductive Medicine and the European Society of Human Reproduction and Embryology concluded that there is no evidence for improved live-birth rates or decreased pregnancy complications associated with the use of metformin either before conception or during pregnancy. Furthermore, women with PCOS who become pregnant may be at increased risk of adverse pregnancy outcomes, especially if obesity, insulin resistance, or both are present.

HIRSUTISM

In patients reporting hirsutism, combined therapy with an ovarian suppression agent and an antiandrogen, such as spironolactone, appears effective, though caution must be used when combining a contraceptive containing drospirenone with spironolactone. Mechanical hair removal with shaving, plucking, waxing, depilatory creams, electrolysis, and laser vaporization are often the first-line treatment options for most women with PCOS.

Bibliography

Azziz R, Carmina E, Dewailly D, Diamanti-Kandarakis E, Escobar-Morreale HF, Futterweit W, et al. Positions statement: criteria for defining polycystic ovary syndrome as a predominantly hyperandrogenic syndrome: an Androgen Excess Society guideline. Androgen Excess Society. J Clin Endocrinol Metab 2006;91:4237–45.

Dunaif A, Givens JR, Haseletine FP, Merriam GR, editors. Polycystic ovary syndrome. Boston (MA): Blackwell Scientific Publications; 1992.

Ehrmann DA. Polycystic ovary syndrome. N Engl J Med 2005;352:1223–36.

Fauser BC, Tarlatzis BC, Rebar RW, Legro RS, Balen AH, Lobo R, et al. Consensus on women's health aspects of polycystic ovary syndrome (PCOS): the Amsterdam ESHRE/ASRM-Sponsored 3rd PCOS Consensus Workshop Group. Fertil Steril 2012;97:28–38.e25.

Polycystic ovary syndrome. ACOG Practice Bulletin No. 108. American College of Obstetricians and Gynecologists. Obstet Gynecol 2009;114:936–49.

Revised 2003 consensus on diagnostic criteria and long-term health risks related to polycystic ovary syndrome. Rotterdam ESHRE/ASRM-Sponsored PCOS Consensus Workshop Group. Fertil Steril 2004;81:19–25.

Resources

American College of Obstetricians and Gynecologists. Polycystic ovary syndrome. Patient Education Pamphlet AP121. Washington, DC: American College of Obstetricians and Gynecologists; 2011.

American College of Obstetricians and Gynecologists. Treating infertility. Patient Education Pamphlet AP137. Washington, DC: American College of Obstetricians and Gynecologists; 2012.

American Society for Reproductive Medicine. Medications for inducing ovulation: a guide for patients. Birmingham (AL): ASRM; 2012. Available at: http://www.asrm.org/uploadedFiles/ASRM_Content/Resources/Patient_Resources/Fact_Sheets_and_Info_Booklets/ovulation_drugs.pdf. Retrieved August 12, 2013.

American Society for Reproductive Medicine. Polycystic ovary syndrome (PCOS). Fact sheet. Birmingham (AL): ASRM; 2012. Available at: http://www.reproductive-facts.org/uploadedFiles/ASRM_Content/Resources/Patient_Resources/Fact_Sheets_and_Info_Booklets/PCOS.pdf. Retrieved August 12, 2013.

Department of Health and Human Services, Office on Women's Health. Polycystic ovary syndrome (PCOS) fact sheet. Washington, DC: HHS; 2010. Available at: http://www.womenshealth.gov/publications/our-publications/fact-sheet/polycystic-ovary-syndrome.pdf. Retrieved August 12, 2013.

SEXUAL FUNCTION AND DYSFUNCTION

Sexuality involves a broad range of expressions of intimacy and is fundamental to self-identification, with strong cultural, biologic, and psychologic components. There is a range of sexual practices that are normal, and different cultures have their own definitions of normal. It is necessary for clinicians to understand the sexual response pattern and the variations of these responses to assist in the identification and treatment of patients with sexual dysfunction.

Sexual Function

Most clinicians are familiar with the traditional human sexual response cycle of Masters, Johnson, and Kaplan. This model depicts a linear sequence of discrete events: desire, arousal, plateau, orgasm, and resolution (see Fig. 4-4). However, the usefulness of this model for depicting women's sexuality is limited. Sexual response in women is complex, and events do

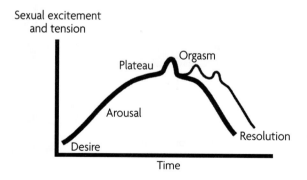

Fig. 4-4. Traditional sexual response cycle of Masters, Johnson, and Kaplan. (Reprinted from Basson R. Female sexual response: the role of drugs in the management of sexual dysfunction [published erratum appears in Obstet Gynecol 2001;98:522]. Obstet Gynecol 2001;98:350–3.)

not always occur in a predictable sequence, as they usually do in men. A woman's sexuality is influenced by her health and emotional well-being; likewise, healthy sexual functioning promotes physical and emotional well-being. An alternate model of women's sexual response (see Fig. 4-5) depicts the many sexual motivations, sexual stimuli, and psychologic and biologic factors that govern the processing of those stimuli, thus determining the woman's arousability.

Studies suggest that fewer than one half of patients' sexual concerns are recognized by their physicians. The obstetrician–gynecologist has an important role in assessing sexual function because many women view their sexuality as an important quality-of-life issue that frequently is affected by reproductive events. Clinicians should not make assumptions or judgments about the woman's behavior and, when counseling patients, should keep in mind the possibility of cultural and personal variation in sexual practices.

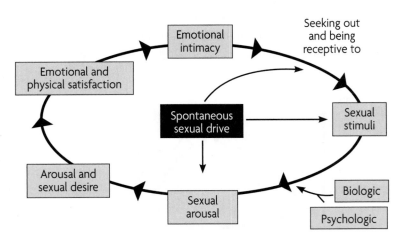

Fig. 4-5. Nonlinear model of female sexual response developed by Basson. Basson's nonlinear model acknowledges how emotional intimacy, sexual stimuli, and relationship satisfaction affect female sexual response. (Modified from Basson R. Female sexual response: the role of drugs in the management of sexual dysfunction [published erratum appears in Obstet Gynecol 2001;98:522]. Obstet Gynecol 2001;98:350–3.)

Sexual Dysfunction

Female sexual dysfunction encompasses a number of conditions that cause disturbance in a woman's sexual response. The adverse effect of female sexual dysfunction on the quality of life of affected women can extend into interpersonal relationships and the workplace. Sexual dysfunction of one type or another is common and experienced by most women at some time in their lives. Although female sexual dysfunction is prevalent, it often is neglected in the health care setting because women are unlikely to discuss it with their health care providers unless asked. Health care providers can convey to patients that it is appropriate to discuss sexual concerns by integrating the topic of sexual dysfunction into office visits.

ETIOLOGY

Sexual dysfunction may be related to emotional issues (eg, relationship difficulties, past sexual abuse), psychologic problems (eg, depression, anxiety, poor body image), physical impairment or illness, medications, alcohol or drug use, or biologic factors (eg, fatigue). The subtypes lifelong or acquired and generalized or situational are used in the *Diagnostic and Statistical Manual of Mental Disorders*, Fifth Edition (DSM-5), to designate the development and course of symptoms.

Numerous medications (both prescription and over-the-counter) and substances (such as illicit drugs and alcohol) have been associated with sexual dysfunction. Psychotropic medications, antihypertensives, histamine blockers, and hormonal contraceptives also have been implicated. The most common medications linked to sexual dysfunction are the selective serotonin reuptake inhibitors. The most frequently reported problems are orgasmic dysfunction, decreased sexual desire, and decreased arousal.

Emotional issues can be the basis for sexual dysfunction. The physician should attempt to identify any factors that could affect sexual function and provide education and counseling about them. Events from the past, such as childhood inhibitions or sexual abuse, can affect sexual function. Patients with complex sexual problems of a psychologic nature may benefit from referral to a mental health professional. When emotional problems clearly are limited to unsatisfactory sexual experiences, referral to a qualified sex therapist is appropriate. If the difficulty involves issues other than sexuality, referral to a counselor skilled in marital and other relationship problems may be preferable. Individuals with sexual dysfunction that results from a history of sexual victimization should be referred to mental health professionals with an expertise in abuse-related problems.

Male factors include low desire and erectile dysfunction, which may be based on organic or psychologic factors. Acknowledgment and support from the woman's physician may assist the patient in helping her partner seek counseling and treatment.

EVALUATION

The initial approach to the evaluation of a patient who presents with a possible sexual dysfunction disorder begins with obtaining a sexual history during the review of symptoms. Taking a thorough sexual history includes recording the patient's medical, surgical, social, and psychiatric history. Information about the use of prescription and over-the-counter medications and other substances should be elicited. If an examination is performed, the patient should be informed of what it will entail. The presence of a chaperone is recommended during examination, regardless of the gender of the health care provider, but privacy during history-taking may elicit more thorough responses.

The clinician should be prepared to discuss patients' concerns about sexual function in a setting of mutual respect and trust. A nonjudgmental and respectful approach by the clinician, as well as awareness by the clinician of his or her own biases—and the active attempt to counteract them—is essential for effective care. Patients are more likely to develop trusting relationships with their health care providers when the issue of confidentiality has been addressed directly. A confidential relationship, in turn, can facilitate the open disclosure of health histories and behaviors. The clinician should not make assumptions about the gender of the woman's partner. Although most women report that their sexual partners are men, some women have sex only with other women, and others may have partners of both sexes. The use of terms such as partner instead of husband and sexual activity instead of sexual intercourse and an understanding of nonheterosexual sexuality will assist in open communication and assessment of any difficulties (see also the "Lesbians and Bisexual Women" section in Part 3).

The use of broad, open-ended questions in a routine history gathering can help disclose problems that require further exploration. The following are examples of basic questions, posed in a gender-neutral fashion:

- "Are you sexually active?"
- "Are you sexually satisfied?"
- "Do you have questions or concerns about sexual functioning?"
- "Do you think your partner is satisfied?"

Inquiry about the partner's sexual function and level of satisfaction may elicit more specific information and give an indication of the couple's level of communication. Deliberate inquiries should be made to assess the quality of the interpersonal relationship between the patient and her partner, including mutual satisfaction with their sexual relationship. After asking general questions, it may be helpful to ask additional pointed questions, such as the following:

- "Do you have orgasms?"
- "Are you satisfied with the frequency of sexual activity?"
- "Does your vagina lubricate enough?"

This will delineate better the exact nature of a patient's dysfunction. Difficulties with prior sexual experience, insufficient foreplay, and attitudes about sexual pleasure can be elicited with careful history taking. For example, difficulties reaching orgasm or markedly reduced intensity of orgasmic sensations may not be a problem unless the patient or partner perceives it to be.

CLASSIFICATION AND DIAGNOSIS

The DSM-5 identifies four specific types of female sexual dysfunction: 1) female sexual interest/arousal disorder, 2) female orgasmic disorder, 3) genito-pelvic pain/penetration disorder (a new classification that merges and expands on the DSM-IV-defined disorders of vaginismus and dyspareunia), and 4) substance/medication-induced sexual dysfunction

(Table 4-5). In addition, the DSM-5 also classifies disorders as other specified sexual dysfunction and unspecified sexual dysfunction, and the authors of the DSM-5 note that other factors, such as inadequate sexual stimulation or nonsexual mental or physical disorders, may explain sexual dysfunction as well. For example, atrophic vaginitis after spontaneous menopause or oophorectomy may cause pain with vaginal penetration and difficulties in lubrication that impair sexual arousal. Women often experience more than one type of sexual function disorder.

A diagnosis of one of the DSM-5–classified female sexual dysfunctions is made when symptoms persist for at least 6 months (except in the case of substance/medication-induced sexual dysfunction) and are sufficient to result in significant personal distress. In addition, diagnosis requires that the symptoms are not better explained by a nonsexual mental disorder, a medical condition, severe relationship distress or other significant life stressors, or the effects of a substance or medication (except in the case of substance/medication-induced sexual dysfunction).

Table 4-5. Types of Female Sexual Dysfunction

Disorder	Definition
Female sexual interest/ arousal disorder	A lack of, or significant decrease in, at least three of the following: 1) interest in sexual activity, 2) sexual or erotic thoughts or fantasies, 3) initiation of sexual activity and responsiveness to a partner's initiation, 4) excitement or pleasure during all or almost all sexual activity, 5) interest or arousal in response to internal or external sexual or erotic cues (eg, written, verbal, visual), 6) genital or nongenital sensations during sexual activity in almost all or all sexual encounters. Symptoms have persisted for a minimum of 6 months and cause clinically significant distress in the individual.*
Female orgasmic disorder	Marked delay in, marked infrequency of, or absence of orgasm, or markedly reduced intensity of orgasmic sensations, in almost all or all occasions of sexual activity. Symptoms have persisted for a minimum of 6 months and cause clinically significant distress in the individual.*

(continued)

Table 4-5. Types of Female Sexual Dysfunction *(continued)*

Disorder	Definition
Genito-pelvic pain/ penetration disorder	The persistent or recurrent presence of one or more of the following symptoms: 1) difficulty having intercourse, 2) marked vulvovaginal or pelvic pain during intercourse or penetration attempts, 3) marked fear or anxiety about vulvovaginal or pelvic pain anticipating, during, or resulting from vaginal penetration, and 4) marked tensing or tightening of the pelvic floor muscles during attempted vaginal penetration. Symptoms have persisted for a minimum of 6 months and cause clinically significant distress in the individual.*
Substance/medication- induced sexual dysfunction	A disturbance in sexual function that has a temporal relationship with substance/medication initiation, dose increase, or substance/medication discontinuation and causes clinically significant distress in the individual.[†]

*A diagnosis of a sexual dysfunction disorder can be made only if the sexual dysfunction is not better explained by a nonsexual mental disorder or as a consequence of severe relationship distress (eg, partner violence) or other significant stressors and is not due to the effects of a substance or medication or another medical condition.

[†]The disturbance is not better explained by an independent sexual dysfunction disorder. Evidence that suggests a nonsubstance/medication-induced sexual disorder includes a history of an independent sexual dysfunction disorder, symptoms that precede the onset of substance or medication use, or symptoms that persist for at least 1 month after cessation of acute withdrawal or severe intoxication.

Data from American Psychiatric Association. Diagnostic and statistical manual of mental disorders: DSM-5. 5th ed. Washington, DC: APA; 2013.

MANAGEMENT

Management of sexual dysfunction will vary with the type of dysfunction, although many types of dysfunction are related. In general, sexual dysfunction involves the couple, and therapy should be with both partners. However, even if an individual has a specific problem, it still may be appropriate for the partner to be involved in therapy. Some treatments for sexual dysfunction may be within the scope of the obstetrician–gynecologist. If not, referrals to mental health practitioners, marriage or relationship counselors, or sex therapists are appropriate.

Female Sexual Interest/Arousal Disorder

For women with a reduced or absent sexual interest or arousal, sensate focus exercises can help couples develop verbal and nonverbal means to communicate with each other to improve satisfaction. Studies have found transdermal testosterone to be effective for the short-term treatment of low sexual desire in women, with little evidence to support long-term use (longer than 6 months). However, testosterone is not approved by the U.S. Food and Drug Administration for this treatment.

Female Orgasmic Disorder

Behaviorally oriented, time-limited treatment programs for previously anorgasmic women have been described. Behavioral treatments include masturbation instruction, communication exercises, sensate focus exercises, and systematic desensitization. Psychotherapy and couples counseling and support groups of women with similar problems may be helpful. After counseling, self-stimulation techniques may be beneficial for the patient. Recently, surgical procedures, such as "vaginal rejuvenation" or "G-spot amplification" have been promoted as a means of enhancing sexual satisfaction. Often, the exact procedure performed is not clear because standard medical nomenclature is not used. Such procedures are not medically indicated, and their safety and effectiveness have not been documented (see also the "Ambulatory Gynecologic Surgery" section later in Part 4).

Genito-Pelvic Pain/Penetration Disorder

Effective treatment of fear of pain with vaginal penetration consists of psychotherapy and behavior modification called desensitization, which gradually allows patients to overcome their fear by using sequential vaginal dilators of increasing diameter. Pelvic floor physical therapy can also effectively address pain and tensing or tightening of the pelvic floor muscles associated with vaginal intercourse.

Sexual dysfunction increases as women age, even in the absence of measurable physiologic changes or a specific diagnosis of genito-pelvic pain/penetration disorder. After menopause, women often report a lack of vaginal lubrication that makes intercourse painful. The use of vaginal estrogen and lubricants can ease the problem. Although more common in the elderly, women of any age may experience this problem, particularly women with relatively lower estrogen levels, such as women who lactate or women who use depot medroxyprogesterone acetate for contraception.

Substance/Medication-Induced Sexual Dysfunction

When medications result in sexual dysfunction, the medication or dosage may need to be changed or eliminated. Couples should be counseled about the effects of illness or medication on sexuality and be encouraged to experiment with alternative forms of sexual expression to accommodate physical limitations. Female sexual dysfunction that is linked to the use of certain medications (eg, selective serotonin reuptake inhibitors) typically resolves when the medication is adjusted. Consultation with a health care provider with expertise in psychiatric medications who can assist in distinguishing baseline female sexual dysfunction from dysfunction that results from treatment of depression may be helpful. A medication adjustment with long-term follow-up may be important for improved sexual functioning.

Bibliography

American Psychiatric Association. Diagnostic and statistical manual of mental disorders: DSM-5. 5th ed. Washington, DC: APA; 2013.

Basson R. Female sexual response: the role of drugs in the management of sexual dysfunction [published erratum appears in Obstet Gynecol 2001;98:522]. Obstet Gynecol 2001;98:350–3.

Basson R. Sexuality and sexual disorders. Clin Update Womens Health Care 2003; II(2):1–94.

Brotto LA, Bitzer J, Laan E, Leiblum S, Luria M. Women's sexual desire and arousal disorders [published erratum appears in J Sex Med 2010;7:856]. J Sex Med 2010; 7:586–614.

Drugs that cause sexual dysfunction: an update. Med Lett Drugs Ther 1992;34:73–8.

Female sexual dysfunction. Practice Bulletin No. 119. American College of Obstetricians and Gynecologists. Obstet Gynecol 2011;117:996–1007.

Hayes RD, Bennett CM, Fairley CK, Dennerstein L. What can prevalence studies tell us about female sexual difficulty and dysfunction? J Sex Med 2006;3:589–95.

Kennedy SH, Rizvi S. Sexual dysfunction, depression, and the impact of antidepressants. J Clin Psychopharmacol 2009;29:157–64.

Resources

American Association for Marriage and Family Therapy, 112 South Alfred Street, Alexandria, VA 22314. (703) 838-9808. http://www.aamft.org. Retrieved August 12, 2013.

American Association of Sexuality Educators Counselors and Therapists. Available at: http://www.aasect.org. Retrieved August 12, 2013.

American College of Obstetricians and Gynecologists, District II. Finding solutions for female sexual dysfunction. Albany (NY): American College of Obstetricians and Gynecologists, District II; 2010. Available at: http://mail.ny.acog.org/website/FSDResourceGuide.pdf. Retrieved September 14, 2013.

American College of Obstetricians and Gynecologists. Your sexual health. Patient Education Pamphlet AP072. Washington, DC: American College of Obstetricians and Gynecologists; 2010.

Association of Reproductive Health Professionals. Clinician competencies for sexual health. Washington, DC: ARHP; 2010. Available at: http://www.arhp.org/upload Docs/SHF_Competencies.pdf. Retrieved August 12, 2013.

Haefner HK, Collins ME, Davis GD, Edwards L, Foster DC, Hartmann ED, et al. The vulvodynia guideline. J Low Genit Tract Dis 2005;9:40–51.

Health care for lesbians and bisexual women. Committee Opinion No. 525. American College of Obstetricians and Gynecologists. Obstet Gynecol 2012;119:1077–80.

Health care for transgender individuals. Committee Opinion No. 512. American College of Obstetricians and Gynecologists. Obstet Gynecol 2011;118:1454–8.

International Society for Sexual Medicine. Available at: http://www.issm.info. Retrieved September 14, 2013.

Kingsberg SA, Iglesia CB, Kellogg S, Krychman ML. Handbook on female sexual health and wellness. Washington, DC: Association of Reproductive Health Professionals; 2011. Available at: http://www.arhp.org/uploadDocs/ARHP_ACOG_SexualityHandbook.pdf. Retrieved September 19, 2013.

Society for Sex Therapy and Research. Available at: http://www.sstarnet.org. Retrieved September 14, 2013.

Vulvodynia. ACOG Committee Opinion No. 345. American College of Obstetricians and Gynecologists. Obstet Gynecol 2006;108:1049–52.

PELVIC ORGAN PROLAPSE

Pelvic organ prolapse occurs with descent of one or more pelvic structures: the uterine cervix or vaginal apex, anterior vaginal wall (usually with bladder, cystocele), posterior vaginal wall (usually with rectum, rectocele), or peritoneum of the cul-de-sac (usually with small intestine, enterocele). However, a specific definition of what constitutes clinically significant prolapse remains elusive. Although almost one half of parous women can be identified as having prolapse by physical examination criteria, most are not clinically affected; the finding of prolapse on physical examination is not well correlated with specific pelvic symptoms.

The prevalence of pelvic organ prolapse has increased as life expectancy has increased. National population-based estimates using validated measures report an overall 2.9% prevalence of symptomatic pelvic organ prolapse. However, other population-based surveys have revealed prevalence estimates as high as 8%. In the United States, an estimated 300,000 surgical procedures are performed annually for prolapse. A woman's lifetime risk of undergoing a surgical intervention for symptomatic pelvic floor disorders is approximately 11–19%. A large percentage of these women, 6–29%, will require additional surgery for recurrent pelvic organ prolapse or urinary incontinence, and those who have undergone at least two prior prolapse procedures have reoperation rates higher than 50%. Pelvic organ prolapse is the leading indication for hysterectomy in postmenopausal women and accounts for 15–18% of hysterectomies in all age groups.

Risk Factors

Possible risk factors for pelvic organ prolapse include genetic predisposition, parity (particularly vaginal birth), menopause, advancing age, prior pelvic surgery, connective tissue disorders, and factors associated with elevated intra-abdominal pressure (eg, obesity, chronic constipation with excessive straining). Women with symptomatic pelvic organ prolapse usually are postreproductive and have had vaginal deliveries or chronic repetitive increases in intra-abdominal pressure, though women who have never been pregnant also may exhibit pelvic relaxation. Weakness of the pelvic floor tissues, which may be congenital, also can cause pelvic floor dysfunction.

Evaluation and Diagnosis

Many patients with prolapse are asymptomatic. Patients who are symptomatic typically have symptoms of vaginal bulging or pressure and may have related bladder, bowel, or sexual dysfunction. It is advisable to examine a symptomatic woman in lithotomy and standing positions before and after a maximum Valsalva maneuver. Urinary or rectal incontinence can be assessed at the same time. One evaluation tool for the assessment of pelvic relaxation is the Pelvic Organ Prolapse Quantification system. It promotes universal standards to determine and measure pelvic floor defects. Further urogynecologic investigation can be helpful if urinary incontinence or fecal incontinence, extensive vaginal prolapse, or voiding difficulty are present (see also the "Urinary Incontinence" section later in Part 4). Urodynamic testing, cystoscopy, and pelvic floor imaging may be useful adjuncts before surgical repair, and the decision to perform these procedures should be individualized.

Management

Clinician knowledge and experience with normal pelvic floor function and its variations are required to initiate treatment. It is important to be fully cognizant of noninvasive treatments (pelvic floor muscle exercises, pessaries) and surgical interventions. Treatment is determined by the following:

- Patient age
- Physical activity level
- Severity of symptoms and physical findings
- Degree of disability
- Coital activity

- Desire for future fertility
- Desire for surgery

Women with pelvic organ prolapse who are asymptomatic or mildly symptomatic can be observed at regular intervals, unless new bothersome symptoms develop.

NONSURGICAL INTERVENTIONS

Pessary use should be considered before surgical intervention in all women with symptomatic prolapse. Although pessary use is the only specific nonsurgical treatment, pelvic floor muscle rehabilitation and symptom-directed therapy may be offered. Supplemental approaches to improve outcomes and decrease failure rates may include weight loss and exercise (to promote general health), intensive pelvic muscle exercises, and treatment of patients with chronic respiratory or metabolic conditions, constipation, and other intra-abdominal disorders.

SURGICAL INTERVENTIONS

Multiple surgical techniques are available to address the various anatomic and functional problems in women with pelvic organ prolapse. Data are evolving regarding the efficacy of available surgical interventions, which include transvaginal native tissue repair; abdominal, laparoscopic, and robotic options; and transvaginal mesh augmentation approaches. Pelvic organ prolapse vaginal mesh repair should be reserved for high-risk individuals in whom the benefit of mesh placement may justify the risk, such as individuals with recurrent prolapse (particularly of the anterior compartment) or with medical comorbidities that preclude more invasive and lengthier open and endoscopic procedures. Surgeons placing vaginal mesh should undergo training specific to each device and have experience with reconstructive surgical procedures and a thorough understanding of pelvic anatomy. The American College of Obstetricians and Gynecologists strongly supports audit and review of outcomes with vaginal mesh implants.

Bibliography

Blandon RE, Bharucha AE, Melton LJ,3rd, Schleck CD, Babalola EO, Zinsmeister AR, et al. Incidence of pelvic floor repair after hysterectomy: A population-based cohort study. Am J Obstet Gynecol 2007;197:664.e1–7.

Bump RC, Mattiasson A, Bo K, Brubaker LP, DeLancey JO, Klarskov P, et al. The standardization of terminology of female pelvic organ prolapse and pelvic floor dysfunction. Am J Obstet Gynecol 1996;175:10–7.

Jones KA, Shepherd JP, Oliphant SS, Wang L, Bunker CH, Lowder JL. Trends in inpatient prolapse procedures in the United States, 1979–2006. Am J Obstet Gynecol 2010;202:501.e1–7.

Nygaard I, Barber MD, Burgio KL, Kenton K, Meikle S, Schaffer J, et al. Prevalence of symptomatic pelvic floor disorders in US women. Pelvic Floor Disorders Network. JAMA 2008;300:1311–6.

Olsen AL, Smith VJ, Bergstrom JO, Colling JC, Clark AL. Epidemiology of surgically managed pelvic organ prolapse and urinary incontinence. Obstet Gynecol 1997;89:501–6.

Pelvic organ prolapse. ACOG Practice Bulletin No. 85. American College of Obstetricians and Gynecologists. Obstet Gynecol 2007;110:717–29.

Rortveit G, Brown JS, Thom DH, Van Den Eeden SK, Creasman JM, Subak LL. Symptomatic pelvic organ prolapse: prevalence and risk factors in a population-based, racially diverse cohort. Obstet Gynecol 2007;109:1396–403.

Smith FJ, Holman CD, Moorin RE, Tsokos N. Lifetime risk of undergoing surgery for pelvic organ prolapse. Obstet Gynecol 2010;116:1096–100.

Tegerstedt G, Maehle-Schmidt M, Nyren O, Hammarstrom M. Prevalence of symptomatic pelvic organ prolapse in a Swedish population. Int Urogynecol J Pelvic Floor Dysfunct 2005;16:497–503.

Vaginal placement of synthetic mesh for pelvic organ prolapse. Committee Opinion No. 513. American College of Obstetricians and Gynecologists. Obstet Gynecol 2011;118:1459–64.

Whiteside JL, Weber AM, Meyn LA, Walters MD. Risk factors for prolapse recurrence after vaginal repair. Am J Obstet Gynecol 2004;191:1533–8.

Resources

American College of Obstetricians and Gynecologists. Pelvic support problems. Patient Education Pamphlet AP012. Washington, DC: American College of Obstetricians and Gynecologists; 2010.

American College of Obstetricians and Gynecologists. Urogynecology: an illustrated guide for women. Washington, DC: ACOG; 2004.

American College of Obstetricians and Gynecologists. Urogynecology: a case management approach [CD-ROM]. Washington, DC: ACOG; 2005.

American Urogynecologic Society. Available at: http://www.augs.org. Retrieved September 18, 2013.

Food and Drug Administration. Update on serious complications associated with transvaginal placement of surgical mesh for pelvic organ prolapse: FDA safety communication. Silver Spring (MD): FDA; 2011. Available at: http://www.fda.gov/medicaldevices/safety/alertsandnotices/ucm262435.htm. Retrieved August 15, 2013.

Hagen S, Stark D. Conservative prevention and management of pelvic organ prolapse in women. Cochrane Database of Systematic Reviews 2011, Issue 12. Art. No.: CD003882. DOI: 10.1002/14651858.CD003882.pub4.

Maher C, Feiner B, Baessler K, Schmid C. Surgical management of pelvic organ prolapse in women. Cochrane Database of Systematic Reviews 2013, Issue 4. Art. No.: CD004014. DOI: 10.1002/14651858.CD004014.pub5.

The role of cystourethroscopy in the generalist obstetrician-gynecologist practice. ACOG Committee Opinion No. 372. American College of Obstetricians and Gynecologists. Obstet Gynecol 2007;110:221–4.

Urinary incontinence in women. ACOG Practice Bulletin No. 63. American College of Obstetricians and Gynecologists. Obstet Gynecol 2005;105:1533–45.

URINARY INCONTINENCE

Urinary incontinence, the involuntary leakage of urine, is a common condition caused by a variety of factors and may result in an assortment of urinary symptoms. The prevalence of incontinence appears to increase gradually during young adult life, has a broad peak around middle age, and then steadily increases in the elderly. The economic costs of urinary incontinence account for more than $20 billion per year in the United States, with 50–70% of the total cost attributed to resources used for incontinence management or "routine care," such as absorbent pads, protection, and laundry. Urinary incontinence has been shown to affect women's social, clinical, and psychologic well-being. It is estimated that less than one half of all incontinent women seek medical care, even though urinary incontinence often can be treated.

Etiology

Among women who experience urinary incontinence, the differential diagnosis includes genitourinary and nongenitourinary conditions (see Box 4-10). Some conditions that cause or contribute to urinary incontinence are potentially reversible (see Box 4-11). The relative likelihood of each condition causing incontinence varies with the age and health of the individual. Detrusor abnormalities and mixed urinary incontinence symptoms are more common among older, noninstitutionalized women with incontinence, whereas stress incontinence is more common among younger, ambulatory women. More severe and troublesome urinary incontinence probably occurs with increasing age, especially in women older than 70 years.

Evaluation and Diagnosis

The history and physical examination are the first and most important steps in evaluation of patients with urinary incontinence.

Box 4-10. Differential Diagnosis of Urinary Incontinence in Women

Genitourinary Etiology
- Filling and storage disorders
  — Urodynamic stress incontinence
  — Detrusor overactivity (idiopathic)
  — Detrusor overactivity (neurogenic)
  — Mixed types
- Fistulae
  — Vesical
  — Ureteral
  — Urethral
- Congenital
  — Ectopic ureter

Nongenitourinary Etiology
- Functional
  — Neurologic
  — Cognitive
  — Psychologic
  — Physical impairment
- Environmental
- Pharmacologic
- Metabolic

Modified from Urinary incontinence in women. ACOG Practice Bulletin No. 63. American College of Obstetricians and Gynecologists. Obstet Gynecol 2005;105:1533–45.

Urologic, bowel, medical, surgical, gynecologic, neurologic, and obstetric histories as well as a complete list of the patient's medications (including nonprescription medications) should be obtained. In addition to patient history evaluation, a 3-day or 7-day bladder diary and pad counts are considered a practical and reliable method of obtaining information on voiding behavior and incontinence severity. A bowel history is

---

Box 4-11. Common Causes of Transient Urinary Incontinence

- Urinary tract infection or urethritis (including from sexually transmitted infections)
- Atrophic urethritis or vaginitis
- Drug adverse effects
- Pregnancy
- Increased urine production
  — Metabolic (hyperglycemia, hypercalcemia)
  — Excess fluid intake
  — Volume overload
- Delirium
- Restricted mobility
- Stool impaction
- Psychologic

Data from Resnick NM, Yalla SV. Management of urinary incontinence in the elderly. N Engl J Med 1985;313:800–5.

---

important because anal incontinence and constipation are relatively more common in women with urinary incontinence and pelvic organ prolapse. Certain medical and neurologic conditions (such as diabetes, stroke, and lumbar disc disease) may cause urinary incontinence. A history of hysterectomy, vaginal repair, pelvic radiotherapy, or retropubic surgery should alert the physician to possible effects of prior surgery on the lower urinary tract.

After a history is obtained, patients with urinary incontinence should undergo a physical examination (of the abdomen, pelvis, and rectum), neurologic examination (of the lower thoracic, lumbar, and sacral nerves), direct observation of urine loss (ie, cough stress test), measurement of postvoid residual volume, and urine dipstick test (with urinalysis and a urine culture as indicated), with initial therapy based on these findings. If the patient has symptoms of dysuria, increased urgency, and frequency of acute onset and has urine dipstick test results positive for leukocyte esterase or nitrites, antibiotic treatment is appropriate, and the patient can be reevaluated in several weeks.

A preliminary diagnosis can be made with simple office and laboratory tests, with initial therapy based on these findings. A trial that assessed the outcomes of mid-urethral surgery in women with uncomplicated stress-predominant urinary incontinence revealed no difference in outcomes in women undergoing only a basic office evaluation versus women undergoing such an evaluation with the addition of urodynamic testing; thus, many women may be spared an expensive and uncomfortable evaluation.

If complex conditions are present, the patient does not improve after initial therapy, or surgery is being considered, definitive specialized studies may be necessary. Supplementary evaluation may include the following:

- Blood testing (evaluation of blood urea nitrogen, creatinine, glucose, and calcium)
- Urodynamic testing (uroflowmetry, cystometry, multichannel urodynamics)
- Cystourethroscopy
- Imaging (eg, radiography, ultrasonography, magnetic resonance imaging)

Management

Many individuals with mild symptoms of urinary incontinence depend on barrier management. For women who desire treatment, physicians should offer conservative therapy as first-line treatment for stress urinary incontinence (including behavioral therapy and pessary use) as well as for urgency urinary incontinence (medications, behavioral therapy, bladder training, and some neuromodulation techniques). Surgery is indicated for the treatment of stress urinary incontinence when conservative treatments have failed to satisfactorily relieve the symptoms and the patient wishes further treatment in an effort to achieve continence.

NONSURGICAL INTERVENTIONS

Behavioral therapy—including pelvic floor muscle exercises, bladder training, prompted voiding, fluid management, and stress and urgency strategies—improves symptoms of stress, urge, and mixed incontinence and can be recommended as a conservative treatment in many women. Pelvic floor muscle training appears to be an effective treatment for adult women with stress, urge, and mixed incontinence. Absorbent products are available for use by women undergoing treatment, for women who choose not to have treatment, or for women for whom treatment is ineffective.

Pharmacologic agents, such as oxybutynin, tolterodine, and others, may have some beneficial effect on symptoms of overactive bladder. The use of sacral and posterior tibial nerve neuromodulation, or intradetrusor injections of botulinum toxin may be considered for those women with urge urinary incontinence refractory to medical therapy, behavioral therapy, or both.

SURGICAL INTERVENTIONS

Many surgical treatments have been developed for stress urinary incontinence, but only a few—retropubic colposuspension and sling (pubovaginal and mid-urethral) procedures—have supporting evidence for recommendations. Long-term data suggest that Burch colposuspension and mid-urethral sling procedures have similar objective cure rates; pubovaginal slings have a slightly higher cure rate than the Burch procedure but are associated with more complications. Because of their feasibility as an outpatient procedure, their relative ease of performance, and comparable cure rates with few complications, standard full-length mid-urethral slings (retropubic and transobturator) have evolved into an acceptable first-line surgical option. Recent meta-analyses suggest that outcomes from single-incision mini-slings may not have the same effectiveness. Selection of treatment should be based on patient characteristics, evolving evidence regarding long-term cure and complication rates, and the surgeon's experience.

Bibliography

Abdel-Fattah M, Ford JA, Lim CP, Madhuvrata P. Single-incision mini-slings versus standard midurethral slings in surgical management of female stress urinary incontinence: a meta-analysis of effectiveness and complications. Eur Urol 2011;60: 468–80.

Hooton TM. Clinical practice. Uncomplicated urinary tract infection. N Engl J Med 2012;366:1028–37.

Hunskaar S, Arnold EP, Burgio K, Diokno AC, Herzog AR, Mallett VT. Epidemiology and natural history of urinary incontinence. Int Urogynecol J Pelvic Floor Dysfunct 2000;11:301–19.

Nager CW, Brubaker L, Litman HJ, Zyczynski HM, Varner RE, Amundsen C, et al. A randomized trial of urodynamic testing before stress-incontinence surgery. Urinary Incontinence Treatment Network. N Engl J Med 2012;366:1987–97.

Nygaard I, Barber MD, Burgio KL, Kenton K, Meikle S, Schaffer J, et al. Prevalence of symptomatic pelvic floor disorders in US women. Pelvic Floor Disorders Network. JAMA 2008;300:1311–6.

Nygaard IE, Heit M. Stress urinary incontinence. Obstet Gynecol 2004;104:607–20.

Resnick NM, Yalla SV. Management of urinary incontinence in the elderly. N Engl J Med 1985;313:800–5.

Richter HE, Albo ME, Zyczynski HM, Kenton K, Norton PA, Sirls LT, et al. Retropubic versus transobturator midurethral slings for stress incontinence. Urinary Incontinence Treatment Network. N Engl J Med 2010;362:2066–76.

Subak LL, Brubaker L, Chai TC, Creasman JM, Diokno AC, Goode PS, et al. High costs of urinary incontinence among women electing surgery to treat stress incontinence. Urinary Incontinence Treatment Network. Obstet Gynecol 2008;111:899–907.

The role of cystourethroscopy in the generalist obstetrician-gynecologist practice. ACOG Committee Opinion No. 372. American College of Obstetricians and Gynecologists. Obstet Gynecol 2007;110:221–4.

Urinary incontinence in women. ACOG Practice Bulletin No. 63. American College of Obstetricians and Gynecologists. Obstet Gynecol 2005;105:1533–45.

Resources

American College of Obstetricians and Gynecologists. Urinary incontinence. Patient Education Pamphlet AP081. Washington, DC: American College of Obstetricians and Gynecologists; 2010.

American College of Obstetricians and Gynecologists. Urogynecology: a case management approach [CD-Rom]. Washington, DC: ACOG; 2005.

American Urogynecologic Society. Available at: http://www.augs.org. Retrieved September 20, 2013.

Dumoulin C, Hay-Smith J. Pelvic floor muscle training versus no treatment, or inactive control treatments, for urinary incontinence in women. Cochrane Database of

Systematic Reviews 2010, Issue 1. Art. No.: CD005654. DOI: 10.1002/14651858. CD005654.pub2.

Duthie JB, Vincent M, Herbison GP, Wilson DI, Wilson D. Botulinum toxin injections for adults with overactive bladder syndrome. Cochrane Database of Systematic Reviews 2011, Issue 12. Art. No.: CD005493. DOI: 10.1002/14651858.CD005493. pub3.

Food and Drug Administration. Update on serious complications associated with transvaginal placement of surgical mesh for pelvic organ prolapse: FDA safety communication. Silver Spring (MD): FDA; 2011. Available at: http://www.fda.gov/medicaldevices/safety/alertsandnotices/ucm262435.htm. Retrieved August 15, 2013.

Food and Drug Administration. Urogynecologic surgical mesh implants. Available at: http://www.fda.gov/MedicalDevices/ProductsandMedicalProcedures/Implants andProsthetics/UroGynSurgicalMesh/default.htm. Retrieved September 30, 2013.

Glazener CMA, Lapitan MCM. Urodynamic studies for management of urinary incontinence in children and adults. Cochrane Database of Systematic Reviews 2012, Issue 1. Art. No.: CD003195. DOI: 10.1002/14651858.CD003195.pub2.

Goode PS, Burgio KL, Richter HE, Markland AD. Incontinence in older women. JAMA 2010;303:2172–81.

Hartmann KE, McPheeters ML, Biller DH, Ward RM, McKoy JN, Jerome RN, et al. Treatment of overactive bladder in women. Evidence Report/Technology Assessment No. 187. AHRQ Pub. No. 09-E017. Rockville (MD): Agency for Healthcare Research and Quality; 2009. Available at: http://www.ahrq.gov/research/findings/evidence-based-reports/bladder-evidence-report.pdf. Retrieved September 20, 2013.

Ogah J, Cody JD, Rogerson L. Minimally invasive synthetic suburethral sling operations for stress urinary incontinence in women. Cochrane Database of Systematic Reviews 2009, Issue 4. Art. No.: CD006375. DOI: 10.1002/14651858.CD006375. pub2.

URINARY TRACT INFECTIONS

More than one half of women will have a urinary tract infection (UTI) sometime in their life, which makes it one of the most common bacterial infections in adults. These infections may include asymptomatic bacteriuria, cystitis, or acute pyelonephritis. Cystitis is an infection limited to the lower urinary tract, whereas pyelonephritis, or upper tract infection, includes the renal parenchyma and renal pelvis calyceal system. Risk factors for urinary infection in premenopausal and postmenopausal women are listed in Box 4-12.

A recurrent UTI is defined as either a relapse (infection with the same organism, usually within 2 weeks of completing treatment) or re-infection (infection with a different organism or the same organism after a negative intervening urine culture). Multiple recurrences occur in 3–5% of women. Most recurrences are re-infections rather than relapses. Risk factors for recurrent infection in premenopausal women include frequent intercourse, long-term spermicide use, diaphragm use, a new sexual partner, and young age (less than 15 years) at first UTI. Risk factors for recurrent UTIs in postmenopausal women differ from those in premenopausal women and include urinary incontinence, presence of a cystocele, vulvovaginal atrophy, and abnormal postvoid residual urine.

Evaluation and Diagnosis

Diagnosing UTIs in a timely manner should be within the purview of all women's health care providers. A woman with acute bacterial cystitis will typically present with symptoms, including painful voiding, frequency, and urgent urination; she also may report suprapubic pain or pressure, hematuria, or discoloration of urine. Bacteriuria (whether asymptomatic or associated with symptoms) is diagnosed with a clean-catch midstream urine sample. Leukocyte esterase or nitrite testing on urine dipstick is a reasonable screening test, but sensitivity is only 75%, so false-negatives may be common. If bacteriuria is accompanied by fever, chills, flank pain, or costovertebral angle tenderness on examination, acute pyelonephritis is likely.

Urine culture is not necessary in all women with acute cystitis but should be performed if the diagnosis is unclear, if there is no clinical improvement

---

Box 4-12. Risk Factors for Urinary Tract Infection in Premenopausal and Postmenopausal Women

Premenopausal Women
- History of urinary tract infection
- Frequent or recent sexual activity
- Diaphragm use
- Use of spermicidal agents
- Increasing parity
- Diabetes mellitus
- Obesity
- Sickle cell trait
- Anatomic congenital abnormalities
- Urinary tract calculi
- Neurologic disorders or medical conditions that require indwelling or repetitive bladder catheterization

Postmenopausal Women
- Vaginal atrophy
- Incomplete bladder emptying
- Poor perineal hygiene
- Pelvic organ prolapse
- Lifetime history of urinary tract infection
- Type 1 diabetes mellitus

Modified from Treatment of urinary tract infections in nonpregnant women. ACOG Practice Bulletin No. 91. American College of Obstetricians and Gynecologists. Obstet Gynecol 2008;111:785–94.

within 48 hours of treatment, in the case of recurrence, and in all cases of upper tract infection. Women with frequent recurrences and prior confirmation by diagnostic tests who are aware of their symptoms may be empirically treated without recurrent testing for pyuria.

Management

Screening for and treatment of asymptomatic bacteriuria is not recommended in nonpregnant, premenopausal women. Asymptomatic bacteriuria has not been shown to be harmful in this population, nor does treatment of asymptomatic bacteriuria decrease the frequency of symptomatic infections.

Treatment of acute cystitis that is uncomplicated (ie, no underlying anatomic issue or medical condition) can be accomplished with 3-day therapy. Numerous studies have shown that 3-day antimicrobial regimens are usually as effective and better tolerated than longer treatment in premenopausal and postmenopausal women. Single-dose therapy is considered less effective and should be reserved only for the lowest-risk women. Recommended agents and dosages for uncomplicated acute bacterial cystitis are listed in Table 4-6. Treatment of complicated UTIs (eg, in patients with diabetes mellitus, abnormal anatomy, prior urologic surgery, a history of renal stones, an indwelling catheter, spinal cord injury, immunocompromise, or in pregnant patients) requires a 7–10-day course of antibiotics.

Pyelonephritis can be treated on an outpatient basis in healthy women who can tolerate oral medication and fluids. Standard therapy is 14 days (total) of oral or parenteral antibiotics; improvement in symptoms should be noted by 48–72 hours after initiating therapy. If the patient is not able to tolerate liquids or medication by mouth, hospital admission is required for intravenous hydration and antibiotics. Regardless of route of antibiotics, urine culture should be obtained before treatment. A urine culture test of cure usually is performed when the 2-week course of antibiotics is completed.

A major consequence of indiscriminate prescribing practices of common antibiotics is the emergence of antimicrobial resistance. Data from areas reporting antimicrobial susceptibility profiles have shown an alarming increase in the prevalence of resistance to amoxicillin and trimethoprim–

sulfamethoxazole. Health care providers should be aware of community-specific or hospital-specific resistance data, and susceptibility testing should be used when needed to determine the choice of antibiotic. *Escherichia coli*

Table 4-6. Recommended First-Line Treatment Regimens for Uncomplicated Acute Bacterial Cystitis*

Treatment	Dosage	Adverse Events
Trimethoprim and sulfamethoxazole	One tablet (160-mg trimethoprim and 800-mg sulfamethoxazole) twice daily for 3 days	Fever, rash, photosensitivity, neutropenia, thrombocytopenia, anorexia, nausea and vomiting, pruritus, headache, urticaria, Stevens–Johnson syndrome, and toxic epidermal necrosis
Trimethoprim	100 mg, twice daily for 3 days	Rash, pruritus, photosensitivity, exfoliative dermatitis, Stevens–Johnson syndrome, toxic epidermal necrosis, and aseptic meningitis
Nitrofurantoin macrocrystals	50–100 mg, four times daily for 7 days	Anorexia, nausea, vomiting, hypersensitivity, peripheral neuropathy, hepatitis, hemolytic anemia, and pulmonary reactions
Nitrofurantoin monohydrate macrocrystals	100 mg, twice daily for 7 days	Same as for nitrofurantoin macrocrystals
Fosfomycin tromethamine	3-g dose (powder) single dose	Diarrhea, nausea, vomiting, rash, and hypersensitivity

*The 2010 Infectious Diseases Society of America guidelines for the treatment of acute uncomplicated cystitis recommend these as first-line antimicrobial treatment agents. The guidelines recommend reserving use of ciprofloxacin, levofloxacin, and norfloxacin for treatment of other important conditions, and thus consider these second-line antimicrobial treatment agents for acute uncomplicated bacterial cystitis.

Data from Gupta K, Hooton TM, Naber KG, Wullt B, Colgan R, Miller LG, et al. International clinical practice guidelines for the treatment of acute uncomplicated cystitis and pyelonephritis in women: A 2010 update by the Infectious Diseases Society of America and the European Society for Microbiology and Infectious Diseases. Infectious Diseases Society of America. European Society for Microbiology and Infectious Diseases. Clin Infect Dis 2011;52:e103–20 *and* Treatment of urinary tract infections in nonpregnant women. ACOG Practice Bulletin No. 91. American College of Obstetricians and Gynecologists. Obstet Gynecol 2008;111:785–94.

has been shown to be the causative pathogen in more than 80% of women. Other common pathogens include *Staphylococcus saprophyticus, Klebsiella pneumoniae, Enterococcus,* and *Proteus mirabilis.*

Recurrent UTIs can result in high utilization of health care services and frustration for the patient. In addition to lifestyle changes and reducing the use of spermicides, continuous prophylaxis for 6–12 months with once-nightly antibiotic treatment is reasonable. Postcoital prophylaxis with a single dose of a single agent also might decrease recurrences.

Bibliography

Gupta K, Hooton TM, Naber KG, Wullt B, Colgan R, Miller LG, et al. International clinical practice guidelines for the treatment of acute uncomplicated cystitis and pyelonephritis in women: A 2010 update by the Infectious Diseases Society of America and the European Society for Microbiology and Infectious Diseases. Infectious Diseases Society of America. European Society for Microbiology and Infectious Diseases. Clin Infect Dis 2011;52:e103–20.

Treatment of urinary tract infections in nonpregnant women. ACOG Practice Bulletin No. 91. American College of Obstetricians and Gynecologists. Obstet Gynecol 2008;111:785–94.

Resources

American College of Obstetricians and Gynecologists. Urinary tract infections. ACOG Patient Education Pamphlet AP050. Washington, DC: ACOG; 2008.

American College of Obstetricians and Gynecologists. Urogynecology: a case management approach [CD-ROM]. Washington, DC: ACOG; 2005.

American Urogynecologic Society. Available at: http://www.augs.org. Retrieved August 15, 2013.

Infectious Diseases Society of America. Infections by organ system: genitourinary. Available at: http://www.idsociety.org/Organ_System/#Genitourinary. Retrieved August 15, 2013.

Jepson RG, Williams G, Craig JC. Cranberries for preventing urinary tract infections. Cochrane Database of Systematic Reviews 2012, Issue 10. Art. No.: CD001321. DOI: 10.1002/14651858.CD001321.pub5.

INFERTILITY

Approximately 12% of women of childbearing age in the United States have received infertility services (including counseling and diagnosis) in their lifetime. Infertility affects women and men and typically is defined as the inability to achieve pregnancy within 1 year of appropriately timed, unprotected intercourse or therapeutic donor insemination. According to the American Society for Reproductive Medicine, earlier evaluation and treatment is recommended for women older than 35 years who fail to conceive after 6 months of unprotected intercourse and may be warranted in other women based on medical history or physical findings (such as a history of oligomenorrhea or amenorrhea; known or suspected uterine, tubal, or peritoneal disease or stage III to stage IV endometriosis; or known or suspected male subfertility). It has long been recognized that infertility increases with advancing age. As today's society emphasizes delay of childbearing, not only are many couples who seek fertility services older, they also have acquired diseases and maintained lifestyles that can adversely affect their fertility. These factors, which include endometriosis, sexually transmitted infections, smoking, and obesity, compound the naturally decreasing fertility associated with age.

Three major potential etiologic factors are assessed to uncover the causes of infertility: 1) male factor dysfunction, 2) ovulation dysfunction, and 3) female anatomic abnormalities. Although the specific causes of infertility differ depending on the population studied, in general, one third of infertility is due to female factors alone, one third is due to male factors alone, and the remaining third either is due to a combination of male and female problems or remains unexplained after evaluation. It is common for couples to have more than one cause of infertility. If so, earlier and more aggressive treatment may be indicated.

It is important for health care providers to understand and accept the emotional and educational needs and demands of patients with infertility.

Physicians should appraise their own interests, personality, training, and experience and be prepared to refer patients to subspecialists when appropriate. A team approach is frequently helpful in ensuring that patients receive an adequate evaluation and appropriate counseling. Counseling of patients with infertility who are treated with assisted reproductive technologies (ART) should include, among other things, information regarding the risk of multiple gestation; the ethical issues surrounding multifetal pregnancy reduction; and obstetric and neonatal risks; as well as alternatives to ART, including adoption. In addition, clinicians should be familiar with any state laws regarding infertility services and treatment or insurance coverage.

Supporting services for couples with infertility may include the following:

- Reproductive endocrinology
- Assisted reproductive technologies
  — In vitro fertilization
  — Intracytoplasmic sperm injection
  — Donors (oocyte, sperm, embryo)
  — Gestational carriers and surrogate mothers
  — Preimplantation genetic testing
  — Oocyte cryopreservation (for women facing infertility that is due to chemotherapy or gonadotoxic therapies and for couples who are unable to cryopreserve embryos)
- Psychologic support
- Legal assistance and support
- Urologic and andrology services
- Adoption agencies
- Infertility support groups
- Family counseling

Bibliography

Adoption. ACOG Committee Opinion No. 528. American College of Obstetricians and Gynecologists. Obstet Gynecol 2012;119:1320–4.

Aging and infertility in women. Practice Committee of the American Society for Reproductive Medicine. Fertil Steril 2006;86:S248–52.

Centers for Disease Control and Prevention, American Society for Reproductive Medicine, Society for Assisted Reproductive Technology. 2011 Assisted Reproductive Technology Fertility Clinic Success Rates Report. Atlanta (GA): U.S. Department of Health and Human Services; 2013. Available at: http://www.cdc.gov/ART/ART2011/. Retrieved January 17, 2014.

Definitions of infertility and recurrent pregnancy loss: a committee opinion. Practice Committee of American Society for Reproductive Medicine. Fertil Steril 2013;99:63.

Diagnostic evaluation of the infertile female: a committee opinion. Practice Committee of American Society for Reproductive Medicine. Fertil Steril 2012;98:302–7.

Effectiveness and treatment for unexplained infertility. Practice Committee of the American Society for Reproductive Medicine. Fertil Steril 2006;86:S111–4.

Elements to be considered in obtaining informed consent for ART. Practice Committee of the American Society for Reproductive Medicine. Practice Committee of the Society for Assisted Reproductive Technology. Fertil Steril 2006;86:S272–3.

Endometriosis and infertility. Practice Committee of the American Society for Reproductive Medicine. Fertil Steril 2006;86:S156–60.

Female age-related fertility decline. Committee Opinion No. 589. American College of Obstetricians and Gynecologists. Obstet Gynecol 2014;123:719–21.

Macaluso M, Wright-Schnapp TJ, Chandra A, Johnson R, Satterwhite CL, Pulver A, et al. A public health focus on infertility prevention, detection, and management. Fertil Steril 2010;93:16.e1–10.

Multifetal pregnancy reduction. Committee Opinion No. 553. American College of Obstetricians and Gynecologists. Obstet Gynecol 2013;121:405–10.

Obesity and reproduction: an educational bulletin. Practice Committee of American Society for Reproductive Medicine. Fertil Steril 2008;90:S21–9.

Oocyte cryopreservation. Committee Opinion No. 584. American College of Obstetricians and Gynecologists. Obstet Gynecol 2014;123:221–2.

Perinatal risks associated with assisted reproductive technology. ACOG Committee Opinion No. 324. American College of Obstetricians and Gynecologists. Obstet Gynecol 2005;106:1143–6.

Reddy UM, Wapner RJ, Rebar RW, Tasca RJ. Infertility, assisted reproductive technology, and adverse pregnancy outcomes: executive summary of a National Institute of Child Health and Human Development workshop. Obstet Gynecol 2007;109:967–77.

Smoking and infertility: a committee opinion. Practice Committee of the American Society for Reproductive Medicine. Fertil Steril 2012;98:1400–6.

Resources

American College of Obstetricians and Gynecologists. Evaluating infertility. Patient Education Pamphlet AP136. Washington, DC: American College of Obstetricians and Gynecologists; 2012.

American College of Obstetricians and Gynecologists. Treating infertility. Patient Education Pamphlet AP137. Washington, DC: American College of Obstetricians and Gynecologists; 2012.

American Society for Reproductive Medicine. Adoption: a guide for patients. Birmingham (AL): ASRM; 2006. Available at: http://www.asrm.org/uploadedFiles/ASRM_Content/Resources/Patient_Resources/Fact_Sheets_and_Info_Booklets/adoption.pdf. Retrieved August 12, 2013.

American Society for Reproductive Medicine. Fact sheets and info booklets. Available at:http://www.reproductivefacts.org/FactSheetsandBooklets. Retrieved August 12, 2013.

Criteria for number of embryos to transfer: a committee opinion. Practice Committee of the American Society for Reproductive Medicine. Practice Committee of Society for Assisted Reproductive Technology. Fertil Steril 2013;99:44–6.

RESOLVE: The National Infertility Association. Available at: http://www.resolve.org. Retrieved August 12, 2013.

EARLY PREGNANCY COMPLICATIONS

The management of early pregnancy complications is within the purview of obstetrician–gynecologists and other providers of women's health care. Clinicians should be aware of local hospital rules and regulations and requirements of their professional liability insurance carrier as to whether this is viewed as obstetric or gynecologic care. The American College of Obstetricians and Gynecologists considers early pregnancy complications to be within the definition of gynecology. Management of conditions such as ectopic pregnancy and spontaneous and induced abortion, including early second-trimester abortion, often are included in such a practice. Liability insurance should cover this role of gynecologists in the management of such early pregnancy-related conditions.

Early Pregnancy Loss

Early pregnancy loss is defined as a nonviable intrauterine pregnancy at less than 13 weeks of gestation. It is the most common complication of the first trimester of pregnancy. Early pregnancy loss is unrelated to induced abortion procedures. In the first trimester, the terms miscarriage, spontaneous abortion, and early pregnancy loss are all used interchangeably, and there is no consensus on terminology in the literature. Later in pregnancy, losses are categorized as either early fetal death (20–27 weeks of gestation) or late fetal death (28 weeks of gestation and later). The term stillbirth also is used to describe fetal deaths at 20 weeks of gestation or more. These types of losses are not addressed in this section.

ETIOLOGY, RISK FACTORS, AND COMPLICATIONS

The most frequent cause of early pregnancy loss is fetal genetic abnormalities. Other rare but possible causes for early pregnancy loss include infection, maternal hormonal factors, immune responses, and serious medical disease of the mother. Among clinically established pregnancies, the rate of early pregnancy loss is approximately 10–20%; it usually occurs between the 7th week and 12th week of pregnancy. Once fetal heart tones are determined, the risk of miscarriage decreases. Overall, 50–60% of early pregnancy losses occur as a result of fetal chromosomal abnormalities, with most of these chromosomal abnormalities or variations occurring as random events. The most common finding is triploid aneuploidy.

The risk of early pregnancy loss is higher in women older than 35 years, in women with systemic diseases, in women undergoing fertility treatment, and in women with a history of repeated early pregnancy losses. Complications of early pregnancy loss are rare but include excessive blood loss, retained fetal tissue, and infection.

DIAGNOSIS AND MANAGEMENT

Possible symptoms of early pregnancy loss include lower back or abdominal pain, vaginal bleeding, abdominal cramps, or tissue that passes from the vagina. In addition to evaluation of the patient's medical history and signs and symptoms, an evaluation to diagnose early pregnancy loss may include the following:

- Interpretation of serum human chorionic gonadotropin (hCG) measurements
- Interpretation of endovaginal ultrasonography
- Interpretation of serum progesterone concentrations
- Physical examination

If an early pregnancy loss occurs, it is important to determine whether any fetal or placental tissue remains in the uterus. Management options for early pregnancy loss may include the following:

- Expectant management and observation
- Uterine curettage
- Medical treatment with misoprostol

- Review of histopathology
- Evaluation to determine causes of recurrent pregnancy loss (see also the "Recurrent Pregnancy Loss" section later in Part 4)
- Grief counseling, as indicated

If any remaining tissue is not passed in a reasonable amount of time, uterine curettage or medical treatment with misoprostol can be used to complete the abortion. Clinicians should be familiar with any state requirements regarding the reporting of fetal death and the disposal of fetal remains.

Ectopic Pregnancy

More than 100,000 ectopic pregnancies occur in the United States every year. Because many patients are now treated in the office, the actual number may be difficult to determine; however, it probably represents approximately 2% of all pregnancies. The number of deaths from ectopic pregnancy has dropped during the past decade. However, it is still the fourth leading cause of maternal mortality in this country.

RISK FACTORS

Because ectopic pregnancy can be life-threatening, women with known risk factors for ectopic pregnancy should seek care early in the gestation to ensure that it is a normal intrauterine gestation. Risk factors for ectopic pregnancy include the following:

- Advanced maternal age
- Prior treatment for infertility
- Pelvic infection
- Previous tubal surgery, including tubal occlusion
- Previous ectopic pregnancy

Most women who have an ectopic pregnancy are unaware of any risk factors and seek care when they experience pain or bleeding.

DIAGNOSIS AND MANAGEMENT

In addition to obtaining a medical history and evaluating signs and symptoms, the evaluation to diagnose an ectopic pregnancy may include the following:

- Interpretation of serum hCG measurements
- Interpretation of transvaginal ultrasonography
- Interpretation of serum progesterone concentrations
- Surgical procedures such as endometrial biopsy, dilation and curettage
- Culdocentesis, laparoscopy, or laparotomy

Ectopic pregnancy is suspected in the presence of the following:

- Hemoperitoneum in the first trimester
- Abnormally low hCG levels or low hCG levels with incremental increases that do not rise appropriately
- Ultrasonography that reveals an empty uterus when the hCG value is above the discriminatory zone, or a gestational sac outside the endometrial cavity

An ectopic pregnancy is confirmed when it can be visualized either laparoscopically or by ultrasonography.

The goal of early diagnosis is to treat the patient before the ectopic pregnancy ruptures and the patient presents as a surgical emergency. Treatment options for ectopic pregnancy include the following:

- Expectant management and observation
- Chemotherapy
- Surgery

The choice of therapy must take into consideration the skill of the clinician and his or her experience with the treatment modalities. One must consider the reproductive desires of the patient and use good clinical judgment in determining whether expectant management is appropriate for select ectopic pregnancies that show signs of possible spontaneous resolution. Intramuscular methotrexate is appropriate for the treatment of selected patients with small, unruptured tubal pregnancies who can be expected to present reliably for posttreatment follow-up. Patients need to be carefully monitored, and successful treatment may require more than one dose of methotrexate. Although expectant management of an ectopic pregnancy is not ideal in most circumstances, there may be a role for it when hCG levels are low and falling.

Molar Pregnancy

A molar pregnancy, also called a hydatidiform mole, is an abnormal pregnancy characterized by the presence of an abnormal growth of cells originating from the placenta. Molar pregnancy is a form of gestational trophoblastic disease that often is diagnosed in the first trimester or early second trimester of pregnancy. The incidence of molar pregnancy is approximately 1 in 1,000 pregnancies, and it is more common in women of Southeast Asian origin. The clinical presentation of a molar pregnancy is similar to other forms of failed pregnancies and can include abnormal bleeding, uterine enlargement greater than expected for gestational age, and absent fetal heart tones. See the "Cancer Diagnosis and Management" section earlier in Part 4 for a description of the management of molar pregnancy.

Bibliography

American Academy of Pediatrics, American College of Obstetricians and Gynecologists. Standard terminology for reporting of reproductive health statistics in the United States: appendix F. Guidelines for perinatal care. 7th ed. Elk Grove Village (IL): Washington, DC: AAP; American College of Obstetricians and Gynecologists; 2012. p. 497–512.

American Cancer Society. What are the key statistics about gestational trophoblastic disease? Available at: http://www.cancer.org/cancer/gestationaltrophoblasticdisease/detailedguide/gestational-trophoblastic-disease-key-statistics. Retrieved August 9, 2013.

Bianco K, Caughey AB, Shaffer BL, Davis R, Norton ME. History of miscarriage and increased incidence of fetal aneuploidy in subsequent pregnancy. Obstet Gynecol 2006;107:1098–102.

Diagnosis and treatment of gestational trophoblastic disease. ACOG Practice Bulletin No. 53. American College of Obstetricians and Gynecologists. Obstet Gynecol 2004;103:1365–77.

Medical management of ectopic pregnancy. ACOG Practice Bulletin No. 94. American College of Obstetricians and Gynecologists. Obstet Gynecol 2008;111:1479–85.

Medical treatment of ectopic pregnancy. Practice Committee of American Society for Reproductive Medicine. Fertil Steril 2008;90:S206–12.

Murphy SL, Xu J, Kochanek KD. Deaths: final data for 2010. Natl Vital Stat Rep 2013;61(4):1–168. Available at: http://www.cdc.gov/nchs/data/nvsr/nvsr61/nvsr 61_04.pdf. September 20, 2013.

National Institute for Health and Care Excellence. Ectopic pregnancy and miscarriage: diagnosis and initial management in early pregnancy of ectopic pregnancy and miscarriage. NICE Clinical Guideline 154. Manchester (UK): NICE; 2012. Available at: http://www.nice.org.uk/guidance/CG154. Retrieved July 14, 2014.

Professional liability and gynecology-only practice. Committee Opinion No. 567. American College of Obstetricians and Gynecologists. Obstet Gynecol 2013;122:186.

Soares PD, Maesta I, Costa OL, Charry RC, Dias A, Rudge MV. Geographical distribution and demographic characteristics of gestational trophoblastic disease. J Reprod Med 2010;55:305–10.

Resources

American College of Obstetricians and Gynecologists. Early pregnancy loss: miscarriage and molar pregnancy. Patient Education Pamphlet AP090. Washington, DC: American College of Obstetricians and Gynecologists; 2013.

American College of Obstetricians and Gynecologists. Ectopic pregnancy. ACOG Patient Education Pamphlet AP155. Washington, DC: ACOG; 2009.

Misoprostol for postabortion care. ACOG Committee Opinion No. 427. American College of Obstetricians and Gynecologists. Obstet Gynecol 2009;113:465–8.

Resolve Through Sharing: Bereavement Services. Gundersen Health System. Available at: http://www.bereavementservices.org/resolve-through-sharing. Retrieved August 9, 2013.

RESOLVE: The National Infertility Association. Available at: http://www.resolve.org. Retrieved August 9, 2013.

RECURRENT PREGNANCY LOSS

Recurrent pregnancy loss, defined by the American Society for Reproductive Medicine as two or more pregnancy losses, occurs in approximately 1% of women who desire to bear children. Thus, patients with two or more spontaneous abortions are candidates for an evaluation to determine the cause, if any, for their pregnancy losses.

Recurrent early pregnancy loss can be a difficult and frustrating problem for patients and clinicians. The following factors should be considered in the evaluation of women with recurrent pregnancy loss:

- Characteristics of prior pregnancy losses
- Exposure to toxins and drugs
- Genetic abnormalities
- Pelvic infections
- Endocrine or metabolic dysfunction
- Immunologic disorders
- Uterine abnormalities
- Psychologic stress of the associated loss
- Age of the patient

For couples with recurrent pregnancy loss, it is reasonable to offer a basic evaluation. Tests commonly offered to couples with recurrent pregnancy loss are as follows:

- Karyotyping of both partners to look for balanced chromosome abnormalities
- Hysterosalpingography, ultrasonography, sonohysterography, or hysteroscopy to look for uterine abnormalities

Couples affected by balanced translocations should be counseled regarding the risk of recurring spontaneous abortion, offered prenatal genetic studies, and offered the use of newer assisted reproductive technologies in future pregnancies. Corrective surgery for uterine defects may be reasonable when such defects appear to interfere with implantation or pregnancy growth.

Other appropriate tests may depend on the timing of the pregnancy loss. For example, antibody testing for antiphospholipid syndrome (lupus anticoagulant, anticardiolipin, and anti-β_2-glycoprotein I antibody testing) are not indicated in most cases of fetal loss. Obstetric indications for antiphospholipid antibody testing include a history of one unexplained loss of a morphologically normal fetus at or beyond the 10th week of gestation or of three or more unexplained consecutive spontaneous pregnancy losses before the 10th week of pregnancy (with maternal anatomic or hormonal abnormalities and paternal and maternal chromosomal causes excluded).

Testing for inherited thrombophilias in women who have experienced recurrent fetal loss in the first trimester is not recommended because it is unclear if anticoagulation therapy reduces recurrence. However, tests for thrombophilia should be considered in cases of otherwise unexplained fetal death in the second trimester or third trimester. Some of the older evaluations and treatments of recurrent pregnancy loss have been based on poorly designed clinical studies and unproven hypotheses. Patients and physicians in search of a solution have sometimes explored less-well-accepted etiologies and empirical or alternative treatments. Although the assessment of luteal phase progesterone production or effect is firmly entrenched in the traditional evaluation of recurrent pregnancy loss, the evidence that supports this is scant. Treatment for luteal phase defect is of unproven efficacy. Cultures for bacteria or viruses and tests for glucose intolerance, antibodies to infectious agents, antinuclear antibodies, paternal human leukocyte antigen status, and maternal antipaternal antibodies are not beneficial. Immunoglobulin and paternal leukocyte therapies are not effective in preventing recurrent pregnancy loss and are no longer routinely recommended in the evaluation of women with recurrent pregnancy loss. There is conflicting literature regarding the role of thyroid abnormalities in recurrent pregnancy loss.

It now appears that more than 50% of couples who complete evaluation will not have an identifiable cause. Informative and supportive counseling plays an important role and may lead to the best pregnancy outcomes. Couples with unexplained recurrent pregnancy loss should be counseled regarding the potential for successful pregnancy without treatment.

Bibliography

Antiphospholipid syndrome. Practice Bulletin No. 132. American College of Obstetricians and Gynecologists. Obstet Gynecol 2012;120:1514–21.

Definitions of infertility and recurrent pregnancy loss: a committee opinion. Practice Committee of American Society for Reproductive Medicine. Fertil Steril 2013;99:63.

Inherited thrombophilias in pregnancy. Practice Bulletin No. 138. American College of Obstetricians and Gynecologists. Obstet Gynecol 2013;122:706–17.

Intravenous immunoglobulin (IVIG) and recurrent spontaneous pregnancy loss. Practice Committee of the American Society for Reproductive Medicine. Fertil Steril 2006;86:S226–7.

Resources

American College of Obstetricians and Gynecologists. Repeated miscarriage. Patient Education Pamphlet AP100. Washington, DC: American College of Obstetricians and Gynecologists; 2013.

Family history as a risk assessment tool. Committee Opinion No. 478. American College of Obstetricians and Gynecologists. Obstet Gynecol 2011;117:747–50.

Preimplantation genetic screening for aneuploidy. ACOG Committee Opinion No. 430. American College of Obstetricians and Gynecologists. Obstet Gynecol 2009;113:766–7.

RESOLVE: The National Infertility Association. Available at: http://www.resolve.org. Retrieved August 9, 2013.

INDUCED ABORTION

The medical definition of abortion is the interruption of pregnancy after nidation (the intrauterine implantation of a fertilized egg). According to data compiled by the Guttmacher Institute, approximately 1.21 million legal induced abortions were performed in the United States in 2008, which is 8% fewer than in 2000. The abortion ratio (the number of abortions per 1,000 live births) and the abortion rate (the number of abortions per 1,000 women aged 15–44 years) have decreased from 1990 to 2005 and remained stable through 2008. Women who obtain legal induced abortions are predominantly white, young, and unmarried.

Access to Care

Termination of pregnancy before viability is a medical matter between the patient and the physician, subject to the physician's clinical judgment, the patient's informed consent, relevant state and federal laws, and the availability of appropriate facilities. The American College of Obstetricians and Gynecologists (the College) supports access to care for all individuals and the availability of all reproductive options, irrespective of financial status. If a termination is chosen, it should be performed safely and as early as possible. The College opposes unnecessary regulations that limit or delay access to care (see also the College's Abortion Policy statement at www.acog.org/Resources_And_Publications/Statements_of_Policy_List).

Legal Issues

Induced abortion remains one of the most regulated medical procedures in the United States. Although the U.S. Supreme Court has determined that state bans on abortion are unconstitutional, it has upheld many state laws that make abortion services less accessible. These laws include specific physician and hospital requirements, gestational age limits, restrictions on use of state funds and private insurance, waiting periods, required parental involvement, specialized facility requirements, and mandatory information requirements. Physicians should be aware of relevant federal and state abortion regulations.

Timing

According to the Centers for Disease Control and Prevention, approximately 64% of abortions are performed before 63 days gestation. Circumstances that can lead to second-trimester abortion include delays in suspecting and testing for pregnancy, delay in obtaining insurance or other funding, and delay in obtaining referral, as well as difficulties in locating and traveling to a health care provider. Poverty, lower education level, and having multiple disruptive life events have been associated with higher rates of seeking second-trimester abortion. In addition, major anatomic or genetic anomalies may be detected in the fetus in the second trimester and women may choose to terminate their pregnancies. Some obstetric and medical indications for second-trimester termination include preeclampsia and preterm premature rupture of membranes, among other conditions.

Methods

Methods of induced abortion include suction (or vacuum) curettage, dilation and evacuation (D&E), medical abortion, and labor-inducing abortion. The type of abortion method chosen depends on several factors, including gestational age, patient health, patient preference, and health care provider experience. Options for first-trimester abortion include suction curettage and medical abortion. Second-trimester abortion methods include D&E, medical abortion, and labor-inducing abortion.

Suction curettage uses cervical dilation (if necessary) followed by a suction device to remove the contents of the uterus. Dilation and evacuation involves cervical dilation followed by the use of grasping forceps to remove the fetus; a final suction curettage often is performed to ensure that the fetus is completely evacuated. Medical abortion involves the use of medications, such as mifepristone and misoprostol, rather than a procedure to induce an abortion. It typically is performed up to 63 days of gestation (calculated from the first day of the last menstrual period), although medical abortion may be used to terminate pregnancies beyond this time. Methods of labor-inducing abortion include the use of one or more of the following: prostaglandin analogues, mifepristone, osmotic cervical dilators, Foley catheters, and oxytocin.

Complications

The mortality rate associated with abortion is low (0.6 per 100,000 legal, induced abortions), and the risk of death associated with childbirth is approximately 14 times higher than that with abortion. Abortion-related mortality increases with each week of gestation, with a rate of 0.1 per 100,000 procedures at 8 weeks of gestation or less, and 8.9 per 100,000 procedures at 21 weeks of gestation or greater. Complications associated with suction curettage, D&E, and medical abortion include infection, hemorrhage, cervical laceration, retained products of conception, and failed abortion (ie, ongoing pregnancy). Uterine perforation can occur with suction curettage and D&E, whereas uterine rupture can occur with medical abortion and labor-inducing abortion.

Patient Counseling

Clinicians are not required to perform abortions. However, they should be prepared to counsel patients fully on their options and to manage complications of induced abortions, as needed. Before an abortion, a patient who is undecided should be counseled on her options for the pregnancy. The patient should be fully informed in a balanced manner about all options, including raising the child herself, placing the child for adoption, and abortion. The information conveyed should be appropriate to the gestational age and must be delivered without personal bias.

The woman should make a firm decision that she wants an abortion before she decides on the abortion technique. Methods that are appropriate based on gestational age and patient health should be discussed, including information about the possible complications associated with each technique. Clinicians should address patient concerns about common misconceptions about abortion. Specifically, patients should be informed that the available evidence concludes that induced abortion is not associated with an increase in breast cancer risk, nor is a patient at increased risk of regret, depression, or infertility after an abortion. Contraceptive counseling is important. The clinician also should evaluate the patient's available psychosocial support and refer her to counseling or other supportive services, as appropriate.

Evaluation and Management

A comprehensive evaluation should be performed before induced abortion and includes the following:

- Complete medical history
- Thorough physical examination
- Screening for vaginitis and sexually transmitted infections, as indicated
- Appropriate laboratory testing, as indicated
  - Pregnancy test
  - Rh determination
  - Complete blood count
- Ultrasonography, as indicated, to diagnose pregnancy, establish gestational age, and localize the placenta, if indicated
- Consideration for cervical preparation
- Prophylactic antibiotics (for suction curettage or D&E)
- Completion of appropriate paperwork and consent forms, as required by state, hospital, and facility

Clinicians who perform abortions in their offices, clinics, or freestanding ambulatory care facilities should have a plan to provide prompt emergency services if a complication occurs and should establish a mechanism for transferring patients who require emergency treatment. Routine pathologic examination of tissue is not necessary after an induced abortion via suction curettage or D&E in which embryonic or fetal parts can be identified with certainty. In such instances, a description of the gross products of conception should be recorded. The United States has no national system for the mandatory reporting of induced termination of pregnancy. However, state health departments vary greatly in approaches to the compilation of these data, and clinicians should be aware of any such reporting requirements.

The following postprocedure care should be provided:

- Immunoprophylaxis with anti-D immune globulin for women who are RhD-negative

- Counseling on signs of hemorrhage, uterine perforation, retained tissue, infection, and failed abortion, as appropriate

- Psychologic or other support service consultation, as indicated

- Provision of contraception, if desired; except for hysteroscopic sterilization, diaphragm, or cervical cap, all forms of contraception can be considered after abortion and initiated on the day of the procedure; however, intrauterine devices should not be inserted in the case of immediate postseptic abortion (see also the "Family Planning" section in Part 3).

Clinical training curricula and additional policy guidelines for abortion care are available from the National Abortion Federation (see Resources).

Bibliography

Abortion access and training. ACOG Committee Opinion No. 424. American College of Obstetricians and Gynecologists. Obstet Gynecol 2009;113:247–50.

American College of Obstetricians and Gynecologists. Abortion policy. College Statement of Policy. Washington, DC: American College of Obstetricians and Gynecologists;2011.Availableat:http://www.acog.org/Resources_And_Publications/Statements_of_Policy_List. Retrieved September 24, 2013.

American College of Obstetricians and Gynecologists. Legislative interference with patient care, medical decisions, and the patient–physician relationship. College Statement of Policy. Washington, DC: American College of Obstetricians and Gynecologists;2013.Availableat:http://www.acog.org/Resources_And_Publications/Statements_of_Policy_List. Retrieved September 24, 2013.

Antibiotic prophylaxis for gynecologic procedures. ACOG Practice Bulletin No. 104. American College of Obstetricians and Gynecologists. Obstet Gynecol 2009; 113:1180–9.

Bartlett LA, Berg CJ, Shulman HB, Zane SB, Green CA, Whitehead S, et al. Risk factors for legal induced abortion-related mortality in the United States. Obstet Gynecol 2004;103:729–37.

Grimes DA. Risks of mifepristone abortion in context [editorial]. Contraception 2005;71:161.

Guttmacher Institute. Abortion. Available at: http://www.guttmacher.org/sections/abortion.php. Retrieved August 15, 2013.

Induced abortion and breast cancer risk. ACOG Committee Opinion No. 434. American College of Obstetricians and Gynecologists. Obstet Gynecol 2009;113: 1417–8.

Jones RK, Kooistra K. Abortion incidence and access to services in the United States, 2008. Perspect Sex Reprod Health 2011;43:41–50.

Jones RK, Zolna MR, Henshaw SK, Finer LB. Abortion in the United States: incidence and access to services, 2005. Perspect Sex Reprod Health 2008;40:6–16.

Medical management of first-trimester abortion. Practice Bulletin No. 143. American College of Obstetricians and Gynecologists. Obstet Gynecol 2014;123:676–92.

Pazol K, Creanga AA, Zane SB, Burley KD, Jamieson DJ. Abortion surveillance—United States, 2009. Centers for Disease Control and Prevention. MMWR Surveill Summ 2012;61:1–44.

Raymond EG, Grimes DA. The comparative safety of legal induced abortion and childbirth in the United States. Obstet Gynecol 2012;119:215–9.

Second-trimester abortion. Practice Bulletin No. 135. American College of Obstetricians and Gynecologists. Obstet Gynecol 2013;121:1394–1406.

U S. Medical Eligibility Criteria for Contraceptive Use, 2010. Centers for Disease Control and Prevention. MMWR Recomm Rep 2010;59(RR-4):1–86.

Update to CDC's U.S. Medical Eligibility Criteria for Contraceptive Use, 2010: revised recommendations for the use of contraceptive methods during the postpartum period. Centers for Disease Control and Prevention. MMWR Morb Mortal Wkly Rep 2011;60:878–83.

Resources

American College of Obstetricians and Gynecologists. Induced abortion. Patient Education Pamphlet AP043. Washington, DC: American College of Obstetricians and Gynecologists; 2011.

Association of Reproductive Health Professionals. Reproductive health topics: abortion. Available at: http://www.arhp.org/topics/abortion. Retrieved August 15, 2013.

National Abortion Federation. Available at: http://www.prochoice.org. Retrieved August 15, 2013.

Paul M, Lichtenbert ES, Borgatta L, Grimes DA, Stubblefield PG, Creinin MD, editors. Management of unintended and abnormal pregnancy: Comprehensive abortion care. West Sussex: Wiley-Blackwell; 2009.

Physicians for Reproductive Health. Available at: www.prch.org. Retrieved August 15, 2013.

Planned Parenthood Federation of America. Available at: http://www.planned parenthood.org. Retrieved August 15, 2013.

Society of Family Planning, Clinical guidelines. Available at: http://societyfp.org/resources/guidelines.asp. Retrieved June 28, 2013.

AMBULATORY GYNECOLOGIC SURGERY

Many invasive procedures that were once routinely performed by the obstetrician–gynecologist in the inpatient setting now can be performed safely, efficiently, and cost-effectively in an appropriately equipped ambulatory setting. Two examples are diagnostic laparoscopy and diagnostic hysteroscopy. In addition, some more complex traditionally in-patient procedures can be replaced, when appropriate, with simpler outpatient procedures, for example, endometrial sampling in place of diagnostic dilation and curettage and loop electrosurgical excision procedure in place of cone biopsy of the cervix. Some of these procedures can be undertaken in the office setting, whereas others are more appropriately performed in a freestanding or hospital-based ambulatory surgical facility. The type of procedure and individual patient factors determine the most appropriate setting.

Ambulatory surgical procedures should be limited to those for which there is a reasonable expectation of discharge within a short time, with traditional recovery occurring at home; that can be performed safely; that are consistent with staff expertise, facilities, and equipment; and that are appropriate relative to the intrinsic risk of the procedure, the patient's condition, and the need for anesthesia.

Regulations

Clinicians should be aware of any federal, state, and local regulations governing surgical procedures, including ambulatory surgical procedures that require anesthesia or conscious sedation. Clinicians should be aware of payers' regulations regarding sites for which professional and facility charges will be paid because they have a bearing on where procedures may be performed.

When the office setting is chosen for the performance of ambulatory surgery, policies, procedures, and practices should be developed to facilitate a safe and effective environment. Box 4-13 includes important considerations for the performance of ambulatory procedures in the office setting. Details on the organization of a freestanding or hospital-based ambulatory care surgical facility and the involvement of the hospital staff in the ambulatory care facility's activities are available from a variety of sources, including The Joint Commission, Occupational Safety and Health Administration, Accreditation Association for Ambulatory Health Care, American Association for Accreditation of Ambulatory Surgery Facilities, Inc., and the Centers for Medicare & Medicaid Services (see Resources).

Box 4-13. Office Set-Up Checklist for Surgical Procedures

Documentation and Systems
- Create a policy and procedure manual (updated with the American College of Obstetricians and Gynecologists' current *Guidelines for Women's Health Care*)
- Create a patients' rights handout
- Create informed consent materials
- Arrange for a transfer agreement with nearby hospital
- Ensure compliance with local building codes, fire codes, and Occupational Safety and Health Administration regulations
- Ensure compliance with state board of pharmacy and Drug Enforcement Administration regulations
- Ensure compliance with state and professional guidelines
- Create an office-based surgery procedure record
- Ensure a procedure outcome reporting system is in place
- Create an adverse-event reporting system

Equipment and Supplies
- Ensure adequate equipment for level of anesthesia and analgesia, including
    — monitors for blood pressure and pulse and heart rate
    — pulse oximeter
    — exhaled carbon dioxide monitor for deep sedation
    — reliable oxygen source

(continued)

Box 4-13. Office Set-Up Checklist for Surgical Procedures *(continued)*

- — suction
- — cardiac monitor
- — resuscitation equipment, including defibrillator
- — auxiliary electrical power source
- — emergency medications
- Maintain, test, and inspect all equipment per manufacturers' recommendations
- Ensure ability to monitor level of sedation
- Ensure ability to rescue patients from excessive sedation

Staff
- Ensure that a physician or other health care provider certified in advanced cardiac life support, pediatric advanced life support, or basic life support is immediately available to provide emergency resuscitation.
- Institute a quarterly mock drill
- Ensure credentialing and privileging of all participating physicians

Patient Selection
Create a checklist that meets the following requirements:
- Meets ASA Physical Status #1 criteria or medically controlled ASA Physical Status #2 criteria
- Contains prescreening verification that the patient is a candidate for an office-based procedure. Contraindications include, but are not limited to, the following:
  - — Personal or family history of adverse reaction to local anesthetic
  - — History of previous failure with local anesthesia or low pain threshold
  - — Need for maximal relaxation
  - — Poor tolerance of pelvic examinations
  - — An acute respiratory process
  - — High-risk airway assessment
  - — Abnormal blood sugars
  - — Extreme obesity
  - — Pregnancy (unless procedure is pregnancy related)

(continued)

Box 4-13. Office Set-Up Checklist for Surgical Procedures *(continued)*

— Failure to understand or cooperate with the procedure (eg, unable to comply with preoperative dietary restrictions)

— Substance abuse

• Documents appropriate workup and patient selection

• Documents informed consent process, noting risks, benefits, and alternatives

---

Abbreviation: ASA, American Society of Anesthesiologists.

Modified from American College of Obstetricians and Gynecologists. Report of the presidential task force on patient safety in the office setting: appendix G. Quality and safety in women's health care. 2nd ed. Washington, DC: American College of Obstetricians and Gynecologists; 2010. p. 91–108.

Facilities

The ambulatory surgical setting should provide the highest quality care in an environment supportive of the patient's individual comfort, rights, and dignity. The following three general levels of ambulatory surgical facility care are recognized by the American College of Obstetricians and Gynecologists:

• Level I—provides for minor surgical procedures performed under topical and local infiltration blocks with or without oral or intramuscular preoperative sedation. Excluded are spinal, epidural, and regional blocks. Simple procedures of limited invasiveness that require only local anesthesia often can be accomplished safely in the ambulatory surgical setting with minimal extra requirements of space, personnel, and backup equipment.

• Level II—provides for minor or major surgical procedures performed in conjunction with oral, parenteral, or intravenous sedation or under analgesic or dissociative drugs. When more extensive procedures are performed using local anesthesia, or when conscious intravenous sedation is used, a more advanced level of training of personnel and more extensive preoperative, intraoperative, and postoperative monitoring are required.

- Level III—provides for major surgical procedures that require general or regional block anesthesia and support of bodily functions. Procedures that may require major emergency laparotomy should not be performed in any ambulatory surgical setting.

The appropriate facility for a given patient will depend on many factors, including the following:

- Condition of the patient
- Type of anesthesia to be used
- Resources of the facility
    - Facility design
    - Safety management
    - Emergency treatment availability
    - Hospitalization services
    - Ancillary services (onsite and offsite)
        - ☐ Pharmaceutical services
        - ☐ Laboratory services
        - ☐ Pathology services
        - ☐ Diagnostic imaging services
        - ☐ Blood product availability

A physician, the surgeon, the anesthesiologist, or a combination of these practitioners determines the appropriate facility based upon the safety and well-being of the patient.

The selection of patients is based on the condition of the patient and the potential risks of the procedure. This evaluation involves clinical judgment based on history, physical examination, and preoperative laboratory studies. The American Society of Anesthesiologists (ASA) has created a system for classifying the physical status of patients before surgery (Box 4-14). Level I facilities usually provide care only for patients who meet ASA

Box 4-14. American Society of Anesthesiologists' Physical Status Classification System

ASA Physical Status 1—A normal, healthy patient

ASA Physical Status 2—A patient with mild systemic disease

ASA Physical Status 3—A patient with severe systemic disease

ASA Physical Status 4—A patient with severe systemic disease that is a constant threat to life

ASA Physical Status 5—A moribund patient who is not expected to survive without the operation

ASA Physical Status 6—A declared brain-dead patient whose organs are being removed for donor purposes

Abbreviation: ASA, American Society of Anesthesiologists.

Reprinted with permission from American Society of Anesthesiologists. ASA physical status classification system. Available at: http://www.asahq.org/Home/For-Members/Clinical-Information/ASA-Physical-Status-Classification-System. Retrieved September 30, 2013.

Physical Status #1 and #2 criteria. Level II and level III facilities in some cases provide care to patients who meet ASA Physical Status #3 and #4 criteria, but documented evidence of preoperative evaluation by a physician is required. When compromise or dysfunction is identified, consultation with an appropriate specialist may be necessary.

Not all patients are good candidates for surgery in the office setting. Box 4-13 lists examples of contraindications for office procedures. For certain patients, it is not practical to use the office setting for procedures that require a level of patient cooperation, such as dilation and curettage or hysteroscopy. The patient's mental or emotional suitability for ambulatory surgery and the social and environmental setting into which she will return also should be taken into consideration.

Selection and Management of Anesthesia

The type and level of anesthesia should be dictated by the procedure with input based on patient preference. The decision regarding type of anesthesia should not be altered based on limitations of equipment or personnel. Such limitations might necessitate performing the procedure in a more acute care facility. The level of anesthesia will dictate the equipment and personnel needed. Box 4-15 and Table 4-7 describe physiologic functioning at various levels of sedation or analgesia.

Box 4-15. Types of Sedation or Analgesia

Minimal Sedation (Anxiolysis)—A drug-induced state during which patients respond normally to verbal commands. Although cognitive function and coordination may be impaired, ventilatory and cardiovascular functions are unaffected.

Moderate Sedation or Analgesia ("Conscious Sedation")—A drug-induced depression of consciousness during which patients respond purposefully* to verbal commands, either alone or accompanied by light tactile stimulation. No interventions are required to maintain a patent airway, and spontaneous ventilation is adequate. Cardiovascular function is usually maintained.

Deep Sedation or Analgesia—A drug-induced depression of consciousness during which patients cannot be easily aroused but respond purposefully* following repeated or painful stimulation. The ability to independently maintain ventilatory function may be impaired. Patients may require assistance in maintaining a patent airway, and spontaneous ventilation may be inadequate. Cardiovascular function is usually maintained.

General Anesthesia is a drug-induced loss of consciousness during which patients are not arousable, even by painful stimulation. The ability to independently maintain ventilatory function is often impaired. Patients often require assistance in maintaining a patent airway, and positive pressure ventilation may be required because of depressed spontaneous ventilation or drug-induced depression of neuromuscular function. Cardiovascular function may be impaired.

---

*Reflex withdrawal from a painful stimulus is not considered a purposeful response.

Reprinted with permission from the American Society of Anesthesiologists. Continuum of depth of sedation: definition of general anesthesia and levels of sedation/analgesia. Park Ridge (IL): ASA; 2009. Available at: http://www.asahq.org/For-Members/-/media/For%20Members/Standards%20and%20Guidelines/2012/CONTINUUM%20OF%20DEPTH%20OF%20SEDATION%20442012.ashx. Retrieved September 30, 2013.

Table 4-7. Continuum of Depth of Sedation*

Physiologic Function	Minimal Sedation (Anxiolysis)	Level of Sedation or Analgesia		
		Moderate Sedation or Analgesia (Conscious Sedation)	Deep Sedation or Analgesia	General Anesthesia
Responsiveness	Normal response to verbal stimulation	Purposeful† response to verbal or tactile stimulation	Purposeful† response following repeated or painful stimulation	Unarousable, even with painful stimulus
Airway	Unaffected	No intervention required	Intervention may be required	Intervention often required
Spontaneous ventilation	Unaffected	Adequate	May be inadequate	Frequently inadequate
Cardiovascular function	Unaffected	Usually maintained	Usually maintained	May be impaired

*Monitored anesthesia care does not describe the continuum of depth of sedation; rather, it describes "a specific anesthesia service in which an anesthesiologist has been requested to participate in the care of a patient undergoing a diagnostic or therapeutic procedure."

†Reflex withdrawal from a painful stimulus is not considered a purposeful response.

Modified with permission from the American Society of Anesthesiologists. Continuum of depth of sedation: definition of general anesthesia and levels of sedation/analgesia. Park Ridge (IL): ASA; 2009. Available at: http://www.asahq.org/For-Members/-/media/For%20Members/Standards%20 and%20Guidelines/2012/CONTINUUM%20OF%20DEPTH%20OF%20SEDATION%20442012.ashx. Retrieved September 30, 2013.

All necessary medication should be in the room and immediately available before the onset of the procedure. Controlled drugs should be logged out from a secure location. A medication administration log (including the use of local anesthetic agents) must be maintained during the procedure.

A person responsible for administration of medication and monitoring the patient must be present in the procedure room. The administration of any anesthetic must be performed or supervised by a qualified physician. Depending on the level of anesthesia, patient monitoring might be assumed by a medical assistant, nurse, certified nurse anesthetist, or anesthesiologist. General or spinal anesthetics must be administered by an anesthesiologist, a physician eligible to take the anesthesiology board examination, or a registered nurse–anesthetist under the direct supervision of an anesthesiologist. Local or regional block anesthesia with or without sedation should be induced by or under the supervision of a qualified physician. Clinicians who induce intravenous conscious sedation must have sufficient training and experience related to the use, administration, adverse effects, and complications of all applicable medications. Knowledge of airway management, advanced life support, and emergency medical management is required.

There should be a designated recovery area adequately staffed and equipped to assure that the patient has the level of monitoring appropriate for the procedure and anesthesia. For all but minimal or light sedation, there should be oxygen and suction available. If it is anticipated that any level of sedation may be needed, staff must confirm that the patient has an escort to drive the patient home before starting the procedure. No patient should leave the office following any level of sedation without an escort.

The level of anesthesia achieved is the primary concern regarding patient safety and not the agents used (ie, oral versus intravenous medications). Whether given orally or parenterally, narcotics and sedatives pose similar risks. The patient should be evaluated for depth of sedation regardless of mode of delivery, including all the recommended monitoring equipment and procedures.

PATIENT RISK FACTORS
The following factors may place a woman at an increased risk of complications from anesthesia and should be communicated to the anesthesia

care practitioner in advance to permit formulation of a management plan:

- Marked obesity
- Severe facial and neck edema
- Extremely short stature
- Difficulty opening her mouth
- Small mandible, protuberant teeth, or both
- Arthritis of the neck
- Short neck
- Anatomic abnormalities of the face or mouth
- Large thyroid
- Asthma or other chronic pulmonary diseases
- Cardiac disease
- History of problems attributable to anesthetics
- Bleeding disorders
- Other significant medical complications

POLICIES ON EMERGENCY MEDICATION, RESUSCITATION, AND ABILITY TO RESCUE PATIENT FROM EXCESSIVE SEDATION

These policies should be based on the ASA levels or other scale according to level of invasiveness. When local anesthesia with minimal preoperative oral anxiolytic medication is used, personnel with training in basic life support should be immediately available until all patients are discharged home. Emergency equipment for cardiorespiratory support and treatment of anaphylaxis must be readily available (and in good working order) for those who are trained to use it.

The use of moderate sedation requires that a minimum of two staff individuals must be on the premises, one of whom shall be a licensed physician with current training in advanced resuscitative techniques (eg, advanced cardiac life support or pediatric advanced life support), until all patients are discharged home. In addition, at least one physician must be present or immediately available any time patients are present. Emergency equipment, advanced cardiac life support medication, and trained personnel for cardiorespiratory support and treatment of anaphylaxis must be immediately available.

According to the ASA, because sedation is a continuum, it is not always possible to predict how an individual patient will respond. Practitioners who intend to produce a given level of sedation should be able to rescue patients whose level of sedation becomes deeper than initially intended. Rescue of a patient from a deeper level of sedation than intended is an intervention by a practitioner proficient in airway management and advanced life support. The qualified practitioner corrects adverse physiologic consequences of the deeper-than-intended level of sedation (such as hypoventilation, hypoxia, and hypotension) and returns the patient to the originally intended level of sedation. It is not appropriate to continue the procedure at an unintended level of sedation. Health care providers who administer moderate sedation or analgesia ("conscious sedation") should be able to rescue patients who enter a state of deep sedation or analgesia, whereas those who administer deep sedation or analgesia should be able to rescue patients who enter a state of general anesthesia.

Preoperative Care

When surgery is being considered, certain criteria should be fulfilled to determine the appropriateness of the surgical procedure. The proposed procedure must be indicated, based on targeted history and physical examination. Alternative treatments should have been considered, and it should be determined that the benefits to the patient outweigh the risks. Known contraindications and risk factors should have been ruled out or considered. Informed consent must have been obtained from the patient or legal guardian. The surgeon and all other participating physicians must have the necessary credentials and privileges to perform the specific procedures required. The facility must have the equipment and staff necessary for the procedure and any anticipated complications.

PREOPERATIVE EVALUATION AND TESTS

The extent of preoperative counseling and testing needed to prepare patients for ambulatory surgery depends on the type of procedure being performed. Preoperative tests and procedures should be individualized based on the patient's age and medical status with respect to the planned surgery. This testing should be aimed at evaluating the patient's known disease and at screening for unsuspected pathologic findings that would warrant further preoperative evaluation or alter the surgeon's planned therapeutic approach. The guiding principle is to determine any contraindications or risk factors that should be known and to establish baselines that may be important in managing the postoperative course.

The following should be completed before outpatient surgery, and the findings should be noted in the medical record:

- A recent general and targeted history and physical examination should be performed, with specific attention to pregnancy status, preexisting or concurrent illness, medications, allergies, and adverse drug reactions that may have an effect on (or contraindicate) the operative procedure or anesthesia, as well as medications and supplements that might affect blood coagulability. Some patients are allergic or sensitive to common operating room materials, such as latex, povidone–iodine, adhesive tape, and metal used for surgical staples. Patients should be evaluated for such allergies during the preoperative examination and during the "time out."

  Because many diagnostic and therapeutic modalities may pose a direct or indirect risk to an embryo, facilities should establish specific procedures, applicable to all services, for identifying unsuspected pregnancies in women of reproductive age. A menstrual history and physical examination can be helpful in this determination. If there is any reason to suspect pregnancy, a pregnancy test should be performed in advance of any such procedure.

- Laboratory data should be collected, as indicated based on the patient's needs and condition and on the procedure. Laboratory testing will vary considerably with the extent of the planned surgery, the patient's age, preexisting conditions, potential complications, institutional policies, and insurance requirements.

- Informed consent should be obtained, including an informed consent form or other documentation indicating that the diagnosis, the reason for the surgery, a description of the planned procedure, the intended benefits, risks, and possible alternatives have been explained to the patient.

- Preoperative written instructions should be given to the patient, if appropriate, and include directions regarding any necessary restrictions on food and fluid intake and warning that failure to heed such directions may result in cancellation of the procedure.

On the day of surgery, the following should be performed, with results noted in the medical record:

- Preanesthetic evaluation, including an interval history, medical record review, and heart and lung examination.
- Careful selection of medications used for preoperative medication and surgical anesthesia, to minimize the risk of major adverse reactions.

Other issues to be considered preoperatively include the following:

- Prophylactic use of antibiotics. Prophylactic antibiotics are recommended for the following procedures: hysterectomy, urogynecologic procedures, hysterosalpingography, chromotubation, and abortion via suction curettage or dilation and evacuation; details can be found in the American College of Obstetricians and Gynecologists' Practice Bulletin No. 104, *Antibiotic Prophylaxis for Gynecologic Procedures* (see Bibliography). The American Heart Association no longer recommends the administration of antibiotics solely to prevent endocarditis for any patient undergoing genitourinary or gastrointestinal tract procedures, even patients with the highest risk of adverse outcomes due to bacterial endocarditis (see Bibliography).
- Skin preparation. The goal of skin preparation is to reduce bacterial counts while minimizing skin irritation. Hair removal should be performed only when necessary for adequate visualization. Clippers should be used to minimize the amount of skin disruption. Razors should never be used because they can cause small cuts and nicks to the skin, which increases the risk of wound infection.

- Prevention of venous thrombosis. Preoperative patients should be classified according to levels of risk of thrombosis to determine the benefits and risks of pharmacologic and physical methods of preventing venous thromboembolism. Factors to consider include patient age; procedure type and duration of surgery; and clinical risk factors, such as prior deep vein thrombosis or pulmonary embolism, malignancy, estrogen therapy, and obesity. Evidence-based recommendations from the American College of Chest Physicians for venous thromboembolism prophylaxis are available (see Resources).
- Jewelry. All body jewelry, including piercings, should be removed before surgery.

PROTOCOLS AND CHECKLISTS

In 2003, The Joint Commission on Accreditation of Healthcare Organizations (now The Joint Commission) initially published the *Universal Protocol for Preventing Wrong Site, Wrong Procedure, and Wrong Person Surgery*. The universal protocol is updated annually and is based on three activities before initiation of any surgical procedure: 1) conducting a preoperative verification process, 2) marking the operative site (as appropriate), and 3) taking a "time out" before the procedure (see also the "Patient Safety" section in Part 1).

The "Safe Surgery Saves Lives" initiative was established by the World Health Organization (WHO) Patient Safety program as part of the WHO's efforts to reduce the number of surgical deaths across the globe. Ten essential objectives for safe surgery were identified and compiled to form the WHO Surgical Safety Checklist. A complement to the Universal Protocol, the WHO checklist involves confirming a set of surgical safety standards before induction of anesthesia, before skin incision, and before the patient leaves the operating room (see also the "Patient Safety" section in Part 1).

An additional resource is the "Office Surgical Safety Checklist" developed by the American College of Obstetrician and Gynecologists' Presidential Task Force on Patient Safety in the Office Setting (see Box 4-16). This tool is not comprehensive and, just as the Universal Protocol and WHO checklist, should be adapted to best suit individual practices.

Box 4-16. Office Surgical Safety Checklist

Preoperative (Before Anesthesia or Analgesia)
- Confirm patient identity, site (marked), procedure, and consent
- Ensure no change in patient's medical condition since last office visit
- Check preoperative vital signs
- Review current history and physical
- Review and record all medications taken previously that day
- Confirm nil per os (NPO—nothing by mouth) status, if appropriate
- Confirm preoperative instructions followed by patient
- Review patient allergies
- Confirm presence of any indicated laboratory results (eg, glucose level in a patient with diabetes)
- Assess airway or aspiration risk
- Complete anesthesia and medication check
- Display essential imaging

Preoperative (Before Initiation of Procedure)
- Perform time-out (confirming correct health care provider, patient, site, and procedure)
- Administer any indicated antibiotic prophylaxis within 60 minutes before incision
- Confirm pulse oximetry is being recorded accurately
- Prepare for anticipated critical events (critical or nonroutine steps, anticipated blood loss, length of case, patient-specific concerns, equipment issues)

Intraoperative
- Count and record number of instruments, needles, and sponges, if appropriate
- Record intraoperative medications
- If sedation is used, monitor and document oxygen saturation, blood pressure, pulse, and level of alertness every 5 minutes
- For hysteroscopic procedures, record cavity assessment per manufacturer's guidelines and document fluid balance

(continued)

Box 4-16. Office Surgical Safety Checklist *(continued)*

Postoperative
- Complete instrument, sponge, and needle counts, if appropriate
- Confirm specimen labeling
- Document equipment problems
- Document key concerns for recovery and management of patient

Discharge
- Record vital signs and ensure return to within 20% of baseline, if appropriate
- Confirm there is no evidence of active bleeding
- Document adequate level of consciousness and ambulation, pain and nausea control, ability to tolerate liquids by mouth, and ability to void (if appropriate for the procedure)
- Provide discharge instruction sheet that includes how to recognize an emergency during the postoperative period and the steps to follow should one occur after discharge (eg, hemorrhage)
- Schedule a follow-up call 24–48 hours after procedure, if appropriate
- Schedule an appropriate postoperative follow-up appointment
- Following any level of sedation, the patient should be discharged in the company of a responsible adult licensed to drive a vehicle or able to accompany the patient home by public transportation
- Record the long-term outcome of the procedure
- Record any complications

Modified from American College of Obstetricians and Gynecologists. Report of the presidential task force on patient safety in the office setting: appendix G. Quality and safety in women's health care. 2nd ed. Washington, DC: American College of Obstetricians and Gynecologists; 2010. p. 91-108.; and Patient safety in the surgical environment. Committee Opinion No. 464. Obstet Gynecol 2010;116:786–90.

Intraoperative Care

Proper positioning of the patient and the retractors are important to prevent nerve injury. Care should be taken to avoid excessive flexion or external rotation of the patient's hips to prevent a femoral neuropathy. Proper positioning of the foot and leg will prevent pressure on the peroneal nerve, and is best achieved by using lateral thigh supports.

Fluids must be monitored carefully. In operative procedures, such as hysteroscopy, in which osmotically active solutions are used for visualization, careful intraoperative management of fluid balance is critical to patient well-being.

In elderly patients, operative management should include minimizing anesthesia doses to promote cognitive recovery. It also should include avoiding dehydration, careful positioning to accommodate joint fragility and minimize pain, and ensuring sufficient padding of bony surfaces and cushioning to prevent ulceration.

With the exception of those specimens exempted by the facility's governing body and The Joint Commission, tissue removed during surgery should be submitted to a pathologist for examination. Routine pathologic examination of tissue is not necessary after an induced abortion via suction curettage or dilation and evacuation in which embryonic or fetal parts can be identified with certainty. In such instances, the physician simply should record a description of the gross products of conception.

The Joint Commission includes unintended retention of a foreign object in a patient after surgery or other procedure as a reviewable sentinel event. The American College of Surgeons recommends consistent application and adherence to standardized counting procedures and documentation of the surgical counts, instruments or items intentionally left as packing, and actions taken if count discrepancies occur. Other protocols to prevent unintentional retention of foreign objects during surgery have been developed (see Resources).

Postoperative Care

The following issues should be addressed as part of postoperative care:

- Staff should monitor the patient carefully for pain and treat her as appropriate.

- Nasogastric tube insertion should not be used routinely because it is uncomfortable, increases the incidence of pulmonary complications, and does not reduce the incidence of wound complications.

- Oral feeding with a regular diet immediately postoperatively is safe for most patients who have undergone an ambulatory surgical procedure.
- The patient should be informed of the operative findings when not under the influence of anesthesia.
- Early mobilization and rapid removal of any restraints are important.
- In the elderly, extra precautions should be taken to prevent falls. Delirium is a serious risk of surgery in the elderly; early investigation for medical causes is important, and treatment should be augmented with frequent auditory, visual, and somatosensory orientation.
- Any complications should be recorded.

Adverse Reactions

Vasovagal reactions are the most common adverse reactions to gynecologic procedures performed in the ambulatory surgical setting. These reactions include a number of cardiovascular and autonomic or central nervous system reactions, such as bradycardia, hypotension, diaphoresis, nausea, and convulsions.

A vasovagal reaction usually is the result of patient anxiety but also may occur with cervical dilation or peritoneal stretching, or as a result of pain. In patients who do not have cardiovascular disease, vasovagal reactions usually terminate spontaneously without the need for specific therapy.

Vasovagal reactions may be prevented by the following measures:

- Preoperative patient counseling
- Reassurance during the procedure
- The administration of preoperative atropine or promethazine hydrochloride

Oxygen should be used in cases of prolonged apnea. Assisted respiration is rarely necessary.

A vasovagal reaction should not be confused with the much less common allergic reactions to a local anesthetic or preoperative medication. True allergic reactions to commonly used anesthetic and preoperative medications do not occur often, but personnel should be familiar with common allergic reactions and their appropriate management. Allergic reactions may include urticaria, hives, edema, asthma, and anaphylaxis.

Allergic reactions may be treated with diphenhydramine intravenously, or epinephrine may be given intramuscularly or subcutaneously. Anaphylaxis, whether it is due to a reaction to latex or another factor, is a life-threatening event. Prompt recognition and treatment are critical. Any patient with an anaphylactic reaction should be monitored for recurrent symptoms after initial treatment and resolution. The World Allergy Organization recommends that the length of observation be individualized based on the type of reaction. Additional guidelines for the diagnosis and management of anaphylaxis are listed in the Bibliography.

Recovery and Discharge

There should be a designated recovery area with staff and equipment to ensure that the patient has the level of monitoring appropriate for the procedure and anesthesia. When local anesthetic agents are used for office surgery, minimum space and services are necessary for proper postoperative recovery. When patients are alert, are oriented, have stable vital signs, are free of major pain, and are able to sit up and dress themselves, they may leave the office. When moderate or conscious sedation is used, an area sufficient for patient recovery should be provided and staffed by personnel who continue monitoring vital signs and level of consciousness.

During the recovery period, a member of the health care team should observe the patient closely. This person should maintain a complete record of the patient's general condition, including vital signs, blood loss, and occurrence of complications. When procedures have been performed in an ambulatory surgical facility, a physician, preferably the anesthesiologist, should be present in the facility until the patient has been discharged. This physician should oversee the postanesthetic recovery area and should share with the surgeon the responsibility for discharging patients or transferring them to the backup hospital.

The patient should remain in the recovery area until recovery is sufficient to permit safe discharge according to the criteria listed in Box 4-16. The patient should be examined by a health care provider with appropriate clinical privileges and be discharged on written order. Alternatively, other practitioners may discharge patients according to approved criteria.

Cosmetic Surgery

As cosmetic procedures receive increased attention from the media and patient requests for such procedures grow, there is a corresponding need to determine the proper role of obstetrician–gynecologists in this evolving field. The scope of obstetric–gynecologic practice includes more than reproductive health care. The specialty's broad focus on women's health may include cosmetic services and procedures, just as this broad focus includes a wide variety of preventive care. The obstetrician–gynecologist may provide services that fill a need not adequately met in commercial offices, provide safer or more efficacious treatments than those available in nonmedical settings, or provide services as a convenience to patients.

However, cosmetic procedures (such as laser hair removal, body piercing, tattoo removal, and liposuction) are not considered gynecologic procedures and, therefore, generally are not taught in approved obstetric and gynecologic residencies. Because these are not considered gynecologic procedures, it is inappropriate for the College to establish guidelines for training. As with other surgical procedures, credentialing for cosmetic procedures should be based on education, training, experience, and demonstrated competence equivalent to other specialists who typically perform these procedures.

As with other women's health care procedures, the health, well-being, and safety of the patient who receives cosmetic services must be paramount, and the obstetrician–gynecologist must be knowledgeable of the ethics of patient counseling and informed consent. Inquiries regarding cosmetic products, services, and procedures must come from the patient, and the patient should feel no pressure or obligation to purchase or undergo any cosmetic services. As many patients look to their physicians, often particularly their obstetrician–gynecologists, to define "normal" anatomy, behavior, or function, any unsolicited comments or innuendo could create a perceived need for alteration when none was considered previously.

Special care must be taken when patients are considering procedures in an effort to enhance sexual appearance or function. Although procedures, such as reversal or repair of female genital cutting and treatment for labial hypertrophy, may be medically indicated, female sexual response has been shown to be an intricate process determined predominantly by brain function and psychosocial factors, not by genital appearance. Other procedures, including "vaginal rejuvenation," "re-virgination," and "G-spot amplification," are not medically indicated, and their safety and effectiveness have not been documented. Clinicians who receive requests from patients for such procedures should discuss with the patient the reason for her request and perform an evaluation for any physical signs or symptoms that may indicate the need for surgical intervention. Women should be informed about the lack of data to support the efficacy of these procedures and their potential complications, including infection, altered sensation, dyspareunia, adhesions, and scarring (see also the "Sexual Function and Dysfunction" section earlier in Part 4).

Bibliography

American College of Obstetricians and Gynecologists. Nongynecologic procedures. ACOG Committee Opinion No. 253. Washington, DC: ACOG; 2001.

American College of Obstetricians and Gynecologists. Report of the presidential task force on patient safety in the office setting: Appendix G. Quality and safety in women's health care. 2nd ed. Washington, DC: American College of Obstetricians and Gynecologists; 2010. p. 91–108.

American College of Obstetricians and Gynecologists. The role of the obstetrician-gynecologist in cosmetic procedures. College Statement of Policy 85. Washington, DC: American College of Obstetricians and Gynecologists; 2012.

American College of Surgeons. Patient safety principles for office-based surgery utilizing moderate sedation/analgesia, deep sedation/analgesia, or general anesthesia. Available at: http://www.facs.org/patientsafety/patientsafety.html. Retrieved September 30, 2013.

American Society of Anesthesiologists. ASA physical status classification system. Available at: http://www.asahq.org/Home/For-Members/Clinical-Information/ASA-Physical-Status-Classification-System. Retrieved September 30, 2013.

American Society of Anesthesiologists. Continuum of depth of sedation: definition of general anesthesia and levels of sedation/analgesia. Park Ridge (IL): ASA; 2009. Available at: http://www.asahq.org/For-Members/~/media/For%20Members/Standards %20and%20Guidelines/2012/CONTINUUM%20OF%20DEPTH%20OF%20 SEDATION%20442012.ashx. Retrieved September 30, 2013.

Antibiotic prophylaxis for gynecologic procedures. ACOG Practice Bulletin No. 104. American College of Obstetricians and Gynecologists. Obstet Gynecol 2009; 113:1180–9.

Elective coincidental appendectomy. ACOG Committee Opinion No. 323. American College of Obstetricians and Gynecologists. Obstet Gynecol 2005;106:1141–2.

Elective surgery and patient choice. Committee Opinion No. 578. American College of Obstetricians and Gynecologists. Obstet Gynecol 2013;122:1134–8.

Haynes AB, Weiser TG, Berry WR, Lipsitz SR, Breizat AH, Dellinger EP, et al. A surgical safety checklist to reduce morbidity and mortality in a global population. Safe Surgery Saves Lives Study Group. N Engl J Med 2009;360:491–9.

Hysteroscopy. Technology Assessment in Obstetrics and Gynecology No. 7. American College of Obstetricians and Gynecologists. Obstet Gynecol 2011;117:1486–91.

Nishimura RA, Carabello BA, Faxon DP, Freed MD, Lytle BW, O'Gara PT, et al. ACC/AHA 2008 Guideline update on valvular heart disease: focused update on infective endocarditis: a report of the American College of Cardiology/American Heart Association Task Force on Practice Guidelines endorsed by the Society of Cardiovascular Anesthesiologists, Society for Cardiovascular Angiography and Interventions, and Society of Thoracic Surgeons. J Am Coll Cardiol 2008;52:676–85.

Patient safety in the surgical environment. Committee Opinion No. 464. Obstet Gynecol 2010;116:786–90.

Practice guidelines for sedation and analgesia by non-anesthesiologists. American Society of Anesthesiologists Task Force on Sedation and Analgesia by Non-Anesthesiologists. Anesthesiology 2002;96:1004–17.

Prevention of deep vein thrombosis and pulmonary embolism. ACOG Practice Bulletin No. 84. American College of Obstetricians and Gynecologists. Obstet Gynecol 2007;110:429–40.

Simons FE, Ardusso LR, Bilo MB, El-Gamal YM, Ledford DK, Ring J, et al. World Allergy Organization guidelines for the assessment and management of anaphylaxis. World Allergy Organization. World Allergy Organ J 2011;4:13–37.

Statement on the prevention of retained foreign bodies after surgery. Bull Am Coll Surg 2005;90:15–6.

The diagnosis and management of anaphylaxis: an updated practice parameter. Joint Task Force on Practice Parameters American Academy of Allergy, Asthma and Immunology. American College of Allergy, Asthma and Immunology. Joint Council of Allergy, Asthma and Immunology [published erratum appears in J Allergy Clin Immunol 2008;122:68]. J Allergy Clin Immunol 2005;115:S483–523.

The Joint Commission. Universal protocol. Available at: http://www.jointcommis sion.org/standards_information/up.aspx. Retrieved August 15, 2013.

Vaginal "rejuvenation" and cosmetic vaginal procedures. ACOG Committee Opinion No. 378. American College of Obstetricians and Gynecologists. Obstet Gynecol 2007;110:737–8.

Wilson W, Taubert KA, Gewitz M, Lockhart PB, Baddour LM, Levison M, et al. Prevention of infective endocarditis: guidelines from the American Heart Association: a guideline from the American Heart Association Rheumatic Fever, Endocarditis, and Kawasaki Disease Committee, Council on Cardiovascular Disease in the Young, and the Council on Clinical Cardiology, Council on Cardiovascular Surgery and Anesthesia, and the Quality of Care and Outcomes Research Interdisciplinary Working Group [published erratum appears in Circulation 2007;116:e376-7]. Circulation 2007;116:1736–54.

World Health Organization. Surgical safety checklist. Geneva: WHO; 2009. Available at: http://whqlibdoc.who.int/publications/2009/9789241598590_eng_Checklist.pdf. Retrieved July 10, 2013.

Yokoe DS, Mermel LA, Anderson DJ, Arias KM, Burstin H, Calfee DP, et al. A compendium of strategies to prevent healthcare-associated infections in acute care hospitals. Infect Control Hosp Epidemiol 2008;29(suppl):S12–21.

Resources

Accreditation Association for Ambulatory Health Care. 2014 Accreditation handbook for ambulatory health care. 2014 ed. Skokie (IL): Accreditation Association for Ambulatory Health Care; 2014.

American Association for Accreditation of Ambulatory Surgery Facilities. Available at: http://www.aaaasf.org. Retrieved August 15, 2013.

American College of Surgeons. Guidelines for optimal ambulatory surgical care and office-based surgery. 3rd ed. Chicago (IL): ACS; 2000.

Americans with Disabilities Act, 42 U.S.C. §12101 (2011). Available at: http://www.gpo.gov/fdsys/pkg/USCODE-2011-title42/pdf/USCODE-2011-title42-chap126.pdf. Retrieved September 20, 2013.

Centers for Medicare and Medicaid Services. Clinical Laboratory Improvement Amendments (CLIA). Available at: http://www.cms.gov/Regulations-and-Guidance/Legislation/CLIA. Retrieved July 10, 2013.

Gould MK, Garcia DA, Wren SM, Karanicolas PJ, Arcelus JI, Heit JA, et al. Prevention of VTE in nonorthopedic surgical patients: Antithrombotic Therapy and Prevention of Thrombosis, 9th ed: American College of Chest Physicians Evidence-Based Clinical Practice Guidelines. American College of Chest Physicians [published erratum appears in Chest 2012;141:1369]. Chest 2012;141:e227S–77S.

Institute for Clinical Systems Improvement. Perioperative protocol. Bloomington (MN): ICSI; 2012. Available at: https://www.icsi.org/_asset/0c2xkr/Periop.pdf. Retrieved August 15, 2013.

Massachusetts Medical Society. Office-based surgery guidelines. Waltham (MA): MMS; 2011. Available at: http://www.massmed.org/officebasedsurgery/. Retrieved September 20, 2013.

Solutions for surgical preparation of the vagina. Committee Opinion No. 571. American College of Obstetricians and Gynecologists. Obstet Gynecol 2013;122: 718–20.

The Joint Commission. Comprehensive accreditation manual for ambulatory care: CAMAC. Oakbrook Terrace (IL): The Commission; 2014.

CODE OF PROFESSIONAL ETHICS OF THE AMERICAN COLLEGE OF OBSTETRICIANS AND GYNECOLOGISTS*

Obstetrician–gynecologists, as members of the medical profession, have ethical responsibilities not only to patients, but also to society, to other health professionals and to themselves. The following ethical foundations for professional activities in the field of obstetrics and gynecology are the supporting structures for the Code of Conduct. The Code implements many of these foundations in the form of rules of ethical conduct. Certain documents of the American College of Obstetricians and Gynecologists also provide additional ethical rules, including documents addressing the following issues: seeking and giving consultation, informed consent, sexual misconduct, patient testing, human immunodeficiency virus, relationships with industry, commercial enterprises in medical practice, and expert testimony. Noncompliance with the Code, including the above-referenced documents, may affect an individual's initial or continuing Fellowship in the American College of Obstetricians and Gynecologists. These documents may be revised or replaced periodically, and Fellows should be knowledgeable about current information.

Ethical Foundations

  I. The patient–physician relationship: The welfare of the patient (beneficence) is central to all considerations in the patient–physician

---

relationship. Included in this relationship is the obligation of physicians to respect the rights of patients, colleagues, and other health professionals. The respect for the right of individual patients to make their own choices about their health care (autonomy) is fundamental. The principle of justice requires strict avoidance of discrimination on the basis of race, color, religion, national origin, sexual orientation, perceived gender, and any basis that would constitute illegal discrimination (justice).

II. Physician conduct and practice: The obstetrician–gynecologist must deal honestly with patients and colleagues (veracity). This includes not misrepresenting himself or herself through any form of communication in an untruthful, misleading, or deceptive manner. Furthermore, maintenance of medical competence through study, application, and enhancement of medical knowledge and skills is an obligation of practicing physicians. Any behavior that diminishes a physician's capability to practice, such as substance abuse, must be immediately addressed and rehabilitative services instituted. The physician should modify his or her practice until the diminished capacity has been restored to an acceptable standard to avoid harm to patients (nonmaleficence). All physicians are obligated to respond to evidence of questionable conduct or unethical behavior by other physicians through appropriate procedures established by the relevant organization.

III. Avoiding conflicts of interest: Potential conflicts of interest are inherent in the practice of medicine. Physicians are expected to recognize such situations and deal with them through public disclosure. Conflicts of interest should be resolved in accordance with the best interest of the patient, respecting a woman's autonomy to make health care decisions. The physician should be an advocate for the patient through public disclosure of conflicts of interest raised by health payer policies or hospital policies.

IV. Professional relations: The obstetrician–gynecologist should respect and cooperate with other physicians, nurses, and health care professionals.

V. Societal responsibilities: The obstetrician–gynecologist has a continuing responsibility to society as a whole and should support and participate in activities that enhance the community. As a member of society, the obstetrician–gynecologist should respect the laws of that society. As professionals and members of medical societies, physicians are required to uphold the dignity and honor of the profession.

Code of Conduct

I. Patient–Physician Relationship

1. The patient–physician relationship is the central focus of all ethical concerns, and the welfare of the patient must form the basis of all medical judgments.

2. The obstetrician–gynecologist should serve as the patient's advocate and exercise all reasonable means to ensure that the most appropriate care is provided to the patient.

3. The patient–physician relationship has an ethical basis and is built on confidentiality, trust, and honesty. If no patient–physician relationship exists, a physician may refuse to provide care, except in emergencies (1). Once the patient–physician relationship exists, the obstetrician–gynecologist must adhere to all applicable legal or contractual constraints in dissolving the patient–physician relationship.

4. Sexual misconduct on the part of the obstetrician–gynecologist is an abuse of professional power and a violation of patient trust. Sexual contact or a romantic relationship between a physician and a current patient is always unethical (2).

5. The obstetrician–gynecologist has an obligation to obtain the informed consent of each patient (3). In obtaining informed consent for any course of medical or surgical treatment, the obstetrician-gynecologist must present to the patient, or to the person legally responsible for the patient, pertinent medical facts and recommendations consistent with good medical practice. Such information should be presented in reasonably understandable terms and include alternative modes of treatment and the objectives, risks, benefits, possible complications, and anticipated results of such treatment.

6. It is unethical to prescribe, provide, or seek compensation for therapies that are of no benefit to the patient.

7. The obstetrician–gynecologist must respect the rights and privacy of patients, colleagues, and others and safeguard patient information and confidences within the limits of the law. If during the process of providing information for consent it is known that results of a particular test or other information must be given to governmental authorities or other third parties, that must be explained to the patient (4).

8. The obstetrician–gynecologist must not discriminate against patients on the basis of race, color, religion, national origin, sexual orientation, perceived gender, and any basis that would constitute illegal discrimination.

II. Physician Conduct and Practice

1. The obstetrician–gynecologist should recognize the boundaries of his or her particular competencies and expertise and must provide only those services and use only those techniques for which he or she is qualified by education, training, and experience.

2. The obstetrician–gynecologist should participate in continuing medical education activities to maintain current scientific and professional knowledge relevant to the medical services he or she renders. The obstetrician–gynecologist should provide medical care involving new therapies or techniques only after undertaking appropriate training and study.

3. In emerging areas of medical treatment where recognized medical guidelines do not exist, the obstetrician–gynecologist should exercise careful judgment and take appropriate precautions to protect patient welfare.

4. The obstetrician–gynecologist must not publicize or represent himself or herself in any untruthful, misleading, or deceptive manner to patients, colleagues, other health care professionals, or the public.

5. The obstetrician–gynecologist who has reason to believe that he or she is infected with the human immunodeficiency virus (HIV)

or other serious infectious agents that might be communicated to patients should voluntarily be tested for the protection of his or her patients. In making decisions about patient-care activities, a physician infected with such an agent should adhere to the fundamental professional obligation to avoid harm to patients (5).

6. The obstetrician–gynecologist should not practice medicine while impaired by alcohol, drugs, or physical or mental disability. The obstetrician–gynecologist who experiences substance abuse problems or who is physically or emotionally impaired should seek appropriate assistance to address these problems and must limit his or her practice until the impairment no longer affects the quality of patient care.

III. Conflicts of Interest

1. Potential conflicts of interest are inherent in the practice of medicine. Conflicts of interest should be resolved in accordance with the best interest of the patient, respecting a woman's autonomy to make health care decisions. If there is an actual or potential conflict of interest that could be reasonably construed to affect significantly the patient's care, the physician must disclose the conflict to the patient. The physician should seek consultation with colleagues or an institutional ethics committee to determine whether there is an actual or potential conflict of interest and how to address it.

2. Commercial promotions of medical products and services may generate bias unrelated to product merit, creating or appearing to create inappropriate undue influence. The obstetrician–gynecologist should be aware of this potential conflict of interest and offer medical advice that is as accurate, balanced, complete, and devoid of bias as possible (6, 7).

3. The obstetrician–gynecologist should prescribe drugs, devices, and other treatments solely on the basis of medical considerations and patient needs, regardless of any direct or indirect interests in or benefit from a pharmaceutical firm or other supplier.

4. When the obstetrician–gynecologist receives anything of substantial value, including royalties, from companies in the health care industry,

such as a manufacturer of pharmaceuticals and medical devices, this fact should be disclosed to patients and colleagues when material.

5. Financial and administrative constraints may create disincentives to treatment otherwise recommended by the obstetrician–gynecologist. Any pertinent constraints should be disclosed to the patient.

IV. Professional Relations

1. The obstetrician–gynecologist's relationships with other physicians, nurses, and health care professionals should reflect fairness, honesty, and integrity, sharing a mutual respect and concern for the patient.

2. The obstetrician–gynecologist should consult, refer, or cooperate with other physicians, health care professionals, and institutions to the extent necessary to serve the best interests of their patients.

V. Societal Responsibilities

1. The obstetrician–gynecologist should support and participate in those health care programs, practices, and activities that contribute positively, in a meaningful and cost-effective way, to the welfare of individual patients, the health care system, or the public good.

2. The obstetrician–gynecologist should respect all laws, uphold the dignity and honor of the profession, and accept the profession's self-imposed discipline. The professional competence and conduct of obstetrician–gynecologists are best examined by professional associations, hospital peer-review committees, and state medical and licensing boards. These groups deserve the full participation and cooperation of the obstetrician–gynecologist.

3. The obstetrician–gynecologist should strive to address through the appropriate procedures the status of those physicians who demonstrate questionable competence, impairment, or unethical or illegal behavior. In addition, the obstetrician–gynecologist should cooperate with appropriate authorities to prevent the continuation of such behavior.

4. The obstetrician–gynecologist must not knowingly offer testimony that is false. The obstetrician–gynecologist must testify only on

matters about which he or she has knowledge and experience. The obstetrician–gynecologist must not knowingly misrepresent his or her credentials.

5. The obstetrician–gynecologist testifying as an expert witness must have knowledge and experience about the range of the standard of care and the available scientific evidence for the condition in question during the relevant time and must respond accurately to questions about the range of the standard of care and the available scientific evidence.

6. Before offering testimony, the obstetrician–gynecologist must thoroughly review the medical facts of the case and all available relevant information.

7. The obstetrician–gynecologist serving as an expert witness must accept neither disproportionate compensation nor compensation that is contingent upon the outcome of the litigation (8).

References

1. Seeking and giving consultation. ACOG Committee Opinion No. 365. American College of Obstetricians and Gynecologists. Obstet Gynecol 2007; 109:1255–60.

2. Sexual misconduct. ACOG Committee Opinion No. 373. American College of Obstetricians and Gynecologists. Obstet Gynecol 2007;110:441–4.

3. Informed consent. ACOG Committee Opinion No. 439. American College of Obstetricians and Gynecologists. Obstet Gynecol 2009;114:401–8.

4. Patient testing: ethical issues in selection and counseling. ACOG Committee Opinion No. 363. American College of Obstetricians and Gynecologists. Obstet Gynecol 2007;109:1021–3.

5. Human immunodeficiency virus. ACOG Committee Opinion No. 389. American College of Obstetricians and Gynecologists. Obstet Gynecol 2007;110:1473–8.

6. Professional relationships with industry. Committee Opinion No. 541. American College of Obstetricians and Gynecologists. Obstet Gynecol 2012;120:1243–9.

7. Commercial enterprises in medical practice. ACOG Committee Opinion No. 359. American College of Obstetricians and Gynecologists. Obstet Gynecol 2007;109:243–5.

8. Expert testimony. ACOG Committee Opinion No. 374. American College of Obstetricians and Gynecologists. Obstet Gynecol 2007;110:445–6.

GRANTING GYNECOLOGIC PRIVILEGES*

Credentialing and granting privileges to members of its medical staff are among the most important responsibilities of any health care facility. Credentialing is a multifaceted process that involves verification of licensure, education and training, malpractice experience, malpractice insurance coverage, and board certification as required by the facility. It requires that reports are requested from the National Practitioner Data Bank and other facilities where the applicant has or has had privileges.

The more difficult, yet critical, aspect of this process is determining which requested privileges will be granted. Privileging defines what procedures a credentialed practitioner is permitted to perform at the facility. The granting of privileges is based on training, experience, and demonstrated current clinical competence. Each staff member must be assessed at the time of initial application as well as every 2 years at the time of reappraisal. In addition to routine requests for privileges, a physician also may request privileges to perform a new technology. The process of assessing current clinical competence and granting privileges is difficult and time-consuming, yet it is a critically necessary activity.

Although the terms "credentialing" and "privileging" often are used interchangeably, they are different processes. Credentialing assures membership and comprises the aforementioned components. For privileging, there have been various approaches to setting criteria, such as the following six methods (1):

1. "Laundry list"—An applicant can specifically request procedures and conditions from a checklist.

---

*Modified from American College of Obstetricians and Gynecologists. Quality and safety in women's health care. 2nd ed. Washington, DC: American College of Obstetricians and Gynecologists; 2010.

2. Categorization—Major procedures or treatment areas are identified and classified based on complexity or the level of training.

3. Descriptive—Allows the applicant to describe the requested privileges in narrative form.

4. Delineation by codes—Privileges are requested based on diagnosis codes (from the current edition of the *International Classification of Diseases, Clinical Modification* system), procedure codes from Current Procedural Terminology, or grouping codes from Diagnosis-Related Group codes.

5. Combination—A hybrid of two or more of the methods described.

6. Core privileging—An alternative to the methods described. This assumes that anyone who has completed an approved residency has sufficient knowledge and technical skills to perform competently within the specialty. This method allows for consistency, flexibility, and objective screening for all applicants.

Privileges often are formatted by levels (eg, Level I, Level II, and Level III obstetric privileges and Level I, Level II, and Level III gynecologic privileges). As new technologies evolve, processes for granting privileges for them will need to be formulated. For a sample application for privileges, which outlines such areas as emergency situations, provisional period, and the performance of new procedures, see Appendix C. Hospitals using these materials may adapt them to conform to the specific situations at these facilities. This information is not intended to be all inclusive or exclusive. It is intended primarily for educational purposes.

Granting Privileges

The following list has been developed to aid in granting privileges to those health care providers within the facility to perform gynecologic procedures. The granting of privileges at any level in obstetrics and gynecology is based on satisfaction of criteria for the specified procedures. Criteria for granting privileges must be applied consistently regardless of the applicant's specialty. As stated, the granting of clinical privileges must be based on training, experience, and demonstrated current clinical competence. The educational requirements assume that applicants have achieved a doctor of medicine or doctor of osteopathy degree. Except as otherwise noted, prerequisites for each category of privileges are listed as follows:

TRAINING

Successful completion of an Accreditation Council for Graduate Medical Education (ACGME)-accredited residency program in obstetrics–gynecology

CERTIFICATION

- Board certification (or active candidate) by the American Board of Obstetrics and Gynecology or the American Osteopathic Board of Obstetrics and Gynecology
- Maintenance of Certification, if applicable

Reappraisal (recredentialing and reprivi;eging) (2-year cycle) should require:

- Review of quality improvement file
  - trending
  - sentinel events
  - other problems with specific procedures
- Review of level of activity
  - total number of cases
  - total number of complications
  - outcomes

If the credentials committee determines that the number of cases performed within the cycle is insufficient for adequately assessing competency, it may recommend that the individual be proctored and evaluated for a designated period until competency is demonstrated. However, if the physician has privileges at another institution for the particular procedure, then the individual must provide credentialing data from that hospital for review by the credentials committee and may not require proctoring.

I. Gynecologic Privileges

A. Level I (Basic) Gynecologic Privileges

    1. Privileges may include the following:

        a. Appropriate screening examination of the female, including breast examination

        b. Obtaining vaginal and cervical cytology

        c. Colposcopy

        d. Cervical biopsy, polypectomy

        e. Endometrial biopsy

        f. Cryosurgery and cautery for benign disease

        g. Microscopic diagnosis of urine and vaginal smears

        h. Bartholin cyst drainage or marsupialization

        i. Dilation and curettage for incomplete abortion

        j. Vulvar biopsy

B. Level II (Specialty) Gynecologic Privileges

    1. Privileges may include the following:

        a. All Level I gynecologic privileges

        b. Dilation and curettage, with or without conization

        c. Laparotomy

        d. Operations for removal of uterus, cervix, oviducts, ovaries (abdominal or vaginal), and appendix

        e. Diagnostic laparoscopy

        f. Diagnostic hysteroscopy

        g. Tubal sterilization

        h. Operations for treatment of urinary stress incontinence, vaginal approach, retropubic urethral suspension, or sling procedure

        i. Fistula repairs (vesicovaginal or rectovaginal)

        j. Tuboplasty

        k. Hernia repair (incisional or umbilical)

        l. Operations for treatment of noninvasive carcinoma of vulva, vagina, uterus, ovary, and cervix

        m. Repair of rectocele, enterocele, cystocele

n. Vaginectomy (total or partial)

o. Colpocleisis

p. Strassman procedure (metroplasty)

q. Myomectomy

r. Node dissection (superficial inguinal, pelvic, or para-aortic)

s. Second-trimester abortion by medical or surgical means

C. Level III-A: Basic Endoscopic Procedures

1. Privileges may include the following:
   a. All Level I and Level II gynecologic privileges
   b. Endoscopic ovarian or endometrial biopsy
   c. Minor adhesiolysis
   d. Management of ectopic pregnancy (linear salpingostomy, partial salpingectomy)
   e. Destruction of endometriosis stage I and stage II as graded by American Society for Reproductive Medicine criteria

2. Training should include successful completion of an ACGME-accredited residency program in obstetrics and gynecology

3. Certification should be required:
   a. Board certification (or active candidate) by the American Board of Obstetrics and Gynecology
   b. Maintenance of Certification, if applicable

4. Experience should be required:
   a. The applicant must possess the proficiency and be privileged to perform the requested procedures in an open (laparotomy) manner
   b. The applicant should have been granted privileges to perform basic (Level III-A) endoscopic procedures and should have demonstrated competency in these techniques

D. Level III-B: Advanced Endoscopic Procedures

1. Privileges may include the following:
   a. All Level I and Level II gynecologic privileges
   b. Laparoscopically assisted vaginal hysterectomy
   c. Ovarian cystectomy

    d. Salpingo-oophorectomy

    e. Adhesiolysis

    f. Management of endometriosis, stage III and stage IV

    g. Division of the uterosacral ligaments

    h. Appendectomy

    i. Operative hysteroscopy requiring use of the resectoscope (division or resection of the uterine septum, surgical treatment of Asherman syndrome, resection of uterine myomas)

    j. Myomectomy

    k. Pelvic lymphadenectomy

    l. Pelvic sidewall dissection

    m. Ureteral dissection

    n. Presacral neurectomy

    o. Dissection of obliterated pouch of Douglas

    p. Hernia repair

    q. Retropubic bladder neck suspension

    r. Sling procedure

    s. Bowel surgery

    t. Total hysterectomy

    u. Supracervical hysterectomy

2. Also required is successful completion of advanced training that includes training in listed procedures, or documented course, including didactic and hands-on laboratory experience, unless included in residency program.

3. Experience should include advanced procedures, which require the following additional training and documentation:

    a. Completion of a postgraduate course, accredited by the ACGME that includes didactic training (must include education on equipment operation and safety factors) and hands-on laboratory experience, and

    b. If the privileges requested were not included in residency training, the applicant must follow the requirements for a preceptorship as discussed under the section for "Requests for New Privileges."

   c. In the event that credentials in advanced endoscopy are already established at a different hospital, the applicant must present evidence of these established credentials in lieu of (a) and (b) above. In addition, the applicant must provide a list of cases performed over the past 24 months, including preoperative and postoperative diagnoses, procedure, type of endoscope used, outcome, and complications of the procedure.

   d. A letter from the director of an approved residency program can substitute for (a) and (b) above. In addition, this new residency graduate must provide a list of advanced endoscopy cases performed over the past 24 months.

E. Level III-C: Gynecologic Oncology

   1. Privileges may include the following:
      a. All Level I and Level II gynecologic privileges
      b. Treatment of malignant disease with chemotherapy
      c. Radical hysterectomy for treatment of invasive carcinoma of the cervix and uterus
      d. Radical surgery for treatment of gynecologic malignancy to include procedures on bowel, ureter, bladder, pelvic or abdominal organs, as indicated
      e. Treatment of invasive carcinoma of vulva by radical vulvectomy
      f. Treatment of invasive carcinoma of the vagina by radical vaginectomy and other appropriate surgery
      g. Pelvic, periaortic, and inguinal lymphadenectomy and reconstructive surgery of pelvis and external genitalia

   2. Training also should include documentation of specialized post-residency training, experience, or subspecialty certification by the American Board of Obstetrics and Gynecology.

F. Level III-D: Assisted Reproductive Techniques

   1. Privileges may include:
      a. Gynecologic Level I, Level II, Level III-A, and Level III-B
      b. In vitro fertilization and gamete intrafallopian transfer

      c. Monitoring of ovulation induction and intrauterine insemination

      d. Management of ovarian hyperstimulation

  2. Training should also include the following:

      a. Documentation of training and experience in reproductive endocrinology and pelvic reproductive surgery, including experience in operative laparoscopic procedures, and

      b. Documentation of training and experience with in vitro fertilization–embryo transfer and gamete intrafallopian transfer procedures.

  3. Subspecialty certification (or active candidate) by the American Board of Obstetrics and Gynecology in reproductive endocrinology and infertility also may be considered.

  4. Experience should require demonstrating knowledge of all aspects of assisted reproductive techniques.

G. Level III-E: Laser Therapy

  1. Privileges may include the following:

      a. Laser therapy for cervix, vagina, vulva, and perineum (colposcopically directed)

      b. Conization of cervix

      c. Lysis of adhesions and photocoagulation (intraabdominal "free hand use")

      d. Lysis of adhesions and photocoagulation (microscopically directed)

      e. Oncologic debulking procedures (intraabdominal "free hand use")

  2. Training should also include the following:

      a. Documentation of laser training from a residency program director, attesting to the completion of at least 8 hours of observation and hands-on involvement, or

      b. Documentation of a laser training course, including laser physics, safety, indications and complications, and hands-on experience

3. Experience should include the following:
   a. Level II gynecologic privileges, and
   b. Laser privileges as defined on the hospital-wide laser privilege request form

H. Level III-F: Endometrial Ablation
   1. Privileges may include the following:
      a. Laser ablation
      b. Electrosurgical ablation
      c. Thermal balloon ablation
      d. Other techniques
   2. Training should also include additional training for the following procedures:
      a. Laser ablation
         (1) Documentation from residency program director, attesting to hands-on involvement and competence, or
         (2) Documentation of an operative hysteroscopy and laser ablation of the endometrium course, including laser physics, safety, indications and complications, and hands-on experience
      b. Electrosurgical ablation
         (1) Documentation from residency program director, including at least 8 hours of observation and hands-on involvement, or
         (2) Documentation of competency and demonstration of hands-on experience in operative hysteroscopy with endometrial rollerball
      c. Thermal balloon ablation
         (1) Documentation from residency program director, attesting to the completion of at least 8 hours of observation and hands-on involvement, or
         (2) Documentation of competency and demonstration of hands-on experience

3. Experience should include proficiency in diagnostic hysteroscopy if laser or electrosurgical ablation is performed

II. Gynecologic Privileges for Family Physicians

A. Privileges may include the following:

1. Appropriate screening examination of the female, including breast examination

2. Obtaining vaginal and cervical cytology

3. Colposcopy

4. Cervical biopsy, polypectomy

5. Endometrial biopsy

6. Cryosurgery and cautery for benign disease

7. Microscopic diagnosis of urine and vaginal smears

8. Bartholin duct cyst drainage or marsupialization

9. Vulvar biopsy

B. Family physicians requesting these privileges must demonstrate the following:

1. Successful completion of gynecologic training as delineated in the special requirements for residency training in Family Medicine by the ACGME

2. If transferring from another institution, documentation of current competence as supported by ongoing clinical practice and quality review data

3. Maintenance of board certification (or active candidate) by the American Board of Family Medicine

Requests for New Privileges

Physicians also may request new privileges for added skills or qualifications or after a period of inactivity. Privileges for new skills should only be granted when the appropriate training has been completed and documented and the competency level has been achieved with adequate supervision. Proof of attendance at a postgraduate training course in a new technology or procedure is not sufficient to demonstrate competence in the performance of such procedures. In addition, the National Practitioner Data Bank must be queried whenever physicians request new privileges outside of the normal reappointment credentialing process.

When physicians request re-entry after a period of inactivity, a general guideline for evaluation would be to consider the physician as any other new applicant for privileges. An underlying assumption is that physicians do not necessarily lose competence in all areas of practice with time. A re-entry program should target those areas in which physicians are more likely to have lost relevant skills or knowledge, or in which skills and knowledge need to be updated (2). It is extremely important for physicians considering a leave of absence or major change in practice activities to think in advance about options should they wish to return. At a minimum, licensure and continuing medical education activities should be maintained. Working part-time during an absence helps to maintain a minimal amount of competency.

For more information on granting privileges for added skills or qualifications or after a period of inactivity, please see the "Evaluating Credentials and Granting Privileges" section in Part 1. See also Appendix C for a sample application for gynecologic privileges.

References

1. Cairns CS. Core privileges: a practical approach to development and implementation. 3rd ed. Marblehead (MA): HCPro; 2005.
2. American Medical Association. Physician reentry. Report 6 of the Council on Medical Education (A-08). Chicago (IL): AMA; 2008. Available at: http://www.ama-assn.org/ama1/pub/upload/mm/377/cmerpt_6a-08.pdf. Retrieved July 10, 2013.

APPENDIX

SAMPLE APPLICATION FOR GYNECOLOGIC PRIVILEGES*†

1. Name: _____

2. Department to which I am applying: _____

3. Other department(s) in which
   clinical privileges are held or sought: _____

4. Subject to consultation requirements and other policies, I understand that in exercising my clinical privileges granted, I am constrained by relevant hospital policies requiring consultations for difficult diagnoses, conditions of extreme severity, and procedures and conditions that are beyond my area of training, specialization, and current competence and experience; by hospital policies concerning types of patients for whom it does not have appropriate resources (facilities, equipment, or personnel) to treat except on an emergency basis; and by such special policies as may from time to time be adopted.

5. Emergency situations:

   I also understand

   (a) that the privileges are being requested for regular use in my practice;

---

*Reprinted from American College of Obstetricians and Gynecologists. Quality and safety in women's health care. 2nd ed. Washington, DC: American College of Obstetricians and Gynecologists; 2010.

†This sample application for privileges is provided for educational purposes only. It may require modification for use in a particular facility.

(b) that it is not necessary to request emergency clinical privileges;

(c) that an emergency is deemed to exist whenever serious permanent harm or aggravation of injury or disease is imminent, or the life of a patient is in immediate danger, and any delay in administering treatment could add danger;

(d) that in such emergency, when better alternative sources of care are not reasonably available given the patient's condition, I am authorized and will be assisted to do everything possible to save the patient's life or to save the patient from serious harm to the degree permitted by my license but regardless of department affiliation or privileges;

(e) and that if I provide services to a patient in an emergency, I am obligated to use appropriate consultative assistance when available and to arrange, when it is my responsibility, for appropriate follow-up care.

General Provisions

BASIS FOR GRANTING PRIVILEGES

1. Applicants requesting clinical privileges must demonstrate satisfactory training, experience, and current competence for the privileges being requested and must agree to comply with the provisions contained in the medical staff bylaws.

2. Each applicant requesting privileges in the department of obstetrics and gynecology should be required to present his or her application and a list of recent cases for review by the department chief. (For physicians who have just completed an ob-gyn residency program, the list could be the senior resident case list.) When family physicians or nurse–midwives request privileges, an equivalent list of recently managed cases, representing the full range of privileges being requested, also must be submitted.

PROVISIONAL PERIOD

1. All new appointees to the department of obstetrics and gynecology must undergo a minimum provisional period of no less than 12 months. The practitioner should have admitted a minimum number of cases to the hospital, completed an equivalent number of surgical procedures, or both, as defined by the institution.

2. At the chair's discretion, any additional documentation deemed necessary to assess an applicant's competency in specific procedures during the provisional period may be requested. This documentation may include evidence of specific education or training in a procedure either during residency training or through postresidency courses.

3. At the conclusion of their provisional period, those individuals who did not meet the minimum criteria stipulated under Number 1, or those who requested other than active staff status, should provide the chair with a detailed listing of each case completed within the department as well as the description, scope, and breadth of their practice at other institutions. In addition to the hospital's quality improvement review, the department chair also may request information from other institutions where the individual practices to assess overall competency for the procedure(s) requested.

4. Those individuals requesting privileges for a new procedure must have successfully completed their initial provisional period and have been appointed to the medical staff without restriction.

They also should submit evidence they have completed an educational or training program in the specific procedure either in a residency program or through postgraduate residency training. In addition, each applicant should submit a letter from the director of a residency program stating that he or she is competent in the respective procedure and has completed the appropriate training.

Individuals requesting privileges for a new procedure must be deemed competent to perform the procedure by an individual currently credentialed for that procedure in the department. However, if this is the first time these privileges have been requested within the department, arrangements should be made to ensure that the applicant is adequately evaluated before granting full, unrestricted privileges. In general, a minimum number of cases with preceptorship or observation, as defined by the institution, are required before full, unrestricted privileges can be granted for a new procedure.

NEW, UNTRIED, UNPROVEN, OR EXPERIMENTAL PROCEDURES AND TREATMENT MODALITIES AND INSTRUMENTATION

Experimental drugs, procedures, or other therapies or tests may be administered or performed only after approval of protocols involved by the committee responsible for the institutional review board function. Any other new, untried, unproven, or experimental procedure or treatment modality or instrumentation may be performed or used only after the regular credentialing process has been completed, and the privilege to perform or use said procedure or treatment modality or instrument has been granted to an individual practitioner. For the purposes of this paragraph, a new, untried, unproven, or experimental procedure or treatment modality or instrumentation is one that is not generalizable from an established procedure or treatment modality or instrumentation that involves the same or similar skills, the same or similar instrumentation and technique, the same or similar complications, or the same or similar indications as the established procedure or treatment modality or instrumentation.

Occupational Safety and Health Administration Regulations on Occupational Exposure to Bloodborne Pathogens*

In 1970, the U.S. Congress enacted the Occupational Safety and Health Act to protect workers from unsafe and unhealthy conditions in the workplace. To oversee this effort, the law also created the Occupational Safety and Health Administration (OSHA) within the U.S. Department of Labor. The Occupational Safety and Health Administration has the responsibility for developing and implementing job safety and health standards and regulations. Its standards and regulations apply to all employers and employees. To promote and ensure compliance with its standards, OSHA has the authority to conduct unannounced workplace inspections. It also maintains a reporting and record-keeping system to monitor job-related injuries and illnesses. Failure to comply with OSHA standards may result in the assessment of civil or criminal penalties.

In December 1991, OSHA issued new regulations on occupational exposure to bloodborne pathogens that are designed to minimize the transmission of human immunodeficiency virus (HIV), hepatitis B virus (HBV), and other potentially infectious materials in the workplace. The regulations cover all employees in physician offices, hospitals, medical laboratories, and other health care facilities where workers could be

---

*Data from Bloodborne pathogens, 29 C.F.R. part 1910.1030 (2013). Available at: http://www.gpo.gov/fdsys/pkg/CFR-2013-title29-vol6/pdf/CFR-2013-title29-vol6-sec1910-1030.pdf. Retrieved September 20, 2013.

"reasonably anticipated" as a result of performing their job duties to come into contact with blood and other potentially infectious materials. The regulations were revised, effective April 2001, to comply with the Needlestick Safety and Prevention Act of 2000.

Approved State Plans

Under the federal law that created OSHA, states are encouraged to develop and operate—under OSHA guidance—state job safety and health plans. Currently, 25 states and 2 other jurisdictions have OSHA-approved plans, which require them to provide standards and enforcement programs that are at least as effective as the federal standards. They are as follows:

- Alaska
- Arizona
- California
- Connecticut
- Hawaii
- Illinois
- Indiana
- Iowa
- Kentucky
- Maryland
- Michigan
- Minnesota
- Nevada
- New Jersey
- New Mexico
- New York
- North Carolina
- Oregon
- Puerto Rico

- South Carolina
- Tennessee
- Utah
- Vermont
- Virgin Islands
- Virginia
- Washington
- Wyoming

A list of these state OSHA offices is available on the OSHA web site at www.osha.gov/dcsp/osp/states.html; call the number listed to receive a copy of the state's standards on occupational exposure to bloodborne pathogens. In Connecticut, Illinois, New Jersey, New York, and the Virgin Islands the state plans cover state and local government employees only; the private sector is covered by the federal OSHA standard. In addition, states with an OSHA-approved state plan must comply with the federal OSHA standard.

Complying With Regulations

EXPOSURE CONTROL PLAN

In order to comply with the regulations, health care employers are required to prepare a written "Exposure Control Plan" designed to eliminate or minimize employee exposure to bloodborne pathogens. This plan must list all job classifications in which employees are likely to be exposed to infectious materials and the relevant tasks and procedures performed by these employees. Infectious materials include blood, semen, vaginal secretions, peritoneal fluid, amniotic fluid, any body fluid visibly contaminated with blood, all body fluids in which it is impossible to differentiate between the body fluids, any unfixed human tissue or organ (living or dead), as well as HIV-containing cell or tissue cultures, organ cultures, and HIV-containing or HBV-containing culture medium or other solutions.

Under the plan, employers are required to adopt universal precautions, engineering and work practice controls, and personal protective equipment requirements. Employers also must establish a schedule for implementing the following controls:

- Housekeeping requirements
- Employee training and record-keeping requirements
- Hepatitis B virus vaccination for employees and postexposure evaluation and follow-up procedures
- Communication of hazards

A detailed discussion of each of these requirements follows. The plan must be accessible to employees and made available to OSHA upon request. The Exposure Control Plan must be reviewed annually and updated to reflect changes in technology that eliminate or reduce exposure to bloodborne pathogens. The employer must document this annual consideration and use of appropriate effective safer medical procedures and devices that are commercially available. In designing and reviewing the Exposure Control Plan, the employer must solicit input from nonmanagerial employees who are potentially exposed to injuries from contaminated sharps. Employers must document, in the Exposure Control Plan, how they received input from employees.

MANDATORY UNIVERSAL PRECAUTIONS

The regulations require that universal precautions must be used to prevent contact with blood or other potentially infectious materials. It is OSHA's intention to follow the Centers for Disease Control and Prevention's guidelines on universal precautions. As defined by the Centers for Disease Control and Prevention, the concept of universal precautions requires the employer and employee to assume that blood and other body fluids are infectious and must be handled accordingly.

ENGINEERING AND WORK PRACTICE CONTROLS

Specific engineering and work practice controls for the workplace must be implemented and examined for effectiveness on a regular schedule. These include the following controls:

1. Employers are required to provide hand-washing facilities that are readily accessible to employees; when this is not feasible, employees

must be provided with an antiseptic hand cleanser with clean cloth or paper towels or antiseptic towelettes. It is the employer's responsibility to ensure that employees wash their hands immediately after gloves and other protective garments are removed.

2. Contaminated needles and other contaminated sharp objects shall not be bent, recapped, or removed unless the employer can demonstrate that no alternative is feasible or that a specific medical procedure requires such action. Shearing or breaking of contaminated needles is prohibited. Recapping or needle removal must be accomplished by a mechanical device or a one-handed technique. Contaminated reusable sharp objects shall be placed in appropriate containers until properly reprocessed; these containers must be puncture resistant, leakproof, and labeled or color coded in accordance with the regulations for easy identification.

3. Eating, drinking, smoking, applying cosmetics or lip balm, and handling contact lenses are prohibited in work areas where there is a reasonable likelihood of exposure to potentially infectious materials.

4. Food and drink must not be kept in refrigerators, freezers, shelves, cabinets, or on countertops where blood or other potentially infectious materials are present.

5. All procedures that involve blood or other infectious materials shall be performed in a manner to minimize splashing, spraying, spattering, and creating droplets; mouth pipetting and suctioning of blood or other potentially infectious materials is prohibited.

6. Specimens of blood or other potentially infectious materials must be placed in closed containers that prevent leakage during collection, handling, processing, storage, transport, or shipping; containers must be labeled or color coded in accordance with the regulations for easy identification. However, when a facility uses universal precautions in the handling of all specimens, the required labeling or color coding of specimens is not necessary as long as containers are recognizable as containing specimens; this exemption applies only while the specimens and containers remain in the facility. If outside contamination of the primary container occurs, it must be placed within a second

container that is leakproof, puncture resistant, and labeled or color coded accordingly.

7. Equipment that could be contaminated with blood or other infectious materials must be examined before servicing or shipping and shall be decontaminated as necessary, unless the employer can demonstrate that decontamination of the equipment or parts of the equipment is not feasible. A visible label must be attached to the equipment stating which parts remain contaminated. The employer must ensure that this information is conveyed to all affected employees, the servicing representative, the manufacturer, or all three before handling, servicing, or shipping so that the necessary precautions will be taken.

PERSONAL PROTECTIVE EQUIPMENT

The regulations also stress the importance of appropriate personal protective equipment that employers are required to provide at no cost to employees whose job duties expose them to blood and other infectious materials. Appropriate personal protective equipment includes but is not limited to gloves, gowns, laboratory coats, face shields or masks, eye protection, mouthpieces, resuscitation bags, pocket masks, or other ventilation devices. As defined by OSHA, personal protective equipment is considered "appropriate" if it prevents blood or other potentially infectious materials from reaching an employee's work clothes and skin, eyes, mouth, or other mucous membranes under normal conditions of use.

Employers must ensure that the employee uses appropriate personal protective equipment unless the employer can demonstrate that the employee temporarily declined to use the equipment, when under rare and extraordinary circumstances, it was the employee's professional judgment that use of personal protective equipment would have prevented the delivery of health care services or would have posed an increased hazard to the safety of the worker or co-worker. When an employee makes this judgment, the circumstances shall be investigated and documented in order to determine whether changes can be made to prevent such situations in the future.

Personal protective equipment in the appropriate sizes must be accessible at the worksite or issued to employees. Hypoallergenic gloves, glove liners, powderless gloves, or other similar alternatives, shall be accessible to those employees who are allergic to the gloves normally provided. The employer shall provide for laundering and disposal of personal protective equipment, as well as repair and replace this equipment when necessary to maintain its effectiveness, at no cost to the employee. If a garment(s) is penetrated by blood or other infectious materials, it must be removed immediately or as soon as feasible. All personal protective equipment must be removed before leaving the work area, whereupon it shall be placed in a designated area or storage container for washing or disposal.

Gloves must be worn when it can reasonably be anticipated that the employee may have hand contact with blood, other potentially infectious materials, mucous membranes, and nonintact skin; when performing vascular access procedures; and when handling or touching contaminated surfaces. Disposable gloves shall be replaced as soon as practical when contaminated or when torn or punctured; they shall not be washed or decontaminated for reuse. Utility gloves may be decontaminated for reuse but must be discarded if a glove is cracked, peeling, torn, punctured, or shows other signs of deterioration.

Masks in combination with goggles or protective eye shields must be worn whenever splashes, spray, spatter, or droplets of blood may be created and eye, nose, or mouth contamination can reasonably be anticipated. Gowns and other protective body clothing such as, but not limited to, gowns, aprons, lab coats, clinic jackets, or similar outer garments, shall be worn in occupational exposure situations. The type and characteristics will depend upon the task and degree of exposure anticipated. Surgical caps, hoods, shoe covers, or all three must be worn in situations in which gross contamination can reasonably be anticipated (eg, autopsies, orthopedic surgery).

HOUSEKEEPING

Employers must ensure that the worksite is maintained in a clean and sanitary condition and shall develop and implement a written schedule for cleaning and method of decontamination based upon the location within the facility, type of surface to be cleaned, type of soil present, and tasks or procedures being performed in the area. All equipment and working surfaces shall be cleaned and decontaminated after contact with blood or other potentially infectious materials.

Contaminated work surfaces shall be decontaminated with an appropriate disinfectant after tasks and procedures are completed; immediately or as soon as feasible when surfaces are contaminated or after any spill of blood or other potentially infectious materials; and at the end of the work shift if the surface may have become contaminated since the last cleaning. Protective covering (eg, plastic wrap, aluminum foil, or imperviously backed absorbent paper used to cover equipment and environmental surfaces) must be removed and replaced as soon as feasible upon contamination or at the end of the work shift if they may have become contaminated during the shift. All bins, pails, cans, and similar containers intended for reuse shall be inspected and decontaminated on a regularly scheduled basis and cleaned immediately or as soon as feasible upon visible contamination.

Broken glassware that may be contaminated must not be picked up directly with the hands; it must be cleaned up using a brush and dustpan, tongs, or forceps. Contaminated reusable sharp objects must not be stored or processed in a manner that requires employees to reach by hand into the containers in which these sharp objects have been placed. Containers for contaminated sharp objects must be closable, puncture resistant, leakproof on the sides and bottom, and labeled or color coded in accordance with the regulations. During use, containers for contaminated sharp objects shall be easily accessible to personnel and located as close as possible to the immediate area where sharp objects are used. Additionally, these containers must be maintained upright throughout use, replaced routinely, and not be allowed to be overfilled. Reusable containers shall not be opened, emptied, or cleaned manually or in any other manner that would expose employees to the risk of percutaneous injury. Containers of contaminated disposable sharp objects and personal protective equipment are defined as regulated waste; such containers must prevent the spillage or protrusion of contents during handling, storage, transport, or shipping.

Contaminated laundry shall be handled as little as possible and must be placed in bags or containers at the location where it was used; it must not be sorted or rinsed in the location of use. Contaminated laundry shall be transported in clearly labeled or color-coded bags or containers in accordance with the regulations. Employers shall ensure that employees who have contact with contaminated laundry wear protective gloves and other appropriate personal protective equipment. When a facility ships contaminated laundry offsite to a second facility that does not use universal precautions in handling all laundry, the facility generating the contaminated laundry must clearly mark or color code the bags or containers with appropriate biohazard labels.

HEPATITIS B VACCINATION

Employers are required to provide HBV vaccination free of charge to all employees who are at risk of occupational exposure. The vaccine must be provided within 10 days of an employee's initial assignment, except in the following cases:

- The employee has previously received the complete HBV vaccination series.
- Antibody testing has revealed that the employee is immune.
- The vaccine is contraindicated for medical reasons.

The regulations prohibit employers from making employees participate in a prescreening program as a prerequisite for receiving the vaccine. Employees who refuse the vaccination must sign a "Hepatitis B Vaccine Declination" form stating that they have declined the vaccine. If the U.S. Public Health Service ever recommends booster doses of HBV vaccine, they also must be provided to employees free of charge. The employee, however, is allowed to change his or her mind and elect to receive the vaccine at any time at the employer's expense.

Postexposure Evaluation and Follow-up

Following a report of an employee exposure incident, the employer must make immediately available to the exposed employee a confidential medical evaluation at no cost to the employee and at a reasonable time and place, and follow-up, including at least the following information and follow-up care:

1. Documentation of the route(s) of exposure and the circumstances under which the exposure occurred

2. Identification and documentation of the individual who is the source of the blood or potentially infectious material, unless the employer can establish that such identification is not feasible or is prohibited by state or local law. The source individual's blood shall be tested as soon as possible and after consent is obtained, in order to determine HBV or HIV infectivity. If consent is not obtained, the employer must document that legally required consent cannot be obtained. If the source individual's consent is not required by law, the source individual's blood if available must be tested and the results documented. However, when the source individual is already known to be infected with HBV or HIV, blood testing for HBV or HIV is not required. Results of the source individual's blood test must be made available to the exposed employee, and the employee shall be informed of all applicable laws concerning the disclosure of the source individual's identity and infectious status.

3. Collection and testing of the exposed employee's blood for HBV and HIV serologic status as soon as feasible after the employee gives consent. If the employee consents to baseline blood collection but does not give consent at that time for HIV serologic testing, the sample shall be preserved for 90 days. Testing of the blood shall take place within the 90 days if the employee decides to do so.

4. Postexposure prophylaxis when medically indicated, as recommended by the U.S. Public Health Service

5. Counseling

6. Evaluation of reported illnesses

The employer must ensure that the health professional responsible for the employee's HBV vaccination is provided a copy of the OSHA regulation on bloodborne pathogens. In the case of a health professional evaluating an exposed employee, the employer shall ensure that the health professional is provided the following information:

- A copy of the OSHA bloodborne pathogens regulations
- A description of the exposed employee's duties as they relate to the exposure incident

- Documentation of the routes of exposure and circumstances under which exposure occurred
- Results of the source individual's blood testing, if available
- All medical records relevant to the appropriate treatment of the exposed employee, including vaccination status, which is the employer's responsibility to maintain

The employer must obtain and provide the employee with a copy of the evaluating health professional's written opinion within 15 days of completion. The health professional's written opinion for HBV vaccination shall be limited to whether HBV vaccination is indicated for the employee and if the employee has received such vaccination. The health professional's written opinion for postexposure evaluation and follow-up shall be limited to the following information:

- The employee has been informed of the results of the evaluation.
- The employee has been told about any medical conditions resulting from exposure to blood or other potentially infectious materials that require further evaluation or treatment.

All other findings or diagnoses must remain confidential and shall not be included in the written report.

COMMUNICATIONS OF HAZARDS TO EMPLOYEES

Warning Labels and Signs

The regulations require warning labels on containers of regulated waste and refrigerators and freezers that contain blood or other potentially infectious materials. Warning labels also must be affixed to containers used to store, transport, or ship blood or other potentially infectious materials. The warning labels must be fluorescent orange or orange-red; however, red bags or red containers may be substituted for labels.

Employee Training

Employers must ensure that all employees at risk of occupational exposure participate in a training program at no cost to employees and during working hours. Training shall take place at the time of an employee's initial assignment to tasks that risk exposure and at least annually thereafter. Annual training for employees shall be provided within 1 year of their previous training. Additional training must be provided when changes, such as modifications of tasks or procedures or introduction of new tasks and procedures, affect the worker's exposure risk. The training must be conducted by a person knowledgeable about the subject matter, and the material shall be presented at an educational level appropriate to the employees. The training program at a minimum must include the following information:

1. A copy of the bloodborne pathogens regulations and an explanation of their contents

2. A general explanation of the epidemiology and symptoms of bloodborne diseases

3. An explanation of the modes of transmission of bloodborne diseases

4. An explanation of the employer's Exposure Control Plan and information on how the employee can obtain a copy of the plan

5. An explanation of the appropriate methods for identifying tasks and other activities that may involve exposure

6. An explanation of the methods that will prevent or reduce exposure (including appropriate engineering controls, work practices, and personal protective equipment)

7. Information on the types, proper use, location, removal, handling, decontamination, and disposal of personal protective equipment

8. An explanation of the basis for selection of personal protective equipment

9. Information on the HBV vaccine (efficacy, safety, method of administration, benefits of being vaccinated, and that the vaccine will be offered free of charge)

10. Information on the appropriate actions to take and individuals to contact in an emergency that involves blood or other infectious materials

11. An explanation of the procedure for follow-up if an exposure incident occurs (including the method for reporting incident and the medical follow-up that may be available)

12. Information on the postexposure evaluation and follow-up that the employer is required to provide for the employee

13. An explanation of the signs and labels, color-coding requirements, or both

14. An opportunity for interactive questions and answers with the person conducting the training session

RECORD-KEEPING REQUIREMENTS

The employer shall maintain an accurate record for each employee at risk of occupational exposure that includes the following information:

- The name and social security number of employee
- The employee's HBV vaccination status (dates and any medical information relative to the employee's ability to receive the vaccination)
- The results of examinations, medical testing, and follow-up procedures
- The employer's copy of the health professional's written evaluation as required following an exposure incident
- A copy of the information provided to the health professional as required following an exposure incident

The employer shall ensure the confidentiality of employee records; information shall not be disclosed without the employee's written consent. The employer is required to maintain records for the duration of employment plus 30 years. The employer also must maintain records of the training sessions that include the dates, the names and qualifications of individuals who conducted training sessions, and the names and job titles of employees who attended sessions. These records shall be maintained for 3 years from the date the training session occurred.

All records shall be made available to the assistant secretary of OSHA for examination and copying, including employee medical records, for which the employee's consent is not needed. In the event of an employer going out of business, these records must be transferred to the new owner or must be offered to the National Institute for Occupational Safety and Health.

Sharps Injury Log

An employer with more than 10 employees shall maintain a "sharps injury log" to record percutaneous injuries from contaminated sharps. The information in the log shall be kept in a way to protect the confidentiality of the injured employee. The log must contain:

- The type and brand of device involved in the incident
- The department or work area where the exposure incident occurred
- An explanation of how the incident occurred

The bloodborne pathogens regulations are just one of the OSHA standards that physician offices must follow to be in compliance. Other OSHA regulations include standards on the hazards of chemicals in the workplace, compressed gases, office equipment, and an action plan in case of fire. An emergency hotline number has been established by OSHA to report emergencies: 1-800-321-OSHA (6742).

Clinical Laboratory Improvement Amendments of 1988*

The Clinical Laboratory Improvement Amendments of 1988 (CLIA) establish quality standards for all nonresearch laboratories, including physician offices that perform tests that examine human specimens for the diagnosis, prevention, or treatment of any disease, impairment of health, or health assessment. All physician offices that conduct any such tests must be certified by the Secretary of the Department of Health and Human Services. The Centers for Medicare & Medicaid Services (CMS) administers the CLIA laboratory certification program for the Secretary in conjunction with the U.S. Food and Drug Administration and the Centers for Disease Control and Prevention.

Most obstetrician–gynecologists' offices have either certificates of waiver or certificates for provider-performed microscopy (PPM) procedures. This appendix provides more information on these two types of certificates.

Certificates of Waiver

Laboratories, including physician offices, performing only waived tests must obtain a certificate of waiver from CMS in order to perform these tests. No additional complex tests may be performed by the laboratory without prior authorization from CMS. Currently, an extensive list of waived tests ("Tests Granted Waived Status Under CLIA") exists and can be

---

*Data from Centers for Medicare and Medicaid Services. Clinical Laboratory Improvement Amendments (CLIA). Available at: http://www.cms.gov/Regulations-and-Guidance/Legislation/CLIA. Retrieved July 10, 2013.

obtained on the CMS web site, available at www.cms.gov/clia/downloads/
waivetbl.pdf. This list is revised periodically, and physicians should check
with CMS to obtain the current list.

Offices performing only waived tests are exempt from the bulk of
CLIA regulatory requirements, including proficiency testing, patient test
management, quality control, personnel, quality assurance, and routine inspections. However, physician offices must follow manufacturer's
instructions for performing the test. Physician offices also are subject to
random announced or unannounced inspections to determine whether
only waived tests are being performed and to collect information about
waived tests. Complaints filed against an office also will be investigated
through an inspection.

The three CLIA requirements for waived laboratories are 1) enroll in
the CLIA program; 2) pay applicable certificate fees biennially ($150);
3) follow the manufacturers' test instructions. Renewal applications for
certificates of waiver must be submitted to the U.S. Department of Health
and Human Services no less than 9 months and no more than 12 months
before the expiration of the certificate.

Certificate for Provider-Performed Microscopy Procedure

A certificate for PPM procedures is issued to a laboratory that conducts tests
that fall under the PPM category. The procedures that are now defined as
PPM are as follows:

- Wet mounts, including preparations of vaginal, cervical, or skin
  specimens
- All potassium hydroxide preparations
- Pinworm examinations
- Fern test
- Postcoital direct, qualitative examinations of vaginal or cervical
  mucus
- Urinalysis; microscopic only

- Urinalysis, by dipstick or tablet reagent for bilirubin, glucose, hemoglobin, ketones, leukocytes, nitrite, pH, protein, specific gravity, urobilinogen, any number of these constituents; nonautomated, with microscopy

- Urinalysis, by dipstick or tablet reagent for bilirubin, glucose, hemoglobin, ketones, leukocytes, nitrite, pH, protein, specific gravity, urobilinogen, any number of these constituents; automated, with microscopy (Note: May only be used when the laboratory is using an automated dipstick urinalysis instrument approved as waived.)

- Urinalysis; two or three glass test

- Fecal leukocyte examination

- Semen analysis; presence and/or motility of sperm excluding Huhner

- Nasal smears for eosinophils

A PPM certificate also permits laboratories to perform waived tests but not other tests of moderate or high complexity. Before performing any other tests in the waived or PPM lists, a laboratory must obtain a registration certificate to cover the additional tests of greater complexity.

A laboratory with a PPM certificate also must have a laboratory director, and, if required by state law, the director must possess a state laboratory director license. The laboratory director must be a physician or a midlevel practitioner authorized to practice independently in the state where the laboratory is located. A midlevel practitioner is defined as a nurse–midwife, nurse practitioner, or physician assistant licensed by the state within which the individual practices, if such licensing is required in the state in which the laboratory is located.

The regulations also require that the microscopic tests be personally performed by a physician, a midlevel practitioner under a physician's supervision, or a midlevel practitioner in independent practice, if authorized by the state. To qualify under the PPM category, the procedure also must occur during the patient's visit on a specimen obtained from the practitioner's own patient or from a patient of the group medical practice, clinic, or other health care practitioner where the physician or midlevel practitioner is a member or an employee.

Laboratories with a PPM certificate do receive significant relief from two of the CLIA regulatory requirements. They are not subject to routine inspections, and the cost of the certificates, $200, is significantly less than the cost of a certificate for a laboratory performing tests of greater complexity. Announced or unannounced inspections may be conducted, however, to determine laboratory compliance in performing only the PPM or waived procedures listed, to evaluate complaints, and to collect data on microscopy procedures.

Other Clinical Laboratory Improvement Amendments Requirements

Laboratories with a PPM certificate also must comply with the proficiency testing, patient test management, quality control, and quality assurance requirements of the CLIA for laboratories performing tests of moderate complexity:

- Generally, the regulations prescribe that each laboratory must enroll in a proficiency testing program. At this time, none of the tests in the PPM category are required to fulfill the proficiency testing requirements. Laboratories with PPM certificates are still required, however, to meet the CLIA quality assurance requirements. Basically, this requires a laboratory to verify the accuracy, at least twice a year, of any test not subject to proficiency testing. This can be accomplished in a number of ways, including splitting specimens with a reference laboratory, evaluating the patient's clinical picture, or enrolling in a non-CLIA-approved proficiency testing program that does proficiency testing for PPM procedures.

- Patient test management requirements state that each laboratory must have available and follow written policy and procedures for specimen submission and handling. A written procedure manual also must be available and followed by office personnel for quality control purposes.

Certificates for PPM are valid for up to 2 years. To renew a PPM certificate, the appropriate renewal paperwork must be returned to the U.S.

Department of Health and Human Services 9–12 months before the expiration of the certificate.

Information about CLIA is available at the CMS web site: www.cms.gov. Information on how to apply for a CLIA certificate is available from local state survey agencies. A listing of state survey agency contacts is available on the CMS web site.

EMERGENCY MEDICAL TREATMENT AND LABOR ACT*

In 1986, Congress first enacted legal requirements specifying how Medicare-participating hospitals with emergency services must handle individuals with emergency medical conditions or women who are in labor. Since then, the Emergency Medical Treatment and Labor Act (EMTALA) has undergone numerous refinements and revisions. Physicians should expect that this law will continue to evolve and that there will be additional modifications to it in the future.

Requirements for an Appropriate Medical Screening Examination

Federal law requires that all Medicare-participating hospitals with emergency services must provide an "appropriate medical screening examination" for any individual who requests an examination or treatment for an emergency medical condition anywhere on the hospital property. This examination must be made within the capability of the hospital's emergency department, including ancillary services routinely available to the emergency department. For example, "[i]f a hospital has a department of obstetrics and gynecology, the hospital is responsible for adopting procedures under which the staff and resources of that department are available to treat a woman in labor who comes to its emergency department."

---

*Data from Centers for Medicare and Medicaid Services. Emergency Medical Treatment and Labor Act (EMTALA). Available at: http://www.cms.gov/Regulations-and-Guidance/Legislation/EMTALA/index.html. Retrieved July 10, 2013.

Medical screening examinations also must "…be conducted by individuals determined qualified by hospital by-laws or rules and regulations." Thus, it is up to a hospital to designate who is a "qualified medical person" to provide an appropriate medical screening examination. The law does not require that physicians perform all screening examinations. Therefore, a hospital can determine under what circumstances a physician is required to provide medical screening and when screening can be done by a non-physician.

Determining Whether a Patient Has an Emergency Medical Condition

The legal definition of emergency medical condition is not the same as the medical one. Under the law, the term is defined as follows:

"A medical condition manifesting itself by acute symptoms of sufficient severity (including severe pain, psychiatric disturbances and/or symptoms of substance abuse) such that the absence of immediate attention could reasonably be expected to result in—

- Placing the health of the individual (or, with respect to a pregnant woman, the health of the woman or her unborn child) in serious jeopardy;
- Serious impairment to bodily functions; or
- Serious dysfunction of any bodily organ or part."

It is important to note that with pregnant women, the health of the fetus also must be considered in determining whether an emergency medical condition exists.

Special Determination of Emergency Medical Condition for Pregnant Women

The definition of emergency medical condition also makes specific reference to a pregnant woman having contractions. It provides that an emergency medical condition exists if a pregnant woman is having contractions and "…there is inadequate time to effect a safe transfer to another hospital before delivery; or that transfer may pose a threat to the health or safety of the woman or the unborn child." An emergency medical condition does not exist even when a woman is having contractions as long as there is adequate time to effect a safe transfer before delivery and the transfer will not pose a threat to the health or safety of the mother or fetus.

The Centers for Medicare & Medicaid Services (formerly, the Health Care Financing Administration) has interpreted the definition of labor as "the process of childbirth beginning with the latent phase of labor or early phase of labor and continuing through delivery of the placenta." A woman experiencing contractions is in true labor unless a physician, certified nurse–midwife, or other qualified medical person acting within his or her scope of practice as defined in hospital medical staff bylaws and state laws certifies after a reasonable time of observation that the woman is in false labor.

Patients With Emergency Medical Conditions

Once a patient comes to an emergency department, is appropriately screened, and is determined to have an emergency medical condition, the physician has two choices as to how to proceed:

1. Treat the patient and stabilize her condition.
2. Transfer the patient to another medical facility in accordance with specific procedures outlined in a later section.

In situations in which the woman is experiencing contractions and meets the other aforementioned outlined criteria for an emergency medical condition, the only way to stabilize the patient is to deliver the child and the placenta.

Patients Can Refuse to Consent to Treatment

If a patient refuses to consent to treatment, the hospital has fulfilled its obligations under the law. If a patient refuses to consent to treatment, however, the following three steps must be taken:

1. The patient must be informed of the risks and benefits of the examination, treatment, or both.

2. The medical record must contain a description of the examination and treatment that was refused by the patient.

3. The hospital must take all reasonable steps to secure the patient's written informed refusal. The written document must indicate that the person has been informed of the risks and benefits of the examination, treatment, or both.

Procedures to Follow for Transferring a Patient to Another Medical Facility

In general, a patient who meets the criteria for an emergency medical condition may not be transferred until the patient is stabilized. There are, however, some exceptions to this prohibition.

The patient may request a transfer, in writing, after being informed of the hospital's obligations under the law and the risks of transfer. The unstabilized patient's written request for transfer must indicate the reasons for the request and that the patient is aware of the risks and benefits of transfer.

An unstabilized patient also may be transferred if a physician signs a written certification that based upon the information available at the time of transfer, the medical benefits reasonably expected from the provision of appropriate medical treatment at another medical facility outweigh the increased risks to the individual or, in the case of a woman in labor, to the woman or the unborn child, from being transferred. The certification must contain a summary of the risks and benefits of transfer.

If a physician is not physically present in the emergency department at the time of the transfer of a patient, a qualified medical person can sign the certification described previously after consulting with a physician who authorizes the transfer. The physician must countersign the certification later.

Patients Can Refuse to Consent to Transfer

If the hospital offers to transfer a patient in accordance with the appropriate procedures and the patient refuses to consent to transfer, the hospital also has fulfilled its obligations under the law. When a patient refuses to consent to the transfer, the hospital must take the following three steps:

1. The patient must be informed of the risks and benefits of the transfer.

2. The medical record must contain a description of the proposed transfer that was refused by the patient.

3. The hospital must take all reasonable steps to secure the patient's written informed refusal. The written document must indicate that the person has been informed of the risks and benefits of the transfer and the reasons for the patient's refusal.

Additional Requirements of the Transferring and Receiving Hospitals

The transferring hospital must comply with the following three requirements to ensure that the transfer was appropriate:

1. The receiving hospital must have space and qualified personnel to treat the patient and must have agreed to accept the transfer. A hospital with specialized capabilities, such as a neonatal intensive care unit, may not refuse to accept patients if space is available.

2. The transferring hospital must minimize the risks to the patient's health, and the transfer must be executed through the use of qualified personnel and transportation equipment.

3. The transferring hospital must send to the receiving hospital all medical records related to the emergency condition available at the time of transfer. These records include available history, records related to the emergency medical condition, observations of signs or symptoms, a preliminary diagnosis, results of diagnostic studies or telephone reports of the studies, reports of treatment provided, results of any tests and the informed written consent or certification, and the name of any on-call physician who has refused or failed to appear within a reasonable time to provide necessary stabilizing treatment. Other records not yet available must be sent as soon as practical.

General Requirements

The following seven general requirements should be met:

1. Medical records related to transfers must be retained by the transferring and receiving hospitals for 5 years from the date of the transfer.

2. Hospitals are required to report to the Centers for Medicare & Medicaid Services or the state survey agency within 72 hours from the time of the transfer any time they have reason to believe they may have received a patient who was transferred in an unstable medical condition.

3. Hospitals are required to post signs in areas, such as entrances, admitting areas, reception areas, and emergency departments, with respect to their obligations under the patient screening and transfer law.

4. Hospitals also are required to post signs stating whether the hospital participates in the Medicaid program under a state-approved plan. This requirement applies to all hospitals, not only the ones that participate in Medicare.

5. Hospitals must keep a list of physicians who are on call after the initial examination to provide treatment to stabilize a patient with an emergency medical condition.

6. Hospitals must keep a central log of all individuals who come to the emergency department seeking assistance and the result of each individual's visit.

7. A hospital may not delay providing appropriate medical screening to inquire about payment method or insurance status.

Enforcement and Penalties

Physicians and hospitals violating these federal requirements for patient screening and transfer are subject to civil monetary penalties of up to $50,000 for each violation and to termination from the Medicare program. Hospitals are prohibited from penalizing physicians who report violations of the law or who refuse to transfer an individual with an unstabilized emergency medical condition.

AMERICANS WITH DISABILITIES ACT

In July 1990, the Americans with Disabilities Act (ADA) was signed into law. It is an ambitious federal measure that safeguards the civil rights of individuals with disabilities.

Who Is Protected by the Americans with Disabilities Act?

The ADA protects individuals with disabilities against discrimination in certain critical areas of daily living. These areas include protections for health services, employment, communication, public accommodations, education, and transportation. Disability is defined broadly to include physical and mental impairments that substantially limit one or more major life activities of an individual. A person who has a record of either a physical or a mental impairment or a person who is regarded as having such an impairment also is considered as having a disability.

Although it is impossible to enumerate all of the impairments that are covered by the ADA, the list includes the following: visual, speech, and hearing impairments; epilepsy; muscular dystrophy; heart disease; cancer; human immunodeficiency virus infection (HIV) (symptomatic or asymptomatic); tuberculosis; mental retardation; cosmetic disfigurement; anatomical loss; alcoholism; or emotional or mental illness. There also are a number of conditions that are specifically defined as not disabilities under the ADA. These include current use of illegal drugs, compulsive gambling, kleptomania, pyromania, and sexual behavioral disorders.

Employment Obligations

The antidiscrimination employment provisions of the ADA apply to all employers who have 15 or more employees on staff. To summarize, employers are prohibited from discriminating against a job applicant or an employee currently on staff who is a "qualified individual with a disability." All aspects of employment practices are covered by the law, including job application procedures, hiring, job advancement, compensation, benefits, and discharge. The ADA specifically prohibits preemployment questions about a disability or the nature or severity of a disability.

Who Is a "Qualified Individual With a Disability?"

A qualified individual with a disability is defined as "an individual who, with or without reasonable accommodation, can perform the essential functions of the employment position that such individual holds or desires." In essence, an employer cannot deny a qualified individual with a disability a job or discharge such an employee based on the individual's disability.

An employer also is prohibited from discriminating against an individual because the person is known to have a relationship with a person with a disability. For instance, an employer cannot reject a potential employee solely on the basis that the applicant's spouse has multiple sclerosis and the employer fears that the applicant may not be able to devote full attention to the position.

What Is a Reasonable Accommodation?

An employer also must make reasonable accommodations to assist an individual with a disability in performing a job, unless such accommodations would impose an undue hardship on the business. What comprises a reasonable accommodation varies with the circumstances. A reasonable accommodation could mean that an employer would have to make the office readily accessible and usable by individuals with disabilities. An employer also may be required to restructure an employee's assignments or modify the employee's work schedule as a reasonable accommodation.

The ADA does not require employers to hire unqualified individuals with disabilities. It permits businesses to use selection criteria or standards that screen out or tend to screen out an individual with a disability as long as the criteria are shown to be job related for the position, are consistent with business necessity, and the job functions cannot be accomplished by reasonable accommodations.

Public Accommodations

A "public accommodation" is defined broadly by the ADA as a privately operated entity that owns, operates, or leases a place of public accommodation. Places of public accommodation include physician offices, hospitals, grocery stores, golf courses, libraries, and day care centers, to name a few. Public accommodations, regardless of the size of the business or the number of people employed, also are prohibited from discriminating against individuals with a disability.

Are Physicians Required to Treat All Patients?

Antidiscrimination protections in the ADA prohibit a business that fits the definition of public accommodations from establishing criteria that would screen out or tend to screen out an individual with a disability. The ADA also requires businesses to make reasonable modifications for individuals with disabilities. This makes it discriminatory for physicians to deny care to an individual based solely on the individual's disability. For example, an obstetrician–gynecologist would be in violation of the ADA if the physician established a rule denying care to obstetric patients with HIV. If, however, this same physician no longer practiced obstetrics and referred all pregnant women to other physicians, the physician would be under no obligation to care for this patient. A physician is not required to treat a patient with a condition outside the physician's area of practice or expertise.

A physician also is not required to provide services to an individual with a disability if the individual poses a direct threat to the health or safety of others. A "direct threat" is a significant risk to the health or safety of others that cannot be eliminated by a modification of policies, practices, or procedures or the provision or auxiliary aids and services. Physicians have to be careful, however, that a decision not to provide care is based on objective criteria relying on current medical evidence rather than stereotypes or generalizations about the effects of a particular disability.

Auxiliary Aids

Physicians also are required to provide and pay for auxiliary aids and services to communicate effectively with patients who have disabilities affecting hearing, vision, or speech, unless such accommodations create an undue burden. This is a flexible requirement, and physicians should consider the patient's needs and consult with the patient before determining what form of auxiliary aids to provide.

Other Provisions

Businesses are required to make readily achievable structural changes to their facilities to make them more accessible to the individuals with a disability. New construction also must be in compliance with the ADA. There are federal tax deductions for some expenses associated with removal of barriers and tax credits for eligible small businesses that make certain accommodations required by the ADA.

Americans with Disabilities Act Resources

Americans with Disabilities Act, 42 U.S.C. §12101 (2011). Available at: http://www.gpo.gov/fdsys/pkg/USCODE-2011-title42/pdf/USCODE-2011-title42-chap126.pdf. Retrieved September 20, 2013.

For more information about or assistance with the ADA contact the following:

ADA National Network
1-800-949-4232 (voice/TTY)
http://adata.org

Equal Employment Opportunity Commission
131 M Street, NE
Washington, DC 20507
202-663-4900
202-663-4494 (TTY)
http://www.eeoc.gov

Federal Communications Commission
Telecommunications Relay Services (TRS)
445 12th Street SW
Washington, DC 20554
1-888-225-5322
1-888-835-5322 (TTY)
http://www.fcc.gov/encyclopedia/telecommunications-relay-services-trs

Job Accommodation Network
1-800-526-7234
http://askjan.org

U.S. Department of Justice
Information and technical assistance on the Americans
   With Disabilities Act
950 Pennsylvania Avenue, NW
Civil Rights Division
Disability Rights Section - NYA
1-800-514-0301
http://www.ada.gov

U.S. Department of Labor
Office of Disability Employment Policy
200 Constitution Avenue, NW
Washington, DC 20210
1-866-633-7365
1-877-889-5627 (TTY)
http://www.dol.gov/odep

United States Access Board
1331 F Street, NW
Suite 1000
Washington, DC 20004
1-800-872-2253
1-800-993-2822 (TTY)
http://www.access-board.gov

TITLE VI OF THE CIVIL RIGHTS ACT*

Title VI of the Civil Rights Act prohibits discrimination based on race, color, or national origin. Protections under the Act have been extended to include prohibitions of discrimination against persons with limited English proficiency (LEP). The Office for Civil Rights (OCR) of the U.S. Department of Health and Human Services (HHS) has a longstanding position that in order to avoid discrimination against LEP individuals, health care providers who receive Federal financial assistance must take reasonable steps to provide meaningful access to ensure that such LEP individuals receive, free of charge, the language assistance necessary to afford them meaningful access to their services. The OCR's position is that physicians who receive reimbursement from Medicaid are recipients of Federal financial assistance, and, thus, must comply with the Title VI requirements for language assistance.

The OCR has policy guidance on Title VI compliance available on its web site at www.hhs.gov/ocr or by calling 800-368-1019. According to the OCR, the type of language assistance that must be provided to patients with LEP depends on a variety of factors, including the following:

- The size of the medical practice
- The size of the LEP population it serves
- The nature of the service
- The total resources available to the medical practice
- The frequency with which particular languages are encountered

*Data from Department of Health and Human Services. Limited English proficiency (LEP). Available at: http://www.hhs.gov/ocr/civilrights/resources/specialtopics/lep/. Retrieved July 10, 2013.

- The frequency with which LEP individuals come into contact with the medical practice

If the medical practice determines that it should provide language assistance services, the practice should develop a plan to address the LEP needs. The OCR suggests five steps for creating a plan: 1) identifying LEP individuals who need language assistance, 2) identifying language assistance measures, 3) training staff, 4) providing notice to LEP individuals, and 5) monitoring and updating the LEP plan.

If implementing accommodations for LEP patients would be so burdensome as to make it difficult for the medical practice to stay in operation, or if there are equally effective alternatives for LEP individuals to have access to the type of services provided, the OCR will not find that the medical practice is noncompliant.

The main role of the OCR is to provide technical assistance to help covered entities, including medical practices, meet their obligations. This can include identifying best practices and strategies, identifying sources of federal reimbursement for translation services, and directing health care providers to other resources.

The OCR will investigate whenever it receives a complaint or other information that indicates possible noncompliance with Title VI. If the investigation results in a finding of noncompliance, the OCR will inform the practice in writing of its findings and will identify the steps that must be taken to become compliant. If the practice will not make corrections voluntarily, the OCR has the authority to terminate Federal assistance after an administrative hearing, and also may refer the case to the Department of Justice for injunctive relief or other enforcement proceedings.

Health Insurance Portability and Accountability Act*

Congress adopted the Health Insurance Portability and Accountability Act (HIPAA) in 1996 to provide stronger health insurance protection for people leaving jobs and people with preexisting medical conditions. The HIPAA legislation has had a significant influence on transactions and code sets, security, and privacy of individually identifiable health information. If a practice stores or transmits patient health information electronically, it must comply with HIPAA regulations. Since 1996, several amendments have strengthened the provisions and penalties of the Act.

Transactions and Code Sets

The transactions and code sets rules implement provisions of HIPAA intended to standardize and simplify how health information is stored and submitted in electronic formats. The goal is to make it easier for physicians to submit health insurance claims and for health insurers to process and pay those claims by having everyone format information in a uniform way.

In the regulations, there are certain standard transactions for Electronic Data Interchange of health care data. These transactions are as follows: claims and encounter information; payment and remittance advice; claims status, eligibility, enrollment and disenrollment; referrals and authorizations; and coordination of benefits and premium payment. Under HIPAA,

---

*Modifications to the HIPAA privacy, security, enforcement, and breach notification rules under the Health Information Technology for Economic and Clinical Health Act and the Genetic Information Nondiscrimination Act; other modifications to the HIPAA rules. Fed Regist 2013;78:5565–702.

if a physician conducts one of the adopted transactions electronically, they must use the adopted standard.

Also adopted under HIPAA are specific code sets for diagnoses and procedures to be used in all transactions. The HCPCS (Ancillary Services/Procedures), CPT-4 (Physicians Procedures), CDT (Dental Terminology), ICD-9 (Diagnosis and Hospital Inpatient Procedures), ICD-10 (as of October 1, 2015) and NDC (National Drug Codes) codes with which health care providers and health plan are familiar, are the adopted code sets for procedures, diagnoses, and drugs.

Finally, the U.S. Department of Health and Human Services adopted standards for unique identifiers for employers, health care providers, and health plans, which must also be used in all transactions. Physicians should make sure claims and other transactions comply with the rules.

Security

Electronic storage of patients' personal health information raises some significant concerns about unauthorized release of that information. If patient health information is stored electronically, the HIPAA security regulations apply. The rules include the following:

- Technical requirements
- Physical safeguards
- Administrative safeguards

There is some flexibility in implementing the rules in a physician's practice. Although implementation of some of the standards is required, other standards are considered "addressable." If a standard is addressable,

- determine whether it is reasonable and appropriate for the practice
- substitute another measure
- document why the standard is not appropriate for the practice

Privacy of Individually Identifiable Health Information

Safeguarding the privacy and confidentiality of a patient's personal health information is an ethical obligation for obstetrician–gynecologists (see Appendix A, "Code of Professional Ethics of the American College of Obstetricians and Gynecologists") and a legal requirement. The HIPAA privacy regulation applies if a physician or physician's practice conducts any of the following activities electronically:

- Submitting claims
- Checking a patient's eligibility or coverage
- Requesting preauthorization or a referral
- Receiving payments, notices of payments, or explanation of benefits

If a physician's practice conducts certain transactions electronically, it is a covered entity. The HIPAA privacy regulations cover all forms of protected health information—paper, electronic, and oral. Covered entities must do the following:

- Develop written privacy policies and procedures for the practice.
- Designate a privacy officer who will be responsible for implementing the privacy policy. If the practice is small, this will probably be an existing staff person.
- Train all practice staff on the privacy policy.
- Provide all patients with a written Notice of Privacy Rights and Practices, which explains a patient's privacy rights and outlines how the practice will use her protected health information.
- Make a good faith effort to obtain the patient's written acknowledgment of receiving the notice.
- Obtain contracts with business associates with whom protected health information is shared that provide assurance the business associate will protect the information.
- Limit disclosures of protected health information to the minimum amount necessary.

- Have a plan to assess and ameliorate potential risks and vulnerabilities to privacy and security and review the plan on a regular basis.
- Take reasonable precautions to prevent accidental disclosure of protected health information.

However, HIPAA does not require a practice to do the following:

- Obtain the patient's consent for disclosures of protected health information related to treatment, payment, or operations.
- Make significant physical modifications to the office.
- Limit the amount of clinically relevant information provided to others caring for the patients.

Under HIPAA, a patient has the right to inspect her protected health information and to request that any inaccuracies be corrected. A physician is not required to honor her correction request, but must provide a written justification for refusal. A patient must consent to disclose her protected health information for purposes other than treatment, payment, or operations. A patient also has the right to obtain a copy of her protected health information. If the information is maintained electronically, the patient may request a copy of the information in an electronic format. The physician has up to 30 days to respond to the patient's request.

The Health Information Technology for Economic and Clinical Health Act, part of the American Recovery and Reinvestment Act of 2009, expanded Privacy and Security provisions. Under the Health Information Technology for Economic and Clinical Health Act, privacy and security breach notification requirements were delineated, new rules for the accounting of disclosures were implemented, and penalties for disclosures were increased. Penalties for violating the HIPAA privacy regulations are listed in Table I-1. Prison sentences of 1–10 years can be added to the fines depending on the circumstances of the breach. Physicians are required to notify individuals whose protected health information has been compromised by a breach, even if the breach was caused by a business associate. If the breach involves more than 500 patients, the Health and Human Services Office of Civil Rights must be notified and under certain circumstances, so must the local media.

Patients have a right to restrict disclosure of protected health information to their health plan when paying in full and out of pocket for the health care item or service. Practices must devise a method of identifying restricted information to ensure that the information is not inadvertently made available to a health plan.

Table I-1. Penalties for Violating HIPAA Privacy Regulations*

Reason for Breach	Minimum Penalty	Maximum Penalty
Done unknowingly	$100 to $50,000 per violation	$1.5 million per year
Had reasonable cause	$1,000 to $50,000 per violation	$1.5 million per year
Willful neglect but corrected	$10,000 to $50,000 per violation	$1.5 million per year
Willful neglect but uncorrected	$50,000 per violation	$1.5 million per year

*Prison sentences of 1–10 years can be added to the fines depending on the circumstances of the breach.

Bibliography

American Congress of Obstetricians and Gynecologists. HIPAA regulations and requirements explained. Washington, DC: American Congress of Obstetricians and Gynecologists; 2013. Available at: http://www.acog.org/About_ACOG/ACOG_Departments/HIPAA. Retrieved July 16, 2013.

Department of Health and Human Services. Health information privacy. Available at: http://www.hhs.gov/ocr/privacy. Retrieved July 10, 2013.

Health Insurance Portability and Accountability Act of 1996, Pub. L. No. 104-191, 100 Stat. 1936. Available at: http://www.gpo.gov/fdsys/pkg/PLAW-104publ191/pdf/PLAW-104publ191.pdf. Retrieved September 20, 2013.

Modifications to the HIPAA privacy, security, enforcement, and breach notification rules under the Health Information Technology for Economic and Clinical Health Act and the Genetic Information Nondiscrimination Act; other modifications to the HIPAA rules. Fed Regist 2013;78:5565–702.

APPENDIX J

STATEMENT ON SCOPE OF PRACTICE OF OBSTETRICS AND GYNECOLOGY

THE AMERICAN CONGRESS OF OBSTETRICIANS AND GYNECOLOGISTS' OPERATIONAL MISSION STATEMENT

The American Congress of Obstetricians and Gynecologists is a membership organization of obstetrician–gynecologists dedicated to the advancement of women's health through education, advocacy, practice and research.

Vision Statement

Obstetrics and gynecology is a discipline dedicated to the broad, integrated medical and surgical care of women's health throughout their lifespan. The combined discipline of obstetrics and gynecology requires extensive study and understanding of reproductive physiology, including the physiologic, social, cultural, environmental, and genetic factors that influence disease in women.

Primary and preventive counseling and education are essential and integral parts of the practice of an obstetrician–gynecologist as they advance the individual and community-based health of women of all ages.

Obstetricians and gynecologists may choose a wide or more focused scope of practice, from primary ambulatory health to concentration in a particular area of specialization. This study and understanding of the reproductive physiology of women gives obstetricians and gynecologists a unique perspective in addressing gender-specific health care issues.

Principles of Evidence-Based Medicine

The purpose of this overview is to review and describe the research methodologies used in the medical literature. These methodologies serve as the scientific basis of evidence-based medicine. Given the limitations of space, this review is far from comprehensive. For a more complete overview, the reader is encouraged to obtain a series of articles published in *The Lancet* (1–11). This epidemiology series provides a readable but more detailed overview, a discussion of various research designs, and articles that specifically focus on randomized trials (7–11).

Epidemiologic Studies

Clinical research can be broadly subdivided into two categories—1) experimental and 2) observational—based on whether or not the investigator assigns the exposures (Fig. K-1). Experimental studies can be divided into randomized and nonrandomized trials. Observational studies can be divided into analytic studies (studies with a comparison group) and descriptive studies. Analytic observational studies include cohort studies, case–control studies, and cross-sectional studies. In cohort studies, groups are compared based on an exposure of interest and participants are tracked forward in time for the outcome of interest. In case–control studies, groups are chosen based on the outcome of interest and are traced back to the exposure. Cross-sectional studies are analogous to a snapshot in time; the researcher observes the exposure and the outcome at one time point. Descriptive studies, by definition, have no comparison group. They include case reports and case-series reports. In descriptive studies, investigators cannot evaluate associations or make causal implications. These reports often are interesting clinical vignettes but have limited scientific merit.

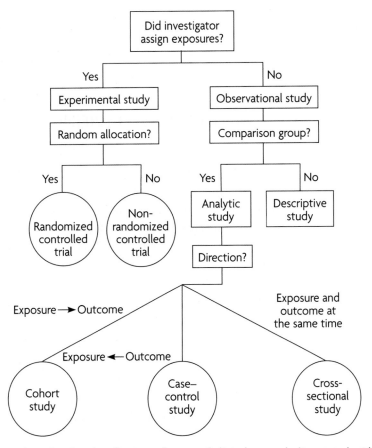

Fig. K-1. Algorithm for classification of types of clinical research. (Reprinted with permission from Grimes DA, Schulz KF. An overview of clinical research: the lay of the land. Lancet Copyright 2002;359:57–61.)

Not all research methods are created equal (Fig. K-2). The randomized clinical trial is the least likely to be subject to serious biases. Cohort, case–control, and cross-sectional studies are common observational analytic studies. In fact, observational studies dominate the women's health literature (12). Observational studies are more susceptible than are experimental designs to many types of bias that can distort the researcher's results and conclusions.

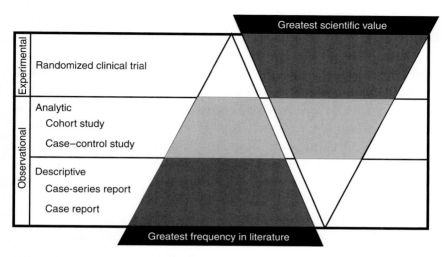

Fig. K-2. A hierarchy of clinical studies.

The choice of research methodology is very important. The reader must first consider the question of whether the study design is appropriate for the specific research question. Descriptive studies are appropriate to describe a highly unusual case or collection of cases. These studies may provide valuable information about the frequency, natural history, or possible determinants of a condition and thus may generate hypotheses. However, descriptive studies cannot test hypotheses on causality or association. Analytic observational studies are particularly appropriate in assessing an association or relationship between an exposure and an outcome when a randomized trial is not feasible or ethical. Cohort studies proceed in a logical sequence in which the exposure precedes the outcome of interest. Cohort studies, however, may require very large sample sizes, especially for outcomes of interest that are rare. A case–control study is a more efficient design with which to address an association between a rare outcome and an exposure of interest, and this type of design may be more feasible when many years are required to develop the outcome of interest. Case–control studies may be counterintuitive to clinicians, because the population under study is selected on the basis of the outcome (ie, these studies "begin at the end") (13).

The randomized trial is the methodology of choice when a researcher or clinician is interested in the effectiveness of a particular therapy or wishes to provide the highest level of evidence for an association. When properly done, the randomized trial approximates the controlled experiment of basic science. The hallmark of this study design is the assignment of participants to exposures based purely on chance. A randomized trial reduces the likelihood of bias when it is properly implemented (with sufficient sample size). Thus, differences in outcomes can be attributed to the exposure or to the arm of a trial rather than to differences in baseline characteristics of the participants.

RANDOMIZED CLINICAL TRIALS

The randomized clinical trial is the standard by which all other methodologies are evaluated. The major advantages of a randomized clinical trial compared with an observational study are its ability to avoid selection bias and its strength of causal inference. The randomized clinical trial is the best design for controlling the influence of known and unknown confounding variables.

In a randomized clinical trial, participants are randomly assigned to an exposure of interest. Performing a randomized clinical trial involves five basic steps:

1. Assemble the study population.
2. Evaluate baseline characteristics.
3. Randomly assign participants to two or more study groups.
4. Apply an intervention or placebo, preferably in a blinded fashion.
5. Monitor the groups and measure outcome variables (blindly, if possible).

Embedded in these five steps are other methodologic issues that should be considered in a properly performed randomized clinical trial. Inclusion and exclusion criteria that are appropriate to the research question must be determined carefully. Participants with a contraindication to the intervention must be excluded. When measuring baseline characteristics, the researcher should consider important predictors of the outcome and confounding variables. In addition, an adequate sample size should be determined, and plans for recruitment should be consistent with these calculations.

As an illustration of the five steps listed previously, consider the following example. In a report published in the American Journal of Preventive Medicine, the U.S. Preventive Services Task Force gave screening young women for *Chlamydia trachomatis* infection an "A" recommendation (see Table K-1) (14). One of the most important studies supporting this recommendation was a large randomized trial of screening in a health maintenance organization in Seattle (15). This trial evaluated the effectiveness of screening and treating unmarried, asymptomatic women (aged 18–34 years) for *C trachomatis*. The study population selected for this trial was believed to be at high risk based on a risk score that incorporated age, race, parity, douching, and having two or more sexual partners in the previous 12 months. Participants were then randomly assigned to two groups: 1) those receiving routine screening and 2) those receiving no routine screening. Baseline characteristics were evaluated to ensure that the two groups were similar at randomization. The intervention was applied, and the outcomes were carefully measured. With routine screening for *C trachomatis*, the incidence of pelvic inflammatory disease (PID) was reduced from 28 cases per 1,000 women-years to 13 cases per 1,000 women-years (relative risk [RR], 0.44; 95% confidence interval [CI], 0.2–0.9).

In randomized trials, it is extremely important to assign patients in a truly random fashion (eg, with a random-number table or computer-generated random assignment), rather than by hospital number or day of the week. It also is important to conceal the assignment (eg, with opaque envelopes) to avoid foreknowledge of the treatment assignment. In this way, investigators are unable to manipulate the randomization to get patients into their preferred treatment groups. It has been demonstrated that trials in which inadequate or unclear allocation concealment was used yielded up to 40% larger estimates of the effect than did trials in which adequate concealment was used (16).

When properly implemented, random allocation and concealment can help avoid bias or imbalances in important baseline factors that can influence the outcome of interest. Blinding the investigator and the participant to the group assignment (the double-blind approach) is a methodological strength. By using this method, the participant follow-up and evaluation of the outcome will be performed in a strictly objective manner, uninfluenced by group assignment. When analyzing a randomized clinical trial,

Table K-1. Standard Recommendation Language of the U.S. Preventive Services Task Force

Recommendation	Language*
A	The USPSTF strongly recommends that clinicians routinely provide [the service] to eligible patients. (The USPSTF found good evidence that [the service] improves important health outcomes and concludes that the benefits substantially outweigh harms.)
B	The USPSTF recommends that clinicians routinely provide [the service] to eligible patients. (The USPSTF found at least fair evidence that [the service] improves important health outcomes and concludes that benefits outweigh harms.)
C	The USPSTF makes no recommendation for or against routine provision of [the service]. (The USPSTF found at least fair evidence that [the service] can improve health outcomes but concludes that the balance of the benefits and harms is too close to justify a general recommendation.
D	The USPSTF recommends against routinely providing [the service]. (The USPSTF found at least fair evidence that [the service] is ineffective or that harms outweigh benefits.)
I	The USPSTF concludes the evidence is insufficient to recommend for or against routinely providing [the service]. (Evidence that [the service] is effective is lacking, of poor quality, or conflicting and the balance of benefits and harms cannot be determined.)

Abbreviation: USPSTF, U.S. Preventive Services Task Force.

*All statements specify the population for which the recommendation is intended and are followed by a rationale statement providing information about the overall grade of evidence and the net benefit from implementing the service.

Reprinted with permission from Harris RP, Helfand M, Woolf SH, Lohr KN, Mulrow CD, Teutsch SM, et al. Current methods of the US Preventive Services Task Force: a review of the process. Methods Work Group, Third US Preventive Services Task Force. Am J Prev Med;20(suppl):21–35. Copyright 2001, with permission from Elsevier.

one should remember the principle of "once randomized, analyze." In other words, once a patient is randomized to an intervention arm, he or she should be analyzed in that group regardless of what happens after randomization. If a patient who was randomized to a group receiving a new antibiotic experiences adverse effects and stops therapy, that patient should be analyzed in the antibiotic group, not dropped from the analysis. This is referred to as intention-to-treat analysis. A randomized clinical trial in which many of the patients have been dropped from the analysis should be scrutinized carefully. Reports of clinical trials should attempt to minimize exclusions after randomization and to perform intention-to-treat analysis.

Randomized clinical trials have many advantages. In the hierarchy of clinical research, the randomized clinical trial provides the greatest strength of causal inference and is the optimal methodology to test the efficacy of treatment programs. If performed properly, randomization protects against confounding and selection bias—error due to systematic difference in characteristics of the study participants and individuals excluded from the study. Double-blinding will help ward off problems of ascertainment bias, diagnostic suspicion bias, and detection bias. Randomized trials with adequate sample size also are the methodology of choice for the evaluation of small or moderate effects. In observational studies, bias might easily explain and account for small to moderate differences (17).

The disadvantages of a randomized trial include expense, feasibility, and ethical issues surrounding the randomization of patients to intervention or placebo. For example, patients with syphilis cannot be randomized ethically to a treatment or a no-treatment group. Another disadvantage is the possible lack of external validity; a randomized trial, when properly done, should have internal validity (ie, it should measure what it sets out to measure), but it might lack external validity. External validity is the ability to generalize the results of a trial to the overall population or to a population of interest. Doing so may not be possible because of the strict inclusion and exclusion criteria of the trial and the fact that patients who consent to participate in a randomized clinical trial may differ from nonparticipants. Finally, randomized trials often are prohibitively expensive to conduct. The cost of large trials can be tens of millions of dollars.

OBSERVATIONAL STUDIES

Observational studies can be divided into analytic studies and descriptive studies. Analytic observational studies include a comparison group and include cohort (longitudinal or follow-up) studies, case–control studies, and cross-sectional studies. Descriptive observational studies include case-series reports and case reports. Descriptive studies have no comparison group. Most epidemiologic studies in the reproductive health literature are observational studies (18). Of original research articles published in the journal *Obstetrics & Gynecology* in 2012, 85% were classified as observational.

Cohort Studies

A cohort study differs from a randomized clinical trial in that it does not have a randomization scheme that determines which patients receive the intervention or exposure. A cohort study is carried out by assembling a group of individuals who have been exposed to an intervention and comparing this group with a control group of patients who have not been exposed. These two groups are monitored over time and evaluated for a specific outcome of interest. An excellent example in the reproductive health literature is the Nurses' Health Study, one of the most comprehensive cohort studies ever performed (19, 20). Thousands of nurses have been monitored over time with comprehensive interviews and medical record reviews to evaluate various risk factors (eg, oral contraceptive use and estrogen therapy) and the development of disease (eg, cancer and cardiovascular disease).

Cohort studies are more subject to systematic (nonrandom) error than are randomized clinical trials and, thus, are weaker than randomized clinical trials in establishing causation. Because a clinician's decision to recommend a specific therapy and a patient's choice to accept therapy are clearly nonrandom decisions, the strength that the two groups are equal at baseline (provided by random allocation in a randomized trial) is lost. For example, women who take oral contraceptives may have very different baseline characteristics than women who use other forms of contraception or no contraception, and these characteristics may be related to the outcome of interest. In cohort studies, women who receive an intervention may be cared for or evaluated differently from women who do not receive the intervention. For example, a woman taking oral contraceptives is more likely to be seen by a physician regularly than a woman who has had a tubal sterilization. As a result, there is an increased chance of detecting an abnormality in the woman taking oral contraceptives. This type of bias is called detection bias.

In all epidemiologic studies, it is extremely important for investigators to identify and control for confounding variables (ie, factors associated with the intervention or exposure and the outcome of interest) (Box K-1, Fig. K-3). Cohort studies can attempt to control for confounding variables and differences in baseline characteristics through stratification and multivariable analysis. However, it is impossible to control for unknown or unmeasured confounding variables. Because of the major sources of bias just described, associations should be interpreted with caution because small or modest effect sizes may be due to residual confounding or bias.

By definition, randomized trials are prospective in design; they start with groups exposed to an intervention and monitor them over time for the outcome of interest. Cohort studies also proceed forward in time, from exposure to outcome, but they may be carried out either prospectively or retrospectively. If patients are enrolled in a cohort study, grouped on the basis of their exposure, and then monitored longitudinally, the study is clearly prospective. However, it also is possible to look back in time (retrospectively) to assemble a group of patients who were and were not exposed

---

Box K-1. What Is a Confounding Variable?

Confounding comes from the Latin word confundere, to mix together; thus, some authorities refer to confounding as a "mixing of effects." A confounding variable is a variable that can cause or prevent the outcome of interest, is not the causal pathway as an intermediate variable, and also is associated with the factor under investigation. Consider the relationship between oral contraceptives and cervical neoplasia. A woman's sexual history (eg, onset of intercourse or new partners) may be a confounding variable in this relationship. Sexual history is related to the outcome (cervical neoplasia) and also may be related to the exposure (oral contraceptives).

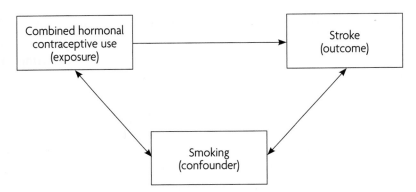

Fig. K-3. Example of confounding. Cigarette smoking may be associated with combined hormonal contraceptive use (exposure) and outcome of interest (stroke). An analysis should control for the effect of smoking on the outcome of interest.

at some time in the past and to monitor them to the present time. This type of cohort study is called a retrospective cohort study. In prospective and retrospective cohort studies, the study moves in the same direction: forward in time. However, data gathering may be prospective (forward in time) or retrospective (backward in time). Prospective cohort studies often require large sample sizes (for uncommon and rare outcomes) and long periods of follow-up. Thus, these studies can be very expensive and time-consuming. The case–control study can overcome some of these logistical obstacles.

Case–Control Studies

It has been said that a case–control study "begins at the end" (Fig. K-4) (13). Cohort studies and randomized clinical trials begin with patients exposed to an intervention or risk factor and monitor these patients for the development of the outcome. Case–control studies select patients on the basis of whether they have the outcome of interest. The outcome could be a disease, if the investigation is evaluating risk factors for the disease, or it may be an ultimate outcome, such as alive or dead in a study of cancer prognosis. Cases, or patients with the outcome, are compared with controls, or individuals without the outcome, to determine whether there is an association between an exposure and the outcome of interest. Therefore, the design in a case–control study is, by definition, retrospective. As a result of the process of selecting individuals based on the outcome or disease,

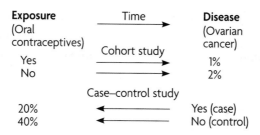

Fig. K-4. Examples of cohort and case-control studies of the relation between oral contraceptives and ovarian cancer.

case–control studies typically study only one outcome, but they may evaluate several exposures.

The major advantage of case–control studies is that they are highly efficient. Often they require the fewest patients to demonstrate an association and can be done in less time and with less money than other studies, especially when the disease in question is rare or takes years to develop (eg, cancer or cardiovascular disease). Consider the following example of a case–control study. Women with hereditary ovarian cancer and a pathogenic mutation in either *BRCA1* or *BRCA2* were compared with a group of controls without ovarian cancer. The investigators assessed the patients' past exposure to oral contraceptives and noted that oral contraceptive use was associated with a 50% reduction in the risk of ovarian cancer (21). If this study was done as a cohort study or randomized trial, it would take decades to evaluate the development of ovarian cancer in a cohort of women taking oral contraceptives.

Despite their advantages, case–control studies are easy to do poorly and are prone to many biases. One of the major challenges in case–control studies is choosing an appropriate control group, which is critical in these studies. For example, the Women's Health Study was a multicenter case–control study to evaluate the relationship between PID and the intrauterine device (22). Barrier contraception protects against sexually transmitted diseases and PID. Thus, the choice of control group (condom users) resulted in an inflated estimate of the relationship between the intrauterine device and PID. In general, the control group should be representative of individuals who are at risk of the disease, and individuals in the control group should have the same opportunity for exposure as case patients. Controls should be similar to the cases in all important respects, except for not having the outcome of interest. Because the health outcome is known at the start in these studies, this knowledge may influence the measurement and interpretation of data (observer bias). In addition, participants enrolled in these studies may have difficulty recalling medical history or exposures. If case participants are more (or less) likely to remember an exposure than control participants (ie, there is differential recall), then the study may be subject to recall bias. As observational studies, case–control and cohort studies are susceptible to many other types of bias. A careful reader of the literature will search for bias and uncontrolled confounding when interpreting the results of observational studies.

Studies also may be "nested," or set within an existing cohort study, such as nested case–control or nested cohort studies. In these nested studies, information previously obtained during the cohort study (eg, blood samples) is evaluated for a subset of participants with and without the outcome of interest. Cases are participants with the outcome or disease of interest. Control participants are selected at random from the population without the outcome of interest (nested case–control). For example, in a nested case–control study of risk factors for uterine rupture, black women were found to have a lower risk of rupture compared with white women (23). In a nested cohort study, exposure groups are selected from within a large, established cohort.

Cross-Sectional Studies

Another type of observational analytic study is the cross-sectional study (also called a prevalence study or frequency survey). The cross-sectional study can be thought of as a snapshot of a group of individuals, some of whom have the disease (outcome) and exposure and some of whom do not. Individuals who have the disease of interest are considered prevalent cases. The difference between prevalence and incidence is important, because these terms often are misused in medical writing. Incidence refers to new cases that have developed over a specified time. Prevalence is the proportion of individuals in a population who have the disease at a specific time.

Using a cross-sectional study design, an investigator can evaluate associations between disease and exposure but cannot establish a temporal relationship between them. As an example, consider a hypothetical cross-sectional study of the relationship between serum prolactin levels and the use of oral contraceptives. A large group of young women are assembled, some of whom are taking oral contraceptives (exposure group) and some of whom are not. Prolactin levels are determined for all the women. The researchers may find an association between oral contraceptive use and elevated prolactin levels. However, they cannot conclude that oral contraceptive use causes elevations in prolactin levels. It is possible that women with elevated prolactin levels are more likely to have irregular bleeding and, thus, are more likely to be prescribed oral contraceptives. Because cross-sectional studies use prevalent cases rather than incident cases, a temporal relationship cannot be established, and the information provided can be misleading.

A cross-sectional study design often is used to evaluate diagnostic tests (24). To illustrate the concepts of diagnostic test performance, consider a cross-sectional study to evaluate the performance of a laboratory test for the diagnosis of PID (25). A group of women with signs and symptoms consistent with upper genital tract infection come to an emergency room to have blood drawn for the test and have a laparoscopy for the definitive diagnosis of PID. The result of the evaluation is summarized in a 2×2 table (Fig. K-5).

Disease

		Present	Absent
Test result	**Positive**	True positives (TP)	False positives (FP)
	Negative	False negatives (FN)	True negatives (TN)

Fig. K-5. Example of a 2×2 table illustrating diagnostic test characteristics of sensitivity and specificity. Sensitivity is defined as TP/(TP + FN); specificity, TN/(TN + FP); positive predictive value, TP/(TP + FP); and negative predictive value, TN/(TN + FN).

Diagnostic test performance is characterized by a test's sensitivity and specificity. Sensitivity is the ability of a test to correctly identify patients with the disease of interest; of all the diseased patients, sensitivity is the proportion of patients who test positive (true positives/diseased = true positives/[true positives + false negatives]). Specificity is the ability of a test to correctly identify patients without the disease of interest (true negatives/nondiseased = true negatives/[true negatives + false positives]). For sensitivity and specificity, one must think "vertically" based on the 2×2 table shown in Figure K-5. These test characteristics deal with the extent to which diseases are diagnosed correctly.

Receiver operating characteristic curves are another way to visualize sensitivity and specificity cutoffs for diagnostic tests. In these curves, test sensitivity is plotted on the Y axis, and (1 – specificity) on the X axis. A test that follows the diagonal line (the line between [0.0] and [1.1]) represents the flip of a coin. An ideal test will have high sensitivity and high specificity. Researchers can measure the area under the receiver-operating characteristic curve to compare two or more tests. As an example, erythrocyte sedimentation rate was compared with C-reactive protein level for the diagnosis of PID (Fig. K-6). Neither test performed very well, but C-reactive protein test had a greater area under the curve (25).

Generally, clinicians are more interested in the likelihood of the disease given a positive or negative test result (the predictive values of the test). Predictive values are calculated by determining the percentage of positive (or negative) tests that correctly predict the presence (or absence) of the disease of interest. For predictive values, one must think horizontally. Positive predictive value is the percentage of women with a positive test who actually have the disease (true positives/ positive tests = true positives/[true positives + false positives]). The negative predictive value is the percentage of women with a negative test result who do not have the disease (true negatives/negative test results = true negatives/[true negatives + false negatives]). Predictive values depend on the prevalence of the disease in a population. For example, if a disease is extremely rare, it will be difficult to have a high-positive predictive value, even if sensitivity and specificity are high. Predictive values can be calculated from the standard 2×2 table based on the formulas listed earlier. Predictive values also may be determined by way of Bayes' theorem.

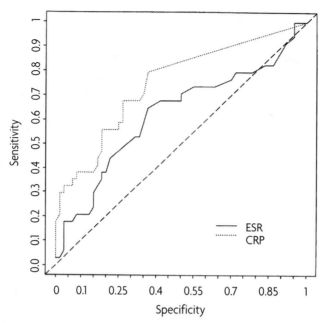

Fig. K-6. Receiver operating characteristic curves for C-reactive protein and erythrocyte sedimentation rate. Abbreviations: CRP, C-reactive protein; ESR, erythrocyte sedimentation rate. (Reprinted from Peipert JF, Boardman L, Hogan JW, Sung J, Mayer KH. Laboratory evaluation of acute upper genital tract infection. Obstet Gynecol 1996;87:730–6.)

Likelihood ratios are an additional way to evaluate information from a diagnostic test. These calculations use sensitivity and specificity to estimate the likelihood of an outcome given a positive or negative test result. The likelihood ratio of a positive test is calculated as sensitivity/(1 – specificity), whereas the likelihood ratio for a negative test is the inverse. Large likelihood ratios (eg, higher than 10) suggest that the diagnostic test may be useful to "rule in" a disease, whereas small ratios (eg, lower than 0.1) may "rule out" a disease. Likelihood ratios also may be used to calculate the posttest probability of a disease (posttest probability = pretest probability x likelihood ratio).

Descriptive Studies

Case reports and case-series reports are types of descriptive studies. These studies represent the least sophisticated of study designs. The purpose of descriptive studies is to assess and describe a finding in a case or group of cases. Descriptive studies are severely limited by the lack of a comparison group and by the potential bias of the investigators.

Establishing cause and effect is not possible in a descriptive study. Because they are hypothesis generating, descriptive studies may serve as the basis for future analytic studies. For example, in a case-series report of seven women who developed functional ovarian cysts while taking phasic contraceptive pills, the authors stated that "phasic contraceptive pills may be a threat to patient health and safety" (26). This report led to further investigation and refutation of these conclusions (27).

Systematic Reviews of Medical Evidence

META-ANALYSIS

In clinical research, meta-analysis is a commonly used tool used in the systematic review and aggregation of data from randomized controlled trials or observational studies. Obstetrics and gynecology has led other medical specialties in attempting to perform a systematic review of all randomized trials conducted in its discipline (28). One example is the Cochrane Library, which includes the Cochrane Database of Systematic Reviews. This electronic database began in England to review perinatal data, and it has expanded to include reviews of many areas of medicine (29). Combining data with meta-analysis can increase statistical power and the ability to evaluate treatment effects and complications in clinical trials, as well as associations between risk factors and disease in etiologic research. In addition, by combining results from several studies, generalizability may be increased. Meta-analysis is especially useful when sample sizes of individual clinical trials are too small to detect an effect or when a large trial is too costly and time-consuming to perform. For example, when investigators performed a meta-analysis to evaluate the efficacy of oral β-agonist maintenance therapy in delaying delivery and decreasing the incidence of preterm birth and its complications, they found no benefit of oral β-agonist maintenance therapy (30). A decision analysis performed to assess the use of magnesium sulfate for seizure prophylaxis in women with mild preeclampsia demonstrated that either strategy (using or not using magnesium) is acceptable because the neonatal and maternal outcomes were nearly identical (31).

A meta-analysis should adhere to specific methodological principles (28). Because the technique is a synthesis of existing studies (most commonly, randomized trials), an explicit study protocol should be developed to outline study inclusion and exclusion criteria. The researchers should provide some assessment of the combinability of the studies, including tests of homogeneity when appropriate. An evaluation and measurement of potential biases should be performed. The statistical methods used, including sensitivity analysis, should be described. Lastly, the authors should provide a discussion regarding the applicability of the results.

DECISION ANALYSIS

Decision analysis is a quantitative approach to evaluate the relative values of different management options (32). The process begins by systematically breaking down a clinical problem into its components and creating a decision tree, or algorithm, to represent the components (parameters) and decision options. Consider the problem of preventing early-onset group B streptococcal disease. A decision analysis was performed to address three different approaches to prevent early-onset neonatal group B streptococcal disease (32).

Probability values for each of the parameters in the decision tree are estimated from a review of the medical literature and expert opinion. The decision tree is then analyzed with statistical methods, and a net value for the different decision options in relation to one another is determined. A technique called sensitivity analysis is used to test how variations in these probabilities can affect the conclusions of the decision analysis. Factors that can be measured, such as mortality, are easier to analyze than are outcomes, such as quality of life.

ECONOMIC ANALYSIS

The use of economic analysis has increased in the medical literature (33). For example, the issue of screening for cystic fibrosis by identifying prenatal carriers has been addressed with this technique (34). Economic analysis, including cost–benefit and cost-effectiveness analyses, is another type of systematic review. Economic analysis is similar to decision analysis but focuses on monetary cost. Once a decision analysis is performed on a specific clinical problem, data on costs of various management options are compared. A cost-effectiveness analysis compares the costs of different options to determine the best care for the least cost. Cost–benefit analysis includes some consequences of the decision options that are nonmonetary, such as years of life saved or disability avoided. For example, using a decision analytic model, investigators demonstrated that a policy of elective cesarean delivery for ultrasonographically diagnosed fetal macrosomia of nondiabetic women is economically unsound (35).

Economic analyses, however, are not without limitations. Often it is difficult to put a monetary cost or a utility on a clinical outcome, and these estimates often are highly subjective. In addition, many cost-effectiveness studies reported in the obstetric and gynecologic literature have been found to have important methodological shortcomings (36). Therefore, the reader must be highly cautious in interpreting some of these findings and should have some basic knowledge about the methodological standards of these reports.

Statistics in Reproductive Health Research

HYPOTHESIS TESTING AND TYPES OF ERROR

The concept of hypothesis testing forms the basis for most statistical testing. The hypothesis of a study often is phrased in the form of a null hypothesis (H_0) that there is no difference present. Research studies should have a clear statement of their hypothesis before the research begins. A hypothetical example of a null hypothesis is as follows: There is no association between the use of low-dose oral contraceptives and the development of endometrial cancer. If one rejects the null hypothesis (H_0), then an alternative hypothesis (H_A) that some association exists is accepted. An alternative hypothesis could be the following: The use of low-dose oral contraceptives reduces the risk of developing endometrial cancer.

An association, however, may be clinically important or trivial. It is important to distinguish between statistical significance (which can be achieved with large sample sizes, regardless of the effect size) and clinical significance. Consider a study of 2,000 women who are randomized to receive antibiotic A or B to be treated for cervical *C trachomatis* infection. If the cure rate in the 1,000 women taking doxycycline is 95%, and the cure rate for the other drug is 97%, then there is a statistically significant difference ($P=.02$). However, this difference of 2% may not be considered clinically significant.

Research studies, like diagnostic tests, are not infallible. Two specific errors are of concern to epidemiologists and researchers: the type I error (α) and the type II error (β). A type I error occurs when a statistically significant difference is found in a study when there truly is no difference. The level of type I error is based on the choice of level of statistical significance. A significance value of $P<.05$ implies that the risk of type I error, or the possibility that a positive study finding was because of chance alone, is 5%. A type II error is the chance that a study finds no difference when a difference truly does exist. A study's power is its ability to detect an association when one truly exists (Power = 1–type II error, or $1-\beta$). Therefore, a 20% chance of a false-negative study translates to 80% power. The chance of a type II error is related inversely to sample size and to the statistical power of the study. Increasing a study's sample size can reduce the chance of a type II error (37).

Investigators should calculate the required sample size before beginning a study to avoid the problem of a type II error. Many clinical trials have described a therapy as ineffective when, in reality, the therapy may have a clinically meaningful effect but the trial was not of sufficient size to detect it (38).

PROBABILITY VALUES COMPARED WITH POINT ESTIMATES AND CONFIDENCE INTERVAL ESTIMATION

Although the use of *P* values and hypothesis testing is firmly entrenched in the medical literature, confidence interval estimation and the use of point estimates are more informative for researchers and readers (39). Many authorities favor the use of point estimates (eg, RR) and their 95% CIs to the calculation of *P* values (40). A relative risk is the risk of the outcome in the exposed population relative to that in the unexposed, or control, population. A relative risk greater than 1 implies an increased risk, and a relative risk less than 1 implies a protective effect. For example, the relative risk of endometrial cancer in women who are more than 22.7 kg overweight is 10, or a 10-fold increased risk. The risk of ovarian cancer in women with pathogenic mutations in the *BRCA1* or *BRCA2* gene is reduced by 60% in women who have used combination oral contraceptives for 6 years or more relative to women who did not use oral contraceptives. When the 95% CI excludes 1, then the results are statistically significant at the *P*<.05 level. In addition, the width of the confidence interval provides some estimate of the precision of the effect size. The narrower the confidence interval, the more precise the point estimate. This concept can be represented graphically, as seen in a meta-analysis evaluating the sensitivity and specificity of liquid-based and conventional cervical cytology (Fig. K-7) (41).

MEASURES OF ASSOCIATION

Another form of point estimate is the odds ratio (OR), which often is confused with relative risk. The major difference between these terms is that relative risks are calculated from prospective data, such as data from a cohort study or a randomized trial, whereas ORs usually are calculated in retrospective case–control studies. Odds ratios also may be calculated from a logistic regression analysis (see later discussion) (42). The OR is the ratio of the odds of being exposed to an agent in the case group relative to the odds in the control group. In general, the odds ratio is a reasonable approximation of the relative risk when the disease under study is rare. However, many investigators are mistakenly using an OR when the outcome of interest is not rare, and doing so can lead to inaccurate estimates of the effect. The main reason RRs or ORs and their confidence intervals often are preferred is that these data provide more than just a test of significance; they also provide a measure of the magnitude of the association, its direction (ie, whether the exposure results in an increased or decreased risk of the disease), and some estimate of the precision of the effect.

A commonly used statistical tool in epidemiologic studies is mathematical modeling, such as multivariable analysis. The most common example of multivariable analysis used in the reproductive-health literature is logistic regression analysis. A confounding variable is associated with the exposure or intervention and the outcome of interest but is not in the causal

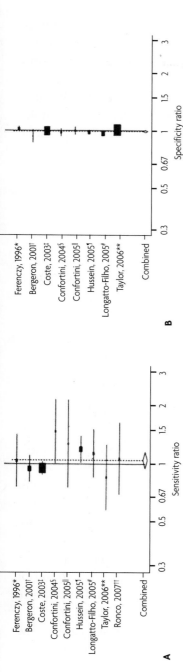

A

Ferenczy, 1996*
Bergeron, 2001[†]
Coste, 2003[‡]
Confortini, 2004[§]
Confortini, 2005[||]
Hussein, 2005[¶]
Longatto-Filho, 2005[#]
Taylor, 2006[**]
Ronco, 2007[††]

Combined

Sensitivity ratio
0.3 0.5 0.67 1 1.5 2 3

B

Ferenczy, 1996*
Bergeron, 2001[†]
Coste, 2003[‡]
Confortini, 2004[§]
Confortini, 2005[||]
Hussein, 2005[¶]
Longatto-Filho, 2005[#]
Taylor, 2006[**]

Combined

Specificity ratio
0.3 0.5 0.67 1 1.5 2 3

*Ferenczy A, Robitaille J, Franco EL, Arseneau J, Richart RM, Wright TC. Conventional cervical cytologic smears vs. ThinPrep smears. A paired comparison study on cervical cytology. Acta Cytol 1996;40:1136–42.

[†]Bergeron C, Bishop J, Lemarie A, Cas F, Ayivi J, Huynh B, et al. Accuracy of thin-layer cytology in patients undergoing cervical cone biopsy. Acta Cytol 2001;45:519–24.

[‡]Coste J, Cochand-Priollet B, de Cremoux P, Le Gales C, Cartier I, Molinie V, et al. Cross sectional study of conventional cervical smear, monolayer cytology, and human papillomavirus DNA testing for cervical cancer screening. BMJ 2003;326:733–6.

[§]Confortini M, Bulgaresi P, Cariaggi MP, Carozzi FM, Cecchini S, Cipparrone I, et al. Comparing conventional and liquid-based smears from a consecutive series of 297 subjects referred to colposcopy assessment. Cytopathology 2004;15:168–70.

[||]Confortini M, Carozzi F, COrtecchia S, Garcia MC, Sani C, Tinacci G, et al. Technical evaluation of the new thin layer device CellSlide (Menarini Diagnostics). Diagn Cytopathol 2005;33:387–93.

[¶]Hussein T, Desai M, Tomlinson A, Kitchener HC. The comparative diagnostic accuracy of conventional and liquid-based cytology in a colposcopic setting. BJOG 2005;112:1542–6.

[#]Longatto-Filho A, Pereira SM, Di Loreta C, Utagawa ML, Makabe S, Sakamoto Maeda MY, et al. DCS liquid-based system is more effective than conventional smears to diagnosis of cervical lesions: study in high-risk population with biopsy-based confirmation. Gynecol Oncol 2005;97:497–500.

[**]Taylor S, Kuhn L, Dupree W, Denny L, De Souza M, Wright TC Jr. Direct Comparison of liquid-based and conventional cytology in a South African screening trial. Int J Cancer 2006;957–62.

[††]Ronco G, Cuzick J, Pierotti P, Cariaggi MP, Dalla Palma P, Naldoni C, et al. Accuracy of liquid based versus conventional cytology: overall results of the new technologies for cervical cancer screening: randomized controlled trial. BMJ 2007;335:28.

Fig. K-7. (A) Relative sensitivity at cutoff high-grade squamous intraepithelial lesion or worse. **(B)** Relative specificity at cutoff high-grade squamous intraepithelial lesion or worse. (Reprinted from Arbyn M, Bergeron C, Klinkhamer P, Martin-Hirsch P, Siebers AG, Bulten J. Liquid compared with conventional cervical cytology: a systematic review and meta-analysis. Obstet Gynecol 2008;111:167–77.)

pathway. Logistic regression is a statistical tool used to evaluate simultaneously the relationship of many variables (including the exposure and potential confounders) to an outcome of interest. With logistic regression, the outcome in question is dichotomous (eg, yes or no, alive or dead). The result is an adjusted estimate of the association that controls for the effect of confounding variables. The expertise of a biostatistician or epidemiologist can be very valuable to a researcher who is interested in the technique of multivariable analysis.

Interpreting the Medical Literature

Although epidemiologic studies cannot prove causation, they can be used to determine the likelihood of causation. The following criteria should be considered when evaluating a cause and effect relationship:

- Strength of the association: The stronger the association, the more likely it is to be real.
- Temporal relationship: Does the cause precede the effect?
- Consistency: Are the study findings consistent over many reports?
- Biologic plausibility: Does the relationship make biologic sense?
- Biologic gradient: Is there a dose–response relationship?
- Evidence: Is there experimental evidence to support or refute the association?

A critical reader of the medical literature should be able to determine a study's methodology and recognize the scientific value of the research. When interpreting the medical literature, the reader should consider not only the methodology (eg, randomized trial or observational study) but also the quality of the study. One way to describe the quality of evidence presented is the rating system used in *Obstetrics & Gynecology*. This level of evidence rating system ranges from level I to level III. Level I evidence is from a randomized controlled trial, level II evidence is from a cohort or case–control study that includes a comparison group, and level III evidence is from an uncontrolled descriptive study, including case series (43, 44).

Readers should no longer unconditionally accept the standard review or the "gospel of the expert." Opinions of authorities and reports of expert committees are no longer regarded as acceptable, high-quality medical evidence. An educated reader should evaluate the evidence available from high-quality studies in the medical literature and recognize when evidence to support a specific practice or association is weak.

References

1. Grimes DA, Schulz KF. An overview of clinical research: the lay of the land. Lancet 2002;359:57–61.

2. Grimes DA, Schulz KF. Descriptive studies: what they can and cannot do. Lancet 2002;359:145–9.

3. Grimes DA, Schulz KF. Bias and causal associations in observational research. Lancet 2002;359:248–52.

4. Grimes DA, Schulz KF. Cohort studies: marching towards outcomes. Lancet 2002;359:341–5.

5. Grimes DA, Schulz KF. Uses and abuses of screening tests [published erratum appears in Lancet 2008;371:1998]. Lancet 2002;359:881–4.

6. Schulz KF, Grimes DA. Case–control studies: research in reverse. Lancet 2002;359:431–4.

7. Schulz KF, Grimes DA. Generation of allocation sequences in randomised trials: chance, not choice. Lancet 2002;359:515–9.

8. Schulz KF, Grimes DA. Allocation concealment in randomised trials: defending against deciphering. Lancet 2002;359:614–8.

9. Schulz KF, Grimes DA. Blinding in randomised trials: hiding who got what. Lancet 2002;359:696–700.

10. Schulz KF, Grimes DA. Sample size slippages in randomised trials: exclusions and the lost and wayward. Lancet 2002;359:781–5.

11. Schulz KF, Grimes DA. Unequal group sizes in randomised trials: guarding against guessing. Lancet 2002;359:966–70.

12. Funai EF, Rosenbush EJ, Lee MJ, Del Priore G. Distribution of study designs in four major US journals of obstetrics and gynecology. Gynecol Obstet Invest 2001;51:8–11.

13. Peipert JF, Grimes DA. The case-control study: a primer for the obstetrician-gynecologist. Obstet Gynecol 1994;84: 140–5.

14. Nelson HD, Helfand M. Screening for chlamydial infection. Am J Prev Med 2001;20(suppl):95–107.

15. Scholes D, Stergachis A, Heidrich FE, Andrilla H, Holmes KK, Stamm WE. Prevention of pelvic inflammatory disease by screening for cervical chlamydial infection. N Engl J Med 1996;334:1362–6.

16. Schulz KF, Chalmers I, Hayes RJ, Altman DG. Empirical evidence of bias. Dimensions of methodological quality associated with estimates of treatment effects in controlled trials. JAMA 1995;273:408–12.

17. MacMahon S, Collins R. Reliable assessment of the effects of treatment on mortality and major morbidity, II: observational studies. Lancet 2001;357:455–62.

18. Funai EF. Obstetrics & Gynecology in 1996: marking the progress toward evidence-based medicine by classifying studies based on methodology. Obstet Gynecol 1997;90: 1020–2.

19. Grodstein F, Manson JE, Stampfer MJ. Hormone therapy and coronary heart disease: the role of time since menopause and age at hormone initiation. J Womens Health (Larchmt) 2006;15:35–44.

20. Tworoger SS, Fairfield KM, Colditz GA, Rosner BA, Hankinson SE. Association of oral contraceptive use, other contraceptive methods, and infertility with ovarian cancer risk. Am J Epidemiol 2007;166:894–901.

21. Narod SA, Risch H, Moslehi R, Dorum A, Neuhausen S, Olsson H, et al. Oral contraceptives and the risk of hereditary ovarian cancer. Hereditary Ovarian Cancer Clinical Study Group. N Engl J Med 1998;339:424–8.

22. Burkman RT. Association between intrauterine device and pelvic inflammatory disease. Obstet Gynecol 1981;57: 269–76.

23. Cahill AG, Stamilio DM, Odibo AO, Peipert J, Stevens E, Macones GA. Racial disparity in the success and complications of vaginal birth after cesarean delivery. Obstet Gynecol 2008;111:654–8.

24. Peipert JF, Sweeney PJ. Diagnostic testing in obstetrics and gynecology: a clinician's guide. Obstet Gynecol 1993;82: 619–23.

25. Peipert JF, Boardman L, Hogan JW, Sung J, Mayer KH. Laboratory evaluation of acute upper genital tract infection. Obstet Gynecol 1996;87:730–6.

26. Caillouette JC, Koehler AL. Phasic contraceptive pills and functional ovarian cysts. Am J Obstet Gynecol 1987;156: 1538–42.

27. Grimes DA, Godwin AJ, Rubin A, Smith JA, Lacarra M. Ovulation and follicular development associated with three low-dose oral contraceptives: a randomized controlled trial. Obstet Gynecol 1994;83:29–34.

28. Peipert JF, Bracken MB. Systematic reviews of medical evidence: the use of meta-analysis in obstetrics and gynecology. Obstet Gynecol 1997;89:628–33.

29. Starr M, Chalmers I, Clarke M, Oxman AD. The origins, evolution, and future of The Cochrane Database of Systematic Reviews. Int J Technol Assess Health Care 2009;25(suppl 1):182–95.

30. Macones GA, Berlin M, Berlin JA. Efficacy of oral beta-agonist maintenance therapy in preterm labor: a meta-analysis. Obstet Gynecol 1995;85:313–7.

31. Cahill AG, Macones GA, Odibo AO, Stamilio DM. Magnesium for seizure prophylaxis in patients with mild preeclampsia. Obstet Gynecol 2007;110: 601–7.

32. Rouse DJ, Owen J. Decision analysis. Clin Obstet Gynecol 1998;41:282–95.

33. Macones GA, Goldie SJ, Peipert JF. Cost-effectiveness analysis: an introductory guide for clinicians. Obstet Gynecol Surv 1999;54:663–72.

34. Doyle NM, Gardner MO. Prenatal cystic fibrosis screening in Mexican Americans: an economic analysis. Am J Obstet Gynecol 2003;189:769–74.

35. Rouse DJ, Owen J, Goldenberg RL, Cliver SP. The effectiveness and costs of elective cesarean delivery for fetal macrosomia diagnosed by ultrasound. JAMA 1996;276:1480–6.

36. Smith WJ, Blackmore CC. Economic analyses in obstetrics and gynecology: a methodologic evaluation of the literature. Obstet Gynecol 1998;91:472–8.

37. Peipert JF, Metheny WP, Schulz K. Sample size and statistical power in reproductive research. Obstet Gynecol 1995;86:302–5.

38. Freiman JA, Chalmers TC, Smith H Jr, Kuebler RR. The importance of beta, the type II error and sample size in the design and interpretation of the randomized control trial. Survey of 71 "negative" trials. N Engl J Med 1978;299:690–4.

39. Grimes DA. The case for confidence intervals. Obstet Gynecol 1992;80:865–6.

40. Rothman KJ. A show of confidence. N Engl J Med 1978;299:1362–3.

41. Arbyn M, Bergeron C, Klinkhamer P, Martin-Hirsch P, Siebers AG, Bulten J. Liquid compared with conventional cervical cytology: a systematic review and meta-analysis. Obstet Gynecol 2008;111:167–77.

42. Peterson HB, Kleinbaum DG. Interpreting the literature in obstetrics and gynecology: II. Logistic regression and related issues. Obstet Gynecol 1991;78:717–20.

43. Scott JR. Adapting to the times [editorial]. Obstet Gynecol 2007;109:2–3.

44. Scott JR. Green journal refinements [editorial]. Obstet Gynecol 2007;109:1264–5.

Resources

American College of Obstetricians and Gynecologists. Reading the medical literature. Washington, DC: ACOG; 1998. Available at: http://www.acog.org/Resources_And_Publications/Department_Publications/Reading_the_Medical_Literature. Retrieved June 28, 2013.

Centre for Health Evidence. Available at: http://www.cche.net. Retrieved August 29, 2013.

Cochrane Collaboration. Available at: http://www.cochrane.org. Retrieved August 29, 2013.

APPENDIX

U.S. Organizations Concerned With Gynecology and Women's Health Care

AAGL
6757 Katella Ave
Cypress, CA 90630
(800) 554-2245
http://www.aagl.org/
The AAGL vision is to serve women by advancing the safest and most efficacious diagnostic and therapeutic techniques that afford less invasive treatments for gynecologic conditions through the integration of clinical practice, research, innovation, and dialogue.

Accreditation Council for Graduate Medical Education
515 North State Street, Suite 2000
Chicago, IL 60654
(312) 755-5000
http://www.acgme.org
The Accreditation Council for Graduate Medical Education is a private professional organization responsible for the accreditation of 8,887 residency education programs. Twenty-six specialty-specific committees, known as Residency Review Committees, periodically initiate revision of the standards and review accredited programs in each specialty and its subspecialties.

American Academy of Physician Assistants
2318 Mill Rd, Suite 1300
Alexandria, VA 22314
(703) 836-2272
www.aapa.org
The American Academy of Physician Assistants is the national professional society for physician assistants. It represents a profession of more than 86,500 certified physician assistants across all medical and surgical specialties in all 50 states, the District of Columbia, most U.S. territories, and within the uniformed services. The American Academy of Physician Assistants advocates and educates on behalf of the profession and the patients physician assistants serve. It works to ensure the professional growth, personal excellence, and recognition of physician assistants. It also works to enhance their ability to improve the quality, accessibility, and cost-effectiveness of patient-centered health care.

American Board of Obstetrics and Gynecology
2915 Vine Street
Dallas, TX 75204
(214) 871-1619
http://www.abog.org
The American Board of Obstetrics and Gynecology is an independent, nonprofit organization that certifies obstetricians and gynecologists in the United States. The American Board of Obstetrics and Gynecology examines and certifies nearly 1,700 obstetrician-gynecologists and subspecialists in maternal–fetal medicine, reproductive endocrinology and infertility, and gynecologic oncology each year. Additionally, more than 18,000 physicians are examined annually for the purpose of maintenance of certification.

American College of Nurse–Midwives
8403 Colesville Road, Suite 1550
Silver Spring, MD 20910
(240) 485-1800
http://www.midwife.org
The American College of Nurse–Midwives is the professional organization for certified nurse–midwives and certified midwives. It reviews research;

administers and promotes continuing education programs; and works with organizations, state and federal agencies, and members of Congress to advance the well-being of women and infants through the practice of midwifery.

American College of Osteopathic Obstetricians & Gynecologists
8851 Camp Bowie West, Suite 275
Fort Worth, TX 76116
(817) 377 0421
http://www.acoog.org
The American College of Osteopathic Obstetricians & Gynecologists is committed to excellence in women's health care and to the education and support of osteopathic health care providers.

American Institute of Ultrasound in Medicine
14750 Sweitzer Lane, Suite 100
Laurel, MD 20707-5906
(800) 638-5352
http://www.aium.org/
The American Institute of Ultrasound in Medicine is a multidisciplinary medical association of more than 9,000 physicians, ultrasonographers, scientists, students, and other health care providers. Established more than 50 years ago, the American Institute of Ultrasound in Medicine is dedicated to advancing the safe and effective use of ultrasonography in medicine through professional and public education, research, development of guidelines, and accreditation.

American Medical Association
515 N. State Street
Chicago, IL 60654
(800) 621-8335
http://www.ama-assn.org/
The American Medical Association is a professional medical society dedicated to promoting the art and science of medicine and the betterment of public health.

American Society for Colposcopy and Cervical Pathology
1530 Tilco Drive, Suite C
Frederick, MD 21704
(800) 787-7227
http://www.asccp.org/
The American Society for Colposcopy and Cervical Pathology is the national organization of health care providers committed to improving health through the study, prevention, diagnosis, and management of lower genital tract disorders.

American Society for Reproductive Medicine
1209 Montgomery Highway
Birmingham, AL 35216-2809
(205) 978-5000
http://www.asrm.org
American Society for Reproductive Medicine is a multidisciplinary organization dedicated to the advancement of the art, science, and practice of reproductive medicine through advocacy, education, and continuing medical education.

American Urogynecologic Society
2025 M Street, NW, Suite 800
Washington, DC 20036
(202) 367-1167
http://www.augs.org
The American Urogynecologic Society is dedicated to research and education in urogynecology and the detection, prevention, and treatment of female lower urinary tract disorders and pelvic floor disorders. Its members are practicing physicians, nurses, physical therapists, health care providers, and researchers from many disciplines, all dedicated to improving the urogynecologic health of women.

Association for Hospital Medical Education
The Council on Continuing Medical Education
109 Brush Creek Road
Irwin, PA 15642
(724) 864-7321
http://www.ahme.org

The Association for Hospital Medical Education is a national nonprofit professional organization involved in the continuum of medical education. The Council on Continuing Medical Education develops professional education programs to enhance the knowledge and skills of continuing medical education providers and administrators and to facilitate the continued development of continuing medical education as a value-added educational activity that provides a positive measurable effect on the quality of health care.

Association of periOperative Registered Nurses, Inc.
2170 South Parker Road, Suite 400
Denver, CO 80231
(800) 755-2676
http://www.aorn.org
The Association of periOperative Registered Nurses, Inc., is a nonprofit membership association that represents the interests of more than 160,000 perioperative nurses by providing nursing education, standards, and clinical practice resources.

Association of Physician Assistants in Obstetrics and Gynecology
563 Carter Court, Suite B
Kimberly WI 54136
(800) 545-0636
http://www.paobgyn.org/
The Association of Physician Assistants in Obstetrics and Gynecology works to improve the health care of women by supporting physician–physician assistant teams who provide cost-effective, quality care to female patients and by promoting a network of communication and education between health care providers dedicated to women's health.

Association of Professors of Gynecology and Obstetrics
2130 Priest Bridge Drive, Suite 7
Crofton, MD 21114
(410) 451-9560
http://www.apgo.org
The Association of Professors of Gynecology and Obstetrics represents academic obstetrician–gynecologists in the United States and Canada. It offers

contemporary, applicable teaching tools and resources for physician–educators, with the ultimate goal of providing optimum health care to women.

Association of Reproductive Health Professionals
1901 L St. NW, Suite 300
Washington, DC 20036
(202) 466-3825
http://www.arhp.org
The Association of Reproductive Health Professionals is a multidisciplinary association of professionals who provide reproductive health services or education, conduct reproductive health research, or influence reproductive health policy. The Association of Reproductive Health Professionals educates health care providers, policy makers, and the public and fosters research and advocacy to improve reproductive health.

Association of Women's Health, Obstetric and Neonatal Nurses
2000 L Street, NW, Suite 740
Washington, DC 20036
(800) 673-8499
http://www.awhonn.org
The Association of Women's Health, Obstetric and Neonatal Nurses (AWHONN) is a nonprofit membership organization that promotes the health of women and newborns through advocacy, research, and education.

Council of University Chairs of Obstetrics and Gynecology
230 W. Monroe, Suite 710
Chicago, IL 60606
(312) 676-3929
http://www.cucog.org
The Council of University Chairs of Obstetrics and Gynecology was established for the charitable and educational purposes of promoting excellence in medical education in the fields of obstetrics and gynecology. Through the unique leadership positions of its members, the organization promotes and encourages excellence in medical student, resident, and fellowship training, clinical practice, and basic and clinical research in women's health.

Gynecologic Oncology Group
Four Penn Center
1600 John F. Kennedy Boulevard, Suite 1020
Philadelphia, PA 19103
(800) 225-3053
http://www.gog.org
The Gynecologic Oncology Group is a nonprofit international organization with the purpose of promoting excellence in the quality and integrity
of clinical and basic scientific research in the field of gynecologic malignancies. The Group is committed to maintaining the highest standards in
clinical trials development, execution, analysis and distribution of results.

Gynecologic Surgery Society
2440 M Street, NW, Suite 801
Washington, DC 20037
(202) 293-2046
http://www.gynecologicsurgerysociety.org
The Gynecologic Surgery Society is a professional medical association
focused on the dissemination of information on advances in gynecologic surgery through conferences, meetings, and the *Journal of Gynecologic
Surgery*.

Infectious Diseases Society for Obstetrics and Gynecology
B327A–4500 Oak Street, Box 42
Vancouver, BC V6H 3N1, Canada
(604) 875-3459
http://www.idsog.org
The Infectious Diseases Society for Obstetrics and Gynecology is a professional society dedicated to improving women's health care through the
advancement of knowledge in infectious diseases and the facilitation of
personal and collaborative relationships among investigators in infectious
diseases related to women's health care.

Jacobs Institute of Women's Health
The George Washington University School of Public Health and
  Health Services
2021 K Street, NW, Suite 800
Washington, DC 20006
(202) 994-4184
http://www.jiwh.org
The Jacobs Institute of Women's Health is a nonprofit organization working to improve health care for women through research, dialogue, and information dissemination.

North American Menopause Society
5900 Landerbrook Drive, Suite 390
Mayfield Heights, OH 44124
(440) 442-7550
http://www.menopause.org
The North American Menopause Society is a nonprofit organization dedicated to promoting the health and quality of life of all women during midlife and beyond through an understanding of menopause and healthy aging.

North American Society for Pediatric and Adolescent Gynecology
19 Mantua Road
Mt. Royal, NJ 08061
(856) 423-3064
http://www.naspag.org
The North American Society for Pediatric and Adolescent Gynecology is an educational society devoted to bringing programs to health care provider groups who medically manage problems related to pediatric and adolescent gynecologic health.

North American Society for Psychosocial Obstetrics and Gynecology
409 12th Street, SW
Washington, DC 20024
(202) 863-2570
http://www.naspog.org
The North American Society for Psychosocial Obstetrics and Gynecology aims to foster scholarly scientific and clinical studies of biopsychosocial aspects of obstetric and gynecologic medicine. The aim is broadly defined

to include the psychologic, psychophysiologic, public health, sociocultural, ethical, and other aspects of such functioning and behavior.

Society for Academic Specialists in General Obstetrics and Gynecology
Sanger Hall, 11th Floor, Room 11-029
1101 East Marshall Street
PO Box 980034
Richmond, VA 23298-0034
(804) 828-7877
www.sasgog.org
The Society for Academic Specialists in General Obstetrics and Gynecology was established to facilitate the exchange of information among specialists in general obstetrics and gynecology who practice in academic settings. The purpose of the Society is to foster excellence in research and education, support career development, and enhance the delivery of clinical care to promote health and prevent disease in women.

Society of Family Planning
255 South 17th Street
Suite 1102
Philadelphia, PA 19103
(866) 584.6758, ext. 301
http://www.societyfp.org/
The Society of Family Planning is dedicated to the scientific study of family planning and to providing an ongoing source of research funding for projects that are underfunded by government and industry. It works to advance family planning research and education by providing evidence-based insight to improve clinical care in the areas of contraception and abortion.

Society of Gynecologic Oncology
230 W. Monroe, Suite 710
Chicago, IL 60606
(312) 235-4060
http://www.sgo.org
The Society of Gynecologic Oncology is the medical specialty society for physicians trained in the comprehensive management of gynecologic cancers. It improves the care of women with gynecologic cancers by encouraging research, disseminating knowledge, raising the standards of practice in

the prevention and treatment of gynecologic malignancies, and collaborating with other organizations interested in women's health care, oncology, and related fields.

Society of Gynecologic Surgeons
7800 Wolf Trail Cove
Germantown, TN 38183
(901) 682-2079
http://www.sgsonline.org
The Society of Gynecologic Surgeons is a select member group of over 250 physicians who are involved in the teaching and practice of advanced gynecologic surgery. The mission of the Society of Gynecologic Surgeons is to promote excellence in gynecologic surgery through acquisition of knowledge and improvement of skills, advancement of basic and clinical research, and professional and public education.

Society for Maternal-Fetal Medicine
409 12th Street, SW
Washington, DC 20024–2188
(202) 863-2476
http://www.smfm.org
The Society for Maternal-Fetal Medicine is dedicated to the promotion and expansion of education in obstetric perinatology and the exchange of new ideas and research in the field of maternal–fetal medicine.

Society for Reproductive Investigation
888 Bestgate Rd., Suite 420
Annapolis, MD 21401
(410) 571-1143
http://www.sgionline.org
The Society for Reproductive Investigation is a scientific organization with members throughout the world. Its mission is to promote excellence in reproductive sciences through research, education, and advocacy.

INDEX

Page numbers followed by letters *b*, *f*, or *t* indicate boxes, figures, and tables, respectively.

A

Abnormal genital bleeding, 573–582
  causes of, 573–574
  diagnosis of, 574–575
  differential diagnosis of, 573–574
  management of, 575
Abnormal uterine bleeding (AUB), 573, 575–580
  causes of, 576–577
  classification of, 575–576, 576*f*
  diagnosis of, 577–579
  evaluation of, 577–579
  management of, 579–580
Abnormal uterine bleeding-leiomyoma (AUB-L), 577
Abnormal uterine bleeding-ovulatory (AUB-O) dysfunction, 577
ABOG. *See* American Board of Obstetrics and Gynecology
Abortion
  defined, 717
  induced, 717–723
    access to care, 717
    complications of, 719
    evaluation before, 720
    legal issues related to, 717–718
    management of, 720–721
    methods of, 718–719
    mortality data, 719
    patient counseling related to, 719–720
    prevalence of, 717
    spontaneous, 707,709
    timing of, 718
Abortion rate, decrease in, 717

Abortion ratio, decrease in, 717
Abuse, 537–553. *See also* Violence; *specific types*
  alcohol, 334–338
  of children, 545–548, 547*b*
  domestic violence, 537–543, 540*b*, 542*b*
  drug, 334–338
  elder, 487, 543–545
  intimate partner violence, 537–543, 540*b*, 542*b*
  prescription drug misuse, prevention of, 338
  rape, 549–550, 551*b*
  reproductive coercion, 548–549
  sexual, in adolescents, 458–459
  sexual, in children, 430–431, 545–548, 547*b*
    adult manifestations of, 545–548, 547*b*
    defined, 545
    evaluation of, 430
    examination findings, 431
    forensic evidence of, 430
    human immunodeficiency virus infection related to, 546
    prevalence of, 430
    reporting of, 431
    screening for, 546, 547*b*
    sexually transmitted infections due to, 431, 546
    support for survivors of, 546, 548
    treatment for, 431
  sexual assault, 549–550, 551*b*
  sexual coercion, 548–549
  substance, 329–341
  types of, 537
  of women with disabilities, 515
ACA. *See* Patient Protection and Affordable Care Act